CHILDHOOD OBESITY
Prevention And Treatment
Second Edition

CHILDHOOD OBESITY
Prevention And Treatment
Second Edition

Jana Pařízková and Andrew P. Hills

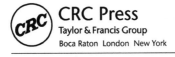

CRC Press
Taylor & Francis Group
Boca Raton London New York

CRC Press is an imprint of the
Taylor & Francis Group, an **informa** business

CRC Press
Taylor & Francis Group
6000 Broken Sound Parkway NW, Suite 300
Boca Raton, FL 33487-2742

First issued in paperback 2019

© 2005 by Taylor & Francis Group, LLC
CRC Press is an imprint of Taylor & Francis Group, an Informa business

No claim to original U.S. Government works

ISBN-13: 978-0-8493-2253-2 (hbk)
ISBN-13: 978-0-367-39331-1 (pbk)
Library of Congress Card Number 2004057047

Library of Congress Cataloging-in-Publication Data

Paŕízková, Jana.
    Childhood obesity : prevention and treatment / Jana Paŕízková and Andrew P. Hills.--2nd ed.
        p. cm.
    Includes bibliographical references and index.
    ISBN 0-8493-2253-7 (alk. paper)
        1. Obesity in children. I. Hills, Andrew P. II. Title.

    RJ399.C6P37 2004
    618.92'398--dc22

                                                                      2004057047

Visit the Taylor & Francis Web site at
http://www.taylorandfrancis.com

and the CRC Press Web site at
http://www.crcpress.com

Preface

The global epidemic of overweight and obesity in adults is now also a major health problem for children and youth (Livingstone, 2001; Kimm et al., 2002; Koletzko et al., 2002; Eriksson et al., 2003b). While childhood obesity has existed since ancient times, there is increasing evidence that prevalence rates today are greater than ever before. This increase in fatness heightens the health risks for later periods of life but also has a substantial impact during the growing years (Klein, 2004).

Over the last decade more research has been devoted to this significant problem. However, the majority of studies have described the various manifestations and consequences of obesity, and few have addressed its causes. Considerable effort has been devoted to the identification of suitable ways to prevent, treat, and manage the condition. However, numerous questions remain unanswered.

This volume summarizes many of the findings on obesity during growth with a particular focus on more recent knowledge and an appraisal of research on treatment and management. Importantly, the volume addresses some potential solutions for the prevention of obesity in childhood. While the major focus of the book considers children and adolescents, some reference is made to relevant research with adults. Significantly more research has been completed with the adult population; therefore, knowledge and understanding of practices with this group may have important consequences for children and youth. Readers are referred to data presented elsewhere — for example, the Proceedings of the International and European Congresses on Obesity (ICO and ECO) that have taken place during recent years.

A number of approaches to prevent, treat, and manage childhood obesity have been presented in the literature to date. The authors of this volume, however, believe that the prevention and management of simple obesity should be promoted with the incorporation of natural factors (appropriate nutrition and physical activity) to rectify energy imbalance and achieve a desirable body composition. This approach has a greater opportunity of success in earlier periods of life when obesity is not fully developed. These comments assume of course, the absence of significant endocrine disorders such as Cushing's syndrome, and hypothyroidism, or genetic syndromes such as Prader-Willi, Bardet-Biedl, and others, which are accompanied by increased adiposity. These genetic anomalies with an impact on body fatness are very rare in children (Chiumello and Poskitt, 2002); however, genetic predisposition plays a significant role and during recent years has been studied extensively. Nonetheless, the contribution of genetics is inconclusive.

Poor lifestyle behaviors are largely responsible for excess fatness in the majority of cases of obesity during childhood. As shown by some authors, for example, Klish (1993), even in such cases an environmental intervention can have a significant impact and help to improve the situation for the child. The management of an appropriate environment for an obese child requires a conscious and consistent attention to diet and physical activity that may be difficult both for the child and his or her family. Importantly, weight loss for an obese youngster is not the sole aim in weight management. Rather, the overall improvement of the physiological, psychological, and social status of the individual should be the goal.

A significant restriction of food intake may be necessary when the degree of obesity is excessive or morbid. Unfortunately, this scenario is necessary for an increasing number of children and youth. This trend may be the result of childhood obesity being underestimated and neglected as a health problem. The best way to manage obesity in the family, school, and the wider environment of the child is to be vigilant and help in the early detection and intervention to minimize excess deposition of fat. The optimal scenario in the management of childhood obesity is not to permit its development at all. Early interventions should be well planned and timely, and follow best practice guidelines to achieve the desired outcomes.

The aim of this volume is to address a broad range of aspects related to the prevention and management of the condition and present current information. The number of studies has increased enormously since the publication of the first edition, and it would be too difficult to analyze and summarize them all at this moment. Definitive analyses and suggestions for the solution of childhood obesity are surely premature. Further research and clinical experience will be needed to contribute to a more positive outcome in the future.

Authors

Professor Jana Pařízková, M.D., Ph.D., D.Sc. is a Senior Scientist at the Centre for the Management of Obesity, Institute of Endocrinology in Prague, and Charles University and Masaryk University, Czech Republic. She earned her medical degree from Charles University in Prague in 1956, where she graduated summa cum laude. She pursued her Ph.D. degree in medical physiology at the Institute of Physiology of the Czechoslovak Academy of Sciences in 1960, and received her D.Sc. degree in nutrition and metabolism ibidem in 1978. She was also given a fellowship at the Laboratoire de Nutrition Humaine, Hôpital Bichat in Paris, France, in 1965–1966.

Dr. Pařízková's main research interests include body composition as related to dietary intake, physical performance and fitness, lipid metabolism variables, development of gross and fine motor skills, and physical activity regimes across a life span, with special focus on the growth and development period. She has also focused on the development of obesity during growth and cardiovascular risks later in life, and on health promotion and the reduction of health risks through early and/or later nutritional and physical activity interventions. Another main area of research is obesity with related metabolic and clinical problems as related to actual physical activity level and diet in all age categories.

Dr. Pařízková is the author of 17 monographs including *Development of Lean Body Mass and Depot Fat in Children* (1962) and *Body Composition and Lipid Metabolism under Conditions of Various Physical Activity* (1974), published in Czech and updated in English by Martinus Nijhoff, B.V., Medical Division (The Hague, 1977) and by Editora Guanabara Dois (Rio de Janeiro, 1982) and titled *Body Fat and Physical Fitness*. In 1996 she published the monograph *Nutrition, Physical Activity and Health in Early Life*, and in 2000 *Childhood Obesity: Prevention and Treatment*, CRC Press (the latter with A.P. Hills). She has co-authored and edited ten other monographs, including *Physical Fitness and Nutrition during Growth* (S. Karger, Basel 1998, co-edited with A.P. Hills). She is also the author of some 500 articles in national and international scientific journals and many proceedings, including international congresses. She has been an invited speaker at more than one hundred international congresses and conferences — for example, the International Union of Nutritional Sciences (IUNS) — where she was a chairperson and/or organizer of symposia and workshops in 1975, 1978, 1981, 1989, 1997, and 2001. Science Citation Index has included more than 1100 references to her articles, monographs, chapters in monographs, etc.

The World Health Organization (WHO) appointed Dr. Pařízková as visiting professor, International Course on Nutrition and Hygiene, Hyderabad,

SEARO 1977; consultant to WHO, Geneva 1978; member of the panel of experts, Food and Agricultural Organization/World Health Organization/ United Nations University (FAO/WHO/UNU; FAO, Rome 1981), on energy and protein requirements, published by WHO, Geneva 1985; and a member of the consultation group on the epidemiology of obesity of the Regional Office of WHO for Europe, in Warsaw, Poland, in 1987. She was also visiting professor at the University of Connecticut (1993, 1995), University of Perugia, Italy (1993, 1995), and others.

Other awards include the Philip Noel Baker Prize, ICSPE by UNESCO in 1977, Memorial Medal from Charles University in 1978, Prize of the Rector of Charles University in 1996, and the International Memorial Medal of Aleš Hrdlička in 1996.

Dr. Pařízková is a member of the Czech Medical Association of J.E. Purkyně, (CzME JEP), the International Commission for Anthropology of Food (ICAF) through the International Union of Anthropological and Ethnological Sciences (IUAES), the European Academy of Nutritional Sciences (EANS), the Czech Association of Nutrition, the Czech Society for the Study of Obesity, and the Czech Anthropological Society. In addition, she is a member of the following organizations: the European Association for the Study of Obesity, International Association for the Study of Obesity, International Society for the Advancement of Kinanthropometry (ISAK), and European Anthropological Association. She previously served as chairperson of the Nutrition and Physical Performance committee through the IUNS, and as a member of the Scientific Committee of the International Council for Sport and Physical Education (ICSPE) through UNESCO. She was also elected a member of the New York Academy of Sciences (1963) and has been conferred with an honorary appointment to the Research Board of Advisors of the American Biographic Institute.

Professor Andrew P. Hills is a prominent exercise physiologist with a primary interest in pediatric obesity and exercise. Dr. Hills trained initially as a physical educator before earning an MSc degree at the University of Oregon, after being awarded a Rotary Foundation Graduate Fellowship in 1981. His Ph.D. was undertaken at the University of Queensland, Australia, in the Department of Anatomy. His thesis was titled "Locomotor characteristics of obese pre-pubertal children." Dr. Hills is a Fellow of Sports Medicine Australia, Secretary–Treasurer of the International Council for Physical Activity and Fitness Research, and the immediate past President of the Australasian Society for the Study of Obesity. In addition he is a series editor of the prestigious Medicine and Sport Science Series published by Karger AG, Basel (2001).

His current appointment is Professor in the School of Human Movement Studies at Queensland University of Technology, where he established and directed a multidisciplinary clinic with a special emphasis on weight management for many years. Dr. Hills has published widely in the fields of physical growth and development and obesity, and has authored or edited

8 monographs, written 18 book chapters, and written over 100 papers and presentations. His books include *Exercise and Obesity* (edited by A.P. Hills and M.L. Wahlqvist), published by Smith-Gordon and Co., London (1994), and recently *Body Composition Assessment in Children* (edited by T. Jurimae and A.P. Hills), published by Karger AG, Basel.

Current research emphases include adaptation to weight loss in the obese, the relationship between the energy cost of walking and adiposity, and the relationship between body composition and body image in the obese and submaximal markers of exercise intensity.

Acknowledgments

The authors wish to thank Ms. Jennie Yeung for her excellent work during the preparation of the manuscript.

Contents

Part 2   Treatment and Management Principles

Part 1

Main Characteristics of Childhood Obesity

1

Introduction

During recent years, and since the first edition of this book, the prevalence of obesity has increased further in the adult population in most Westernized countries. A particularly problematic feature of this general trend is that the condition is also developing at much earlier stages in life than was the case in the past. Further, this situation is no longer limited to the industrialized countries with a sound food supply and high standard of living. This is a major concern, not only in affluent countries such as the United States, European countries, and others. In the Third World (Kimm, 2002), the trend is for upper socioeconomic classes to be more predisposed to the condition (Mirtipati et al., 1998). This is evidenced by a plethora of scientific articles from numerous regions of the world, reports in lay journals, and the mass media generally. Irrespective of the setting, there is an urgent need for a collective approach to the prevention, treatment, and management of obesity, particularly with respect to the problems of the condition during the growing years (Barlow and Dietz, 1998; Brooke and Abernathy, 1985; Koletzko et al., 2002).

The increasing prevalence of obesity is, however, a component of the bigger general health situation of increasing diseases of "affluence." These health problems have resulted from an unsuitable and unhealthy lifestyle. The obesity problem appears to be magnified in the United States, perhaps due to the country's overall level of development, with among the greatest increases in obesity prevalence, including during childhood. With increasing obesity has come a corresponding increase in accompanying health risks such as type 2 diabetes, atherosclerosis, and hypertension. This may indicate that children in the current generation are at risk of dying at a younger age than their parents.

Genetic factors and environmental conditions play a central role in the early development of obesity, but the situation varies in different countries. This topic will be treated in greater detail in later chapters. The prevalence of obesity in all age groups, however, has increased so fast that significant changes in the gene pool cannot be considered as the only explanation. Prevalence varies significantly in different parts of the world, especially when comparing some populations in Asia or Africa with Western populations. For example, the prevalence of obesity using the standard criteria of a body mass index (BMI) greater than 30kg/m² in a group of Japanese aged 15 to 84 years, followed between 1990 and 1994, was quite low compared with the data in Western populations (Yoshiike et al., 1998). But more recently, due to increased prosperity not only in Asia — for example in India (Subramanyam, Jayashree and Rafi, 2003a,b) — but also in Africa, childhood obesity has also increased in countries such as Cameroon (Pasquet et al., 1999) and the Republic of South Africa (Cameron, 1998).

Some would argue that because there are so many children in the world who are hungry and starving, why should we care too much about obesity, the health problem of affluence and a poor lifestyle? One never sees an obese child from a poor Asian or African village! However, when the economic situation in such countries improves, the prevalence of obesity increases, as is the case in India, Brazil, Paraguay, Venezuela, South Africa, and so forth. In most of these countries, including Mexico, obesity and malnutrition coexist (Jimenez-Cruz, Bacardi-Gascon, and Spindler, 2003). Thus, when problems such as malnutrition, decreased immuno-resistance, infectious diseases, and other health outcomes are improved, new health problems appear. Childhood obesity has also been identified in lower socioeconomic groups in the industrially developed countries, which suggests that obesity is due mainly to poor lifestyle behaviors, such as the consumption of cheaper fats and sugar products, commonly combined with reduced physical activity. Given the widespread nature of obesity, particularly under conditions of an improving economic and social situation, the adequate management of the condition during growth is an urgent challenge for most countries of the world (Florencio et al., 2001).

The "Westernization of the diet," including increased consumption of total and saturated fat intake, has also changed other health risks, such as the blood cholesterol level in children in the United States. In Spain and Japan, statistics indicate that their population has reached the 75th percentile of the United States. This cannot be explained by adiposity alone, and changes in fat intake have predicted changes in Spain but not in Japan. Differences in genetic response to higher fat intake may explain the elevated cholesterol levels in Japanese children, even when fat intake is lower than in the United States (Couch et al., 2000). This example provides clear evidence of the interplay of genetic and environmental factors, and potentially, interactions between multiple environmental factors.

According to recent data from the United States, 65% of U.S. citizens are overweight, and almost one-third are severely obese, double the number 20 years ago. Fifteen percent of children aged 6 to 19 years, or three times the number in 1980, top the weight charts. If the U.S. population continues to gain weight at the same rate, some experts predict that nearly every person in North America could be overweight by the year 2030. This situation may worsen given the current scenario.

The situation, however, can vary in the same country, as it does in big U.S. cities and rural areas, or depending whether it is the north or south of the country. For example, preschool children living in the north and central regions of Mexico have higher obesity prevalence rates than those living in the southeast (Jimenez-Cruz, Bacardi-Gascon, and Spindler, 2003). The risk of obesity in these regions was positively associated with the educational level of the head of the household (Hernandez et al., 1996) and also with the social and economic situation. This variability will be described and analyzed in detail in subsequent chapters.

An analysis of the variability in the prevalence of obesity, and the effect of the environmental conditions, both in the past and at present, is important. In addition, an understanding of the characteristic features of obesity in various parts of the world could help to elucidate and define the most important factors and mechanisms that promote the development of marked obesity during growth and therefore provide some assistance on how to treat and prevent the condition.

However, it must be acknowledged that an analysis of the available data from well-controlled studies on childhood obesity, along with comparisons of this work, are far more difficult than comparable between-study analyses of adults. Differences exist in the aims, research design, criteria for assessment, protocols, and methodology, but there is an additional significant problem. This relates to comparisons confounded by differences in chronological age and maturational status, which are self-evidently much larger during growth than in the adult years. Further, the stage of development and maturation differs according to gender but may also be different in various countries, especially when comparing children from different economic and social situations. This can also be reflected in body adiposity and local criteria for its normality. Therefore, differences in the age of onset and duration of obesity as related to the critical periods of growth in subjects evaluated in various studies must also be considered.

Obesity in a growing organism is not the same as obesity present in a fully mature adult or aging organism. The same diversity applies to approaches to prevention, treatment, and management with differences according to age, stage, character, and duration of obesity, and the type of treatment and its duration.

The relationships between various factors and variables in growing subjects are therefore largely peculiar to the specific study population. As such, it may not be surprising that the synthesis of findings and conclusions from available publications are often controversial. However, in spite of a degree of pessimism surrounding the successful management of childhood obesity, there is a developing body of knowledge that augurs well for a favorable outcome and solution to this major health problem.

In summary, despite some of the common features and characteristics of the condition, each child is an individual with a distinct personality, health and nutritional status, and physical fitness background, so each individual should be evaluated and treated recognizing these inherent unique characteristics. A failure to recognize this uniqueness may contribute to an oversimplification and generalization of the situation of a particular child. This may be one of the main reasons for the lack of success to date in the treatment of childhood obesity.

1.1   Evaluation of Obesity and Its Causal Factors during Growth

Obesity may be defined as a multifactorial syndrome that consists of anthropological, physiological, biochemical, metabolic, anatomical, psychological, and social alterations. The condition is characterized by an increased level of adiposity and a corresponding increase in body weight, which has to be evaluated according to the standard values for the individual age categories of girls and boys.

The precise level of fatness that defines obesity is somewhat arbitrary. Himes (1980) suggested that excessive fatness should be determined according to some health-related criteria. At that time, he indicated that there was limited definitive knowledge regarding specific health implications of various levels of fatness and that this void was particularly evident for the childhood population. Since the early 1980s, there has been a progressive accumulation of health-related implications of higher levels of adiposity.

A useful start is to make a distinction between overweight and obesity. Overweight refers to an increase in body weight above an arbitrary standard, usually defined in relation to height. Obesity, on the other hand, refers to an abnormally high proportion of the body composition as body fat (Bray, 1987), or a surplus of adipose tissue (Kannel, 1983) as related to other tissues of the body (Wahlqvist and Hills, 1994b). A more precise definition of what constitutes problematic obesity in all individuals is a challenge as there is no universally accepted classification system or completely satisfactory numerical index of obesity. This is particularly the case for children and the immature adolescent (Parry-Jones, 1988). The utilization of the BMI using the criteria and cutoff points suggested by Cole and Rolland-Cachera (2002; see Chapter 4) and measurements of body composition, including skinfolds, has contributed to an improvement in the evaluation of childhood obesity.

The definition of factors contributing to the development of obesity is also a major challenge. As the processes of growth, development, and maturation during childhood and adolescence do not proceed at the same pace in various countries, it is also not easy to evaluate the adequacy of changes in growth status, for example in height, weight, BMI, and body composition.

However, considerable effort has been made to standardize measurement criteria with work undertaken by researchers and also by the World Health Organization (WHO), the International Obesity Task Force (IOTF), the Food and Agricultural Organization (FAO), the United Nations University (UNU), and the European Child Obesity Group, or ECOG (1985). From an anthropometric perspective, a number of groups are responsible for the progression of a standardized approach to measurement, for example, the International Society for the Advancement of Kinanthropometry (ISAK).

Obesity has commonly been defined in relation to certain limits of body fatness. For example, for prepubertal children, acceptable percent body fat levels are 17–18%, 15–18% for young adult males (aged 18 years), and 20–25% for young females of a similar age (Gray and Bray, 1988). However, the values for the individual age categories of girls and boys vary from year to year, and in addition, are related to the level of sexual development (Pařízková, 1977). There is also considerable merit in relating weight to weight for height values of the reference population being sampled, and as such, definitions of obesity in children have also taken the form of weight-for-height distributions (percentiles; see Chapter 4).

As in other disciplines, publication bias appears to exist in the literature, particularly regarding the evaluation of obesity and also the results of weight management. Therefore, it is necessary to evaluate the results of available studies with caution. Suggestions for the management of such bias once it has been identified, or reducing its likelihood, are also discussed in the literature (Allison, Faith, and Gorman, 1996). This also applies to the results of various scientific meetings on this topic (e.g., Critical Reviews of Food Science, 1993; New York Academy of Science, 1993; ECOG, 1996; 1998; 2003; 2004).

A continuing theme is the paramount role of nutrition in the form of energy intake — both absolute and relative — caused by a range of factors. In relation to an increased intake of food, a possible higher metabolic efficiency or energy utilization in certain subjects predisposed to obesity has been considered. The role of genetics, manifested, for example, by family clustering, has been the focus of extensive research more recently (Bouchard, 1993; Bouchard, 1997; Magnusson and Rassmussen, 2002; Treuth, Butte, and Herrick, 2001; O'Rahilly et al., 2003). Composition of the diet has also received considerable attention, particularly a high intake of fat and/or sugar. Energy output resulting from various levels and types of physical activity and exercise has also been considered, along with the interplay of all of these parameters.

A further problem is the reliability of methods and procedures used in the individual studies to date. For example, more recent studies using advanced techniques have revealed a clear discrepancy between self-reported and actual energy intake and self-reported and actual physical activity or energy expenditure in obese subjects. This is of particular concern for obese individuals who have had difficulties losing weight by dietary adjustment (Forbes, 1993). The same applies to food choice and habits, food aversions and preferences.

Limitations in the assessment of dietary energy intake using self-report have been reported by other authors (Schoeller, 1995) with the most common shortcoming being underestimation (underreporting) of energy intake. Therefore, self-reported dietary intake data must be interpreted with caution unless independent methods of assessing validity are included in the experimental design. In addition, intercorrelations between measures of body composition and adiposity are generally highly significant but the data do not necessarily correspond.

Findings on the effects of genetics and inherited factors have focused attention especially on children of obese parents where not only metabolic, hormonal predispositions but also dietary and physical activity habits play a role. Reasons for discrepancies have also been considered and analyzed according to the family situation. The obesity status of the mother, father, or other family members did not have an effect on the accuracy of the information recalled. However, the results indicated that the lack of differences consistently observed in dietary intake between obese and normal-weight children could not be explained by differential accuracy of recalled information on food intake (Klesges et al., 1988). The same applies to reports on physical activity, as shown clearly by Mayer (1974), who followed obese and normal-weight children during various physical activities. Mayer found marked differences in self-reported levels of physical activity among normal-weight and obese children in spite of the same report in both groups. An evaluation of the level of physical activity with the help of simple methods such as triaxial accelerometers has yielded more reliable estimates of the level of physical activity in obese children aged 8 to 15 years than self-report instruments (Coleman et al., 1997). This means that much of the information available on the level of physical activity in obese children may not be objective.

There is evidence that energy intake, certainly in the United Kingdom, declined between the 1950s and 1970s, and this was explained by the reduction of physical activity and increase in inactive behaviors. Moreover, sedentary behaviors have increased even more during recent years, particularly pursuits such as the use of computers, television, and video games. Another explanation for some of the differences was that higher factors were used to calculate the energy derived from protein, fat, and carbohydrate in the 1930s and 1940s than were used later. If the later factors are applied to the results of earlier surveys, the values for energy are reduced by about 10%. This correction brings the results of the earlier surveys into line with those of the later ones for boys up to 14 years and girls up to 10 years (Widdowson, 1983). However, older boys and girls as well as adults do appear to eat less than was the case in the past. This has also been confirmed by other comparisons (Durnin, 1984).

In addition, more recently the role of the "thrifty genotype" has been considered as important (Flodmark, 2002; Neel, 1999; James, 2002). This genetic programming was necessary during human phylogeny; metabolism was asymmetric with energy accumulation. It was a necessary condition of survival during the course of history. In the more developed Middle East, Europe, or China, there was never an extended period of uninterrupted food abundance, as famines were regular and frequent. Therefore fat accumulation, when food was available, meant survival in times of shortage, while the possible detrimental effects of abundant food intake and being overweight expressed in unrealistically old age were not relevant.

All of these issues are of concern for all periods of life, but commence with the fetal period. A predisposition for the later development of obesity may start as early as during pregnancy. One of the key questions is whether women should increase their intake of food during this time. It is postulated that metabolic economies enable women during pregnancy to produce on the average 4 kg of fat and a fetus weighing on average 3.5 kg without any increase in energy intake. However, a number of pregnant women "eat for two," which might be one of the main reasons for the development of obesity in both mother and child (Widdowson, 1983). The role of factors influencing the organism from the very beginning of life has been considered due to increasing evidence of the importance of the mother's dietary intake and nutritional status during pregnancy (increased in both a positive and/or a negative way), weaning practices, and eating habits since the first months of life (see Chapter 3). The early genesis of adult diseases, including obesity, has become a topic of consideration and research, and some scientific meetings have been devoted to this issue (for example, recent meetings on fetal origins of adult diseases in Mumbai, 2001 and Brighton, 2003). The phenomenon is still the topic of much discussion; however, there is some evidence of the importance of the delayed consequences (James, 2002).

Following youngsters from the early years of life is also essential from the point of view of the marked delayed consequences of increased adiposity, which present a serious risk for the development of co-morbid conditions. For example, the Framingham Study followed secular trends and risk factors for cardiovascular disease and showed that compared with 1957 to 1960, mean BMI and prevalence rates for overweight and hypertension were higher in 1984 to 1988, despite higher levels of reported physical activity (Posner et al., 1995). Some evidence has also been provided by several other longitudinal studies such as the Bogalusa Heart Study (Srinivasan, Mayers, and Berenson, 2001), the Fels Longitudinal Growth Study, and others. Closer cooperation between nutritionists, dietitians, exercise physiologists, and other clinicians (which is currently insufficient) could also help to solve the obesity problem and its early beginnings in children.

Risk factors for childhood obesity are similar in various parts of the world. In a group of Chinese children it was found that parents' weight (as evaluated by Kaup's Index), birth weight, and breastfeeding were risk factors (see Chapter 3). The obesity prevalence in China and Taiwan, including in childhood, is increasing significantly (Chu, 2001; Guillaume and Lissau, 2002; Tudor-Locke, Ainsworth, and Adair, 2003). Despite the reported increase in childhood obesity, basal metabolic rate is often not different in obese children compared to normal-weight individuals (Chapter 5). However, the earlier the appearance of overweight and obesity, particularly before 4 years of age, the more severe the condition is likely to be (provided no intervention is undertaken). The earlier onset of the condition may be due to a different etiology; for example, earlier obesity has been linked with prenatal factors, while later obesity has been related to the type of feeding in early life (Xu, 1990). Such results strongly underline the necessity of early interventions as consistently recommended by a wide range of experts in the area (Pařízková, 1977; Widhalm, 1985; Dietz, 1986, 1993; Epstein, 1993; Epstein et al., 1998; Korsten-Reck et al., 1990, 1994). Generally, the earlier the commencement of treatment for childhood and adolescent obesity, the higher the likelihood of long-term success.

Factors contributing to obesity may not always be the same in both genders. For example, in boys, physical inactivity measured both in terms of television viewing time and registrations of participation in sports activities contributed independently to body fat mass. In girls, there was a weaker or no contribution by physical inactivity (the Belgian Luxembourg Child Study II, Guillaume et al., 1997).

1.2   Main Problems in the Treatment of Childhood Obesity

A number of ways to manage obesity have been defined, and these options provide a very useful guide to management of the obese child or youth. However, this is not the main problem. The most difficult challenge is for the individual to adhere to the principles of the treatment and permanently maintain a desirable weight and body composition. The ideal treatment and management of obesity must involve a range of health professionals in a team approach. Williams, Bollella, and Carter (1993) have suggested that the process should involve pediatricians and other specialists who could play a significant role in addressing increased adiposity in children during the growing years.

A more fundamental starting point is for all health professionals to be aware of the condition. Given the lack of understanding of obesity by many people, this process must involve education regarding the actual and future risks of obesity, especially when the condition develops during the early phases of growth. Advances in the treatment of obesity during childhood (Suskind and Sothern, 1993) have been presented at many scientific meetings, including those of the New York Academy of Sciences (1993); ECOG in 1997, 1998, 2003, and 2004; the European and International Congresses on Obesity (e.g. 1994, 1998, and 2002); the International Nutrition Congresses (IUNS, 2001, in Vienna); and others during recent years.

Some suggest (Price et al., 1989) that the pediatrician's perception of the problem of childhood obesity is usually adequate and results in an appropriate approach to management. However, some medical practitioners still underestimate the health risks of obesity and potential accompanying problems. The eating habits that are employed across the lifespan are established in infancy. During this period, pediatricians can have a significant impact on young mothers and their children by encouraging a diet low in saturated fat, sugar, and sodium. The diet should be adequate in energy and meet the recommended dietary allowances (RDAs) for all macro- and micronutrients corresponding to the needs of the growing child (Kashani and Nader, 1986). Parents may also underestimate the problem of obesity in their children and delay the time of desirable intervention, with negative consequences for the child later on.

Placing personal responsibility with regard to all dietary intake and lifestyle practices solely on a child brainwashed by scientifically prepared TV commercials and in other mass media is unrealistic. However, this could also be the case with mature adults who are very well aware of their problems. The creation of an "obesogenic environment" in our contemporary society is a significant health and also economic risk for any government. More attention and involvement of political, administrative, economic, and public health-care sectors should occur. It would be highly desirable if more economic profit came from healthy food production and publicity, and advertisements should be at least similarly aggressive as for unhealthy foodstuffs. The same applies (along with the necessary propaganda) to the promotion of an active lifestyle, including increased exercise above that undertaken previously. The economic imperatives must also be stressed, and it is encouraging to see some recent evidence of efforts in this respect.

In addition to counseling for dietary moderation, pediatricians, other medical doctors, and health professionals should encourage the incorporation of regular physical activity. Such an approach would not only assist in the prevention of obesity but also the cardiovascular and metabolic diseases, especially coronary heart disease. However, it is unfortunate that we still encounter a lack of comprehension of the childhood obesity problem in those who could manage it best: pediatricians and general practitioners.

As mentioned earlier, a poor child in a developing country never becomes obese. Similarly, a young track-and-field athlete or long-distance runner does not generally have excess body fat. This does not mean, however, that the recommendation of such an activity level should be made for everybody, but rather to display that under certain conditions, increased adiposity can be avoided. Common sense would suggest that the employment of a highly restricted energy intake or excessively hard physical training as a means of managing childhood obesity is inappropriate; however, an adequate prescription of both could influence the growing organism significantly. In spite of the potential contribution of genetic factors, the laws of the conservation of energy cannot be avoided or excluded. This provides some guidance on the management of obesity and especially the prevention of obesity in many children.

Nevertheless, the illustrative example of a young adequately active youngster is an appropriate model to highlight the role of physical activity and exercise in the prevention of obesity. This approach has been repeatedly considered (Gutin and Manos, 1993; Pařízková, 1977, 1996a,b). The implementation of "old truths" has also applied to other areas, especially those concerning the desirable parent, emotional, and pedagogic influence on the child. Unfortunately for too many people, an interest in physical activity and exercise does not extend beyond the exertion of being a spectator of sporting events either in person or by watching on television. Too few people of all ages have a personal commitment to physical activity and exercise, and therefore are not active participants.

On the occasion of a recent International Life Sciences Institute (ILSI) Europe Mini-Workshop on Overweight and Obesity in European children and adolescents, it was concluded that a consensus on the definition of child obesity on the basis of BMI was not sufficient, especially for monitoring of the secular increase in obesity prevalence. In most European countries, there is significant variation in the prevalence of childhood obesity. Evidence presented at this meeting showed that dietary patterns rather than simple energy intake may be responsible for children's obesity. In this respect more research is necessary. Regarding physical activity, more longitudinal studies are needed as changing demographic and social characteristics also play an important role in the changes in children's obesity (ILSI Europe, 1998).

1.3 The Role of Lifestyle and the Mass Media in the Development and Prevention of Childhood Obesity

The lifestyle of most people in industrially developed countries is significantly influenced by the mass media. Due to the changing economic, social, and cultural situation in many countries of the Third World, the same factors may apply, especially those in the higher social strata. However, economic improvements have also enabled some in the lower social strata to develop a lifestyle more commonly connected with more affluence.

Paradoxically, the mass media, and particularly television, can play an important role in the management of obesity (Cheung, 1993), including during the growth period. Many children and adolescents spend more time in front of the television and with computers and video games than in any daily activity other than sleep. A number of studies have confirmed that obesity is directly related to the number of hours spent watching television (Dietz and Gortmaker, 1985, 1993; Gortmaker et al., 1990). For many children, the world as displayed on television represents a greater reality than their wider "real world." Television stars are rarely obese, and generally represent the other end of the size and shape spectrum.

The inactive behavior of television viewing is often combined with frequent, very attractive commercials advertising food and drink (Bar-Or et al., 1998; James, 2002). Rather than promoting sound eating practices, these advertisements more commonly promote foods that are not recommended for the optimal development of health and fitness of children. Unfortunately, the power of advertising is such that young people are a captive audience and readily associate with the unfavorable practices that are presented, most commonly of highly processed and energy-dense foods. Inadequate composition of food intake has become something of an irresistible addiction.

The consumption of simple sugars may be especially risky from an obesity point of view; however, the consumption of sugar has to be considered individually, and in relationship to energy output, physical activity, and overall energy turnover in the organism. Active athletes consume not only more energy and fat but also more sugar without risk of increased adiposity, provided their activity is permanently increased. A similar situation exists, for example, in hardworking sugar cane cutters in Haiti, who have a high sugar intake, but this is in conjunction with intense daily workloads and overall generally lower energy intake.

Running in tandem with food advertisements is the portrayal and subsequent adoration of the ultra-slim, lean, and very tall "beautiful people" with bodily characteristics that approximate plastic dolls. Individuals of this shape represent an extremely small proportion of the normal population. Unfortunately, such images are powerful in the portrayal of an idealized shape. Those who attempt to make wholesale changes to size and shape in order to emulate a societal ideal may be at risk of serious nutritional problems such as anorexia nervosa, bulimia, bulirexia, and obesity. The extent of eating and weight disorders is poorly understood, but the situation is clearly cause for concern in some places. For example, in the Czech population, about 5% of adolescent girls suffer from an eating disorder, and in some other, especially Western countries, the prevalence is higher and increasing.

Therefore, television reflects a cultural contradiction by promoting both food consumption and leanness (Dietz, 1990, 1991, 1993). However, there is an enormous reservoir of potential stimuli available for the wide spectrum of television viewers, both in the promotion of optimal nutrition for growing children as well as for the ecological sustainability of food supply in the future.

The association between television viewing as a marker of sedentarism and obesity has been analyzed from the data collected during cycles II and III of the NHANES study in the United States. In all samples, significant associations between time spent watching television and the prevalence of obesity were revealed. The relationships were consistent even after controlling for a number of possible intervening factors studied simultaneously, such as race, socioeconomic class, region, population density, family variables, and season (Dietz and Gortmaker, 1985). Television viewing was also positively associated with relative weight in Argentinian children and predicted the development of obesity two years later (Faozof, Saenz, and Gonzales, 1999).

An active lifestyle is certainly preferable as there is also a better chance of minimizing marginal or more serious vitamin and mineral deficiencies that could result if food intake was restricted (Pařízková, 1993b). There is enormous potential for the media to portray attractive idols and their way of life. Celebrities could be used to great effect to promote appropriate lifestyle practices such as optimal nutrition and exercise. Such people are able to perform at a high level and look attractive or glamorous, but at the same time also achieve outstanding professional, economic, and social success.

1.4   The Position of an Obese Child

The image of the obese child as "fat, friendless, and unhealthy" is best to prevent as soon as possible. Societal perceptions of thinness and overweight echo the prejudices against the obese condition, even in very young children (Hill and Silver, 1995). It is common for young girls to inappropriately judge their size and shape and have a greater than desirable perceived relevance of weight. Healthy eating is often confused with dieting, which is indicative of the need for better instruction on adequate eating and a more consistent presentation of the health implications of overweight in health promotion. Obese children are likely to be victims and perpetrators of bullying behaviors than their normal-weight peers. This can hinder their social and psychological development at present and also in the future (Janssen et al., 2004).

The conduct of research and the treatment of pediatric obesity have a long tradition in some countries (Cheek, 1968; Mayer, 1974; Pařízková, 1963a,b; 1966; Vamberová, Pařízková, and Vaněčková, 1971), but some new ideas and approaches have appeared as the situation has worsened during the last decades. A large number of approaches to treatment and management have been developed to suit different contexts and psychosocial and economic costs (Covington, 1996). New findings on selected factors such as insulin-like growth factor (IGF) and leptin may provide further possibilities for future success in the management of childhood obesity (Schonfeld-Warden and Warden, 1997). However, until now no marked positive results of leptin application have been found in obese children. Studies on genetic factors such as melanocortin or TrPg/Ag genes with regard to children are more rare than in adults, but new information about these effects has also contributed to the understanding of the obesity problem from this point of view (Chapter 3 and Chapter 9).

One of the main challenges in obesity management is that no comprehensive and fully accepted explanations have been given for the significant increases in the condition across recent decades (Taubes, 1998). Therefore, there is no definite consensus on the main approaches to the treatment of obesity during growth. Major issues are the individuality of the particular obese child and the multifactorial origin of the condition.

The best approach is the prevention of obesity by closely monitoring energy intake, output, and turnover, mainly by monitoring diet and physical activity levels from as early as possible in childhood, especially in children at risk (Davison and Birch, 2001). Such individuals may include, for example, children with obese parents or with a strong family history of obesity (Dietz, 1986; Epstein et al., 1998; Pařízková, 1977; 1996a,b).

1.5   Long-Term Consequences of Childhood Obesity

The association of long-term health risks with child and adolescent adiposity has been reviewed by numerous authors (Power, Lake, and Cole, 1997; Caroli and Burniat, 2002; Zwiauer et al., 2002). On the basis of large epidemiological studies, the child-to-adult adiposity relationship is now well documented, although methodological differences can hinder meaningful comparisons (Dietz, 1998a,b; Guillaume and Lissau, 2002). Fatter children are at a higher risk of becoming overweight or obese adults in spite of the findings that the correlation between, for example, BMI assessed at an age younger than 18 years and adult values is often only mild or moderate.

A study of Japanese youth showed that among obese subjects aged 17 years, most had tracked from primary school or preschool. The earlier the commencement of overweight or obesity, the higher was the BMI at 17 years (Sugimori et al., 1999). Other longitudinal studies have also documented this finding as outlined in subsequent chapters.

The interference of many other factors along with increasing age may be responsible for this limited relationship. Therefore, more long-term studies are necessary to confirm the suggestion from some studies that adult disease risks are associated with a change in adiposity from normal weight in childhood to obesity in adulthood. However, population-based approaches to prevent and treat obesity are necessary for all age categories as it is not only obesity that starts during childhood that is problematic. Obesity that originates and develops at any period of life increases morbidity and mortality in all stages of the human ontogeny, and it should be prevented and treated at any age. There are individuals who were obese during childhood and did not become obese as adults; however, childhood obesity is always a risk for later years of life.

The prediction of adiposity in French adults from anthropometric measurements, including four skinfolds and BMI during childhood and adolescence, was completed after two decades of follow-up. The best correlation between childhood and adulthood values in this population was found for BMI. Correlations between child and adult values of skinfolds were better in males than in females, especially for trunk skinfolds. In females, arm skinfold thickness, especially the biceps, showed a better predictive value than trunk skinfolds. Trunk skinfolds, which are more often associated with metabolic complications of obesity than limb skinfolds, are predictive from childhood measurements in males, but not in females (Rolland-Cachera, Bellisle, and Sempé, 1989).

The assessment of BMI and skinfold thickness may facilitate the identification of children at greater risk of later obesity and the commencement of some preventive measures as early as possible. The utilization of natural approaches such as the improvement of diet and physical activity are recommended in childhood and adolescence, as they are far more preferable than the drastic approaches for weight reduction when obesity is fully developed in later life. Epstein et al. (1995b) have suggested that targeting physical inactivity (such as television viewing and similar activities) along with an increase in vigorous activity are important approaches in the promotion of health and the prevention of obesity.

Contradictory opinions exist regarding whether obesity is preventable (Garrow, 1990). However, it is undisputed that it is possible to limit the deposition of excess fat by various procedures and therefore reduce additional health risks that may be even more dangerous. Finally, it must be stressed that starting a preventive approach as early as possible is always best (Dietz, 1986, 1993; Epstein et al., 1998; Leung and Robson, 1990; Lissau et al., 2002; Pařízková, 1977, 1996a, 1998a,b,c, 2003). The information on childhood obesity in different parts of the world is still scattered and incomplete, and the description and analysis on a global scale using comparable valid criteria as well as methodology have not yet been conducted. This is a task for future international cooperation.

2

Geographical, Historical, and Epidemiological Aspects

2.1 Changes in Obesity Prevalence and Accompanying Variables in Children over Recent Decades in Various Countries

The prevalence of childhood obesity varies in different populations. Some previously published results are difficult to interpret due to such issues as varying definitions of obesity, cutoff points for obesity being derived from differing (local or national) populations, and the oftentimes nonrandomized samples employed. It was only recently that comparisons between studies and populations have become easier, and this trend has corresponded with the utilization and widespread acceptance of the body mass index (BMI) as an indicator of body fatness (Bouchard and Blair, 1999; WHO, 1998; Lobstein, James, and Cole, 2003). In addition, cutoff points for BMI have been established, and this has enabled the differentiation of overweight and obesity into various age categories. Older studies did not use this criterion for the evaluation of obesity, but morphological characteristics of individuals' obesity were commonly used to categorize the condition.

The global prevalence of obesity has become the focus of attention for numerous countries and their respective professional and scientific bodies (Koletzko et al., 2002; Lobstein, James, and Cole 2003; Maffeis, 2000). Changing demographic and social circumstances — in Europe, for example — are linked to childhood obesity. However, it is highly unlikely that these factors interact in the genesis of obesity in a similar way in different individuals and population groups. The understanding of all mechanisms is still limited (Livingstone, 2000). Childhood obesity and its resultant unfavorable outcomes underlie the necessity for a timely diagnosis and subsequent management (Florencio et al., 2001; Wabitsch, 2000).

The World Health Organization (WHO) paid special attention to this problem some years ago (Gurney and Gorstein, 1988; WHO, 1998), but the situation has worsened considerably in the recent past. An International Obesity Taskforce (IOTF) has been established, and the initiative has the full support of the WHO and the International Association for the Study of Obesity (IASO). As a consequence of this interest, an increasing number of clinicians, general practitioners, nutritionists, dietitians, physiologists, and anthropologists are now working in the area of obesity prevention, treatment, and management. A major goal has been to define childhood obesity.

The confusion in the international literature has been substantially reduced since the acceptance in 1997 of the IOTF Childhood Obesity Working Group's decision to use BMI as an indicator of fatness in children and to develop a BMI-for-age reference chart, including cutoff points of BMI for overweight and obesity. These were established on the basis of measurements in six advanced nations (Cole and Rolland-Cachera, 2002) but have been criticized as being not objective for populations with different characteristics (Vígnerová, Lhotská, and Bláha, 2001; Misra, 2003).

The results of studies on the prevalence of obesity, physical activity, and preventive efforts have been compared recently between some countries such as the United States and Europe (Guillaume and Lissau, 2002; Van Mil, Goris, and Westerterp, 1999). As shown for MONICA (WHO monitoring of cardiovascular diseases project) populations, age-standardized proportions of BMI also vary for adults from country to country.

In males, the highest rates of obesity were found in Malta; the region of Bas-Rhin in France; Kaunas (the former USSR, now Lithuania); the former Czechoslovakia (now the separate countries of the Czech Republic and Slovakia); and Germany. On the other hand, the lowest rates of obesity were found in China, Sweden, New Zealand, and Australia. For adult females, the highest prevalence of obesity (BMI > $30\text{kg}/\text{m}^2$) was also found in Kaunas, the Novosibirsk region, and Moscow (all former USSR); Poland; the former Czechoslovakia; and Italy. The lowest prevalence rates for females were found in China. Otherwise, the obesity prevalence was similar for both genders (WHO, 1998). It should be noted, however, that these examples apply to the years 1983 to 1986 (WHO, 1988) and that for places such as China, the situation has been in a process of change recently (Chu, 2001; Iwata et al., 2003).

Gurney and Gorstein (1988) evaluated the prevalence of obesity in preschool-aged children in selected countries and found that the lowest rates were in Papua New Guinea, Bangladesh, the Philippines, Burkina Faso, and other developing countries. The highest rates were found in the islands of Trinidad and Tobago, Iran, Mauritius, Canada, Jamaica, and Chile. In those places the economic situation may have changed recently, leading to a significant increase in obesity rates. Only selected countries not included in MONICA studies were evaluated, in particular the industrially developed countries.

More than 30% of the population in the Caribbean, the Middle East, Northern Africa, and Latin America is overweight. Populations living on the Pacific and Indian Ocean islands have among the highest prevalence of obesity in the world. In Asia and black Africa, the overall incidence of overweight is still low, but it is high in urban areas. In most of these countries, the increase in the number of overweight people has occurred within the last few years. Excess weight appears first among the affluent and then among low-income classes, including young children and teenagers.

More recently, 160 nationally representative cross-sectional surveys from 94 countries were analyzed; overweight was defined as weight-for-height > 2 SD (standard deviation) from the National Center for Health Statistics/ World Health Organization international reference median. The global prevalence of overweight was 3.3%. Some countries and regions had considerably higher rates, and overweight was shown to increase in 16 of 38 countries with trend data. Countries with the highest prevalence of overweight are located mainly in the Middle East, North Africa, and Latin America. Rates of wasting (reduced weight related to height) were higher than those of overweight, with the wasting rates in Africa and Asia 2.5 to 3.5 times higher than those of overweight (de Onis and Blossner, 2000). The obesity problem and the economic costs of its management create an extra burden along with the existing malnutrition in these countries (Delpeuch and Maire, 1997).

International comparisons of social situations in countries such as Brazil, China, and Russia showed that over- and underweight exist simultaneously. The underweight/overweight ratio was highest in the urban environment of all three countries, and there was no clear pattern in the prevalence of the underweight/overweight household type by income. The underweight child coexisting with an overweight nonelderly adult was the predominant pair combination in all three countries (Doak et al., 2000). More trends in overweight and obesity were identified in the United States, Brazil, China, and Russia; regarding nutritional problems, there was indication of a shift from energy deficiency to an excess intake in China and Brazil. In Russia, obesity decreased slightly and overweight increased, while in the United States there has been a marked shift to excess weight in all age categories (Wang, Monteiro, and Popkin, 2002).

2.1.1 North America

Obesity is most widespread in countries with the highest economic standards. For example, in the United States a significant increase (by up to 30%) in the prevalence of obesity in children and adolescents has been evident in recent times. A comparison of the results of National Health and Nutrition Examination Surveys (NHANES) I and II showed an increase in the average values of BMI of the adult population and also an increase in the ratio of subjects with a BMI higher than 30. The problem is not limited to adults but is also an issue for young children. Most observations over time have not shown an increase in food intake (Durnin, 1984; Gortmaker, Dietz, and Cheung, 1990; Pařízková, 1996b), including comparisons through the 1970s and 1990s. Similar conclusions have been made on the basis of observations in other countries, for example in Sweden (Sunnegardh et al., 1986). An energy imbalance is due to both a reduction of energy output and restrictions in physical activity. This applies to the growing subjects of most socioeconomic levels in the industrially developed countries. The essential roles of an inadequate macronutrient intake have been defined (Kimm, 1993), and the etiology of obesity is also related to intake of individual macronutrients (Gibney, 1995). An imbalance between the intake of protein, fat, and carbohydrate does not correspond to the RDAs of the WHO, the European Union (EU), and also of the particular countries.

Secular changes in the trends for obesity prevalence were demonstrated by the Bogalusa Heart Study at the end of the 1980s. Height and weight were assessed in 5- to 14-year-old children, from 1973 to 1984. The age- and gender-specific 85th percentile were used as the cutoff point for the ponderal index (weight/height^3). Secular trends for the increase of weight (2.5 kg) and ponderosity (0.5 to 0.7 kg/m^3) were revealed. Gains in ponderosity over the 11-year period were greater at the 75th percentile than at the 25th percentile. The prevalence of overweight increased from 15 to 24% (Shear et al., 1988). Further assessments in the Bogalusa Heart Study (Srinivasan, Mayers, and Berenson, 2001; Frontini et al., 2001) and others have confirmed this trend. Data from national surveys in the United States indicate that the prevalence of obesity has increased during the last decades. As a criterion for overweight and/or obesity, the 85th (obesity) and 95th (super-obesity) percentiles of triceps skinfold have been used. Compared with skinfold data from the 1963 to 1965 National Health Examination Survey (NHES), the 1976 to 1980 NHES indicated a 54% increase in the prevalence of obesity among children aged 6 to 11 and a 98% increase in the prevalence of super-obesity.

Compared with skinfold data from the 1966 to 1970 NHES, cycle 3 skinfold data from the second NHES indicated a 39% increase in the prevalence of obesity among children 12 to 17 years old, and a 64% increase in the prevalence of super-obesity. The increase in the obesity prevalence was apparent in all age categories and both genders, and was also the same for white and black subjects. Blood pressure data from the four surveys mentioned suggest that the share of pediatric hypertension associated with obesity in children has also increased. According to the speed of changes in the prevalence of obesity, environmental causes are likely to be responsible rather than changes in genetic and hereditary factors (Gortmaker et al., 1987).

The National Health Examination Surveys were executed in five representative cross-sectional studies with face-to-face interview and medical examination from 1963 to 1991. The periods were 1963 to 1965, 1966 to 1970, 1971 to 1974, 1976 to 1980, and 1988 to 1991. From 1988 to 1991, the prevalence of overweight according to BMI was 10.9% based on the 95th percentile, and 22% based on the 85th percentile. Overweight prevalence increased during the period examined among all age and gender groups. Similar to findings reported previously for U.S. adults, the increase was greatest between the years 1976 and 1980 (Klish, 1995; Troiano et al., 1995). Associated negative phenomena in the growing population include the decline of fitness in American children as discussed by others.

Numerous observations have confirmed that overweight during childhood and adolescence is associated with overweight during adulthood. Previous reports have documented an increase in the prevalence of overweight among growing subjects and adults during the periods 1976 to 1980 and 1988 to 1991. NHANES III showed an increase in obesity (BMI > 85th percentile) between 1988 and 1994 by 11.2% in 6- to 11-year-old white subjects, and by 12.2% in 12- to 17-year-old white subjects (Troiano et al., 1995). An increase in childhood weight also occurred in a New York WIC population (Nelson, Chiasson, and Ford, 2004).

During the last 20 years, the prevalence of overweight has also increased in U.S. children aged 4 to 5 years whereas a comparable finding was not seen in children aged one to three years. In 1971 to 1974, a total of 5.8% of 4- to 5-year-old girls were obese, in contrast to 10% in 1988 to 1994. During the period 1988 to 1994, the prevalence of overweight among children from 2 months through to 5 years of age was consistently higher in girls than boys. Mexican-American children had a higher prevalence of overweight than non-Hispanic black and non-Hispanic white children.

These results parallel those reported for older children and adults in the United States (Ogden et al., 1997). The prevalence of overweight among low-income U.S. preschool children in the follow-up studies of the Centers for Disease Control and Prevention Pediatric Nutrition Surveillance System indicated an increase. Increases were from 18.6% in 1983 to 21.6% in 1995 (based on the 85th percentile cutoff point for weight-for-height), and from 8.5 to 10.2% for the same period (based on the 95th percentile cutoff point).

Analyses by single age, sex, and race or ethnic group (non-Hispanic white, non-Hispanic black, and Hispanic) all show increases in the prevalence of overweight although changes were greatest for older preschool children (Mei et al., 1998). The level of economic and social class had no significant effect on the increasing prevalence of overweight in 4- to 5-year-old children in this study.

With reference to young black and white girls, baseline data of the National Heart, Lung and Blood Institute (NHLBI) Growth and Health Study (NGHS) population, compared with data of NHANES I and II, also revealed secular trends of obesity prevalence. Anthropometric measures, height, weight, triceps, and subscapular skinfolds were assessed and BMI calculated. Compared with age-similar girls in the 1970s, girls in the present study were taller and heavier and had thicker skinfolds. The differences in body size were most apparent in black girls, who had a greater body mass than white girls, as early as 9 to 10 years of age.

The prevalence of obesity also appears to be increasing among younger girls, especially black girls (Campaigne et al., 1994). This situation is interpreted as an imminent health risk for these individuals in later life. In conjunction with these findings, poor childhood nutrition resulting in overweight and obesity, and adult cardiovascular diseases are considered to be closely related (McGill, 1997). According to a 1995 National Center for Health

Statistics study, 4.7 million American children aged 6 to 17 years were severely overweight. Another estimate from the New Jersey Department of Health and Senior Services indicated that one in four children weigh too much (Noonan, 1997). In addition to the increasing prevalence of obesity in adults, these results are a disturbing trend. If obesity commences in childhood there are more serious health consequences than if obesity developed during adulthood.

In Falkner's study (1993), black and white 9- and 10-year-old U.S. females were followed longitudinally each year during a 5-year period. Parents were seen in the first year and responded to a questionnaire in the third and fifth years. Initial values for height, weight, BMI, and skinfold thickness were higher in black compared to white girls. On the basis of dietary history, black females consumed a greater amount of energy and a larger proportion of it was fat. White females were physically more active and spent less time watching television than black females. More black than white females expressed a desire to be "on the fat side," and body weight of black mothers was approximately 20 pounds higher than that of white mothers. Findings from studies in the 1980s revealed that nearly half of the black American females were obese and that adolescence is a critical period for the development of obesity. It was also revealed that general and central obesity was developing from childhood to young adulthood in African American and European American subjects with family histories of cardiovascular disease (Dekkers et al., 2004).

The influence of sex and socioeconomic status (SES) is significant with respect to the development of obesity from childhood to adulthood in African American and European American subjects with family histories of cardiovascular disease; however, race, sex, and SES have joint effects on degree of adiposity (Dekkers et al., 2004). An increase in obesity in U.S. subjects is often accompanied by metabolic syndrome since childhood, which further highlights the importance of regular population surveillance of this problem (Eisenmann, 2003).

The prevalence of obesity in Native Americans was 13.7% for men and 16.5% for women. Obesity rates for Native American adolescents and preschool children were higher than the respective rates for all races combined (Broussard et al., 1991). In the native population — for example, Navajo adolescents — 33% of girls and 25% of boys were obese, according to the BMI criterion. Navajo youth tended to have larger skinfolds than their white (NHANES II) and Mexican-American (Hispanic Health and Nutrition Examination Survey) counterparts.

A greater difference in subscapular skinfold measurement is indicative of greater deposits of truncal versus peripheral fat. In girls, BMI was positively related to both systolic and diastolic blood pressure. In boys, systolic blood pressure was higher only in subjects with a higher BMI (Gilbert et al., 1992). This study indicates the urgent need for interventions in Navajo children and youth, because obesity is a significant health risk for blood pressure, as is the case for the white population. Similar conclusions have been drawn for other Native American (Davis et al., 1993c) and Mexican-American children (Foreyt and Cousins, 1993). In third- and fifth-grade Mexican-Indian children on the U.S.–Mexican border, the overall prevalence of obesity was 38%; however, the coexistence of obesity, hunger, and undernutrition was also revealed.

The Hispanic Health and Nutritional Examination Survey (1982 to 1984) provided data on BMI, triceps, and subscapular skinfolds and showed that in the United States, Hispanics had a higher prevalence of overweight and obesity than whites. The prevalence in children was assumed to be similar to that in adults. In Mexican-American preschool children, obese subjects had a significantly higher birth weight and the mothers of obese children had a significantly greater BMI.

Analyses of responses to the ideal infant body habitus scale revealed that mothers of obese children selected a chubby baby as ideal significantly more often than mothers of non-obese children (Alexander, Sherman, and Clark, 1991). This attitude could influence the feeding habits and food intake of obese children early in their lives.

Attitudes and behavior related to nutrition vary significantly in white and black American adolescents and contrast with those of adolescents in other countries. For example, Russian adolescents prefer a larger body size, are less likely to diet, and are less concerned about being overweight. A study of Moscow students (using questionnaires) showed that the ideal weight was higher in Russian and black American boys and girls than in white American boys and girls. After controlling for BMI, black American girls were less than half as likely to report dieting compared with white American girls. There were significant differences among white American girls and Russian girls and no ethnic difference among boys in the prevalence of dieting. White American girls and black American girls were much more likely to identify being overweight as an important nutritional concern than Russian girls. No ethnic differences were evident among boys (Stevens et al., 1997).

The NHLBI Growth and Health study showed that black girls at an early age were more likely to engage in eating practices associated with weight gain (McNutt et al., 1997). This included eating in front of the television, eating while doing homework, and skipping meals. Such practices may have implications for obesity development. Along with the differences in the prevalence of obesity — for example, among Caucasian and African-American girls — it has also been shown that children who suffered neglect or abuse are also more likely to become overweight (Dietz, 1998c).

A follow-up on children from affluent Mexican families showed that 24.2% were obese. Children were more likely to be obese if they were male and from small households with few or no other children and with more permissive parents. TV viewing and diet did not explain gender differences in obesity. Parents considered fatness as a sign of good health (Brewis, 2003).

The increase in the prevalence of overweight and obesity in North America varies according to the individual population groups. Secular changes in

Navajo youth from 1955 to 1997 showed no gender differences. In both sexes, mean age-specific stature appeared to be relatively stable around the 50th percentile of U.S. reference values. Mean age-specific mass appeared to be relatively stable between the 50th and 90th percentiles. Approximately 41% of Navajo boys and girls at the age of 6 to 12 years had BMI greater than the 85th percentile of U.S. reference data. The estimated rate of secular change in body mass was about 1.5 kg per decade in younger boys and girls, and about 3 kg per decade in older boys and girls between 1955 and 1997. BMI changed by about 0.5 to 1.0 units per decade during the same period. Thus, overweight and obesity is a serious risk and health problem in U.S. Navajo children (Eisenmann et al., 2000). Even in the youngest schoolchildren, overweight and obesity according to BMI are highly prevalent in American Indian youth (Story et al., 1999). Overweight is more than twice as likely, and obesity is more than three times as prevalent as national patterns (Zephier, Himes, and Story, 1999). The epidemic of obesity in Pima Indians is paralleled by diabetes (Krosnick, 2000). Also, in a study of Hopi children approximately 23% were classified as overweight and an additional 24% as obese (Eisenmann et al., 2000, 2003).

In Canada, the prevalence of obesity is higher in low-income and multiethnic Montreal schoolchildren. Diet and physical activity assessment in these children showed different patterns related to the environmental conditions. Johnson-Down et al. (1997) evaluated children's height, weight, dietary intake, physical activity records, and lifestyle and demographic characteristics and found that 39.4% of children were overweight, higher than the 85th percentile of NHANES II. Dietary fat intake was significantly higher in children from single-parent families and those with mothers born in Canada. The intake of vitamins was related to income level. Children who were more active had a higher intake of energy, calcium, iron, zinc, and fiber but were not heavier. Overweight children systematically underreported their food intake, and their reported intakes did not meet calculated energy needs. This situation makes it difficult to define the reason for energy imbalance and an enhanced deposition of fat. It must be stressed that inadequate reporting is also possible in relation to the specific frequency, intensity, duration, and type of physical activity. An increase in overweight and obesity was further observed in young schoolchildren from the early to late 1990s in multiethnic, low-income, inner-city Montreal (O'Loughlin et al., 2000).

2.1.2 Latin America

Excessive fatness was found in 6.4% of the population of Argentinian children aged 6 to 12 years; these children were evaluated using local standards and Frisancho's norms for U.S. children. In this population, the prevalence of obesity was generally below the expected values. However, the frequency of excessive fatness was significantly higher in both the 8- to 11-year-old male group (8.9%) and in the girls (10.8%). The prevalence of fatness increased with age in girls and from the age of 8 years onward exceeded the expected percentage (Agrelo et al., 1988). A BMI > 85th percentile was found in 33% of children of both genders in 1995; the U.S. reference for adolescents was 21% at the same time.

An anthropometric survey in Cuba revealed that the prevalence of over-weight in preschool children 0 to 5 years of age was identified as the most frequent nutritional problem, with a prevalence of 5.2%. The prevalence of malnutrition, both chronic and acute, was reduced significantly (by 44.4%) in Cuba between the years 1972 and 1993 (Esquivel et al., 1997).

The prevalence of obesity in Chile is also relatively high and is increasing at a rapid rate. As reported by some observers, girls show higher rates than boys. Young children in first grade have a higher prevalence of obesity, probably due to their higher socioeconomic background (Kain, Uauy, and Diaz, 1998).

The nutritional status of children in an area of São Paolo (Brazil) was assessed using the distribution of z-scores of weight-for-age, height-for-age, and weight-for-height, in relation to growth charts of the National Centre for Health Statistics (NCHS) reference population. Children were further subgrouped according to socioeconomic status. Twenty-two percent of chil-dren were stunted, 15% were wasted, 22% were underweight, and 5% were overweight. Data were further analyzed by age, gender, ethnic group, and socioeconomic level. Thirty-two percent of the very low socioeconomic group were both stunted and had a low weight-for-age. A total of 11.6% from the high socioeconomic strata were obese. These results emphasize the need for a range of programs to deal with nutritional problems in different groups of the population, such as in Brazil (Barros et al., 1990).

The stage of nutrition transition can also significantly influence the nutri-tional status in all age categories. In Brazil, malnutrition is the main problem, yet obesity is the leading health issue among both adults and children in the urban areas of the south, southeast, and rural south. Only in the rural northeast, the poorest region in the country, was malnutrition the main problem in children (Mondini and Monteiro, 1997). Similar to other coun-tries, the economic situation has an important effect. However, this applies only within the framework of a certain range of nutrition and malnutrition.

A study in Rio de Janeiro showed the prevalence of overweight and risk for overweight in 37.8% of girls and 36.4% of boys (Ramos De Marins, et al., 2002). Another study in Rio de Janeiro analyzed the associations between low stature as a marker of early malnutrition, obesity, and abdominal fatness among adults. Increased adult fatness in stunted women was not explained by racial and socioeconomic conditions, energy intake, or age at menarche (Sichieri, Siqueira, and Moura, 2000).

2.1.3 Europe

Understanding of the increasing prevalence of obese youth and the variabil-ity in susceptibility for its development in Europe is still limited, though it has been accepted that the new environmental challenges are contributory (Livingstone, 2001).

The Belgian-Luxembourg Child Study was executed in an area with a cluster of obesity as well as other risk factors for cardiovascular diseases and non-insulin-dependent-diabetes (NIDDM) (Guillaume et al., 1993). This study confirmed the important role of an increased BMI at a young age on later health. In the initial phases of the study, children aged 6 to 12 years showed that BMI was significantly related to birth weight in boys but not in girls in the same age groups.

Blood pressure, fasting plasma triglycerides (TG), and insulin but not blood glucose and total cholesterol (TC) increased significantly with higher BMI quintiles. These relationships were most pronounced for the fifth BMI quintile. No significant relationship was found for BMI and breast-feeding, social or educational status of the parents, or estimated physical activity (Guillaume et al., 1993). The continuation of the above-mentioned study with children from 6 to 12 years of age revealed that BMI was strongly correlated between the children and both parents, and between the parents and grandparents (Guillaume et al., 1995). In Brussels, 20% of 12-year-old boys and 19% of 12-year-old girls had a BMI > 120% of the median. In the same sample, 5% had a BMI > 140% of the median (De Spiegelaere et al., 1998a,b). The Belgian-Luxembourg Child Study IV revealed a changed pattern of food intake and an increase in the prevalence of overweight (Guillaume, 1998). Other Belgian studies have showed an increase in BMI from 1969 to 1996 (Hulens et al., 2001).

Similar results have been reported in other industrially developed countries. For example, in Switzerland one study noted a doubling in the proportion of obese children of both genders in the pre- and post-pubertal periods (Woringer and Schutz, 1998). From 1975 to 1989 there was an increase in the prevalence of obese pupils in Hamburg, Germany, from 4 to 11%. In addition, an age differentiation was reported. Overweight was diagnosed in 6.3% of preschool children, 17.2% in children aged approximately 10 years, and 17.3% in children aged approximately 14 years. The effect of social class was apparent both in the prevalence of obesity and in the enrollment in regular exercise. In the low socioeconomic districts the reverse was noted; the rate of overweight and obese children was higher and enrollment in sports activity was low. In high social class districts the rate of overweight and obese children was lower and the rate of sporting children higher (Petersen, 1998).

In Germany the increasing prevalence of obesity shows considerable regional differences. Moreover, obesity increased in 5- to 6-year-old children, with prevalence at an unexpected 7%, and in 13- to 15-year-olds, prevalence reached 8%. These changes were accompanied by many obesity-related morbidities (Wabitsch et al., 2002). An increased prevalence of obesity in preschool children during the period 1982 to 1997 was also revealed in a study by Kalies, Lenz, and Von Kries (2002). This is comparable to other European findings, but the values are lower relative to U.S. and Australian data. Overweight and obesity already appears in German preschool children manifested by higher BMI values (Herpertz-Dahlmann et al., 2003).

Frye and Heinrich (2003) also confirmed an increase of overweight and obesity in children from former Eastern Germany. Higher parental education, low birth weight, and breast-feeding were protective with regard to obesity. In the eastern part of Germany (the former German Democratic Republic), significant changes in subcutaneous fat and BMI occurred, especially from 1985 to 1995. Height increased less than body weight; BMI therefore increased significantly. The amount of subcutaneous fat increased, along with changes in distribution: the ratio of trunk to extremity skinfolds decreased significantly in both genders between 1975 and 1985 but increased significantly between 1985 and 1996. Changes in the nutritional habits and lifestyle, evidently related to the reunification of Germany in 1989, may be the reason for these changes (Kromeyer-Hauschild and Jaeger, 1998; Kromeyer-Hauschild et al., 1999).

Marked increases in obesity prevalence have also occurred in the adult English population (Prentice and Jebb, 1995) when values are compared between 1980 and 1991, or 1989 and 1998 (Hundred, Kitchiner, and Buchan, 2001). Lack of physical activity was considered one of the most important causes; however, on average energy intake decreased during the same period. Trends in weight-for-height and triceps skinfold thickness were followed for English and Scottish children from 1972 to 1982 and from 1982 to 1990, in the framework of the National Study of Health and Growth. Data from 1972, 1982, and 1990 for children aged between 4.5 and 11.99 years were compared. All measurements increased from 1972 to 1990 except for weight-for-height in English boys, and were generally greater when comparing the measurements between 1982 and 1990 than 1972 and 1982. Approximately one-third of the increase in weight-for-height and triceps skinfold thickness from 1972 to 1990 was associated with increases in parental BMIs and decreases in family size. No consistent differences in trends were found between social groups. Greater trends were found for girls and for Scottish children. Scottish boys are now heavier and fatter than their English counterparts (Chinn and Rona, 1994). A steady increase in the prevalence of overweight and obesity in U.K. children was also revealed in further research by Chinn and Rona (2001b) in three cross-sectional studies of British children between 1974 and 1994. Increasing levels of excess weight of some 13 to 20% were noted among British children during the period 1994 to 1998 (Lobstein, James, and Cole, 2003).

Obesity prevalence also increased in younger children, as shown by a follow-up of subjects measured first at the age of 1 to 3 months, and then at the age of 2.9 to 4.0 years. From 1989 to 1998 there was a highly significant increase in the proportion of overweight children, from 14.7 to 23.6%, and of obese children, from 5.4 to 9.2%. There was also a significant increase in the mean BMI and in the mean SD score for weight but not height. Infants showed a small but significant increasing trend in mean SD for weight score (Hundred, Kitchiner, and Buchan, 2001).

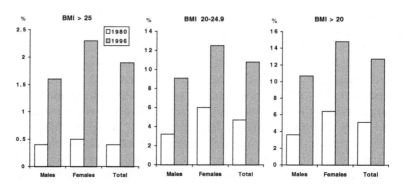

FIGURE 2.1
The changes in the prevalence of obesity (%) in French children during the period from 1980 to 1996. (Based on data from Vol, Tichet, and Rolland-Cachera, 1998.)

A study among Plymouth primary schoolchildren in the United Kingdom also provided evidence for an association between deprivation in early life and childhood obesity. The obesity prevalence increased with age and nearly doubled in the oldest children compared with the youngest. There was a significant trend for higher rates of obesity related to increasing deprivation in both boys and girls (Kinra, Nelder, and Lewendon, 2000).

The values of height, weight, and body fat measured by bio-impedance analysis (BIA) were compared in Scottish children between baseline and 12 months (Fomon et al., 1982). All measures increased; the mean change in the percentage of body fat was +2.8% in girls and +1.8% in boys, though in 21% of girls and 25% of boys the percentage of stored fat decreased over the 12 months of observation. No gender differences in height and weight were observed at either measurement. Compared with the values assessed by Fomon et al. (1982), children were taller and heavier, and had a similar percentage of stored fat at the age of 7 years but a greater percentage of fat at the age of 8 years (Ruxton et al., 1998).

During the last quarter of the past century, childhood obesity also increased in Swiss children born in 1980 and followed longitudinally between 5 and 16 years, when compared with a cohort born in 1954 to 1956. The BMI thresholds of Cole were used; overweight increased more than obesity and was more significant in boys than girls (Woringer and Schutz, 2002).

A study of the prevalence of obesity in French children showed an increase from 5.1 to 12.7% (Figure 2.1). In both adults and children, very severe obesity was about five times as frequent in 1996 as it was in 1980. The prevalence of obesity is still lower in France compared to other industrially developed countries. This increase in prevalence and the overall trend in this respect have raised the level of interest in this serious health problem (Vol, Tichet, and Rolland-Cachera, 1998).

An increase in pediatric obesity in French children from 1980 to 1990 (> 90th percentile of BMI) was 17% and for super-obesity (> 97th percentile of BMI), it was 20% (Rolland-Cachera, Spyckerelle, and Deschamps, 1992).

From 1976 to 1995, the prevalence of obesity in 10-year-old children increased from 6.3 to 14.4%. In addition, fatness and food intake and the composition of food have become more important issues (Rolland-Cachera and Bellisle, 1986; Rolland-Cachera et al., 1995).

These increased trends in the prevalence of obesity are consistent with those noted in the United States and Denmark. In France severe obesity increased more than mild obesity. These changes are derived from an altered skewness of the distribution (Rolland-Cachera, Spyckerelle, and Deschamps, 1992). The prevalence of obesity in Danish recruits increased 50 times during the postwar period, from 0.15 to 5% (Astrup, Lundsgaard, and Stock, 1999). The INCA study conducted from 1998 to 1999 revealed an inverse relationship between overweight and obesity and SES. For example, 6.5% of children in the higher SES were either overweight or obese compared to 23.9% of those from the lower SES (Lioret et al., 2001).

The prevalence of obesity has also increased in other European countries such as Poland (Charzewska and Figurska, 1983; Koehler et al., 1988). In Russian adolescents, a different attitude to the overweight and obese condition has been reported (Stevens et al., 1997). Observations in 23,462 Bulgarian children and adolescents (BMI, skinfolds) showed several peaks in the prevalence of obesity at different ages. The first peak occurred between the ages of 3 to 6 years and reached 10%. The second peak occurred from 10 to 12 years, reached 12–14%, and coincided with the beginning of puberty. The third peak was between 15 and 17 years of age and was more obvious among boys. In more than 80% of cases, obesity started to develop at an early age, commonly during the first 7 years of life (Stanimirova, Petrova, and Stanimirov, 1993).

In the Czech Republic, BMI values increased from 1945 to 1952. From 1961 to 1991, and up to 1995, the prevalence of obesity based on average values of basic morphological parameters had not changed (Vígnerová et al., 1999). In girls, a continued trend overweight reduction was observed. A recent comparison of BMI values of Czech and English children did not show any significant differences (Bláha, Vígnerová, and Lisá, 1999).

In Austria, Elmadfa et al. (1994) showed that the prevalence of obesity increased from 19% at the age of 7–9 years to 29% at the age of 15–19 years in boys. In girls, the prevalence of obesity decreased from 16 to 13% in the same age intervals. Later it was revealed that the prevalence of obese children was approximately 5 to 8% (Widhalm, Sinz, and Egger, 1998) and that overweight in children and adolescents accounted for about 8% of the entire population. There was no marked change in the percentage of subjects who could be classified as overweight or obese in the different age categories. Another estimate for Austrian children is 12 to 15% in 11- to 18-year-old youth (Widhalm, Sinz, and Egger, 1998).

The prevalence of obesity also varies in different parts of individual countries where the environmental conditions are more homogenous. For example, in a small rural community of Lazio (Italy), prevalence was 17.7% and the food intake of children 7 to 14 years old showed an imbalance of nutrients

(Pantano et al., 1992). On the other hand, the prevalence of obesity in Roman adolescents was 6.9% and of hypertension, 6%. This was not particularly high compared to other localities in Italy as well as other industrially developed countries (Menghetti et al., 1993). However, food composition was inadequate, with a high fat intake compared to carbohydrates and starches. If continued, this trend may have a negative effect later in life.

A high prevalence of obesity was also found in the childhood population (mean age of 9.6 years) living in Naples, Italy (Esposito-Del Puente et al., 1996). The percentile values for the triceps skinfold were similar to those reported for other populations of children, but BMI values were different. Children in Naples have the highest BMI values at the 50th, 75th, 90th, and 95th percentiles. The prevalence of obesity among Neapolitan children was estimated using the BMI value at the 90th percentile as a cutoff. The prevalence of obesity in Neapolitan girls was a staggering 5.2 times higher than in France, 3.3 times higher than in Holland, 1.7 times higher than in the United States, and 2.5 times higher than in Milan, Italy. Similar trends were seen for boys: 4.3 times higher than in France, 4.0 times than in Holland, 2.1 times higher than in the United States, and 2.5 times higher than in Milan (Esposito-Del Puente et al., 1996).

An update of obesity in childhood has also been completed in a district of Rome (Visali et al., 1998). Obesity was more common in 8- to 9-year-old children, and when pooled with overweight youngsters, the total represented more than 50% of all children followed in the study. These results underline the alarming extent of the problem of pediatric obesity in city areas in Italy (Visali et al., 1998).

A cross-sectional epidemiological study that included anthropometric measurements and dietary surveys was undertaken with Spanish children aged 6 to 13 years. The prevalence of obesity in this community was 26%, considerably higher than the national average (6 to 15% in 1991 using the same criteria). The most important factors contributing to the development of obesity were low levels of physical activity and genetic and environmental factors influenced by conditioned eating behavior (Mumbiela Pons, Sanmartin Zaragoza, and Gonzales Alvarez, 1997). A comparison of BMI in Aragonese children from 1985 to 1995 showed significant increases in the prevalence of overweight that differed by age and gender. The increasing skewness of BMI in the upper percentiles of the population, especially in boys, suggests that not only do children get fatter but that the fatter individuals are becoming more obese (Moreno et al., 2001b).

A study of Catalonian adolescents showed that 15% were obese. Some 13.5% presented with Grade I obesity (BMI 25 to 29.9 kg/m^2), and 1.3% with Grade II obesity (BMI 30 to 40 kg/m^2). In addition, obese subjects were more likely to show concern for their diet. The results of this study revealed a lower prevalence of obesity in Spain than in the United States. No linear relationship existed between the degree of excess weight and the restraint boundary with regard to eating behavior (Sanchez-Carracedo, Saldana, and Domenech, 1996). However, in some Spanish communities the prevalence of obesity in growing subjects can be higher — for example 26%, which exceeds the national average mentioned earlier.

In Yugoslavia, overweight (that is, +1 to +2 SD) was registered in 19.4% of children in a sample of the national survey of children under 5 years of age (Plecas et al., 1998). Of the children included in the study, 12.9% were above +2 SD relative to the reference weight-for-height value, and 5% above +3 standard deviations. The prevalence of obesity was highest in children aged 2 to 3 years (17.8%), while variations by gender were not significant. Regional distribution showed the highest prevalence of overweight (16.7%) and obese children (17.2%) in the Belgrade area, where 8% of the total sample had a weight for height +3 SD and over the reference values (Plecas et al., 1998).

In representative samples of children aged 6 to 18 years from three cities in northern Yugoslavia, a relatively high prevalence of overweight and obesity was revealed when using different standards as criteria (WHO/NCHS standards and BMI NHANES using the software CHILD). Using BMI criteria, the prevalence of overweight was 12.9% in boys and 12.0% in girls, and the prevalence of obesity was 8.76% in boys and 9% in girls (Pavlovic et al., 1999b). Imbalanced nutrition had an effect on the nutritional status of these children that was also reflected in an increased ratio of health risks; there was an increased level of serum TC in 11.9%, low high-density lipoprotein (HDL-C) in 16%, high low-density lipoprotein (LDL-C) in 21.7%, and hyper-triglyceridemia in 30% of subjects (Pavlovic et al., 1999a).

A statistically significant difference between urban and rural children in the Skopje region of Macedonia was found, with a greater prevalence of overweight in the urban area. In both groups, serum triglycerides were higher in obese children. The same trend was identified in the observed association between the nutritional status and HDL-C levels, where a greater percentage of the obese urban children had lower values of HDL-C (Tasevska et al., 1999). The increasing prevalence of obesity has also been shown in Greek school children (Krassas et al., 2001).

Environmental conditions in the Arctic region of Finland may be the cause of an early maturation. This factor is associated with a higher BMI and proportion of body fat with a greater amount of trunk fat during adolescence, which contributes to overweight and obesity. However, it is unclear whether early maturation is a causal factor or the result of the conditions in this region (Rummukainen and Rasanen, 1999). Adolescent obesity has also been associated with adverse social outcomes such as unemployment, especially in Finnish women (Laitinen et al., 2002).

In Denmark, the prevalence of obesity defined by the 99th percentile of BMI has increased in boys born in the 1940s and since the mid-1960s. This occurred without corresponding changes in the central part of the BMI distribution. When the cutoff for obesity was the 95th percentile, there was a distinct age-dependent increase in the late 1940s (Thomsen, Ekstrom, and Sorensen, 1999). These results indicate that the obesity epidemic is a heterogenous phenomenon resulting from environmental effects starting with preschool age and influencing various sets of the population in a different way. This may be due both to the various sensitivities and predispositions of particular individuals as well as different exposure to the effect of the environment, including nutrition and physical activity level (PAL).

The first evaluation in a representative sample in Cyprus revealed that the prevalence of childhood obesity is comparable to that observed in North America; however, the rate of increase differs significantly depending on the method of estimation (Savva et al., 2002).

2.1.4 Asian Countries

Childhood obesity is also a fast-emerging problem in Asia (Hara, 1988; Takahashi et al., 1999) and is associated with increased health risks (Yajnik, 2004). Obesity prevalence in Chinese children living in Beijing was 2.1% in 1985 and 5% in 1998. A significant relationship between infantile obesity, consumption of junk food, and physical inactivity ($p < 0.05$, $p < 0.01$) has also been noted. In China, television viewing is not yet associated with obesity (Iwata et al., 2003).

The patterns and correlates of obesity in China were also considered in the framework of a national longitudinal survey (the China Health and Nutrition Survey) conducted in 1989 and 1991. In adults, BMI was positively correlated with energy and fat intake, household income, and physical activity. Those living in an urban environment with a higher income displayed a lower energy intake, higher fat intake, and lower physical activity levels compared to those in rural settings and other income categories (Popkin et al., 1995).

The China Health and Nutrition Survey showed that the prevalence of obesity increased from 4.2% in 1989 to 6.4% in 1997 among 2- to 6-year-old Chinese children. This increase occurred mostly in urban areas, where the prevalence of obesity increased from 1.5 to 12.6% in 1997 and the prevalence of overweight increased from 24.6 to 28.9% during the same period. Longitudinal analyses showed BMI increased by 0.2 kg/m^2 per year in urban areas and by 0.1 kg/m^2 per year in rural areas. In a multivariate analysis, overweight at the age of 2 to 5 years, parental overweight, high income, and urban areas independently predicted overweight at the age of 10 to 14 years (Luo and Hu, 2002). Greater increase of fatness with unfavorable central distribution was also confirmed in urban Chinese children in another study in central Beijing (Iwata et al., 2003).

A cross-sectional growth survey of boys and girls from birth to 18 years in Hong Kong enabled the refinement of weight-for-age and weight-for-height percentile charts. There was an average increase of 8.5 kg and 5.1 kg in the 18-year-old boys and girls, respectively, compared to those surveyed 30 years ago. The percentile curves between 6 and 18 years were similar to those for Singaporean and American pre-pubertal children (Leung et al., 1996) with health risks of obesity comparable to those in other parts of the world (Ho, 1990).

According to an island-wide survey in Taiwan, the prevalence of obesity varied from 4.3 to 17.4% in children aged 3 to 19 years. The weight-for-length index was used as local BMI standards were not available. Obese children had a high prevalence of hypertension, hyperlipidemia, and abnormal glucose metabolism with colored striae predominantly located on the thighs, arms, and abdomen (Chen, 1997). A study by Chu (2001) of changes from 1980 to 1994 showed that the mean value of body weight in Taiwanese children increased significantly over increases in body height, especially among boys. Although the percentage of overweight children remained steady during the period for both genders, the prevalence and trends of obesity increased significantly, especially among boys and older girls. The prevalence of obesity was also reported as higher in 2002 than in 1997 by Huang, Wu, and Yang (2003).

In countries where food insecurity and malnutrition have had detrimental effects on child growth and metabolic processes, the increased accessibility and choice of various foodstuffs (including those with high fat and energy), along with sedentary lifestyles introduced during recent periods, may promote obesity development (Richards and Marley, 1998). This also applies to the stunted children suffering from malnutrition during earlier periods of growth (Subramanyam, Jayashree, and Rafi, 2003b).

Elementary schoolchildren in Tokyo were examined for nutritional status and obesity prevalence. The intake of lipids exceeded the recommended levels, and mean BMI and Rohrer's Index scores were slightly higher than Japanese standards. Triglycerides (TG) and the atherogenic index were positively correlated with these obesity parameters, and HDL-C and HDL-C/TC negatively correlated with obesity (Hongo et al., 1992). Further studies have confirmed the increase in childhood obesity in Japan (Murata, 2000; Yoshinaga et al., 2004). Comparisons of the prevalence of overweight (BMI > 21 kg/m^2) in Japanese and Korean junior high school pupils showed a higher prevalence in Korean girls. No differences were found in boys. Body fat measured by BIA in Japanese children was significantly higher than that of Korean children due to a greater lean body mass in Korean subjects, especially in girls. Further observation in younger age categories showed a lack of differences in certain food habits (such as intake of snacks and sweet drinks), but Korean preschoolers spent more time playing outdoors than their Japanese peers (Yoshino et al., 1998). Rapid increases in obesity prevalence were revealed in Japanese boys as well as insignificant increases in girls from elementary schools (Yoshinaga et al., 2004).

In urban India, childhood obesity increased as a marker of diabetes and cardiovascular disease prevalence, and this trend continued until adulthood, when obesity correlated with that apparent at an earlier age. The reasons are the same as in other countries: changes in lifestyle, and diet and physical activity. Age-adjusted percentages of overweight were 17.8 in boys and 15.8 in girls; an increase was noted with age, and the percentages were higher in the lower tertiles of physical activity and in higher socioeconomic groups. Birth weight and current BMI were positively associated (Ramachandran et al., 2002). In Chennai, the prevalence of child overweight in 1981 was 9.6 and 9.7% in 1998. In contrast, the prevalence of obesity was 5.8% in 1981 and 6.2% in 1998. BMI levels for the corresponding age increased during the same period (Subramanyam et al., 2003b).

In Bombay (Mumbai), the prevalence of obesity was related to age group, income, diet type, family history, and occupation. The usual criterion of BMI underestimated the prevalence of obesity, and body fat content overestimated it. These findings highlight the variable character of the morphological development of obesity in different parts of the world. Students had the lowest (10.7%) and medical doctors the highest (53.1%) prevalence of obesity, with prevalence positively associated with financial income and family history. The study underlined the extent of the obesity problem in Bombay and provided directions for nutritional planning in the future (Dhurandhar and Kulkarni, 1992). Some comparisons have showed that the prevalence of obesity in Asian countries in the higher socioeconomic groups is very similar to rates found in the United States and other industrialized countries. Positive energy balance, i.e., higher energy intake and lower output, was suggested as a cause of the increasing obesity in Bengali children in Dhaka (Rahman et al., 2002).

Malaysian preschool children aged 3 to 6 years showed significantly more of the severe grades of obesity compared to Chinese and Japanese children of the same age in Singapore (Ray, Lim, and Ling, 1994). In other Asian countries such as Thailand, with their rapidly growing economies and changing lifestyles, obesity has also become a serious problem. A study was completed of 6- to 12-year-old children, and the prevalence of obesity (as defined by weight-for-height greater than 120% of the Bangkok reference) rose from 12.2% in 1991 to 13.5% in 1992 and to 15.6% in 1993. In another study, it was also concluded that obesity had emerged as a health problem, especially in urban areas. Marked relationships were noted between childhood obesity and parents' educational level and household income (Sakamoto et al., 2001).

In a study by Mo-suwan, Junjana, and Puetpaiboon (1993), increases in body weight and triceps skinfold thickness in obese children who attended a weight control program were significantly less than in the nonattendees in the first year, and also during the second year when the differences were less pronounced. The effect of changes in nutrition due to the transition and acculturation to a different lifestyle has been significant, as is the case in other similar countries.

2.1.5 Middle East, Africa, Oceania

Measurements in Israeli high school girls showed that 17% were obese. A much larger percentage expressed dissatisfaction with their body weight and shape. Comparisons with earlier studies in Israel indicate a large increase in concern for weight and dieting behaviors, with prevalence rates similar to those reported in other Western countries (Neumark-Sztainer, Palti, and Butler, 1995).

The assessment of BMI in Lebanese adolescent girls showed that the mean BMI value in each age range was between the corresponding 90th and 97th percentile of the French reference population. The mean percentage of adolescent girls with severe obesity was 11% (Pharaon, El Metn, and Frelut, 1998). A study of secondary school students in Bahrain, aged 15 to 21 years, revealed the overweight or obese prevalence of boys and girls according to BMI to be 15.6 and 17.4%, respectively. Family size, parents' education, and family history of obesity were also significantly associated with obesity among boys; family history was the only socioeconomic factor significantly related to obesity among girls. Patterns such as eating between meals, the number of meals per day, and the method of eating were not associated with obesity in Bahraini subjects. Boys who ate alone were three times more likely to be obese than those who ate with family members (Musaiger et al., 1993).

Schoolchildren in Cairo aged 11 to 16 years were evaluated for nutritional status using measurements of weight, height, and skinfold thickness. A triceps skinfold greater than 18 mm in boys and 35 mm in girls was considered as a low level of obesity. Age at menarche, birth order, social class, obesity in other members of the family, food habits, and dietary intakes were also examined. The results showed that the prevalence of obesity in Egyptian children living in the capital was comparable to that in the United States. The study also emphasized the importance of social and cultural factors in the development of childhood obesity in Egypt (Darwish et al., 1985); however, the situation may be very different in rural areas. Further measurements in Egyptian children showed a greater prevalence of obesity in urban girls compared with those in rural areas, and in those girls with a higher socioeconomic status (Jackson, Rashed, and Saad-Eldin, 2003).

In Saudi Arabia, children from 1 to 18 years were evaluated using the international sex-specific cutoff points for BMI. The overall prevalence of overweight was 10.7 and 12.7% for the boys and girls, respectively; the prevalence of obesity was 6.0 and 6.74%, respectively. The prevalence varied in different provinces and according to age until after 13 years, when the prevalence rate increased (El Hazmi and Warsy, 2002). In Iran, the prevalence of childhood obesity is significantly higher than would be expected and increases with age (Dorosty, Siassi, and Reilly, 2002). An increase of obese children has also been observed in Kuwait.

In Cameroon, the level of urbanization is one of the highest in sub-Saharan Africa. Dramatic demographic changes facilitate modifications in lifestyle, notably in nutritional patterns. Rapid shifts in the composition of diet and activity patterns along with subsequent changes in body composition are likely to have contributed to the increased prevalence of obesity and related adverse health effects. In a Youandee population, 18.2% of girls and 1.7% of boys aged 12 to 19 years were obese. In children aged 9 to 11 years, 3.3% of boys and girls were overweight, lower than for France and the United States. Menarche in this population appears to be linked to the increased prevalence of overweight, with a dramatic increase from premenarcheal to postmenarcheal status (Tichet et al., 1993; Oppert and Rolland-Cachera, 1998).

A survey of anthropometric profiles expressed in terms of the NCHS standards conducted in the Cape Town metropolitan area in 1990 revealed growth retardation and wasting in this population. These features coexisted with an emergent obesity among 3- to 6-year-old children (Bourne et al., 1994).

A dramatic increase in the prevalence of obesity was also seen in Western Samoa during the period 1978 to 1991. Substantial differences in the prevalence of obesity (BMI > 30 kg/m^2) were found between urban and rural populations in 1978. In 1991, the prevalence of obesity was greater in urban than in rural areas. By contrast, waist/hip ratio (WHR) varied little between each area. Even in subjects aged 25 to 34 years, more than 50% of women from each location and 45% of men from urban areas were obese. Increased physical activity in men but not in women was associated with lower BMI values. Increased levels of education and professional work were associated with increasing BMI, but only significant in men. Multivariate analysis showed age, location (urban), occupation (high status, women) and in men, physical inactivity, to be independently associated with increased risk of obesity. It can be speculated that a comparable increase in obesity prevalence may also be a concern in this country for children and adolescents (Hodge et al., 1994).

Similar changes were described in coastal and highland Papua New Guinea (Hodge et al., 1995), where the association between obesity and the individual degree of modernization was investigated. A modernity score was gained based on the area of origin, father's employment, type and duration of the individual's employment, education, years spent in an urban center, housing type, and spouse score. More "modern" subjects had a higher mean BMI and lower levels of physical activity. Mean WHR also varied with modernity in men but not in women. In a linear regression analysis, the total modernity score was significantly associated with both BMI and WHR in men and women (Hodge et al., 1995). When components of modernity were examined, younger age, more sophisticated housing, and increasing number of years in an urban center were independently associated with BMI in both genders, and education level and reduced physical activity were also significant predictors in men. Associations with WHR were weaker. Additionally, in the French West Indies an excess of overweight and obesity was observed in adolescents (Caius and Benefice, 2002); similar findings were noted for children in the Seychelles with values as high or higher than in some industrialized countries (Stettler et al., 2002).

A substudy of dietary intake suggested that the lowest intake occurred in the least modern subjects of both genders. Children and adolescents were not included in this study, but a similar situation with regard to the effect of modernity may be assumed during the growth period. The adoption of Western ways, which are associated with physical inactivity and increased availability of energy-dense Western food, has already promoted obesity in this rapidly developing Pacific region (Hodge et al., 1995).

2.1.6 Australia

There is growing evidence that the prevalence of obesity in Australian children is increasing. Trend data support substantial increases in BMI between 1985 and 1997 consistent with the situation in other parts of the world. Secular trends of the increase in obesity prevalence were found in Australian children (using a comparison of reanalyzed values of BMI with the new standard international definition in children) for the years 1985 and 1995 (Magarey, Daniels, and Boulton, 2001). The work of Lazarus et al. (1995, 1996) contributed significantly to the decision making regarding the measurement of childhood obesity. During the period 1987 to 1997, the population prevalence of overweight and obesity combined doubled and that of obesity trebled in young Australians. The increase during the period 1969 to 1985 was much smaller (Booth et al., 2003).

The New South Wales Schools Fitness and Physical Activity Survey showed no difference between anthropometric measures when comparing urban and rural boys and girls. Only the WHR ratio was higher in urban girls. Among boys, there were no differences between the SES tertiles in any of the parameters measured (height, weight, waist and hip girths, skinfolds). Among girls, each of the anthropometric measures except skinfolds was negatively related to socioeconomic status. Girls from the highest SES group tended to be less fat than those from the lowest tertile (Booth, Macaskill, and Baur, 1999). At the beginning of the 21st century, at least 20% of Australian youths were overweight or obese, with rapid rises in prevalence apparently continuing (Baur, 2002; Gordon et al., 2003).

The extremely high levels of general and truncal obesity were also shown in 3- to 7-year-old New Zealand children (Gordon et al., 2003). An increase in BMI over an 11-year period was observed in all ethnic groups in New Zealand, and Maori and Pacific island children showed higher percentages of overweight and obesity compared to those with a European background (Turnbull et al., 2004).

2.2 Problems of Obesity in Third World Countries

2.2.1 Prevalence

As previously mentioned, obesity among youngsters and smaller children is increasingly more common in Third World countries. These findings have traditionally been seen in children from families in higher socioeconomic categories — for example, children in Cairo (Darwish et al., 1985) and elsewhere (Chen, 1997). The lifestyle characterizing these individuals is very similar to the situation in industrially developed countries (Pařízková and Hainer, 1989).

Generally, children in developing countries have different problems compared with children in developed countries because they are subjected to poor nutrition and health care. Traditionally, such children have exhibited a relatively low prevalence of obesity irrespective of the criteria used. According to WHO and NCHS 50th percentiles, 20 to 30% of children are stunted at the age of 2 to 3 years. While childhood obesity is not usually associated with such growth patterns, a high prevalence of female adolescent obesity has been reported. Unfortunately, obesity and undernutrition now coexist in many developing countries (Bacardi-Gascon et al., 2003; Rahman et al., 2002).

2.2.2   Obesity and Stunting

An excess deposition of fat can occur in individuals whose height was delayed by early malnutrition and who became stunted. If the availability of food improved and children resumed a more consistent energy intake, they could become quite obese and have a shorter stature that fails to "catch up." This phenomenon has been seen in growing subjects in China, Brazil, and Cameroon, to name a few (Cameron, 1998; Pasquet et al., 1999; Popkin, Richards, and Montiero, 1996). An increased risk of obesity in stunted children has also been reported in Hispanic, Jamaican, and Andean populations.

A study by Popkin, Richards, and Montiero (1996) analyzed the relationship between stunting and the overweight status of children aged 3 to 6 and 7 to 9 years using nationally representative samples in Russia, Brazil, and the Republic of South Africa. In addition, a nationwide survey was conducted in China and identical cutoff criteria for BMI were used for each of the populations studied. The prevalence of overweight in these countries ranged from 10.5 to 25.0% (based on the 85th percentile). The most recent NHANES III results indicate that the prevalence is around 22% in the United States.

Stunting was common in the surveyed countries and affected 9.2 to 30.6% of all children with a significant association between stunting and overweight. The income-adjusted risk ratios for overweight for a stunted child ranged from 1.7 to 7.8. When sufficient food is available, an important association between stunting and increased weight-for-height can appear that applies for a variety of populations of ethnic, environmental, and social backgrounds. This association can have serious public health implications, especially for lower-income countries that have recently experienced significant changes in dietary and activity patterns (Popkin, Richards, and Montiero, 1996).

The underlying mechanisms have not been fully explored. Results of experiments in animals (pigs) malnourished *in utero* and/or over one, two, or three years were retarded in growth and became smaller adults. The longer the period of undernutrition, the greater the impact on the subsequent length of the body. Limb lengths were progressively smaller the fatter the animals became. The standard measurements of the thickness of the subcutaneous fat layer in these animals did not provide a true picture of level of fatness. The muscles in the animals rehabilitated after two and three years of undernutrition were so infiltrated with fat that the muscle fibers were completely embedded within it (Widdowson, 1974).

This raises an important question regarding the development of fat cells. It has been suggested that overfeeding in infancy causes rapid multiplication of cells in the adipose tissue, which in turn leads to an excessive number of fat cells and can result in adult obesity (Brook, 1972; Brook, Lloyd, and Wolf, 1972; Hirsch and Knittle, 1970; Knittle, 1971). The finding in pigs suggests that the opposite can also be true. The animals studied had cells full of fat at ten days of age when undernutrition began, but these cells became completely empty and remained so for the whole of the period of undernutrition whether it lasted one, two, or three years. The pigs began to deposit fat rapidly in their bodies as soon as plentiful food was supplied, and the longer the period of deprivation, the fatter they tended to become.

Marasmic children may also become fat when they are rehabilitated, but there is little information on the number of adipose tissue cells before and after rehabilitation. Brook's (1972) hypothesis on the sensitive period for fat cell multiplication during the first year of life in humans could lead to the conclusion that children who are severely malnourished during the first year of life develop less than the average final number of fat cells. Alternatively this may occur but, similar to the way pigs do, they may lay down fat rapidly when rehabilitated. Deposition of fat during such a situation is more rapid after the period of severe malnutrition than the rehabilitation of other tissues of the body as shown in adults (Minnesota experiment, Keys et al., 1950).

Problems concerning the effects of early nutrition on the deposition of fat in the body and the number of cells in the adipose tissue produced to accommodate this fat have yet to be resolved. The area deserves some primary attention by scientists. Delayed effects of early nutritional factors can explain some of the contradictions concerning, for example, obesity prevalence under comparable conditions, which was impossible to interpret until the present time. The effect of malnutrition during pregnancy with following increased food intake during the postnatal period is also considered a possible factor in the subsequent development of obesity later in life (James and Wallace, 2001).

Studies on children living in a shantytown in São Paolo, Brazil, showed that nutritional stunting may increase the risk of obesity. To elucidate the mechanism of the relationships between stunting and obesity, a 22-month longitudinal study was undertaken in 2 groups of girls aged 7 to 11 years, one with mild stunting but normal weight-for-height and a control group with normal weight and height. The energy and macronutrient intake and energy output were comparable in both groups. The same applied to their insulin-like growth factor (IGF-1) levels, which were below the normal range. A significant positive relationship between baseline IGF-1 and the change in height-for-age during the study was found in all subjects combined.

Another significant association was found between the baseline percentage of dietary energy supplied by fat and the gain in weight for height during the follow-up in girls with mild stunting but not in the normal control girls. The slope of these relationships was not significantly different. These results raise the question of whether the mildly stunted children would be more susceptible to excess fat deposition when given a high fat diet. The etiological role of low levels of IGF-1 should be also considered in this respect (Sawaya et al., 1998).

In industrially developed countries similar associations are shown. For example, there was a high prevalence of overweight and short stature among children involved in the Head Start program in Massachusetts (Wiecha and Casey, 1994). The prevalence varied by race and ethnicity, with a statistically significant upward trend in overweight among Hispanic children. Children 4 years of age or older were more likely than younger children to become overweight, and the prevalence of short stature did not vary significantly by year, gender, or age (Wiecha and Casey, 1994).

In a study of the association between stunted children and an increased risk of obesity, the following factors were included in the measurements in São Paolo children: anthropometric characteristics of the subjects and their parents; fasting and postprandial energy expenditure; respiratory quotient (RQ); substrate oxidation (using indirect calorimetry in a 3-day resident study in which all food was provided); and body composition (dual-energy x-ray absorptiometry [DXA]). Stunted children showed normal resting energy expenditure relative to body composition and also had normal post-prandial thermogenesis. Fasting RQ was significantly higher in stunted children; consequently, fasting fat oxidation was significantly lower (Hoffman et al., 2000). In a study of South African children, no association was found between stunting and obesity, but high levels of mild stunting were observed (Jinabhai, Taylor, and Sullivan, 2003).

2.2.3   The Effect of Acculturation on Obesity in Children

The trend of obesity development due to acculturation seems to be changing in some developing countries. However, obesity accompanying stunting has also been revealed in the countries that previously demonstrated a low prevalence of childhood obesity. Although there are still unsatisfactory data for a comprehensive investigation, it would appear that the documented increases in obesity are associated with both dietary change and altered physical activity patterns. In turn, these changes occur as a result of social, cultural, and psychological processes related to economic and nutritional transitions.

Increasing fat consumption due to the availability of cheap vegetable oils and fats in low-income nations and social classes may easily result in increased childhood obesity, including stunted children in the developing countries (Cameron, 1998).

The effect of acculturation is significant in the obesity patterns of ethnic subpopulations living in the United States. Changes in the second and third generations were analyzed within the framework of the National Longitudinal Study of Adolescent Health. Height and weight data collected in the second wave of the survey in a nationally representative sample of 13,783 adolescents were used. Multivariate logic techniques were used to analyze the interactions between age, gender, and intergenerational patterns of adolescent obesity. The results were compared with those of NHANES III. The smoothed version of the NHANES I, 85th percentile cutoff was used for the measure of obesity in this study. For the whole sample, 26.5% of adolescents were obese.

The rates in the individual ethnic groups were as follows: white non-Hispanics 24.2%; black non-Hispanics 10.9%; all Hispanics 30.4%; and all Asian-Americans, 20.6%. The Chinese (15.3%) and Filipino (18%) samples showed markedly lower obesity than non-Hispanic whites. All groups showed more obesity among males than among females, except for blacks (27.4% for males and 34.0% for females). Asian-American and Hispanic adolescents born in the United States are more than twice as likely to be obese as are the first-generation residents of all 50 states (Popkin and Udry, 1998).

There has been an upward shift in both weight-for-height and height-for-age distributions since 1968, indicating that Mescalero children today are, on average, heavier and taller. However, no secular trends in obesity (weight-for-height above the 95th percentile) were found in Mescalero Apache Indian preschool children from 1968 to 1988. The prevalence throughout the 21-year period was as much as two to four times higher than expected when compared with the CDC/WHO reference (Hauck et al., 1992).

Similar changes have also been found in populations transferred to developed countries that are undergoing significant modifications in their lifestyle, especially with regard to nutrition and physical activity regimes. However, this also concerns tribal populations living permanently in their territories where the conditions of life have changed markedly. For example, the Canadian Inuits after a certain period since the 1970s have showed significant changes in dietary intake and daily workload. As a result, an increase in BMI and percentage of stored fat along with a significant decrease in functional capacity — i.e., aerobic power (measured as maximum VO_2) — occurred. Diabetes and other health problems have appeared simultaneously in the whole population (McElroy and Townsend, 1996; Shephard, 1991). Obesity and a central deposition of fat have also been reported in the Inuit population in Greenland (Jorgensen et al., 2003).

Children of immigrants from countries of the Third World who move to better social conditions may become overweight or obese. For example, nutritional status and obesity prevalence was followed in resettled refugee children from Chile and the Middle East. Obesity was common in Chilean children on arrival in Sweden and increased further after resettlement (Hjern et al., 1991). However, obesity does not necessarily result from significant overeating under these new conditions. Rather, the increased availability of food in subjects adapted to a restricted energy intake and diet with a different composition of macronutrients (especially saturated fats) early in life could be one of the reasons for the increased prevalence.

In children born to Maghrebian immigrants in the Parisian area of France in the 1970s and 1990s, there was an increase in body mass (Rovillé-Sausse, 1998). Compared to the nonimmigrant children, the prevalence of obesity in children of Maghrebian origin was 11% in boys and 19% in girls at the age of 3 years. Obesity occurred more frequently in girls. Between 1970 and 1990 the frequency of obesity increased from 9.5 to 29.5% in girls at the age of 3 years. Nutrition and the method of feeding during the first weeks of life did not influence the BMI values after one year of age.

Adiposity rebound (AR, or the subsequent increase in BMI in young children) was precocious with 27% of the obese children experiencing AR between 36 and 48 months. It can be concluded that two types of adiposity appeared in the measured subjects. The first occurred among very young children before one year of age and is transitional in relation to hyperphagia of the newborn. The second obesity increase began after one year and continues, in relation to biological factors (such as parent to children correlation) and to diet and nutritional habits resulting from migration. The migrants adapt their traditional diet to the new food patterns (Rovillé-Sausse, 1998).

Another example of the impact of markedly changed social and economic conditions are the transitional changes in nutrition and changed prevalence of overweight and obesity in children from the former East Germany (German Democratic Republic) (Kromeyer-Hauschild and Jaeger, 1998; Kromeyer-Hauschild et al., 1999). Within this population there were significant changes in subcutaneous fat and BMI, especially from 1985 to 1995. Height increased less than body weight; BMI therefore increased significantly. The amount of subcutaneous fat increased along with changes in distribution; the ratio of trunk to extremity skinfolds decreased significantly in both genders between 1975 and 1985 but increased significantly between 1985 and 1996. Changes in the nutritional habits and lifestyle, evidently related to the reunification of Germany in 1989, may be the reason for these changes.

2.3 Summary

Obesity has become a global health problem that is no longer limited to the industrially developed countries but that is also present in countries of the Third World. The prevalence of childhood obesity has been increasing in nearly all parts of the world, especially in the industrially developed nations such as the United States, Canada, and countries of Western Europe. In addition, from the perspective of social strata, the economic level in developing countries is higher than ever before, which has occurred with an increasing prevalence of obesity. This phenomenon has been explained as being the result of changing conditions of life, especially changed diet (increased intake of fat and simple sugars), reduced physical activity, and smaller workloads. For this reason, marked differences appear even in the same country, where obesity exists along with malnutrition. This concerns not only developing countries, but also developed countries such as the United States. Obesity is increasing in countries such as China and India and also in some African countries such as Cameroon. A special case of obesity is excess fat deposition in stunted children who experienced malnutrition during early periods of life but were later exposed to an abundance of food. This phenomenon was found in countries such as Brazil. In addition, in countries where there were marked changes in social and economic conditions (e.g., in the former German Democratic Republic), childhood obesity prevalence increased.

Present BMI cutoffs, as mentioned in this chapter, have been considered as having a very low sensitivity and thus may underestimate the prevalence of childhood obesity. Therefore, population-specific measures rather than international cutoffs are recommended. This especially concerns Asian ethnic groups (Misra, 2003), and revisions of the cutoffs for BMI to define overweight and obesity are necessary. However, it is noted that ethnic-specific revisions for particular BMI cutoffs are not considered warranted by some authors, because it is believed that simple and uniform definitions are necessary for evaluations across populations (Stevens et al., 2003). In spite of the lack of homogeneity of results, it can be concluded that obesity in children has increased.

Exact international comparisons are only possible if a number of conditions are met by individual studies. These include using the same or comparable methods, sampling techniques, protocols, choice of parameters and criteria, apparatus, statistical treatment, evaluation, and, where possible, data gained from comparable populations.

3

Main Factors Associated with Obesity in Various Periods of Growth

3.1   Attitudes toward Obesity in Different Periods of Life

The different ways in which obesity is viewed at various stages during the growing years is an interesting phenomenon. For example, many people commonly view a degree of fatness in young children as acceptable. In many cultures fatness is desirable and a sign of healthiness. Such an attitude may stem from the long-held belief that a degree of fatness helps, due to increased energy reserves, to guarantee an enhanced survival rate through greater resistance to disease, most commonly respiratory and gastrointestinal infections. In previous centuries, little angels in the paintings of the great masters were always presented as chubby rather than thin. Such images of young children were commonplace and presented the ideal of a small child.

Today, with advances in medical knowledge and technology, drugs such as antibiotics and other advanced treatment modalities, additional fat is no longer essential to the survival of the young child. On the contrary, in the developed nations of the world, there may be a substantial increased risk for the young person who carries a higher level of body fat (Klein, 2004). Excess fatness in childhood may jeopardize the health status of an individual by increasing the risk of contracting the "diseases of modern living" later in life but potentially as early as during adolescence. In sharp contrast to this scenario, many young people living in Third World countries could benefit substantially from greater fat deposits, particularly the most disadvantaged in the lower social strata.

It is commonplace, particularly in families with obese children, to fail to perceive excess weight and fatness in youngsters as a serious problem until approximately puberty. At this time or earlier, the bigger and fatter child starts to recognize and feel his or her position among the peer group and very commonly reports concerns in relation to fatness, lack of friends, and a belief that one is unhealthy ("fat, friendless and unhealthy") (Hill and Silver, 1995). Parents of obese children often believe that their offspring will grow out of their childhood body fatness and that they will be of "normal" size and shape later in life. Unfortunately, in far too many cases this does not happen. Even after a temporary reduction of weight and fatness and an overall amelioration of the status of the child during the time of sexual maturation, excessive fatness is often a continuing problem. The problem of obesity may become more pronounced following the cessation of growth or after some other major life-changing event during adolescence or adulthood. For example, pregnancy (or repeated pregnancies) in women or a change in employment or marriage may be catalysts for increased body fatness for many people at different times during their adult years.

A consistent message throughout this volume is that fat children more easily become obese adolescents and adults, especially when overweight or obesity has commenced early in life. Even though it is always possible to improve body composition status and lose excess fat later during growth or young adulthood, such changes are progressively more difficult as one ages. Commonly, despite great effort, a sustained reduction of weight and fat is difficult to maintain and in many cases weight is regained. An all-too-common occurrence is that weight regain often surpasses the earlier starting weight.

The prevalence of obesity varies markedly with age. In preschoolers it is relatively low compared to the older age groups, and prevalence increases along with chronological age. In a population study of children and youth aged 3 to 18 years in Milan, Italy, the prevalence of obesity was highest in older students (aged 11 to 18 years), 17.9% compared with 4.7% of nursery school pupils (Ceratti et al., 1990). Similar results have been reported for Czech children (Pařízková, 1996b); however, the prevalence rate has increased to a higher level since (Kimm and Obarzanek, 2002). "Feeding our children to death: the tragedy of childhood obesity in America" has been a recent complaint (Freeman-Fobbs, 2003).

Compared with other chronic diseases such as cardiovascular disease, diabetes, and related metabolic problems, the prevention, treatment, and management of obesity are different. Each of the common chronic diseases is recognized as having their genesis in childhood. As a result, for example, appropriate targeted interventions have been very successful in preventing and treating atherosclerosis. However, it should be recognized that improvements have taken an extended period of time to materialize given that Kannel and Dawber (1972) identified that atherosclerosis was a pediatric problem over 30 years ago. This was also demonstrated by findings in the Bogalusa Heart Study (Berenson, Srinivasan, and Nicklas, 1998).

Interestingly, many of the chronic diseases are interrelated. For example, obesity is a significant risk factor for cardiovascular problems and is also the common denominator in many of society's other chronic health problems, including type 2 diabetes. The same is true of the modalities of regular physical activity and appropriate nutritional practices (Hills and Wahlqvist, 1994a; Wahlqvist and Hills, 1994b). In the late 1960s, Fanconi (1969) considered the nutritional situation of children in his definition of health and stressed the importance of an adequate nutritional status that should exclude overeating from the earliest periods of life (Stang and Bayerl, 2003).

The dramatic increase in childhood obesity — over 30% in the recent decades in some countries — has focused attention on various factors and their interactions during growth that may result in the deposition of excess fat. A genetic analysis of weight and overweight in 4-year-old twins was recently conducted (Koeppen-Schomerus, Wardle, and Plomen, 2001). Some studies have tracked the effect of individual factors; however, most have considered a range of factors and their interplay over time in relation to the development of obesity. The variability in studies on children and adolescents makes comparative analyses of all data much more difficult than is the case with adults.

Because of the speed and magnitude of change in the prevalence of obesity in so many populations, a significant modification in the gene pool cannot be considered as a main cause. Rather, the environmental factors that may influence the genetic predisposition of an organism to be or not to be expressed are now considered the main contributing factors to the surge in obesity prevalence. The role of "thrifty genes" (Neel, 1999; James, 2002) enabling one to better economize ingested food has been suggested as a contributing factor. Another hypothesis is that an increased rate of assortive mating may have contributed to the recent rise in obesity rates in some countries, particularly the rates of very severe and more extreme obesity. However, the latter hypothesis has not been well documented and therefore further work is required to assess its potential impact on obesity prevalence through both genetic and nongenetic mechanisms (Hebebrand et al., 2000). The major consideration in subsequent sections is on further environmental factors that may predispose the overweight and obese condition.

However, even in countries with relatively stable social conditions the prevalence of obesity and thinness has changed over time as compared with previous French data. For example, the International Obesity Task Force (IOTF) data on the prevalence of obesity in 2000 in French children (7 to 9 years of age) showed that it was similar to the prevalence recorded in the late 1980s in the United States. Data in France are comparable to those reported in other studies conducted in Western Europe (Rolland-Cachera and Bellisle, 2002). Time trends are apparent and the changing conditions of life, including diet, obviously contribute to these similarities.

3.2   Familial Clustering of Obesity and the Effect of Heredity

As indicated earlier, the importance of genetic factors cannot be underestimated (Bouchard, 1993; Treuth et al., 2001) even when the determination of the differentiation between environmental and genetic factors is extremely difficult. Moreover, familial clustering of obesity was followed in a number of studies, which were mostly conducted with nonhomogenous design and different methods.

One of the more common reported trends is that having overweight parents (particularly the mother) increases the likelihood of being overweight later (Hui et al., 2003; Trudeau et al., 2003; Williams, 2001). The effect of heredity was mainly demonstrated by the resemblance of level of fatness in parents, children, and siblings, especially in monozygotic and dizygotic twins (Hainer et al., 2000). Such studies have now been undertaken in a range of populations and ethnic groups — for example in Taiwan (Wu et al., 2003), the United States (Faith et al., 2002), and Iran (Mirmiran, Mirbolooki, and Azizi, 2002).

It has also been suggested that heredity does not only concern the genes but also resulting dietary habits, food intake, and lifestyle, including physical activity level and spontaneous interest in exercise. In summary, where there is a family risk of obesity it is even more critical to pay close attention to the growth and development of the child involved (Faith et al., 2002; Hui et al., 2003; Magnusson and Rasmussen, 2002).

Substantial advances in the genetic underpinning of obesity have emerged during recent years (Bouchard, 1997), but behavioral genetic methods are used more rarely. Obesity is largely determined by a mix of environmental factors directly related to human behavior in regard to eating and physical activity. In relation to behavior, the eating and physical activity habits of a family have become the special focus of attention in recent research. There are compelling reasons why this aspect of the development of obesity should be studied in more detail. Behaviors that result in the increased deposition of body fat are also genetically conditioned (Bouchard, 1997). For example, the volume and character of physical activity during defined periods of time are more similar in mono- than in dizygotic twins (Ledovskaya, 1972; Sklad, 1972).

Genetic factors, or more specifically, *polygenic factors*, may be the most important for the development of obesity. This aspect of obesity has been addressed recently but mainly in adult populations. The aggregation of additional environmental factors at the family level may be very decisive, particularly when the family lives together (Sorensen and Lund-Sorensen, 1991). Similarly, the delayed effects of the factors influencing the growing organism in the early stages of development may not be manifested until later periods of life. The situation is further complicated by additional factors outside the family environment, factors that may be equally important in the establishment and maintenance of later-onset obesity.

The Quebec Longitudinal Study revealed familial aggregation of BMI and subcutaneous fat measurements (including fat distribution) over 12 years. Measurements were taken twice in this period. Simple univariate familial correlation analysis of the change scores and bivariate analysis of the longitudinal measures were appropriate for the evaluation of the factors leading to both change and stability across this period (Rice et al., 1999).

Familial behavior indicators such as parental physical activity may also be predictors of the activity levels of prepubertal children (Brock et al., 1999). In this study, respiratory quotient (RQ) and energy expenditure (EE) correlated significantly in mothers and a cohort of children as well as in mothers and girls in terms of percentage of moderate physical activity. In contrast, the only variable that correlated significantly in fathers and children was time spent in low-level activity. The strong relationship between activity habits of parents was also evidenced by the results of this study. Boys in the highest tertile for EE were 2.4 times more likely to have parents in the top EE tertile. A similar trend for RQ was not significant. However, the parent-child relationship of physical inactivity appeared to be stronger than that of vigorous activity (Fogelholm et al., 1999). Therefore, fat deposition in children may be reduced by changing the lifestyle of the parents — for example, increasing physical activity to serve as a model. Involving the family is the best approach for a positive intervention involving both physical activity and diet (Pinelli et al., 1999). Most parents fail to recognize the health risks of obesity in their children (Etelson et al., 2003); parental recognition of these problems can play a major role in obesity management and prevention.

Mother and child correlations in anthropometric parameters are significant in preschool children (Pařízková, 1996a). Also, statistically significant relationships have been found between infant feeding practices and obesity in preschool children. The educational level of the mother varied inversely with children's weight for height. The parents' child-feeding attitudes had no obvious relationship with the anthropometric parameters of children of preschool age (Patterson et al., 1986).

A longitudinal study in 504 obese Norwegian children over a 40-year period showed that the degree of overweight in the family and at puberty were the determinants of adult weight level. The mean level of persistent overweight in the adults was 35% (20 to 60%). Body weight was increased even when food intake was within the recommended range. Additionally, excessive overweight in puberty was associated with greater adult morbidity and mortality (Mossberg, 1991). Obesity commencing before puberty is associated with persistence of visceral fat during adolescence (Brambilla et al., 1999).

The Belgian-Luxembourg Child Study evaluated children from 6 to 12 years of age and showed that BMI is strongly correlated between children and both parents (Guillaume et al., 1993). The familial link extended beyond one generation as the obesity problems of grandparents were related to the BMI of parents and also to obesity in the children. In addition, the correlation between birth weight and current BMI of the children was confirmed in the youngest age group in girls, and birth weight also correlated with the BMI of the mother. In these children, the energy intake was high and energy output low due to low levels of physical activity. These results indicate that obesity can be traced through three generations in familial clustering in this area and is already evident at birth. Statistical analyses suggest that familial factors have a more significant effect on obesity in children than other broader environmental factors (Guillaume et al., 1995; Frisancho, 2000; Fuentes et al., 2002).

The results of a study by Locard et al. (1992) showed that parental overweight and birth overweight are closely related to the degree of a child's obesity at the age of 5 years. In this study, the environmental factors that contributed to childhood obesity were: southern European origin of the mother, snacks, excessive TV viewing and, more interestingly, short sleep duration. A logistic regression model, after taking parental obesity into account, showed that the relationship between obesity and short sleep duration persisted independently of TV viewing (Locard et al., 1992).

A number of factors that can predispose an individual to obesity were assessed in preadolescent girls with varying risks of obesity. The girls were obese or nonobese children of parents with or without obesity. Total energy expenditure (TEE) was measured by doubly labeled water (DLW) and resting metabolic rate (RMR) by indirect calorimetry. After adjusting for age, body composition, and degree of pubertal development, there were significant differences in RMR between the groups. The lowest RMR values were revealed in obese girls born to two overweight parents. However, the largest differences in adjusted RMR were found between the normal-weight and obese girls with two obese parents each. Neither TEE nor non-basal energy expenditure (TEE–RMR) as an indicator of energy spent on physical activity differed between the groups. Height and weight development up to the age of one year did not differ. However, at the age of 2 and 4 years, obese girls whose parents were both obese had significantly higher BMI values. Therefore, preadolescent girls at risk of obesity are not generally predisposed to overweight and obesity because of RMR differences. Furthermore, obese girls seem to spend less time engaged in exercise and physical activity (Laessle, Wurmser, and Pirke, 1998).

A 4-year longitudinal study of Italian children who at the beginning of the study were 8.6 ± 1.0 years, confirmed that the main risk factor for obesity was parental obesity. Sedentary behavior such as TV viewing was independently associated with overweight at the age of 8 years. Physical activity plus energy and nutrient intakes did not significantly affect the change in BMI over the 4-year period of observation when the parents' obesity was taken into account (Maffeis, Talamini, and Tato, 1998).

A study of risk factors in a transitional society in Thailand found that the prevalence of obesity among school children was 14.1%. Statistically significant associations with obesity were found for the family history of obesity, a low exercise level, and obesity in both parents. Increased risk was associated with higher family income and smaller family size. Specifically, the highest population-attributable fraction was for family history of obesity, followed by a low level of physical activity and exercise, and then an obese or overweight mother (Mo-suwan and Gaeter, 1996).

To elucidate the role of genetic factors, measurements of BMI and percentage of body fat by BIA and skinfolds in mono- and dizygotic twins (MZ, DZ) was conducted. Pearson's correlations revealed a stronger association among MZ than DZ twins for BMI and also for percentage of stored fat, suggestive of a consistent genetic influence. Considering the percentage of body fat, the model of best fit included additive genetic and unique environmental influences. Using a more precise measure of adiposity than BMI confirmed a substantial genetic influence. As was the case for adults (Hainer et al., 2000), the mix of environmental determinants of pediatric adiposity was "unique" rather than "common" in nature (Faith et al., 1998).

Allison et al. (1994) studied the heritability of BMI in pairs of adolescent black and white male and female twins. The BMIs were adjusted for age and transformed to approximate normality. Hierarchically nested structural equation models were tested. These analyses showed that both the genotype and the environment exerted greater influence on the BMI of black than white adolescents. Variance in BMI was greater for blacks, but the heritability was the same for both black and white adolescents.

The findings of the Stanislas Family Study emphasized that weight is a composite phenotype reflecting different components that evolve in distinct ways during the whole life span. In research related to susceptibility genes in obesity, the evaluation of fat mass should be the preference over weight or BMI values (Lecomte et al., 1997).

In another study of Italian children, the association between obesity and parental and perinatal factors was evaluated. After an adjustment for age, significant relationships between the risk of obesity and body weight at birth and the mother or father's BMI were found in both boys and girls. When parental and perinatal variables were included as independent variables in a multiple logistic regression model controlling for the effect of age, parental BMI and children's birth weight remained independently associated with childhood obesity. In females, an interaction between birth weight and the mother's BMI was found. Thus, parental obesity and birth weight were the most important risk factors for obesity among children in northeast Italy (Maffeis et al., 1994c). It is important to acknowledge the mixture of contributing factors that result in variability in size and shape.

Metabolic rate and somatic development were evaluated in a longitudinal study of children of obese (group O) and normal-weight (group N) parents, who participated in a study of metabolic rate and food intake when 3 to 5 years old. When the final measurements were conducted 12 years later, a marked gender difference was revealed. In boys, parental obesity predicted a more rapid growth but not adiposity, along with an earlier decline in resting metabolic rate (RMR/kg weight). Childhood energy intake/kg body weight was not predictive. In girls, the reverse was found — that is, childhood energy intake/kg predicted both body size and adiposity, while parental obesity had limited predictive value. These gender differences are consistent with the earlier sexual maturation of girls. Growth differences are consistent with the hypothesis that a low BMR/kg body weight is associated with a precocious pattern of growth and development in children and youth with a predisposition for obesity (Griffiths et al., 1990).

The familial risk of obesity was examined in another study of children 4.4 to 5.0 ± 0.5 years old. Children were subdivided according to parental weight status; the high-risk group had one or both parents overweight, the low-risk group had both parents of a normal weight. The initial body weight of children was the same, but after one year the high-risk group gained marginally more weight. The total energy intake was similar, but the high-risk group consumed a larger percentage of energy from fat and a smaller percentage from carbohydrate. Only slight differences were observed in the level of physical activity of both groups. In summary, a distinctive pattern that may lead to increased weight gain may have been present in the high-risk group (Eck et al., 1992).

Obese children in Taiwan were about five times as likely to have an obese parent as control children. There was also a significantly greater chance of members of the obese group having an obese sibling compared to the control group (Chen, 1997).

In Scandinavia, a 40-year longitudinal follow-up of children treated for obesity from 1921 to 1947 was undertaken in Sweden. Questionnaires at 10-year intervals showed that 47% of patients were still obese in adulthood. Of these, 84.6% were two standard deviation scores (SDS) above the norm for BMI than in childhood. The family history of obesity (in grandparents and parents) and the degree of obesity during puberty were the most important markers for obesity in adulthood. Food intake in the study population corresponded to RDAs, but this was not sufficient to prevent the development of obesity in adulthood. Excess overweight in puberty (SDS greater than +3) was associated with higher than expected morbidity and mortality in adulthood (Mossberg, 1989).

Measurement of energy expenditure in parents and children did not support the hypothesis that the obesity of children of obese parents is caused by major defects in energy expenditure. TEE was measured over 14 days in children aged 5 ± 0.9 years and in their parents. The study utilized DLW to measure total energy expenditure of the subjects and physical activity energy expenditure (AEE) was derived by subtracting resting energy expenditure (REE) under postprandial conditions. Fat and fat-free mass (FFM) was measured by bioelectrical impedance (BIA). There were no significant relationships between TEE and AEE in children after adjustment for FFM and body fat content in children or body fat in mothers or fathers. A three-way analysis of covariance, with FFM as the covariate, showed a significant effect of gender in children, obesity in mothers, or obesity in fathers on TEE or AEE in children. There was a significant effect of gender and a significant interaction between obesity in mothers and fathers on REE values. Relative to children with two nonobese or two obese parents, REE was approximately 6% lower in children when mothers only, or fathers only, were obese. Results of this study did not show any effect of parents' obesity on energy expenditure of children (Goran et al., 1995).

The challenge of obesity along with insulin-dependent diabetes mellitus (IDDM) is also paramount in Native Americans. The specific reasons for this have not yet been elucidated, but it has been hypothesized that Native Americans have a genetic predisposition to overweight under conditions of a "Westernized" environment of abundant food and decreased levels of energy expenditure. Most studies show a high prevalence of overweight in this population in all age categories. Historical comparisons have shown that this is a relatively recent phenomenon. Preliminary evidence for two formative school-based programs in the southwest United States suggests that Native American communities are receptive to such interventions. Targeted programs specific to the particular native culture may slow the rate of excess weight gain and lead to improved fitness in school children (Broussard et al., 1995).

A 3-year longitudinal study to investigate the dietary, physical activity, family history, and demographic predictors of relative weight change was undertaken in a group of preschool children (Klesges et al., 1995). Results showed that boys of normal-weight parents, or those who had only one parent overweight, had the usual reduction in BMI values (Pařízková, 1996a,b,c; Rolland-Cachera et al., 1984) while those with both parents overweight displayed BMI increases. Girls with overweight fathers showed BMI increases while others experienced usual decreases of BMI during this period of growth. Parent reaction has been shown to be related to weight status and self-perception in 5-year-olds (Davison and Birch, 2001a,b).

As shown by Rolland-Cachera (1993, 1995; Rolland-Cachera et al., 1984), the earlier-than-normal rebound of BMI (the so-called adiposity rebound –[AR]) predisposes the individual to the later development of obesity. This was also confirmed in the study of Klesges et al. (1995), especially for children of overweight parents. In addition, baseline intakes of energy from fat as well as decreases in fat were related to BMI decreases. At higher levels of baseline aerobic activity, subsequent changes of BMI decreased. There was also a trend to changes in leisure activity, with increases in children's leisure activity associated with decreases in subsequent weight gain. To date there has been no study concerning AR in both parents and their children and the relationship to eventual obesity.

Modifiable variables, namely diet and physical activity, accounted for more of the variance in child BMI change than nonmodifiable variables — for example, the number of obese parents (Klesges et al., 1995). This result indicates that at an early age, the role of genetic factors might be weaker than that of environmental factors, including energy output from exercise. However, this might not be true during later periods of development; therefore, an early intervention in lifestyle, especially in children of overweight parents, is plausible. Klesges et al. (1990) investigated parent-child interaction correlates of physical activity in preschool children. Activity levels were evaluated with a system that directly quantified physical activity in the natural environment. Significant relationships were revealed using regression-modeling procedures between: 1) the child's relative weight, parental weight status, and percentage of time spent outdoors; and 2) the child's activity levels. Parental obesity was associated with lower levels of physical activity in children.

Children's relative weight was associated with slightly higher levels of physical activity, and more outdoor activity was associated with higher activity levels. The participation of parents in the activities of children also significantly interacted with levels of parental obesity in predicting activity levels. Those children with a 50% risk of obesity (as defined by both, one, or neither parent being overweight) had small changes in activity across levels of parent–child interaction, whereas those at high risk for obesity responded with increased activity as parent–child interactions increased (Klesges et al., 1990).

A review of the existing literature on the role of the genetic determinants in daily physical activity, sports participation, and RMR indicated variability from low to moderately high. Transmission and heritability coefficients were calculated from twin and family data. Heritability coefficients for sports participation varied between 0.35 and 0.83, and for daily physical activity between 0.29 and 0.62. If one of the parents or co-twins is active in sports, it is more likely that the child or co-twin is also active in sports. Twin and parent–child correlations for RMR also indicate a moderate genetic effect. At present, only a linkage between RMR and uncoupling protein 2 markers (UCP2) has been reported (Beunen and Thomis, 1999).

Parental overweight or obesity may identify children at risk as related to a range of unhealthy behaviors such as inactivity, fat intake, alcohol consumption, and smoking (Frelut, 2001; Bandini et al., 2002). Over the 9 years of a survey of Australian families, BMI was consistently higher in offspring of overweight or obese father or mothers. Physical fitness at 12, 15, and 18 years of age was negatively related to fathers' obesity in daughters and mothers' obesity in sons. Obesity in fathers was associated with a fourfold increase in risk of obesity at 18 years of age in both sons and daughters, with an independent eightfold increase in risk for daughters if mothers were also obese (Burke, Beilin, and Dunbar, 2001).

Research has also revealed that parents, especially those who are overweight, select environments that promote overweight among their children. This consists of parents' own eating behaviors and child-feeding practices, controlling their own food intake, parental control attempts that may interact with genetic predispositions to promote the development of problematic eating styles, and children's overweight. Guidance for parents is needed, and this should include more complete knowledge and understanding on how children develop patterns of food intake in the family context (size of portions, timing and frequency of meals and snacks, etc.). Early and middle childhood are special periods for the development of food preferences, patterns of food intake, eating styles, and the development of physical activity interests. The impact of stress on family members' eating styles may also play a significant role (Birch et al., 2001a,b).

Differences in diet and activity preferences that would place more susceptible individuals at risk of positive energy balance in the permissive environment in the present industrialized society (including family) may be part of the genetic influences that transmit obesity to the next generation. Children from overweight/obese families had higher preferences for fatty foods in a taste test, less of a preference for vegetables, and a more "overeating type" eating style. They had also stronger preferences for sedentary activities and spent more time in sedentary pastimes. However, there were no differences in speed of eating or reported frequency of intake of high-fat foods (Wardle et al., 2001a,b).

Familial clustering of obesity has also been observed in the east of Tehran, where familial obesity patterns were associated with family dietary intakes (Mirmiran, Mirbolooki, and Azizi, 2002). In another study, parental BMI showed only a weak correlation with their children, but the children's risk of becoming overweight increased with parental overweight (Danielczyk et al., 2002).

There is also a difference between BMI resemblances with regards to full or half-siblings; the almost twice as strong BMI correlation between maternal half-brothers compared to paternal half-brothers illustrates the importance of factors of nonadditive genetic origin. The significant BMI association found between biological unrelated individuals from the same family emphasizes that assortative mating, perhaps linked with regional clustering, should be considered when the heritability of BMI is estimated (Magnusson and Rasmussen, 2002). A study in international adoptees showed differences in prevalence of overweight between various groups of adoptees and differences between adopted and nonadopted subjects that are probably due to the variability in genetic individual susceptibility to overweight (Johansson-Kark, Rasmussen, and Hjern, 2002). Studies show differences in overweight between various groups of adoptees and between adopted and nonadopted subjects, which seem to be related to the diversity in genetic susceptibility to increase of weight (Johansson-Kark, Rasmussen, and Hjern, 2002). Spousal resemblance with regard to obesity has also been analyzed (Katzmarzyk, Hebebrand, and Bouchard, 2002).

Parents who use food to satisfy their children's emotional needs or to promote good behavior may promote obesity by interfering with their children's ability to regulate their own food intake (Baughcum et al., 1998). Interventions in child-feeding practices should not only include parents but also grandmothers and/or any care providers of children. Observations in a Brazilian population has also suggested a positive relationship between maternal and child obesity (Engstrom and Anjos, 1996).

The longitudinal Framingham Children's Study showed that paternal eating style — characterized by dietary restraint, disinhibition, and perceived hunger evaluated by the Three-Factor Eating questionnaire (Stunkard and Messick, 1985) — along with anthropometric characteristics of parents and children, showed that parents who display high levels of disinhibition eating, especially when coupled with high dietary restraint, may foster the development of excess body fat in their children. Parents modeling unhealthy eating behaviors or other more indirect behaviors (probably unconsciously) can suppress the child's innate regulation of dietary intake (Hood et al., 2000). As defined in terms of parents' activity and dietary patterns, children from obesogenic families can be considered at a greater risk of obesity development (Davison and Birch, 2002).

A study comparing the effect of parent and child characteristics as predictors of BMI in daughters aged between 5 and 7 years showed that girls' BMI at the age of 5 years, mothers' change of BMI, fathers' energy intake, fathers' enjoyment of activity, and girls' percentage of energy from fat are best correlated to risk of overweight (Davison and Birch, 2001b). Insulin resistance in children seems to be a function of excess weight rather than other factors (e.g., birth weight, or change of weight), underlining that childhood obesity enhances health risk (Wilkin et al., 2002). Because heredity can influence a number of factors and characteristics in offspring, any obesity intervention should always involve the whole family in order to maximize the health development of the next generation.

A study of obese adult female monozygotic twins during long-term reduction treatment showed greater similarity in the reaction of morphological, hormonal, biochemical, and clinical variables than in unrelated subjects (Hainer et al., 2000). Similar studies in growing twins have not been reported. As mentioned earlier, familial predisposition may also influence how subjects react to particular life events, such as special diets (especially with a high fat content), or to a sedentary lifestyle. However, there is still considerable uncertainty about the role of the interactions between specific genotypes and exposure to various environmental stimuli in both the short-term and long-term development of obesity.

Also, the rare cases of obesity based on identified mutations in single major genes — for example, the leptin gene and the leptin gene receptor — may be considered examples of specific genotype/environment interactions (Sorensen, 1999).

3.3   The Role of Genes on Obesity

Information from both genetic and molecular epidemiology suggests that genetic factors are involved in determining the susceptibility to gaining or losing fat in response to diet and physical activity treatment. The same applies to the risk of developing some of the co-morbidities of obesity. New advanced methods have enabled the description and analysis of various genes and their mutations, considering their effect on the development of early obesity.

Substantial advances in the genetic underpinning of obesity have emerged during recent years (Bouchard, 1997; Chen et al., 2004; O'Rahilly et al., 2003; Li et al., 2003), but behavioral genetic methods are used more rarely. People can get severely obese as a result of genetic disruption of a single element of a homeostatic system regulating energy balance. It is notable that all of the known genetic defects resulting in severe human obesity do so largely through disruption of the normal control in ingestive behavior (O'Rahilly et al., 2003).

Genetic influences on body weight for, say, infants may be independent of those that influence BMI in adults. This can complicate the search for the genetic determinant(s) of obesity in children (Stunkard et al., 1999). Noninvasive methods of measurement are recommended for use in genetic studies. For example, the protocol for the study of the beta3-adrenergic receptor gene polymorphism included sampling of buccal mucosa (76%), hair (44%), cerumen (only 4%) in infants, which caused no anxiety in children and enabled the researchers to gain information on infant polymorphism in the mentioned percentages (Takadoro et al., 2000).

In recent years several single gene disorders resulting in early onset of obesity have been characterized (Farooqui and O'Rahilly, 2000). The discovery of these genetic defects has biological and clinical implications that are greater than the rarity of the health problems that might be expected. Genetic studies following members of the same families and populations offer information on genes and mutations associated with or linked not only to obesity but also fat distribution and other relevant phenotypes (York and Bouchard, 2000). It is also possible to specify mutations that contribute to the development of obesity in humans based on the knowledge of the chromosomal location of genes identified originally in animal studies.

Despite the limited but increasing number of studies, the information on gene-diet interactions in obesity is convincing. This concerns the role of genes in the response of obesity phenotypes to the changes in energy balance and diet composition, especially fat intake.

Various mutations have been studied that could be linked to childhood obesity. One of the frequently followed is Melanocortin 4 receptor (MC4R) and its heterozygous mutations in its coding region as one of the most common genetic causes of human obesity. It has been shown that 81.3% of childhood obesity–associated heterozygous MC4R leads to the intracellular retention of the receptor, which has implications for the pharmacological intervention and treatment of childhood obesity–associated MC4R mutations (Lubrano-Berthelier et al., 2003). Screening of 431 obese children and adults for mutations in the coding sequence and the minimal core promoter of MC4R showed that genetic variation in the transcriptionally essential region of the MC4R promoter is not a significant cause of human obesity (Lubrano-Berthelier et al., 2003). A pathogenic MC4R mutation was found among subjects with severe early-onset obesity, but not among morbidly obese adults (Valli-Jaakola et al., 2004). Another study stressed the importance of characterizing the properties of MC4R variants associated with early-onset severe obesity (Tao and Segaloff, 2003).

A mutation in the MC4R gene causing obesity syndrome is inherited in a codominant manner; its mutations that lead to complete loss of function are associated with a more severe phenotype. The association between the signaling properties of these mutant receptors and energy input underlines the key role of this receptor in the control of eating behavior and the development of obesity (Farooqui et al., 2003). A study of French children showed that MC4R mutations may not be a negligible cause of serious obesity in children, with variable expression and penetrance. Mutations in agouti-related protein (AGRP) and α-melanocyte–stimulating hormone (αMSH) genes did not result in obesity in the study by Dubern et al. (2001). In some populations MC4R mutations are infrequent in the obese population — for example, in the Mediterranean child population (Miraglia-del-Giudice et al., 2002b) or others (Mo et al., 2001).

The role of melanocortin 3 receptor (MC3R) was also studied with respect to the differences in phenotypes between two related heterozygotes, obese siblings, and the observation of obesity in other family members without mutation. It was suggested that obesity results from a varying combination of environmental, behavioral, and multiple genetic factors other than MC3-R, even in the same family (Lee, Poh, and Loke, 2002).

The contribution of propiomelanocortin (POMC) gene variants (Cirillo et al., 2001; Del Giudice et al., 2001) seem to increase the sensibility to develop obesity in early age, but may be limited for childhood obesity as shown by the lack of differences in BMI-SD scores. No significant associations have been identified between any of the polymorphisms and body composition in African-American subjects (Feng et al., 2003). Further studies are suggested on the polymorphism of POMC and its relationship to obesity as an important factor in its development (Miraglia-del-Giudice et al., 2002a). Leptin has been characterized as a satiety factor that acts through the hypothalamus; the α-melanocyte-stimulating hormone derived from POMC and MC4R has been reported to be involved in the effect of leptin in the area.

The influence of the beta3-adrenergic receptor Arg 16 Gly polymorphism on longitudinal obesity changes from childhood to adulthood was followed in a biracial cohort (Bogalusa Heart Study) (Ellsworth et al., 2002). Trp64Arg mutation of the beta3-adrenergic receptor gene was also followed in Japanese obese children. Results suggested that it might affect obesity and HDL metabolism in boys. In contrast, C161T mutation of the PPAR-γ gene by itself is unlikely to influence obesity (Arashiro et al., 2003). Another study in Japanese children showed that Trp64Arg polymorphism of the β3-AR gene appears to be a genetic risk for Japanese children, but Gln223Arg polymorphism of the Ob-R gene does not appear to be associated with obesity (Endo et al., 2000).

Trp64Arg mutation of the beta3-adrenergic receptor gene may also predict the result of dietary intervention in obese children. However, this was not a major factor affecting body weight in Chinese children (Xinli et al., 2001).

The effect of the mentioned polymorphism was also studied simultaneously with the –3826 A-G nucleotide variant of the uncoupling protein-1 (UCP-1) gene with regard to the association to obesity (Urhammer et al., 2000). The study failed to demonstrate an additive or synergistic effect of the Trp64Arg variant of the BAR gene and the –3826 A-G variant of the UCP-1 gene on obesity development.

In the etiology of human obesity, uncoupling protein 3 genetic variants also plays a role. The effect of its genetic variation was followed in children but the mutations of the coding sequence of UCP-3 were deemed unlikely to be a common monogenic cause of human obesity (Halsall et al., 2001). The Quebec Family Study revealed that some alleles of UCP-3 are involved in the origin and development of human obesity (Lanouette et al., 2001). A certain polymorphism (the exon 8 ins/del) of UCP-2 appears to be associated with childhood-onset obesity. The UCP-2/UCP-3 genetic locus seems to play a role in body weight development during growth (Yanovski et al., 2000). A study in Mexican-Americans suggested that variations in UCP-2 and UCP-3 genes are unlikely to have a significant effect on the expression of obesity-related phenotypes in this population (Comuzzie et al., 2003). The association between obesity and the G-allele of the −866 polymorphism in the promoter region of UCP2 gene was reported. A study by Schauble (2003) showed no evidence for transmission disequilibrium in obesity following analyses in obese and underweight subjects. Allele and genotype frequencies did not differ between the extremely obese and never-obese subjects. An association study pertaining to alleles of two polymorphisms of glucose transporter 4 gene in youth with extreme obesity and reduced weight has also been conducted (Friedel et al., 2002).

The Bogalusa Heart Study showed a linkage in an autosomal genome scan for loci influencing longitudinal burden of BMI from childhood to young adulthood white siblings that might harbor genetic predisposition affecting the propensity to develop obesity (Chen et al., 2004). A significant linkage on chromosome 6q22.31-q23.2 for childhood obesity-associated traits in a genome-wide scan in French families was revealed (Meyre et al., 2004).

Some other genes (such as SIMI, CART, SORBS 1) have also been followed. In spite of stressing their role, however, their description of their mutations did not reveal completely the exact mechanisms of obesity development until now, despite the increasing number of publications (Farooqui et al., 2003; Clement and Ferre, 2003; Valli-Jaakola et al., 2004). Changes in adiposity are related to glucocorticoid receptor polymorphism in a long-term study of young females (Tremblay et al., 2003).

Research concerning the role of genes in obesity development in children has developed markedly during recent decades. For example, associations between a polymorphism in the 11-beta hydroxysteroid dehydrogenase type I gene and body composition were studied in overweight and normal children (Gelernter-Yaniv et al., 2003). Monogenic forms of obesity in humans have been defined, and results from mutations in genes involved in the central pathways of food intake regulation have been revealed. These cases, however, are extremely rare. Interaction between the environment and genes is further considered when defining obesity as a complex polygenic disease involving interactions of "susceptibility" genes with environmental factors in children. Analyses are still inconclusive and variable as mentioned earlier as the relative risk associating a specific gene allele and obesity remains low. Therefore, it seems premature to genotype obese patients on a large scale of predictive testing (Clement and Ferre, 2003). Genetic testing may help to discriminate between subtypes of obesity in the future, and define, for example, an adequate pharmacological as well as other treatments. Further research in this area is necessary and is continuing on a large scale. The effect and relationships of various genes with regard to some biochemical, hormonal, and other characteristics are mentioned further in subsequent chapters.

3.4   The Role of Nutrition in Early Periods of Life

Numerous factors influence and interact with the nutrition of children. These factors include the family environment and status, heredity, nutritional knowledge, and feeding behavior (including food choice and values). Additionally, demographic, geographic, climatic, social, economic, and cultural parameters may play a role at different times in the development of a child. In addition, the perception of obesity as a positive or negative characteristic during growth also plays an important role in the growth and later development of the child in his or her family and school environment.

During the first 2 to 3 years of life, humans acquire basic knowledge of what foods are safe to eat (Cashdan, 1994). A willingness to eat a wide variety of foods is greatest between the ages of 1 and 2 years, and this declines to lower levels at the age of 4. Infants introduced to solid food unusually late have a more restricted dietary choice throughout childhood. These data indicate that various factors can change the food preferences and aversions to food during this early period of growth, which may result in an early predisposition to the development of obesity at that young age or later.

A considerable amount of experimental data on obesity has been accumulated in relation to growth and development. The greatest attention has focused on the critical periods of the preschool and prepubertal years. Adolescence is also a period during which the effect of certain factors could result in significant physical changes (Dietz, 1994).

Studies of obese children or adolescents who became obese adults have suggested that obesity that begins in childhood is more severe than obesity that begins in adulthood. The primary reason cited for this increased severity is the longer time frame in which the individual carries additional body fat and the consequent increased risk of co-morbidities and enhanced mortality.

Increased weight in the early years of life (as opposed to increased adiposity) appears to have little effect on adult obesity. But parental obesity represents an essential risk factor for the young person to develop adult obesity. At the time of the adiposity rebound, parental and child obesity carry a comparable risk for the subsequent development (or maintenance) of adult obesity (Dietz, 1998a). By the time of adolescence, parental obesity has a more powerful influence on the risk of adult obesity in comparison to the adolescent's body weight.

The variable effects of parental and childhood obesity during the growing years on the risk of adult obesity suggests an interaction and, potentially, the changing relative influences of heredity and environmental factors (Dietz, 1998a,b). However, not enough is known about the interrelationships between genetic and environmental factors. Nevertheless, results from longitudinal projects such as the Fels Longitudinal Study indicate that those who were overweight early in life (up to 5 years of age) represented the majority of obese adults later in life (Wisemandle, Siervogel, and Guo, 1998).

3.4.1 Fetal Period, Birth Weight, Breastfeeding, and Maternal Practices

The intrauterine environment plays a critical role in the growth and development of the child. Malnutrition during early stages of pregnancy is a likely cause of obesity later in life. Also, children exposed to hyperglycemia *in utero* are more likely to develop insulin intolerance and obesity during childhood (Barker, 1994, 1998). To date, the mechanisms underlying these changes have not been fully explained. Processes of neurohumoral regulation of body weight gain since fetal and newborn period can contribute to the definition of the role of intrauterine adaptations for later obesity predisposition and development (Devascar, 2001).

Animal experiments suggest that stimuli such as a markedly increased or decreased food intake during pregnancy may affect hypothalamic development or pancreatic beta-cell development (Strauss, 1997). Apart from the immediate intrauterine environment, the health status of the prospective mother, maternal practices during her pregnancy, and subsequent breastfeeding (or lack of breastfeeding) can significantly influence the nutritional status of the child.

Birth weight and weight gain during the first month of life were independent factors correlating with BMI at 3 years (Tanaka et al., 2001). A study in Brazilian children showed that birth size, attained size during childhood, and particularly growth velocity in early life were associated with increased prevalence of overweight and obesity during adolescence. However, the vast majority of overweight and obese adolescents were not overweight children (Monteiro et al., 2003). Factors influencing early life and their interplay over time are surely important, but it seems that some additional interventions that were not controlled may have occurred, resulting in obesity later in life (Gunnarsdottir and Thorsdottir, 2003; Guo and Chumlea, 1999). It was also found that birth weight and growth during childhood were associated with blood pressure at 43 years (Hardy et al., 2004). A 20-year longitudinal study from birth showed a relationship of childhood to adulthood obesity. BMI at the age of 3 years was strongly related to BMI in young adulthood (Tsukuda et al., 2003).

A study in Jamaica showed that children stunted in early childhood had less fat and a lower BMI, but had more of a central fat distribution, partially explained by their lower birth weight. The latter association developed between the ages of 7 to 11 years (Walker et al., 2002).

In the early 1970s, the prevalence of obesity in British infants was attributed to early weaning and feeding practices such as overfeeding. However, this cannot provide a complete explanation since fat deposition in early infancy is succeeded by a lean body mass development, and then again, a further acceleration of fat accretion (Poskitt, 1986).

Breastfeeding is considered one of the important factors influencing the nutritional status and body composition of children. Most studies that have examined the effects of breastfeeding on later obesity have found an insignificant effect; e.g., an adjustment for confounders in an attempt to minimize the effect the differences between breastfeeding and formula-feeding mothers was done to varying extents across studies, which might obliterate the effect of breast feeding. However, breastfeeding was positively associated with later body fatness in two studies, and a protective effect of breastfeeding on childhood obesity was seen in four studies (Butte, 2001). The effect of breastfeeding is probably weaker than genetic and other environmental factors, and therefore its effect still remains controversial, as considered by Butte (2001). In British subjects breastfeeding and BMI in childhood was unrelated; breastfeeding was protective against increased BMI at ages 16 and 33 years in females, and at 33 years in males. This effect was markedly reduced and no longer significant after adjustment for confounding factors (Parsons, Power, and Manor, 2003).

However, a study by Koletzko and Von Kries (2001) of Bavarian children showed that overweight and obesity at school age was significantly less prevalent in previously breastfed children, with a clear relation to duration of breastfeeding. Significant confounders were parental education, maternal smoking during pregnancy, low birth weight, and lifestyle factors. Breastfeeding, however, remained a significant protective factor against later overweight and obesity after correction for confounders. Other studies have also showed positive effects of breastfeeding (Armstrong and Reilly, 2002; Nommsen-Rivers, 2004). An inverse association between overweight and breastfeeding in children was also found (Liese et al., 2001).

Therefore, early imprinting of later obesity risk can help to define efficient nutritional interventions favoring longer breastfeeding. Similar conclusions follow from a study of U.S. children, which showed that infants who were breastfed more than formula fed, or who were breastfed for longer periods, had a lower risk of being overweight during older childhood and adolescence, after adjustment for age, gender, sexual maturity, energy intake, time watching TV, physical activity, mother's BMI, and other variables reflecting social, economic, and lifestyle factors (Gillman et al., 2001). A Scottish study revealed a significantly lower prevalence of obesity in children who were breastfed, and the association persisted after adjustment for socioeconomic status, birth weight, and gender (Armstrong and Reilly, 2002). A study of Czech children showed that reduced prevalence of obesity due to breastfeeding is not confounded by socioeconomic status (Toschke et al., 2002).

In German children it was shown that maternal BMI, greater than or equal to $27kg/m^2$, bottle feeding, maternal smoking during pregnancy, and low social status are risk factors for overweight and adiposity at the age of 6 years. Early formula feeding advances the AR that is predictive of obesity later in life (Bergmann et al., 2003).

Studies on the relationship between infant milk feeding and adiposity have provided inconsistent results. Children aged 3 to 4 years from 3 ethnic groups who experienced different infant-feeding practices were assessed using anthropometric parameters. Although a weak relationship was detected between the duration of breastfeeding and body weight, none of the measures of infant feeding was related to the 3 indicators of obesity, namely body weight, BMI, and sum of 7 skinfolds. African-American girls had smaller skinfolds than Anglo- and Mexican-American girls, with no ethnic group differences evident among boys. Concerns about adiposity due to methods of infant feeding can be allayed, at least for young children (Baranowski et al., 1990).

As independent factors, increased birth weight, massive weight gain in the first months after birth, and the level of overweight of the mother or both parents appear to be the major risk factors likely to promote the development of childhood obesity (Robertson et al., 1999). Children with an increased birth weight become fat adolescents only when their mother or father is also overweight or obese (defined by a high BMI or large skinfold thickness). This followup suggests that increased fatness during adolescence is related to parental fatness but not to prenatal fatness (Frisancho, 2000). The risk factor for high blood pressure in children with low birth weight was found only in overweight children in the upper quartile of BMI at age 5 to 9 years (Bergel et al., 2000). Weight gain from birth to 12 months as a ratio to birth weight positively correlated with BMI at the age of 6 years in boys and girls. Boys in the highest quartile of protein intake as a percentage of energy at the age of 9 to 12 months had significantly higher BMI at 6 years as compared to lowest two quartiles. Weight gain during the first year and protein intake explained 50% of the variance in BMI at 6 years (Gunnarsdottir and Thorrsdottir, 2003).

As an important environmental influence, the effect of family situation, including the mother's child-feeding practices and perceptions of their daughter's risk of overweight, were considered. These influences were modest but comparable to the direct association between maternal and child weight, which indicates that measuring family environmental factors can increase the understanding of the etiology of childhood overweight (Birch and Fisher, 2000). Another study, however, did not suggest that there is a particular feeding style that is associated with overweight in young children. Differences were found in feeding behaviors between mothers with either high or low income (Baughcum et al., 2001).

Dietary intake has a significant effect on the catch-up growth during the first two years and can manifest later — for example, at the age of 5 years. Size at birth was representative of the national reference values. To illustrate, 30.7% of children showed a gain in SD scores greater than 0.67 units between 0 and 2 years, indicating clinically significant catchup in growth. These children had lower weight, length, and ponderal index at birth than other children, and were more often from primiparous pregnancies. But children who showed catch-up growth during this period were heavier, taller, and fatter according to BMI, percentage of body fat, and waist circumference (indicating more central distribution of fat) at 5 years than other children. Catch-up growth was predicted by factors relating to intrauterine restraint of fetal growth (Ong et al., 2000; Ong and Dunger, 2002). Mechanisms that signal and regulate early catch-up growth during the postnatal period may influence the association between small size at birth and risks for obesity and diseases in later periods of life. This was also shown in another study by the association of birth weight and BMI, which may have implications for the early origins of both obesity and accompanying co-morbidities (Singhal et al., 2003).

During recent years, the psychosocial domain has also received consider-ably more attention. This is particularly important as physiological or met-abolic consequences should not be considered in isolation but rather a broader perspective needs to be taken. Nutrition in early childhood and fat cell hyperplasia and hypertrophy induced by nutritional factors probably do not imply persistence of obesity but may promote obesity and worsen the prognosis of therapeutic interventions (Zwiauer and Widhalm, 1984). Certainly, experiences in the treatment of adolescent obesity are such that many individuals show poor results and potentially a predisposition to the yo-yo effect of weight cycling (Pařízková, 1977, 1998c). Such results provide more concrete evidence for the importance of early interventions.

An observational twin study, independent of genetic factors that tracked the size and shape of individuals from birth to adulthood, had the following results. The correlation of birth weight with adult body height was r = 0.236, and with adult weight, r = 0.188 (all p-values < 0.0005). Further analyses of these data indicated that intrauterine influences on birth weight have an enduring impact on adult height but not on adult relative weight. These results suggest that the intrauterine period may be considered critical for height but not for weight and adiposity (Allison et al., 1995).

The role of birth weight and body habitus during the early periods of life was also followed in a longitudinal study of Japanese children. Changes in weight and height at birth, 3, 6, 11, 14, and 17 years of age were evaluated using BMI, which was calculated at birth, 3, and 17 years, and the Rohrer index (weight.height^{-3}), which was calculated at 6, 11, and 14 years of age. In girls, obesity at the age of 17 years was related to habitus at birth, and in boys it was related to body habitus at the age of 3 years. According to these results, the recommendation for the prevention of obesity is that interven-tions be commenced as early as possible (Maramatsu et al., 1990).

Adult obesity can be predicted from BMI values assessed at an earlier age: results from the Fels Longitudinal Study showed that a child or adolescent with a high BMI percentile has a high risk of being overweight or obese at the age of 35 years. This risk increases with age; for example, the probability of adult obesity at the 85th percentile for young males was less than, or equal to, 20% up to 17 years of age, which increases to 20 to 59% afterward; this is similar for females (Guo, Chumlea, and Roche, 2002). Childhood BMI and insulin were significant predictors of adult clustering, with BMI being the strongest and showing a curvilinear relationship (Srinivasan, Mayers, and Berenson, 2002). Early menarche is characterized by excess body fatness and a higher BMI and fasting insulin beginning in early childhood, and is also accompanied by higher clustering of adverse risk variables of metabolic Syndrome X in young adulthood (Frontini, Srinivasan, and Berenson, 2003). Adult obesity was related to childhood obesity as shown by a 20-year longitudinal study from birth (Tsukuda et al., 2003). However, this does not apply in all cases (Wang, Ge, and Popkin, 2003).

The trajectory of fat gain in New Zealand girls appears to be established at a young age (there are data to indicate as early as 4 to 5 years of age), and there is a strong tracking before puberty (Goulding et al., 2003a). A multiple regression analysis of BMI data in Canadian children predicted adult BMI from the individual's BMI at the age of 10, 11, and 12 years, plus maternal and paternal BMI measures. The BMI at 12 years was a better predictor of adult BMI than the parental BMI for both genders in an Australian study (Magarey et al., 2003; Trudeau et al., 2003).

Nutrition is a key factor at any stage in life, but at a critical or sensitive period in early life, it influences future metabolism, performance, and morbidity in experimental models with laboratory animals. This also relates to the development of adipose tissue that can significantly influence the animal's later development (Hirsch and Knittle, 1970). Similar data have been collected in humans, but the methodologies of these studies may be questioned. Preliminary results from a prospective multicenter, randomized longitudinal study has provided some results that suggest that the way a preterm infant is fed in the early weeks postpartum may have a major impact on later growth and development, including predisposition to overweight (Hainer et al., 1999; Lukas, 1990).

A study in infants showed that the time of doubling and tripling of birth weight occurs later now compared to 2 to 3 decades ago. The group of children who tripled their weight had a higher percentage of fatter children, but the type of feeding was not significant (Jung and Czajka-Narins, 1985). Also, other studies showed that tracking of BMI from six years was the best predictor of later BMI; tracking was stronger for shorter periods and for subjects with both parents overweight (Abbott et al., 2002). Weight status at an earlier stage was a more important predictor of weight at 20 years than parental weight (Magarey et al., 2003).

With regard to family situation, a dose-dependent association between overweight/obesity and maternal smoking during pregnancy was observed that could not be explained by a wide range of confounders (Toschke et al., 2003). Intrauterine exposure to inhaled smoke products rather than lifestyle resulting from maternal smoking accounts for the increased prevalence of childhood obesity (Von Kries et al., 2002a). Infants of mothers who smoked during pregnancy were lighter at birth than infants of nonsmokers, but from adolescence (age 11 for females, 16 for males) they had an increased risk of being in the highest decile of BMI. This risk for obesity increased with age until 33 years, which suggested strengthening of the relationship over time, and was not accounted for by other known influences. These results are consistent with a long-term effect of intrauterine environment of obesity, possibly through fetal nutrition, and also some other mechanisms (Power and Jafferis, 2002). Five- to six-year-old German children of mothers who smoked had a higher prevalence of obesity than children whose mothers did not smoke (Toschke et al., 2003).

Mother–child feeding patterns did not relate to child overweight status, as shown in the National Longitudinal Survey of Youth conducted in Hispanic, African-American, and non-Hispanic/non–African-American children (Faith et al., 2003). Maternal perception with regard to the weight status of the child can be unrealistic: nearly one-third of them misclassify overweight children as being lower than their weight status, which applies more to sons (Maynard et al., 2003). A child is more likely to be overweight if his or her mother worked more hours per week over the child's life. Further analysis also revealed that a higher SES of the mother is associated with a high work intensity, which is particularly deleterious for her children's overweight status (Anderson, Butcher, and Levine, 2003).

3.4.2   The Effect of the Relative Composition of the Diet

3.4.2.1   *The Intake of Protein and Adiposity Rebound (AR)*

The relative composition of the diet early in life is important. Longitudinal studies (from 0.8 to 10 years of age) in children born in 1955 and 1985 revealed that upper arm muscle/fat area estimates (calculated from arm circumference –[C] and triceps skinfold –[TS]; UFE = C × [TS/2]) increased during this period (Rolland-Cachera, Deheeger, 1997). This result indicates a significant change in body composition. As energy intake has decreased in many places and the percentage of protein in the diet of children has increased, an excessive intake of energy has not been considered as the main cause of increased adiposity. Rather, decreased physical activity is considered responsible (Rolland-Cachera and Bellisle, 1986; Rolland-Cachera et al., 1995).

One of the most important simple markers of the predisposition to later obesity is the AR in children. Individual adiposity curves, assessed by BMI scores, were drawn for a group of children from the age of 1 month to 16 years. Changes in BMI indicate that adiposity increases during the first year of life and then decreases. Another increase occurs at about 6 years of age. In a longitudinal follow-up of French children, it was shown that the individual BMI curves differed regarding their percentile range level and age when AR occurred. Results of this study also showed that there is a significant relationship between the age of AR and adiposity later in life. An early AR, that is, before 5.5 years, was followed by a significantly higher adiposity level than when AR occurred after 7 years of age. This phenomenon was observed independent of the individual's adiposity at 1 year of age (Rolland-Cachera et al., 1984).

Food intake data, along with anthropometric measures, were gathered from 10 months to 8 years of age in French children (Rolland-Cachera et al., 1995). The BMI at the age of 8 years was found to be positively correlated with energy intake at the age of 2 years, but this correlation became nonsignificant after an adjustment for BMI at two years. Protein as a percentage of energy at the age of 2 years was positively correlated with BMI and subscapular skinfold at 8 years, after adjustment for energy intake at 2 years, and also for parental BMI values. The percentage of protein at 2 years was negatively associated with age at AR — that is, the higher the protein intake at 2 years, the earlier the AR and the higher the subsequent BMI level. Protein intake at 2 years was the only nutrient intake related with fatness development during later growth. High protein intake enhanced body fatness at 8 years of age (via the early AR) and a higher BMI were also found later in life.

The association between protein intake and obesity is consistent with the increased body height and accelerated growth in obese children. A high-fat, low-protein diet such as human milk corresponds to the needs for growth during the early growth period (Rolland-Cachera et al., 1995). Bottle-fed children exposed to various milk formulae that contain a higher amount of protein can be at an increased risk of obesity and other pathologies later in life.

As shown by assessments of 10-year-old French children, along with an increased prevalence of obesity, an increased intake of proteins (especially animal protein) together with a lower intake of carbohydrates, sucrose, vegetable proteins and saturated fatty acids was found. The intake of monounsaturated (MUFA) and polyunsaturated fatty acids (PUFA) remained the same while the P/S ratio increased (Figure 3.1) (Rolland-Cachera and Bellisle, 1986; Rolland-Cachera et al., 1995). The increased proportion of protein in children's diets during recent decades may have also affected hormonal status. Nutrient imbalances are particularly apparent in early childhood when a low-fat and high-protein diet is not justified because of the high energy needs for growth and because that is a period characterized by a high rate of myelination of the nervous system (Widhalm, 1996).

At older ages, the proportion of fat exceeds the recommended level with protein intake remaining high (Rolland-Cachera, Deheeger, and Bellisle, 1997). An increased ratio of proteins can have an effect on insulin-like growth factor 1 (IGF1), which results in an increased cellularity of all tissues, including adipose tissue. Generally, accelerated growth and temporarily increased height have been observed in obese children. Therefore, a diet that includes more vegetable products is recommended in order to decrease metabolic risks during growth. Adiposity rebound in the early school years is thus an essential developmental marker. In summary, the earlier AR occurs, the greater the chance that obesity will be experienced later in life.

In a study of Czech children, it was shown that the intake of protein during the first month of life in preterm girls (born at 32 weeks) was significantly associated with later somatic development. A tendency for higher weight, BMI, sum of skinfolds, waist circumference. and sagittal diameter at the L 4/5 level was revealed at the age of 7 years in girls who consumed more protein during the first month of life. Serum leptin levels, assessed at the age of 7 years, reflected fat stores.

A significant correlation of protein intake during the first postnatal month with body weight ($r = 0.430$, $p < 0.05$), and fat-free mass ($r = 0.480$, $p < 0.05$) at the age of 7 years was observed. Birth length and height at the age of

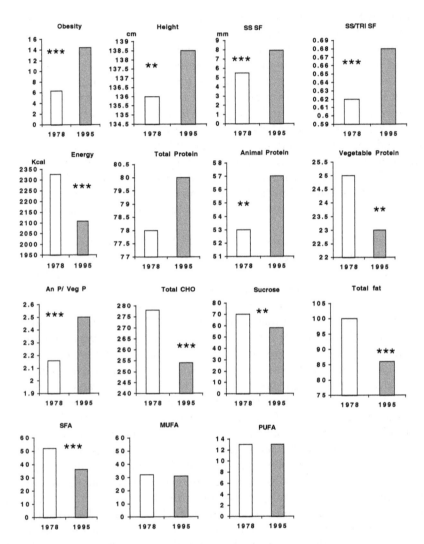

FIGURE 3.1
Comparison of obesity prevalence (% of obesity), average stature (cm), subscapular skinfold (mm) and centrality index (the ratio subscapular/triceps), and intake of energy, protein (animal and vegetable, g) and their ratio, total carbohydrates (CHO), sucrose, total fat, saturated (SFA), monounsaturated (MUFA) and polyunsaturated fatty acids (PUFA, g), and the ratio between PUFA and SFA in French children evaluated in 1978 and 1995. **(p<0.01), ***(p<0.001). (Based on data from Rolland-Cachera, Deheeger, and Bellisle, 1995.)

7 years correlated significantly. It was concluded that the first postnatal month in preterm infants represented a critical nutritional period that affects body weight and body composition (FFM) at the age of 7 years (Hainer et al., 1999). Similar conclusions were derived from the observations of Hoppe et al. (2004).

Retrospective analyses of the data of Dutch children treated for obesity showed that the mean age at which obesity begins is 5.5 years but that the mean age at which medical help is sought is 9.5 years. Seventy-eight percent of these children had one or both obese parents. The average energy intake of these children in pretreatment feeding was 924 kJ less than the recommended dietary allowances for children of the same age category (Wit et al., 1987).

Mother–child anthropometric correlations were significant, as were relationships between infant-feeding practices and childhood obesity. Further, the educational level of the mother was inversely related to the children's weight for height (Patterson et al., 1986).

As confirmed by other studies, parental obesity, high levels of body weight at the age of one year, and time of the BMI rebound are the main risk factors for obesity. The severity of obesity was negatively correlated with AR age, and was not related to spontaneous intake of energy (Girardet et al., 1993).

In the area of development of food preferences, children can be strongly influenced by the family environment, particularly very early in life. It has been determined that food habits are established at the age of 2 to 3 years (Birch et al., 1991; Cashdan, 1994; Strauss and Knight, 1999). The impact of the family environment can have a decisive effect in either a positive or negative way, that is, by introducing and reinforcing good or poor food and physical activity habits. The role of the environment is also manifested by the effect of food advertisement on food consumption, often of undesirable composition. With regard to eating behavior of the obese child, the "obesogenic environment" is significant (Halford et al., 2004a,b). In China, considerable changes in children's overweight and obesity seems to be due mainly to changed dietary patterns, particularly diet composition (Wang and Popkin, 2003).

One might suggest, therefore, that the strict distinction between genetic influence as opposed to environmental impact, especially early in life, is a difficult one to make. Where does one factor begin and end? Does genetics encompass both the inherited biological features that are undisputed, plus a characteristic way of life? Certainly, the strength of the impact of the "way of life" of the family in which a child is raised has a profound impact on all facets of growth and development.

By way of illustrative example, factors associated with obesity in preschool-age children have been analyzed simultaneously with their parents. Familial aggregation of obesity, socioeconomic status, and parents' attitude toward the use of food for non-nutritive purposes was followed up using questionnaires and compared with children's health status, specifically through height, weight, and skinfold thickness measurements. NHANES percentile rankings were used for the evaluation.

3.4.2.2 Fats and Carbohydrates

Fat represented 30% or less of dietary energy in the United Kingdom until the 1930s, when it began to increase (Stephen and Sieber, 1994). This rise was curtailed by rationing during World War II, but afterward fat intake continued to increase, reaching a plateau of about 40% of energy in the late 1950s. There was little subsequent change until the late 1970s. Increased intake of fats has been related to an increase in adiposity (Maffeis et al., 1993b, 1998b).

Trends were similar in all age groups, including children, which might be one of the reasons for the increasing adiposity during growth. Interestingly, these results for change in fat intake differ from those in the United States, where the individual intake has fallen steadily since the mid-1960s. However, during the corresponding period, the prevalence of obesity has also been increased dramatically in the United States, and a high ratio of fats in children's diet has been assumed to be one of the reasons for increasing obesity in this country.

The relationships between fat intake and body fatness were examined in subjects from a representative birth cohort of healthy children recruited in 1975 and followed over 15 years (Magarey et al., 2001). Energy-adjusted fat and carbohydrate intakes were directly and inversely (respectively) related to subscapular skinfold measures but not to BMI or triceps skinfold. In this study, the best predictor of fatness was previous adiposity, with the effect strengthening as the age interval shortened.

The composition of the diet and the frequency and energy distribution in the individual meals during the day also play an important role in the development of obesity (Maffeis et al., 1999a,b; 2000). When the percentage of the daily energy intake contributed by carbohydrates (ECH) equaled or was greater than 51.5%, this was associated with a greater leanness in prepubescent children aged 5 to 11 years. This result was reflected in skinfold thickness measurements, waist/hip ratio, and relative weight differences between children whose ECH was less than 51.5%.

When the frequency of meals increased from three to six per day, relative weight increased from 94.3 to 101.3%. This relationship was not seen in children whose ECH was equal to or greater than 51.5%. In addition, children who had a ratio of energy intake ascribed to the two main meals (that is, lunch and dinner) to a value equal to or greater than 55% were leaner than those who had a higher ratio. These results highlight the importance of an increased ratio of carbohydrates in children's diets and the relevance of reducing the energy intake at each of the main meals to prevent obesity (Maillard et al., 1998).

3.5   The Role of Physical Activity

Children in the United States were recently evaluated as fatter, slower, and weaker than counterparts from other industrially developed countries. This finding may be the result of the adoption of a sedentary lifestyle earlier in life than was commonplace in previous decades.

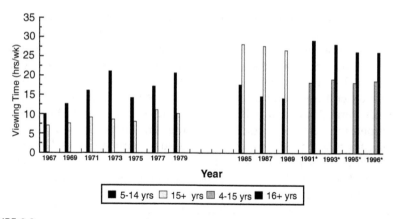

FIGURE 3.2

Changing trends in television viewing time (hrs.week[-1]) of children aged 5 to 14 years and 15+ years. *Based changed to 4- to 15-year-olds and 16+ years in 1991. (Data from *Social Trends*, 1998. With permission.)

Nutrient intake data of the past decade show that the energy and fat intakes of children in the United States may have reduced slightly but have been fairly constant. However, data also indicate that the level of physical activity has declined. Such data strongly suggest that the apparent prevalence of pediatric overweight and obesity may not be as much a function of nutrition as a reduction of physical activity and exercise from the levels that existed in the past (Schlicker, Borra, and Regan, 1994).

In spite of the trends to a decreased fat consumption in the diet in recent times, the increased prevalence of obesity might reasonably be considered to have increased due to the lack of health and dietary instruction, including an adequate exposure to and opportunity for physical activity and exercise. There is still a limited understanding of physical activity levels and energy expenditure in children, but particularly obese children (Maffeis, 1998; Maffeis et al., 1993a,b; Maffeis, Zaffanello, and Schutz, 1997). Reduced physical activity may be considered risky as is the case with an increased intake of simple sugars. However, the impact of the latter may have less of an effect on adiposity in active individuals.

The effect of the level of physical activity in the early periods of life has also been studied but somewhat spasmodically. A study of 4- to 6-month old infants considered body size, rate of growth, energy intake, subcutaneous fat (triceps skinfold), and physical activity (measured by actometer). The energy intake of these infants was more closely related to the degree of activity than to their body size and was not at all related to growth.

Obese children tended to be hypoactive and they consumed correspondingly less energy. The reverse was found in thin infants. Significant negative correlations were found between activity and the triceps skinfold ($r = -0.80$) (Rose and Mayer, 1968). It was recommended that energy intake be adjusted to suit the individual child's needs, his or her body build, degree of activity, and inclination for food.

The influence of the mass media on children and youth has already been mentioned. The impact of TV viewing on nutrition, physical activity (inactivity), and subsequent size and shape (Dietz and Gortmaker, 1993) has been considered an important issue for some time (Rössner, 1991). Generally, the time spent TV viewing has increased markedly since the 1960s (Figure 3.2). In German children aged 5 to 6 years, 34% of boys and 44% of girls spent between 1 and 3 hours watching TV daily (Kortzinger and Mast, 1997).

Competition between attractive TV programs and exercise is too difficult a choice for many children and youth because many are not adapted to any form of increased physical activity or workload. In this respect, children throughout the industrially developed world are similar, with comparable risks of obesity (Bernard et al., 1995). Moreover, children consume a significant proportion of their energy intake during TV viewing, often with high fat proportion (Matheson et al., 2004).

A longitudinal study was undertaken to examine the relationships between hours of TV viewing as a marker of sedentarism, adiposity, and physical activity in female Californian multiethnic adolescents in the sixth and seventh grades (Robinson et al., 1993). After-school TV viewing was not significantly associated with either baseline or longitudinal change in BMI or triceps skinfold thickness. Baseline hours of after-school TV viewing was weakly but negatively associated with level of physical activity in cross-sectional analyses, but not significantly associated with change in level of physical activity over time. Adjustment for age, race, parent education, and parent fatness had no significant effect on the results of this study. Only limited associations with the present level of adiposity, physical activity, or change in either variable over time were revealed (Robinson et al., 1993).

Another study also showed a weak negative association between TV watching and physical activity levels. Physical activity was lower during TV watching than during non-TV watching time (DuRant et al., 1994). Viewing behavior was not associated with body composition status. However, as the range of physical activity of youth, especially girls, is generally low in the industrially developed countries, it is possible to speculate that more marked relationships might appear when more extreme differences in all parameters of physical activity measured were present. It is also important whether TV viewing is compensated or not by increased exercise during the remaining time, which is always possible but not checked in most studies.

Obese children have been shown to have a larger decrease in metabolic rate during TV watching than normal weight children, but this was not statistically significant (262 kcal/day versus 167 kcal/day, respectively) (Klesges, Shelton, and Klesges, 1993). Television viewing has a marked and profound effect on the reduction of metabolic rate, and this might have additional implications for the development of obesity during childhood. In adults, energy expenditure during TV viewing is higher compared to resting energy expenditure and is similar to other sedentary activities. Similarly, obese adults spend more time viewing TV than nonobese individuals (Buchowski and Sun, 1996).

What is the relationship between the nature of TV programming and metabolic rate or energy expenditure? Inactivity represents a wide spectrum of "activities," a so-called continuum of inactivity. At one end of the spectrum, gross inactivity or immobility may be combined with the overconsumption of snack foods. At the other end, TV may be combined with low levels of activity, including fidgeting, but be significantly different from the former example in terms of energy expended.

A study by Salbe et al. (1998) showed that after eight years, subjects who spent a longer time viewing TV and less time with more vigorous sporting activities at the baseline of one year of age (hrs/wk engaged over the past year) had a higher BMI increase. These longitudinal observations also confirmed the role of inactivity in the development of adolescent obesity. However, in other countries such as China, TV viewing is not yet associated with obesity (Takamura et al., 1998).

With respect to the effect of TV viewing on food choice and food intake, weekly viewing hours in a group of children correlated positively with reported requests by children and purchases by parents of foods influenced by TV, and with the energy intake of children. However, the requests of children for sport items and physical activities did not significantly correlate with the number of hours of TV viewing (Taras et al., 1989). It must not be necessarily assumed that all TV viewing is counterproductive; it is necessary to also consider the duration and character of other remaining activities of the subjects followed, which was mostly not controlled.

The role of lack of physical activity in the development of obesity was also examined in a group of obese and nonobese African-American girls. Participation in vigorous (greater than or equal to 6 METs) or moderate physical activity (greater than or equal to 4 METs) was inversely associated with BMI and triceps skinfold thickness. PWC_{170} and isometric strength tests gave similar or better results in both obese and nonobese girls. This did not apply when these parameters were related to body weight. In this case, obese girls demonstrated significantly lower values. These results support the hypothesis that lack of physical activity and low levels of physical fitness are important contributing factors in both the development and the maintenance of obesity (Ward et al., 1997).

The use of DLW for the determination of free-living energy expenditure has shown that obese children underreport intake significantly more than lean children. When measurements are appropriately adjusted for the differences in body size, there are generally no major differences in energy expenditure between lean and obese groups. However, in some cross-sectional studies, a low level of physical activity has been related to current body fatness. Also, some longitudinal studies have shown that a low level of energy expenditure, particularly the energy spent in physical activity and exercise, is associated with both increasing body weight and fatness (DeLany, 1998; Goran and Sun, 1998).

Other potential contributors to the development of pediatric obesity have been considered. For example, the possible association between low levels of exercise and exposure to high-fat foods was analyzed in a group of Texan children aged 8 to 10 years. The prevalence of obesity in these children was 100% higher relative to national normative standards. Neither a high-fat food intake nor reported levels of physical activity were independent risk factors for this condition. However, it was speculated that high fat and inactivity might exert a synergistic effect when both are present in the same child (Muecke et al., 1992).

3.6   The Effect of Social Class

The effect of social conditions is apparent, especially in the countries of the Third World. Under conditions of significant change in the economic, social, and cultural situation, obesity may manifest even more markedly than in other countries. Some of the studies in industrially developed countries have focused on this topic.

Social and economic conditions have a significant relationship to nutrition and dietary intake; therefore the relationships between social class and obesity have also been analyzed (Vígnerová et al., 2004). The influence of social class on the development of obesity was examined in a 1958 longitudinal study. In childhood, the social class differences in the prevalence of obesity were negligible but were quite marked in early adulthood, with a greater percentage of overweight and obesity in lower social classes (provided a certain level of economics usual in industrially developed countries existed). This difference was threefold among obese men and twofold in obese women when respondents were classified on the basis of their own occupation (Power and Moynihan, 1988). The prevalence of obesity was associated with social class in prepubertal youth (Langnase, Mast, and Muller, 2002).

Perception of mothers with regard to the obesity of their children can vary according to SES and income. Low-income mothers do not worry about their children's obesity and were more likely to consider being teased about weight or developing limitations in physical activity as indicators of their children being overweight. Mothers did not believe that their children were overweight if they were active and had a healthy diet; mothers described overweight children as thick and solid, and did not consider environmental factors as decisive. It was also difficult for mothers to deny children food despite having just eaten. The definition of overweight on the basis of growth charts may not have the same meaning for mothers with different income and SES (Jain et al., 2001).

A lower social class position, a lower level of social support, and whether the primary caregiver is unmarried are all associated with a high food intake and higher weight for height score of children (Gerald et al., 1994). A long-term effect of early class background was also manifested. Children from families with fathers involved in a manual profession were more likely to become overweight, and obese young adults compared with peers from families with a nonmanual profession. These subjects were also more likely to remain overweight or obese through early adulthood (Power and Moynihan, 1988).

Another study showed that children from low-income families who were exposed to less cognitive stimulation and who had an obese mother showed an increased risk of obesity independent of other demographic factors. In contrast, the increased rates of obesity in black children, and those with a low family education and nonprofessional parents, may be mediated through the confounding effects of low income and lower level of cognitive stimulation (Strauss and Knight, 1999).

Measurements of children in New York State showed that those who tended to be fatter were members of low SES and from two-parent households than those with few or no siblings and those who ate school lunch or skipped breakfast. Overweight was revealed as a problem among many elementary schoolchildren in this locality (Wolfe et al., 1994). The identification of sociodemographic characteristics may be particularly useful in targeting preventive efforts against later obesity development.

The effect of low SES, regardless of ethnicity or gender, exhibited extremely large increases in adiposity over time in U.S. children, which enhances the risk of co-morbidities (Moore, Howell, and Treiber, 2002). An inverse social gradient — i.e., highest fatness in lowest SES — was apparent also in German children. Parental overweight enhanced the inverse social gradient: the prevalence of overweight was 37.5% in low- and 22.9% in high-SES children of overweight parents (Langnase, Mast, and Muller, 2002). The study reported a much higher prevalence of obesity in the adolescent Mexican-American population than that by the NHANES III; the prevalence was even higher than that specific to Mexican adolescents in the NHANES III, highlighting the effect of SES and the changing social environment (Lacar, Soto, and Riley, 2000).

The association of SES and obesity can be misleading and obscure the influence of the socioeconomic conditions during childhood as it varies in different ages in both genders: SES at 7 years of age predicts obesity in adult females and at birth and 23 years predicted obesity in males at 33 years. Lower education was also associated with adult obesity (Power, Manor, and Matthews, 2003). The effect of unemployment with regard to obesity in young adults from a 1966 birth cohort was also evaluated (Laitinen et al., 2002).

3.7 The Role of Sudden Changes in Lifestyle

Commonly, childhood obesity has its genesis during recovery from illness or accident (for example, a fracture or major sprain) when anxious parents or other carers allow an increased food intake (including delicacies) while the child is limited by a reduced regime of physical activity. Sometimes the child succeeds in reducing his or her body weight and fatness after recovery, but too often, this is the beginning of a long-lasting increase of weight.

Under such circumstances it is very difficult to follow an optimal regime as a high-quality diet and sufficient energy, along with a degree of rest, is necessary. However, the maintenance of an optimal energy balance is possible, but this depends on the environment of the child. Medical care, exercise, and/or dietetic support are highly desirable under these circumstances in order to limit unnecessary health risks resulting from the previous pathological situation and also to reduce the risk of obesity.

There was a rapid increase in the prevalence of obesity in former East German children after the reunification of the country (Jaeger and Kromeyer-Hauschild, 1999). Between 1975 and 1995 the prevalence of overweight (BMI over 90th percentile) of Jena children increased in boys from 10.0 to 16.3%, and in girls from 11.7 to 20.7%. The prevalence of obesity (BMI over 97th percentile) increased from 5.3 to 8.2% in boys, and from 4.7 to 9.9% in girls. The peak of the increase of overweight as well as of obesity can be found for both genders between 1985 and 1995. Using logistic regression, statistically significant associations with overweight were found for occupation of the father, birth weight in both sexes, and amount of fat in girls (Kromeyer-Hauschild et al., 1999). Increasing intake of fast food, soft drinks, and TV and video programs plays a role. Changes in the nutritional situation resulting from social, economic, market, and living conditions after reunification are considered as the main factors in the changing prevalence of obesity in German children (Jaeger and Kromeyer-Hauschild, 1999). This result was something of a special contrast with growth characteristics since 1880, when secular changes started to be studied (Zellner, Kromeyer, and Jaeger, 1996). Special attention should be paid to the further social development in the society and to the link between low social class and overweight and changes of lifestyle, which is mostly not the same for all.

In another country with rapid economic and epidemiological transition, the Seychelles, the prevalence of overweight and obesity in schoolchildren was as high or higher than in some industrialized countries. Obesity was related to a rapid change in weight during the first year of life as found also in other studies (Stettler et al., 2002). Similar results were observed in Inuit children in Canada (Shephard, 1991).

Obesity is also a risk in growing subjects who have adapted to a high level of energy output — for example, young athletes who, for whatever reason, stop their sports training. Some would contend that after an interruption to training, fat is deposited excessively. A number of practical examples (see Chapter 12) exist to portray the sudden effect of a decrease in workload and exercise causing a reduced level of energy expenditure (Gutin, 1998; Pařízková, 1977, 1995.)

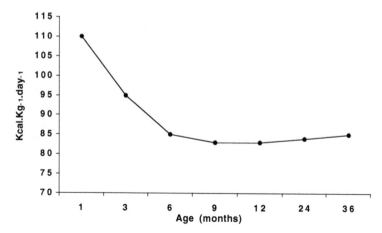

FIGURE 3.3
Estimates for the energy requirements of young children obtained by using doubly labeled water ($^2H_2{}^{18}O$). Values are lower than the present RDAs. (Based on data from Prentice et al., 1988.)

3.8 Recommended Dietary Allowances during Growth

Observations of Prentice et al. (1988) showed that the recommended dietary allowances (RDAs) for energy for infants and young children were too high, and that normal growth has been demonstrated in children who had an energy intake of approximately 10% lower than RDA values. Measurements of total energy expenditure (TEE, using DLW) in healthy normal babies also showed that the current RDAs for energy were considerably higher than the estimates calculated from the direct measurements of total energy expenditure (Davies, 1998). This excess of energy might play a significant role in predisposing an individual to obesity later in childhood (Figure 3.3).

New estimates for energy requirements of young children have been derived by combining the energy deposited during growth with measurements of total energy expenditure obtained using the DLW ($^2H_2{}^{18}O$) method in healthy infants aged 0 to 3 years. The resultant values of energy from 1 to 36 months (Figure 3.4) are substantially lower than current Department of Health and Social Security and FAO/WHO/UNU RDAs. Therefore, it is recommended that dietary guidelines be revised to avoid overfeeding of infants.

A modification of the estimations for the energy requirements of infants and children were then proposed as the basis of new FAO/WHO energy requirements. These were also validated by the measurements of energy intake in both breast- and bottle-fed infants. In addition, this occurred in 1- to

3-year-old children in the Dortmund Nutritional and Anthropometric Longitudinal Designed Study, the results of which showed considerably lower values of energy intake compared to the energy allowances recommended by FAO/WHO/UNU in 1985. Height and weight development of children measured corresponded to suitable standard values (the Netherlands' third nationwide survey). To avoid early overfeeding and predisposition to childhood obesity, new estimations should be mentioned and would be preferable from the perspective of health promotion (Alexy et al., 1998). The WHO and FAO have suggested that there always be a consideration of energy output (see Chapter 5).

Nutritional knowledge plays an important role in dietary intake with regard to recommended allowances in adolescents. However, a followup in obese and nonobese adolescents did not reveal any significant differences in nutrition knowledge or behaviors and food preferences, with the exception that the obese students were better able to identify high-fiber foods. Obese students were also more likely to report infrequent meals with their family (Thakur and D'Amico, 1999). A more detailed questionnaire, "Eating Behavior and Weight Problems Inventory for Children" (EWI-C, which includes 60 items) has been developed. Individual scores enable the formation of six groups that range from underweight to severe obesity. In both gender groups, selected mean scores significantly increase with increasing weight, while others decrease. Norm tables were established that make it possible to define the position of the child in relationship to his or her weight category, and then to evaluate the child's responses (Diehl, 1999). Obviously, knowledge of appropriate diet and physical activity is not a guarantee of behavior.

3.9   Summary

Factors that have a significant effect on obesity development during growth are not only the usual ones — i.e., the imbalance between energy intake and output. Family clustering of obesity reveals significant hereditary factors, including both genes and lifestyle. The sensitivity to weight gain due to genetic predispositions (the role of "thrifty" genes), polymorphism of most genes studied up to now (e.g., melanocortin, Trp64Arg) in their mutual interplay, as well as with further endogenous and exogenous factors of the environment, has been considered and analyzed. In addition, the special role of stimuli such as the nutrition during early life starting with pregnancy, resulting in various birth weight (both increased or decreased), or nutrition at the beginning of postnatal life (breast- and/or bottle-feeding), and later food intake resulting in different speeds of weight gain after birth, or different time of adiposity rebound, seem to play a significant role with regard to the delayed consequences concerning either easier, more difficult, or impossible development of obesity later in life. Composition of food and the ratio of the individual components of the diet (fat, protein) were found to be important for obesity development, most often more than simple overfeeding.

There has not been a general consensus on the effect of the abovementioned factors; however, their essential importance was recognized. Adding further to the complexity in interpretation of findings is the presence of confounders. This includes, for example, the effect of breastfeeding, or increased ratio of proteins in the diet of the early years. The recommended dietary allowances should be reduced as it has been shown by energy expenditure measurements to be unnecessarily high. The level of physical activity and/or inactivity is another factor in the focus of attention due to the changes in lifestyle in all countries. This includes developing countries where life conditions, both diet, its composition, and workload, have changed significantly and relatively fast during recent periods. Sedentarism and the change of diet, including in particular its composition (high saturated fats, simple sugars, lack of vegetables and fruit, etc.) are therefore considered as the most frequent reason for increased fatness, especially in genetically predisposed subjects.

In all instances, obesity cannot develop without sufficient energy being available, a consistently high level that exceeds the base needs of the growing organism. The fact that genetics contribute to the inter-individual differences in the population where energy is available may in itself be considered a gene/environment interaction.

4

Physical Characteristics
of the Obese Child and Adolescent

4.1 Basic Morphological Characteristics, Criteria, and Methods

Anthropometric methods have enjoyed widespread acceptability for the evaluation of overweight and obesity (Huang and Chiang, 1987). However, comparisons of the prevalence of obesity in various parts of the world to date have been difficult as the criteria for classification has not been homogeneous (Widhalm, 1985) and the reference values have varied. What is deemed to be overweight in one country may be normal weight in another. Substantive efforts have resulted in the ability to define more accurately the level of development and nutritional status during growth (Sundaram, Ahuja, and Ramachandran, 1988). Despite considerable recent progress, global consent on selected approaches for the evaluation of overweight and obesity has not been reached due to some discrepancies between classification systems (Neovius et al., 2004).

Tables of standard reference values of body weight and height in individual age categories have been widely used as criteria for the evaluation of overweight and obesity in different populations. Grids that enable a quick orientation to the degree of overweight of an individual during growth have also been used. Some of the more common growth grids used extensively in the past includes those of Wetzel (1942), Tanner, Whitehouse, and Takaishi (1966), and Kapalin (1967), among others.

In recent decades, growth charts for height and weight, prepared for individual children, have also been in widespread use. However, there has been considerable discussion as to whether percentiles and/or standard deviation (SD) values should be used for the evaluation of populations during growth. The World Health Organization (WHO) uses cutoffs based on SD scores rather than percentiles, which are more suitable for the extremes of growth status in the developing world. However, this approach is not compatible with charts based on percentiles. A proposition for a unified growth chart was advanced with nine rather than seven percentiles, and spaced two-thirds of a SD score apart, rather than the more usual unit spacing. The 0.4th percentile is a more practical cutoff for screening purposes than the third or fifth percentiles (Cole, 1994).

Weight-for-age, height-for-age, weight-for-height, and their standard values have also been widely used in the evaluation of children and youth (Waterlow et al., 1997; Falorni et al., 1999). These approaches provide a better approximation of the evaluation of children's growth and nutritional status. Retardation of growth in height and weight, stunting (shorter stature related to age), and wasting (reduced weight related to height) can be differentiated. This approach is considered the most important for the evaluation of children's development in Third World countries, especially where malnutrition exists and commonly affects the child population. This approach has enabled the comparison of different growing populations living under conditions of various levels of nutrition and malnutrition (WHO, 1985, 1997). The same procedure is also suitable for the evaluation of childhood obesity.

Obese children commonly have higher values of height and weight for age than normal weight children. Falorni et al. (1999) showed that more information on the growth of obese subjects may be obtained when evaluating the height and height velocity according to the specific reference standards from the same population of origin. When adopting this modality, no significant variations in height during the reduction therapy are apparent. Slowing down of growth during weight loss in obese children appears only when standards for normal weight children are used. More appropriate information on the growth of obese children may be obtained when evaluating the height and height velocity according to obese-specific reference standards from the same population. This may influence, for example, conclusions on the effect of weight reduction on growth — that is, no significant variation in heights during reduction treatment (Falorni et al., 1999).

The prevalence of obesity based on height and weight data was shown in the Fourth Dutch Growth Study (1997), which used international criteria to compare recent data to that from 1980. Prevalence was higher in girls (8.2–16.1%) than in boys (7.1–15.5%) and therefore reference growth diagrams based on the 1997 Dutch Growth Study were established to enable the diagnosis of overweight and obesity (Hirasing et al., 2001).

According to the measurement of 12 anthropometric characteristics, including BMI (> 97th percentile of reference population), parental characteristics, and lifestyle, it appeared that the prevalence of obesity was related, for example, to the size of the community (6.9% in smaller and 2.3% in large towns). Further, more obese children had mothers with a low level of education (Kovárová et al., 2002).

4.2   Body Mass Index (BMI)

The most widely used method for defining obesity at present, particularly in population studies, is the Body Mass Index (BMI = kg.m^2, or Quetelet's index) (Dietz and Bellizzi, 1999). Some believe that the index is more suited to adults than children and adolescents unless alternative values for p are used at different ages (Wt/Ht^p). The major limitation cited is the inability of BMI to distinguish weight from adiposity (Eto et al., 2004). Additionally, BMI tends to misclassify individuals at the extreme ends of the height spectrum, with very short and very tall individuals often misclassified as obese (Freedman et al., 1999). In very muscular individuals without high levels of fat, BMI values are also commonly very high (Pařízková, 1977). Nevertheless, support for the use of the index with children and adolescents is widespread.

BMI has been widely used for the evaluation of children's growth and development (Rolland-Cachera et al., 1982). A certain lack of precision is unavoidable using this technique because of the different stages of growth observed at any given age. Therefore, in children, the evaluation of size and shape is not easy because the proportionality of the growing organism is changing significantly during various periods of growth. Greater linearity is a natural phenomenon — for example, during the preschool age, and/or prepuberty and puberty. On the other hand, greater bulkiness and predisposition to adiposity appears in infants, toddlers, and those in the early years of schooling. This is also reflected in the changes in BMI (Rolland-Cachera et al., 1982; Rolland-Cachera, Spyckerelle, and Deschamps, 1992).

The utilization of the BMI to categorize under- or overweight is not a problem for adults as the criterion is the same for all age periods — that is, 25 kg/m². The BMI value of 25 to 30 kg/m² defines overweight or preobese status, 30 to 35kg/m² moderate obesity (Obesity Class I), 35 to 40 kg/m² severe obesity (Obesity Class II), and higher than 40 kg/m², a very severe or morbid obesity (Obesity Class III) (WHO, 1998). Nevertheless, the cutoff point for either category or grade of overweight or obesity can vary according to different authors. For example, an adequate BMI for some may be extended to 26kg/m² while for others it would be only 24 kg/m².

The first developmental BMI grids for children and youth were prepared by Rolland-Cachera et al. (1982) and were based on data from a longitudinal study of French children published in 1984 (Rolland-Cachera et al., 1984) (Figure 4.1 and Figure 4.2). Other developmental curves for BMI have been produced in many countries (Hammer et al., 1991; Must, Dallal, and Dietz, 1991; Rolland-Cachera et al., 1991; Bláha et al., 1993, 1997). Some of these BMI grids are based on older data or cover only certain age ranges. Newer BMI grids have been derived for the United Kingdom (Cole, Freeman, and Preece, 1995), Sweden (Lindgren et al., 1995), Italy (Luciano, Bressan, and Zoppi, 1997), and other populations of children. In the preparation of these grids the least mean square (LMS) method elaborated by Cole (1994) was used. This enables the adjustment of the BMI distribution for skewness and allows the expression of an individual's BMI to be an exact percentile or SD score.

It should be noted, however, that the BMI classification method is still deemed to be contentious by some researchers. For example, it can be argued that BMI standards apply mainly to the populations whose data were used

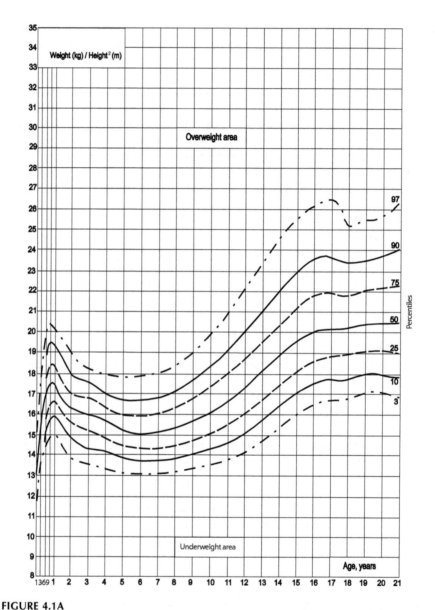

FIGURE 4.1A
Growth grid with percentiles for body mass index (BMI, kg.m⁻²) for girls. (Based on data from Rolland-Cachera and Bellisle, 1986, and Rolland-Cachera et al., 1995.)

for the definition of cutoff points (Fu et al., 2003; Misra, 2003). Others defend the present cutoffs and contend that they are simple, uniform definitions of overweight and obesity that hold across populations (Stevens, 2003). Despite the ongoing debate regarding cutoff points to define obesity, in agreement with Cole et al. (2000) the choice to use the BMI cutoff percentiles passing through the adult BMI cutoff point of 30 seems to be reasonable (Luciano et

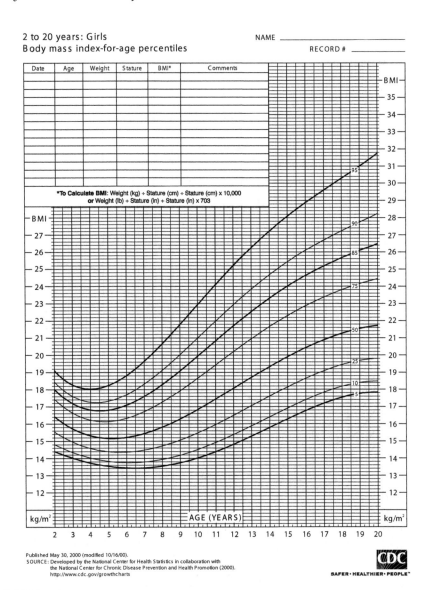

FIGURE 4.1B
Body mass index-for-age percentiles 2 to 20 years: Girls.

al., 2003). The use of population-specific cutoff points would clearly be the preferable choice where available.

In contemporary children, fat-free mass (FFM) and fat may contribute in the same way to the values of BMI compared to the reference child (Wells et al., 2002). BMI correlates with other parameters — for example, there is a slightly higher correlation between BMI and subscapular skinfold than weight-for-height index and the same parameter, as well as with other cardiovascular risk factor variables (blood pressure, serum lipids, and lipoproteins) regardless of

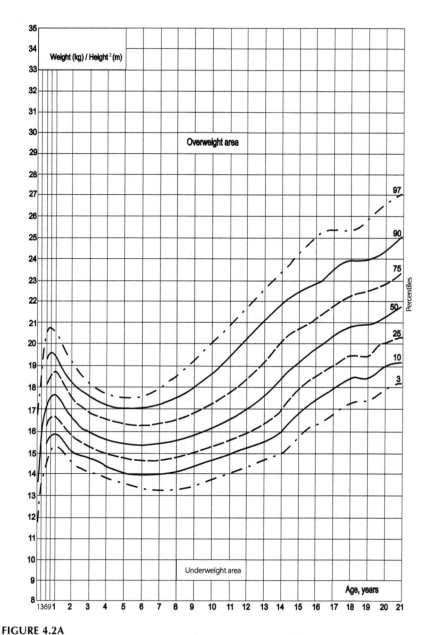

FIGURE 4.2A

Growth grid with percentiles for body mass index (BMI, kg.m⁻²) for boys. (Based on data from Rolland-Cachera and Bellisle, 1986, and Rolland-Cachera et al., 1995.)

age-for-sex groups. However, weight-for-height measures are not superior to BMI as an indicator of obesity (Frontini et al., 2001). A study by Wright et al. (2001) found BMI at age 9 was significantly correlated with BMI at 50, but not with percentage of body fat. After adjustment, BMI correlated with selected health risks. Results of a study in Chinese children and adolescents reported

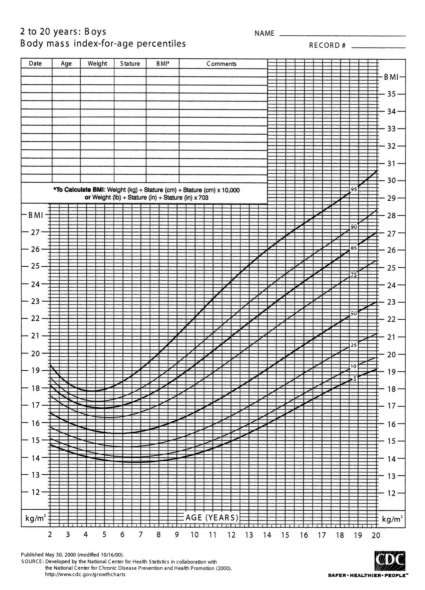

FIGURE 4.2B
Body mass index-for-age percentiles 2 to 20 years: Boys.

an obvious dose-effect relationship between BMI and lipid profiles, which accounted for some rationality of the BMI cutoff points recommended by the Working Group of Obesity in China (Zhai et al., 2004).

4.2.1 Grids for the Evaluation of BMI and Its Rebound in Children

As can be seen from Figure 4.1 and Figure 4.2, BMI increases significantly during the first year of life and then decreases until approximately 6 to 7 years, at which point it increases again. This return and further increase of BMI is defined as the adiposity rebound (AR) of BMI. Standardized percentile curves of BMI for children and adolescents have also been used for U.S. (Hammer et al., 1991) and Czech children (Bláha et al., 1993, 1997; Hajniš, 1993).

As mentioned previously, AR that occurs earlier than 6 years of age is a marker of later adiposity. That is, subjects who increase their BMI at an earlier age are more prone to becoming fatter and potentially obese later in life (Rolland-Cachera, 1993). The results of the Fels Longitudinal Growth Study concur with this contention (Siervogel et al., 1991). Therefore, it appears that the age of AR and the BMI at that age is significantly associated with BMI in early adulthood. Williams, Davie, and Lam (1999) found that the correlations between BMI at the age of 7 years and BMI at ages 18 and 21 were similar in magnitude. This result indicates that it may be possible to predict BMI in early adulthood from BMI values at 7 years of age.

Early AR is considered a risk factor for later obesity and accompanying comorbid conditions. Eriksson et al. (2003a) found that this applied especially when it was preceded by a low weight gain between birth and one year of age. The researchers also found that the incidence of type 2 diabetes decreased progressively from 8.6% in subjects whose adiposity rebound occurred before the age of 5 years to 1.8% in those in whom it occurred after 7 years (Eriksson et al., 2003a). The longitudinal Bogalusa Heart Study indicated that although an early BMI rebound was related to higher relative weight in adulthood, the association was not independent of childhood BMI levels (Freedman et al., 2001a). According to Cole (2004), early adiposity rebound predicts fatness and identifies children with a high BMI percentile and/or crossing upward. Such subjects are likely to have a higher BMI later in life. But BMI percentile crossing is more direct than the timing of adiposity rebound for predicting later increased adiposity. Adiposity rebound, early growth, and menarche may all be associated (Williams and Dickson, 2002).

4.2.2   Variation of BMI in Various Countries

The development of BMI varies in different populations. For example, in the former Czechoslovakia, a cohort of children was followed longitudinally from birth with measurements taken at 3, 6, 9, and 12 months then twice per year from 1 to 20 years of age. An inverse relationship between age at AR and later BMI was confirmed. In the leanest adults, AR had occurred by 7.6 years, and in the heaviest adults, age at AR was around 5 years. Many lean (44%) and fat (58%) infants were adults of average size. The risk of becoming obese as an adult (as compared to an infant who was not fat) was 31/22, or 1.8 (Prokopec and Bellisle, 1992, 1993). Individual growth curves of children with very high or very low adult BMI values convincingly demonstrated the relationship between BMI at 12 months, age at AR, and adult BMI value. Another study demonstrated a correlation between high BMI in childhood and overweight at the age of 21 years and thus the ability to predict adult

BMI from the values in childhood (Williams, 2001). However, many of those who were overweight at 21 years had a BMI below the 75th percentile or even median values in childhood and early adolescence.

In the Czech population, obesity later in life is a more common phenomenon than in countries of Western Europe. Similarly, the prevalence and morbidity from cardiovascular diseases is significantly higher than in Western Europe, the United States, Japan, and others but has been decreasing during the past 15 years. The genesis of such chronic diseases may occur in early childhood and be related to body size and composition but mainly to dietary intake, both total energy and the composition and ratio of macronutrients (Pařízková and Rolland-Cachera, 1997). For example, Czech Recommended Dietary Allowances (RDAs) for children aged 4 to 6 years are higher (65 g per day of protein) compared to European or U.S. RDAs (24 g per day) and the actual intake of protein is often higher in Czech children (Pařízková, 1996a). This is in agreement with the hypothesis of Rolland-Cachera (1995) that an increased ratio of protein in the childhood diet is an important factor for greater weight and earlier AR.

The values of BMI at the 50th and other percentiles not only vary during growth when they express the developmental changes from relative bulkiness-adiposity with linearity and leanness but also during the adult years until the ninth decade (Rolland-Cachera et al., 1990a,b). Changes in BMI between the ages of 20 and 65 years cannot be explained by an increase in energy intake; on the contrary, a reduction in energy intake has been commonly observed from 30 to 35 years onward. The sex and age variations in energy intake were similar to the variations of lean, fat-free body mass, and opposite to fat mass (Rolland-Cachera et al., 1991; Ailhaud and Guesnet, 2004). This may be related to the reduction of physical activity observed in most aging individuals.

A comparison of BMI curves from countries with different nutritional environments shows that the U.S. (Cronk et al., 1982), Swedish (Dahlström et al., 1985), and French curves are very similar. Data from Senegal (Massé and Moraigne, 1969), Burundi (Lemaire and De Maegd, 1969), and India (Subash and Chuttani, 1978) indicate that BMI values are not very different from those of the industrially developed countries up to 6 years of age. Adiposity is relatively low during this period of development irrespective of the nutritional conditions in a given country, with differences more apparent later in the growing years. In the more affluent countries, BMI values usually increase after the age of 6 years, but in Burundi, this increase is delayed to 7 years. In Senegal an increase occurs at approximately 8 years of age whereas in India no increase in BMI is evidenced. The individual age at which BMI increases correlates with bone age (Rolland-Cachera et al., 1984). The increase in BMI values occurs earlier in obese children — for example, as early as 3 years of age (Rolland-Cachera et al., 1988). Differences in BMI trends reflect the notion that increased dietary intake accelerates growth but restricted food intake retards it (Forbes, 1987). When comparisons of the individual percentiles of BMI for children in different industrially

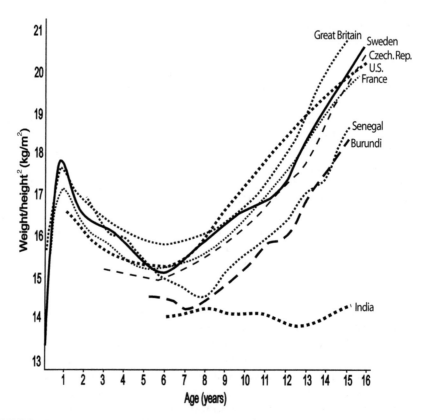

FIGURE 4.3
Development of BMI in different countries. (Based on data from Rolland-Cachera and Bellisle, 1986, and Rolland-Cachera et al., 1984, 1988, 1995.)

developed countries are made, they show considerable similarity that is not found for percentiles of children from the countries of the Third World (Figure 4.3).

Therefore, choosing an appropriate developmental grid for BMI evaluation is a critical issue. At present, it is recommended that national standards suited to the particular situation of the country be used, especially in the developing countries. It is preferable to use those that were derived on the basis of the measurements of the healthy and normal local children rather than of those living under quite different environmental (especially more favorable nutritional) conditions.

4.2.3 BMI Validation

Body mass index has been validated as a measure of size and shape and displays significant correlations with percent body fat (measured by densitometry) and/or by skinfolds in children and adolescents ($r = 0.86$, $p < 0.001$) (Pařízková, 1977, 1998a,b) and similarly in adults (women $r = 0.934$, $p <$

0.001, men r = 0.85, p < 0.001) (Pařízková, 1996b). Therefore, it is possible to estimate percent body fat from BMI values; however, BMI can only approximate body adiposity (Widhalm and Schonegger, 1999). The BMI of obese prepubertal boys is significantly correlated with the percentage of total, extracellular, and intracellular body water, calculated using the multifrequency bioelectrical impedance method and using relevant equations (Yiannakou et al., 1998). In a study of children 2 to 19 years of age, BMI-for-age measures were better at predicting under- and overweight than the Rohrer index (RI)-for-age measures, but the predictive power of BMI-for-age was similar to that of weight-for-height (Mei et al., 2002).

Further validations of BMI have been conducted with simultaneous measurements using the following methods. A significant relationship between body composition measurements by total body conductivity measurements (TOBEC) and BMI was demonstrated in obese children and adolescents aged 6 to 17 years (Schonegger and Widhalm, 1998). The screening performance of BMI with respect to adiposity was also tested using dual-energy x-ray absorptiometry (DXA) in Australian subjects aged 4 to 20 years. Receiver-operating characteristic (ROC) curves were prepared for detecting total body fat percentage at or beyond the 85th percentile. Screening performance was slightly but not significantly better for girls than for boys. The analysis showed that screening for excess adiposity using an appropriate percentile cutoff for BMI is acceptable. The design of screening programs can be facilitated by ROC curves by allowing an explicit trade-off between true-positive and false-positive rates. Although large sample sizes are necessary for precise estimates, the cutoff points that have been recommended appear to offer a reasonable compromise (Lazarus et al., 1996). These, however, must be used with caution in populations other than those used to define the cutoffs.

Despite high correlations between BMI and body fat (Pařízková, 1989; Pietrobelli et al., 1998), further analyses have revealed that BMI is not appropriate as an exact evaluation of body composition, especially in obese youth. The high correlations between BMI and absolute (TBF) and relative amounts of stored fat measured by DXA (PBF -%) concerned both genders (girls PBF r = 0.84, boys r = 0.56, p < 0.0001; TBF girls r = 0.93, boys r = 0.85, p < 0.0001) (Boot et al., 1997). Further, correlations between BMI and skinfold thickness measurements have been reported as follows: girls r = 0.84, boys r = 0.58 (Scharfer et al., 1998).

Widhalm and Schonegger (1999) measured body fat in obese children using TOBEC, and these values were significantly correlated with DXA measurements (r = 0.948, p < 0.0001). The relationships were similar for girls and boys (r = 0.65, r = 63, respectively, p < 0.0001). However, when the obese children were divided into groups with different values of BMI, the groups with the lowest and/or highest values of BMI displayed poor correlations, while in the group with medium values of BMI no correlation was seen. The curvilinear relationship, which starts to incline at a BMI of approximately 25 to 27kg/m^2, demonstrated that an increasing BMI is not necessarily linked to a higher relative amount of fat. When the same children were divided according to age, the highest correlation for BMI and percent body fat was found for subjects aged 6 to 9 years ($r = 0.79$, $p < 0.0001$). Despite remaining significant, the correlation decreased in the higher age groups.

Therefore, interpretation of BMI results for obese children across different age groups should be treated cautiously. Direct measurements of fat and lean body mass are preferable for the evaluation of obesity whenever possible. A significant relationship between body composition measurements by TOBEC and BMI in obese children and adolescents aged 6 to 17 years has also been reported. These results indicate that BMI can be a useful standard for defining obesity in children and adolescents, but only to a moderate degree of adiposity. In cases of severe or morbid obesity in this age group, BMI does not reflect the real degree of fatness (Schonegger and Widhalm, 1998).

In short, the degree of adiposity can vary significantly in subjects with the same BMI, and the percentage of body fat (%BF) associated with BMI classifications of overweight and obesity can differ markedly with age in growing children. A further illustration is as follows: although the predicted %BF of young females was similar to that of young males, female values rose steadily with age, such that an 18-year-old female with a BMI of 30 had an estimated %BF of 42 and a male an estimated %BF of 27 (Taylor et al., 2002). It was also revealed that contemporary children have a different level of fatness for a given BMI compared to the reference child of two decades ago. Contemporary Cambridge children, for example, had BMIs similar to the reference child; but, in both genders, greater fatness and lower mean FFM was found compared to the reference child after taking into account body height. From this it follows that using BMI to assess nutritional status and overweight may underestimate the degree of the child's true adiposity (Wells et al., 2002). Therefore, not only population-specific but also time-adjusted reference values should be used.

The study of Widhalm et al. (2001) using TOBEC revealed that BMI might be a useful parameter for epidemiological studies, but in individual pediatric care, BMI evaluation provides only a limited insight to the degree of obesity, especially from 10 years on. However, the widespread use of BMI has been criticized as cutoffs in the current international standard were derived on the basis of measurements in six child populations from developed countries, and therefore may not be valid for other populations (Fu et al., 2003; Misra, 2003; Vígnerová, Lhotská, and Bláha, 2001). Moreover, variability in the timing of the pubertal growth spurt, the increase in height velocity in the year prior to menarche, plus the earlier menarche in taller and heavier children may contribute to distortions in weight-for-height measurements around puberty (Cole, 1998).

4.2.4 Critical BMI Values as Cutoff Points for Obesity

Until recently there has not been a general consensus regarding the cutoff points of overweight and obesity in children and adolescents. The 85th percentile has often been used to operationally define obesity and the 95th percentile as gross, or severe, obesity. Race-specific and population-based 85th and 95th percentiles of BMI and also of triceps skinfold for humans aged 6 to 74 years were derived from the anthropometric data gathered in the National Health and Nutrition Examination Survey I (NHANES I). Racial differences in these extremes of the distribution do not emerge until adult-hood. On the basis of this outcome it is possible to choose population-based, race-specific, or age-specific criteria for obesity on the basis of assumptions underlying their specific research or clinical aims (Must, Dallal, and Dietz 1991; Rolland-Cachera, Deheeger, and Bellisle, 2001).

However, more cutoff points have been used, including the 95th for over-weight, 97th for obesity, and/or 99th percentile for gross obesity. The cutoff points used in different countries to define obesity range from the 85th (Australia) to the 90th (Finland, France, Greece, Hungary, Japan, U.K.), 95th (U.S., Canada, Saudi Arabia), and 97th percentile (Belgium, Netherlands) (Guillaume, 1999).

At the age of 14 years, the NHANES I 95th percentile cutoff would mis-classify 3.5% of children as "overweight" instead of "at risk of overweight" (Lazarus et al., 1995). These results indicate some variability in the cutoff points that might appear among various populations. The differences may be even greater among growing populations that vary more markedly with regard to environment, way of life, and cultural conditions.

As mentioned in the previous section, some studies have confirmed that the cutoff points for the evaluation of obesity should be derived from the measurements of the local population. For example, smoothed Australian cutoffs for BMI were similar to those derived from the first NHANES I values for whites. However, the NHANES I cutoffs would result in systematic misclassification, for example, among 7-year-olds. The NHANES I 85th per-centile cutoff would wrongly classify 4.6% of normal males and 9.1% of normal females as "at risk of overweight" (Lazarus et al., 1995). BMI cutoff points using age and stage of pubertal development compared with BMI cutoff points using age alone were used for the identification of obesity in adolescents (Taylor et al., 2003). The elaboration of BMI grids for individual parts of the world should be one of the important issues for pediatric research in future years.

A study of Italian adolescents showed different results, especially when underweight, overweight, and obesity are identified. BMI was a useful indi-cator to define obesity but should be used with caution when comparing results based on different references — that is, the percentiles of Rolland-Cachera, Cole, and Cacciari, among others (Turconi et al., 2003).

A study of the predictive value of BMI during growth for overweight in adulthood (defined as BMI > 28kg/m^2 in males and > 26kg/m^2 in females) was conducted during a 35-year longitudinal study. Analyses of data in white children indicated that overweight at the age of 35 years could be predicted from BMI at younger ages. The prediction is excellent at age 18 years, good at 13 years, but only moderate at ages younger than 13 years (Guo et al., 1994).

In summary, BMI is most often used as a guide to levels of adiposity in population studies and also for monitoring change in the obese as a function of treatment for overweight (Bellizzi and Dietz, 1999; Dietz and Bellizzi, 1999; Smith et al., 1997; Stevens, 2003). The shift of BMI over time in French children and the prevalence of obesity as compared to the United States points to a gradual change of diet (particularly carbohydrate and sugar intake) in Western Europe and the United States (Lioret, 2001). The index has proved to be most useful in these respects and particularly in field studies where more accurate measurements are not possible. The growth charts for children 2 to 20 years of age developed by the Centers for Disease Control in the United States have also been widely used in many countries, particularly where normative information is not available.

Plotting BMI with international standard values and cutoff points suggested by Cole and Rolland-Cachera (2002) enables evaluations of the degree of childhood adiposity (see Table 4.1). Categorization of BMI according to age only was shown to be sufficient, and adding stage of puberty does not produce cutoffs that would be superior for children with high adiposity as measured by DXA (Taylor et al., 2003). For children in Verona, the corresponding percentiles are appreciably higher than the IOTF cutoffs, especially for girls. This is due to the unusual pattern of variability (the reason for which has not been elucidated), with the BMI coefficient of variation falling sharply after puberty, a pattern seen only in Singapore among the six studies making up the IOTF cutoffs (Cole, 2003). However, this is the basis of criticism for the present cutoffs (Fu et al., 2003; Misra, 2003), but at the same time, the reason for their defense (Stevens, 2003). Differences in the evaluation of BMI in adolescents may result when using different reference standard curves (Turconi et al., 2003).

The international cutoffs are significantly related to health risks in youth: in the Quebec Family Study the overweight participants had between 1.6 and 9.1 times the risk of elevated cardiovascular disease risk factors (blood pressure, fasting total cholesterol — TC, LDL-C, HDL-C, C/HDL-C, triglycerides, glucose, and physical work capacity) compared to normal-weight participants. Further, boys and girls with four or more risk factors were 19 and 43 times, respectively, more likely to be overweight compared to participants with no risk factors (Katzmarzyk et al., 2003).

However, as mentioned earlier these points were based only on six national studies, and on the assumption that in the population of 18-year-olds 10% of individuals have BMI values above 25, and 3% of subjects have values above 30kg.m^2. The suggested standards thus raise the level of the 90th and 97th percentile, as compared with BMI reference data of 1991, which are used in the Czech Republic. Therefore, the ratio of obese children in the Czech Republic and in many others would be small (Vígnerová, Lhotská, and Bláha, 2001). When testing BMI in various populations, including Singaporean children, it was revealed that cutoff values recommended by the IOTF had low sensitivity and may underestimate the local prevalence of childhood obesity. For screening purposes, population-specific measures

TABLE 4.1

BMI International Cutoffs for Overweight and Obesity

Age (years)	Body Mass Index 25 kg m^{-2}		Body Mass Index 30 kg m^{-2}	
	Males	Females	Males	Females
2	18.41	18.02	20.09	19.81
2.5	18.13	17.76	19.80	19.55
3.5	17.69	17.40	19.39	19.23
4	17.55	17.28	19.29	19.15
4.5	17.47	17.19	19.26	19.12
5	17.42	17.15	19.30	19.17
5.5	17.45	17.20	19.47	19.34
6	17.55	17.34	19.78	19.65
6.5	17.71	17.53	20.23	20.08
7	17.92	17.75	20.63	20.51
7.5	18.16	18.03	21.09	21.01
8	18.44	18.35	21.60	21.57
8.5	18.76	18.69	22.17	22.18
9	19.10	19.00	22.77	22.81
9.5	19.46	19.45	23.39	23.46
10	19.84	19.86	24.00	24.11
10.5	20.20	20.29	24.57	24.77
11	20.55	20.74	25.10	25.42
11.5	20.89	21.20	25.58	26.05
12	21.22	21.68	26.02	26.67
12.5	21.56	22.14	26.43	27.24
13	21.91	22.58	26.84	27.76
13.5	22.27	22.98	27.25	28.20
14	22.62	23.34	27.63	28.57
14.5	22.96	23.66	27.98	28.87
15	23.29	23.94	28.30	29.11
15.5	23.60	24.17	28.60	29.29
16	23.90	24.37	28.88	29.43
16.5	24.19	24.54	29.14	29.56
17	24.46	24.70	29.41	29.69
17.5	24.73	24.85	29.70	29.84
18	25	25	30	30

Source: Adapted from Cole et al. (2000)

rather than international cutoff values should be used (Fu et al., 2003; Misra, 2003).

Japanese pre- and postmenarcheal girls presented with lower weight and height than Caucasian girls, and also with less fat and FFM during the premenarcheal period in a study by Sampei et al. (2003). After menarche, more fat was found in Japanese girls, a finding that adds further support for separate growth curves for different ethnic groups.

In Germany it was recommended that data on height and weight be used to assess German children 0 to 18 years from 17 regions, and derive percentiles for under- and overweight. In the German guidelines, the calculated 90th and 97th BMI percentiles are suggested as cutoff points for the definition of overweight and obesity in local children (Kromeyer-Hauschild et al., 2001).

4.3   Body Composition and Depot Fat

An essential characteristic of obesity is an excess of fat relative to body mass. Therefore, the most important criterion of obesity is a measurement of the amount of adipose tissue represented in either absolute (kg) or relative (%) values. A number of methods exist for the evaluation of body composition. For clinical research purposes for example, a five-compartment model may be preferred (Heymsfield et al., 1993) as this allows a more detailed tracking of changes in body composition.

Body composition studies vary greatly with respect to approaches and methodologies, and numerous reviews describing these characteristics have been published in recent decades. The development of new methodologies has enabled more sophisticated body composition measurements in healthy and pathological subjects (Ellis and Eastman, 1993; Forbes, 1987; Heymsfield et al., 1991; Lohman, 1982; Jebb and Elia, 1993), including infants and young children. Increases in adiposity, regardless of the initial status of body fatness, intensify cardiovascular risk, and this unfavourable trend focuses attention on the need to prevent excess adiposity in childhood (Srinivasan, Mayers, and Berenson, 2001). Prevention could commence with a timely diagnosis and measurement of stored fat.

The evaluation of the total amount of fat and other components in a two-compartment model may be sufficient for the evaluation of simple obesity without the complication of other co-morbidities. Lean body mass (LBM) — which includes lipid particles in cells, etc. and is the stored adipose tissue-free body mass — or FFM is often used as a reference standard for the evaluation of the level of various variables. Measurements in obese children have showed that along with an increased weight, BMI and stored fat there is often a significantly larger LBM when compared to normal-weight children (Pařízková, 1977, 1993a). There has also been considerable discussion regarding the usefulness of more definitive body composition data as a range of benefits may be derived from this information. For example, it has been suggested that medication doses should be related to body composition status such as lean, FFM.

Lean, FFM, along with total body weight, is also used as a reference characteristic to which various functional parameters are related (Gutin et al., 1993, 1998, 1999a). This applies mainly to aerobic power, to other functional characteristics, and also to the food intake and individual macronutrients. Methodological improvements have made it possible to complete a number of studies that were not possible previously, especially in diseased subjects (Ellis and Eastman, 1993; Jebb and Elia, 1993).

However, with respect to children and adolescents during various periods of growth, the selection of exact methods is more limited, and/or results in less reliable findings. Generally, direct validation of available procedures by

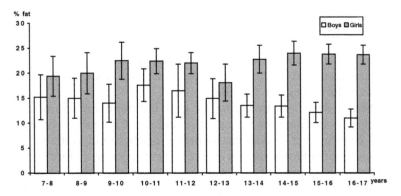

FIGURE 4.4
Body composition changes in normal boys and girls aged 7 to 17 years (hydrodensitometry with simultaneous measurements of the air in the lungs and respiratory passage). Age and gender differences are statistically significant except for ages 10 to 12. (Based on data from Pařízková, 1961a,b; 1977.)

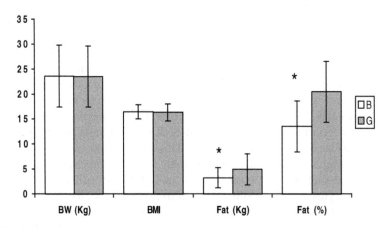

FIGURE 4.5
Body composition characteristics in boys and girls aged 6.4 ± 1.7 years. (Based on data from Taylor et al., 1997.) * indicates ($p < 0.05$).

anatomical or biochemical methods is still lacking. Some "reference methods" such as densitometry are either difficult to use in young children or have a small health risk.

Changes in body composition follow a certain pattern during growth from childhood to adulthood (Figure 4.4) (Pařízková, 1977). Similar gender differences are apparent as early as 6 years of age (Figure 4.5) (Taylor et al., 1997). These changes have been demonstrated in a range of studies such as the Fels Longitudinal Study of children aged 8 to 20 years. This study revealed that there are gender-associated differences in the patterns of change of the percentage of body fat and lean FFM, but not for total body fat. The percentage of fat and FFM were higher with increased rates of maturation (Guo et al., 1997), and these findings may also apply to the early tracking of obesity development during growth. Similar trends in total adiposity have also been reported in later studies, including age trends in males and females (Dai et al., 2002). Body composition development varied significantly according to age and gender.

A particular drawback involving the growing population is that it is not always easy to evaluate the degree of sexual development, very important for body composition evaluation, including of obese individuals. Methods for self-assessment have been developed; however, these methods are somewhat inaccurate. Using self-assessment in overweight girls overestimations were found for Tanner's breast stage, but pubic hair development evaluation was sound. In both overweight and normal weight boys, however, pubic hair was overestimated, which is indicative of the lack of reliability of the method (Bonat et al., 2002). Evaluation of sexual development is often poorly accepted even when executed by a medical doctor or researcher of the same gender.

Figure 4.6 shows differences in height, weight, BMI, and percentage of fat (measured by hydrodensitometry) in normal and obese children aged 11, 12, and 16 years (Pařízková, 1977).

Regarding the cellularity of adipose tissue, there is a poor proliferation in nonobese children until 10 to 12 years. In contrast, in the obese there is a constant proliferation from one year of age. As a result, the number of fat cells at the end of growth is significantly higher in obese subjects (Burniat, 1997). Both early, high-fat adipocyte content and hyperplasia in these children could account for the early AR in BMI in the obese before the age of 5.5 years (Rolland-Cachera et al., 1984). This is significantly associated with increased weight at the end of the growth period. Wabitsch et al. (1997b) demonstrated that in *in-vitro* fat cell cultures, IGF-1 stimulated fat filling of the preadipocytes and the proliferation of mature adipocytes. An excessively voluminous "fat storehouse" could be formed early in life and then later be filled by an inadequate food intake as related to energy needs. However, a positive excessive fat balance, more than a chronic positive energy balance, has been considered recently as a major factor contributing to the increase of the fat deposits (Swinburn and Ravussin, 1993).

4.3.1 Methods

There are numerous advanced methods for the measurement of body composition recommended for children (Lobstein, Baur, and Uauy, 2004; Goran, 1998). The results of the measurements using different methods correlate significantly but commonly do not give identical results. Methods include dual energy x-ray absorptiometry (DXA), bioelectrical impedance analysis (BIA), deuterium (D_2O), total body conductivity (TOBEC), densitometry, and magnetic resonance imaging (MRI). However, equipment is generally expensive

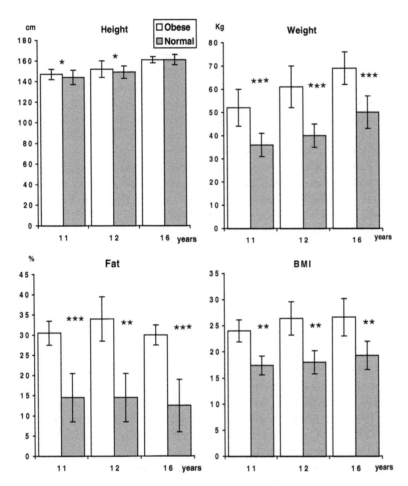

FIGURE 4.6
Differences in height, weight, fat percentage (assessed by hydrodensitometry), and body mass index (BMI) in obese and normal boys. * (p < 0.05); ** (p < 0.01); *** (p < 0.001). (Based on data from Pařízková, 1977.)

and therefore is limited to a number of laboratories, or hospitals and other institutions. If such equipment is used more for diagnostic and clinical purposes, it may be less accessible for physiological measurements.

For measurements of large experimental groups, or for checking the effects of different weight management approaches, more accessible and cheaper methods include bioelectrical impedance analysis (BIA), deuterium (D_2O), and anthropometric methods. The application of these techniques has been described in a number of studies following normal and obese children.

Other body composition methods include volumetric techniques. In addition to water and air displacement, the anthropometric estimation of body volume can also be used (Elia and Ward, 1999). Further, the use of inert gas absorption or dilution methods to assess the content of body water using various items (antioyrine, urea, various isotopes, D_2O or tritiated water, T_2O), are also available. Lean body mass can be estimated using creatinine excretion, 3-methyl-histidine, or ^{40}K measurement.

Many methods are too demanding to expect the cooperation of young subjects, or may be considered too risky for small children even though only slight doses of radiation are provided — for example, with the DXA method. However, technological advances are such that risk reduction has been maximized in many areas, and an increasing number of these methods are now available for use with children and adolescents.

In the past, densitometry measures using hydrostatic weighing with the simultaneous measurement of air in the lungs and respiratory passages were traditional. The method has a very long tradition (Behnke, Feen, and Welham, 1942; Brozek et al., 1963; Lohman, 1982; Pařízková, 1961a, 1963a, 1977) and for many years was recognized as the gold standard criterion measure. The technique is still widely used in laboratories throughout the world; however, it is often very difficult for younger children to cope with being underwater so the procedure has been more commonly used with school-aged children and older participants (Pařízková, 1963a, 1977). At present, DXA is more often commonly used as a reference standard method as is the case for MRI and computerized tomographic scanning (CT).

4.3.1.1 *Anthropometric Methods*

Anthropometric measurements have been considered too simplistic by some researchers. Nevertheless, anthropometry still represents the best opportunity for the evaluation of the nutritional status and degree of obesity in children. This is especially the case when evaluations are conducted under field conditions, or in more modest clinical settings. The common measurements, circumferences, breadths, lengths, skinfolds, and ratios between individual measures have shown high correlations and sound predictive ability when compared with "reference methods" such as densitometry and DXA. In addition to its relative ease of use, another advantage of anthropometry is the price of the equipment and its portability for use in field settings. However, despite the apparent simplicity of anthropometric techniques, researchers must be well trained (Hills and Byrne, 1998c). Finally, anthropometric measurements are generally not too demanding for participants and therefore have a high acceptance level.

Commonly, skinfold thickness measurements are used as a more direct index of body fat. While the technique is arguably simple to perform, considerable attention to detail is imperative to avoid inter- and intraobserver errors (Durnin and Rahaman, 1967; Pařízková, 1963a, 1977; Hills and Byrne, 1998c). Subcutaneous fat measured by skinfolds correlates significantly with the amount of total body fat assessed by other methods. Thus, the total amount of fat can be calculated from various sets of skinfold measurements (for example at 2, 4, 5, or 10 sites) (Pařízková, 1961a; 1963a,b; 1977).

The most common skinfolds are the triceps and subscapular, followed by suprailiac, calf, and biceps sites. The measurement of a larger number of sites can give more reliable results as the measurements are more representative of a wider cross section of the body surface over which the subcutaneous fat layer can vary substantially (Pařízková, 1961b, 1977). The maximum number of skinfolds measured as reported in the literature is 93 (Keys and Brožek, 1953).

The evaluation of body composition from various anthropometric parameters, including skinfolds, have used the *regression equations* derived in 1933 by Matiegka (1929) (Pařízková, 1977; Bláha, Lisá, and Krásnicanová, 1997). The results of the estimated values of body composition using these equations correlate well in adults with the results from densitometric measurements (r = 0.75 – 0.97) (Pařízková, 1977). Age, gender, and other factors have a significant effect on the character of these relationships; therefore, regression equations and any nomograms developed vary in different age groups of males and females. This also applies for growing individuals with marked differences between prepubertal and pubertal subjects and different regressions available for boys and girls before and after 12 to 13 years of age.

However, the relationships can vary during shorter time periods of growth and development. This has been shown by the comparison of regression lines between both the sum of ten skinfolds, and/or abdominal skinfold, and the total amount of fat measured by densitometry in a longitudinal study of boys from 11 to 15 years of age (Pařízková, 1968a, 1970).

Regression equations are only available for growing individuals and then for adults of both genders, but not for individual categories year by year. For more specific evaluations, additional factors such as the degree of sexual maturation, nutritional status, and adaptation to various workloads and exercise can influence the character of the relationships between total and subcutaneous fat. In this respect it may be preferable to characterize fatness on the basis of individual skinfolds and/or the sum of various skinfold measurements. A number of regression equations exist that enable the evaluation of the percentage of body fat from skinfolds in children; however, this should be a secondary consideration (Brook, 1975; Pařízková, 1961b, 1977).

Skinfold measurements are also often used to evaluate the development of adiposity, and the triceps and subscapular sites are the most commonly used. For example, the triceps skinfold was used for the evaluation of fatness in Indian children aged 11 to 18 years. In this population, the trends for these ages, gender differences, and the relationship to socioeconomic status were similar to the results in studies of other child populations. The triceps skinfold also correlated significantly with weight and BMI (Kapoor et al., 1991). A study comparing BMI, triceps skinfold, and arm circumference measurements showed that triceps skinfold gave the best results for obesity screening in adolescents aged 10 to 15 years (Sardinha et al., 1999).

Under field conditions it is generally preferable to measure the smallest number of representative sites, particularly those that are readily accessible.

Recently, the submandibular skinfold measurement was recommended for children aged 3.0 to 15.1 years given the high correlation of this measure with other indices, especially BMI and circumferences (Fleta Zaragozano et al., 1997). The submandibular skinfold was previously included in the above-mentioned sum of ten skinfolds (Pařízková, 1961b, 1977).

Somatotyping has been also used for the estimation of body composition. Somatotype of an individual is expressed by a three-digit evaluation comprising three consecutive numbers (rated from lowest to highest, 1–7) and always listed in the same order. Each number represents the evaluation of a basic component, *endomorphy* (relating to relative adiposity), *mesomorphy* (relating to skeletal muscle development), and *ectomorphy* (relating to the relative linearity of the body) (Carter and Phillips, 1969; Pařízková and Carter, 1976).

4.3.1.2   Methods for the Measurement of the Individual Body Components

Body composition can also be evaluated from the broader perspective of gross components such as fat and FFM, LBM, or the subcomponents of fat-free tissue such as water, mineral, and protein. Other methods can evaluate the mass of the individual tissues, organs, or body segments. The choice of specific method(s) for a particular study depends on the research question, the accuracy and precision required, the availability of the apparatus, subject acceptability, convenience, cost, the need for trained personnel, and health issues such as radiation exposure (Hills and Byrne, 1998c).

As mentioned earlier, reference methods such as densitometry, isotope dilution methods (D_2O), DXA, CT, MRI, and *in vivo* neutron activation analysis (IVNAA) are in use. In the category of bedside or field methods, anthropometry — including skinfold thickness, impedance/resistance (BIA), near-infrared interactance (NIRI), and 24-hour creatinine excretion — can be used (Jebb and Elia, 1993). Various methods have been described and analyzed in extensive reviews by a number of authors (Forbes, 1987; Keys and Brozek, 1953; Lohman, 1993; Shephard, 1991; Lohman, Roche, and Martorell, 1988; Roche, 1992; Roche, Heymsfield, and Lohman, 1996).

The suitability of these techniques for the evaluation of body composition in children varies a great deal; therefore, only some have been used for measurement during growth. In most recent studies the trend has been to use a range of methods for the evaluation of body composition simultaneously. Some of these methods are briefly described in the remainder of this chapter, with examples provided of the results of the measurements in growing individuals.

4.3.1.3   Densitometry

Body density is assessed by hydrostatic weighing and is based on the Archimedean principle, ideally with the simultaneous estimation of the volume of the air in the lungs and respiratory passages (Brozek, 1963; Keys and

Brožek, 1953; Pařízková, 1961a,b, 1977). For the assessment of air in the respiratory passages, the nitrogen dilution method (Pařízková, 1977) or helium dilution method can be used. Body density is then calculated using the formula of Brozek et al. (1963):

Body Density = Weight in air × 0.996/Weight – weight under the water
   – volume of the air LRP × 0.996
   (LRP = respiratory passages and the lungs; 0.996 = density of the
      water during weighing, that is 37°C)

Percent of body fat is calculated using the formula (Keys and Brozek, 1953):

Percent fat (% fat) = (4.201/density – 3.813) × 100

Brozek et al. (1963) later used another constant in the formula — that is, = (4.950/density – 4.50) 100. There are also a number of other equations in use (Shephard, 1991). Lean body mass can also be calculated: LBM = 100 – % fat, kg fat = % fat × body weight/100 (Pařízková, 1977). During repeated measurements the results varied by 0.5% and during the day the variations in body density were minimal.

Some researchers measure the volume of the air separately in the normal atmosphere under similar conditions after a maximal expiration; however, this may cause some imprecision. Also, a certain proportion of the vital capacity (24% of VC) can be subtracted from the value of the volume ascertained by underwater weighing (volume of the body = weight in the air – weight under the water).

This method requires a great deal of cooperation of the subject and a lack of fear when submerging the whole head during the underwater weighing. The method has been used for schoolchildren and adolescents, but it has not always been easy for obese youth as the measurements may require a longer preparation and training time (Pařízková, 1977). Therefore, air displacement plethysmography or body line scanners employing the principles of three-dimensional photography have been suggested because they also have the potential to measure body surface and body volume (total, segments) (Elia and Ward, 1999), which can also be used for the derivation of body density.

4.3.1.4 Dual-Energy X-Ray Absorptiometry (DXA)

Dual-energy x-ray absorptiometry (DXA, or DEXA) is a relatively new scanning technique that measures the differential attenuation of two x-rays as they pass through the body. It differentiates bone mineral from soft tissue and subsequently divides the latter into fat and lean FFM. The method provides information on total body composition, and also on the composition of individual body segments, which is an advantage over densitometry, [40]K measurements, or water dilution. The method has excellent reproducibility as shown in adults; however, the machine is very expensive.

Comparison of boys and girls aged 3 to 8 years of age with the same age, height, weight, BMI, or bone mineral content showed that boys had a lower percentage of fat, lower fat mass (kg), and higher bone-free lean tissue mass than girls. These measurements revealed that girls had approximately 50% more fat than boys (Taylor et al., 1997). The measurement also confirmed that gender differences in body composition are present significantly earlier than the onset of puberty.

The accuracy of body composition measurements (DXA) has been assessed experimentally by comparing the method with total carcass chemical analysis in 16 pigs with a weight range of 5 to 35kg. All estimates of body composition were highly correlated with the results of direct chemical analysis. For the absolute mass of body fat, one DXA analysis underestimated the reference chemical method by 9.5%, whereas an alternate software package resulted in overestimates, averaging 15.5%. Conversely, the average fat-free compartment was initially overestimated by 968 g then underestimated by 892 g. The impact of these differences in the body composition measurements using DXA were also examined in a group of 18 young boys aged 4 to 12 years (Ellis et al.. 1994). When using this method, results need to be interpreted with caution.

Another study using DXA followed both genders from 4 to 26 years and showed that LBM and bone mineral content (BMC) increased with age in females until 13.4 and 15.7 years, respectively, and in males until 16.6 and 17.4 years. Significant correlations between LBM and BMC were found for both genders ($r = 0.98$, $p < 0.0001$ for females, and $r = 0.98$, $p < 0.0001$ for males). The body fat percentage according to DXA measurements (%BF DXA) increased with age in females ($r = 0.52$, $p < 0.001$), but not in males, and was higher in females than in males at all ages.

Using DXA, the trunk-to-leg fat ratio (TLFR) has been calculated as trunk fat/leg fat. After puberty, the TLFR was higher in males than in females, which was not the case during younger ages when no gender differences in TLFR were found. The trunk-to-leg fat ratio, as measured by DXA in Brazilian children, was almost twice that in obese than in normal children (Fisberg et al., 1998). The DXA method underestimated body weight measured by scales by a mean of 0.83 kg. The %BF DXA correlated with %BF derived from skinfold thickness measurements. The results corresponded well in males but overestimated the %BF by skinfold thickness in females. Therefore, the measurements of body composition using DXA confirmed the findings on age changes and gender differences gained by densitometry (Pařízková, 1977) and other methods.

4.3.1.5 Bioelectrical Impedance Analysis (BIA)

Tetrapolar BIA is now widely used in clinical practice but also in experimental growth studies in both normal and obese children (Jurimae et al., 2003). The tetrapolar BIA method applies a small ($800\mu A$) alternating (50 kHz) current that is mainly conducted by the body water and its dissolved electrolytes. The resistance of the current is theoretically inversely proportional to the amount of conductive material —that is, to total body water (TBW) and its dissolved electrolytes. The specific resistivities of intracellular (ICW) and extracellular water (ECW) vary according to differences in the type and amount of dissolved electrolytes in the intra- and extracellular spaces. Therefore, the relationship between body impedance and total body water will be theoretically different between subjects who differ in the proportion of extra- and intracellular water (Deurenberg, 1993).

The BIA method has been validated against reference methods such as densitometry, deuterium oxide dilution (D_2O), and ^{40}K (Lukaski et al., 1985, 1986; Segal et al., 1988) in adults and later for children and adolescents. Total body water was measured using the stable isotope $^2H_2$ ^{18}O and body resistance measured using a tetrapolar technique with a constant 50 kHz, $800\mu A$ alternating current. Total body water was highly correlated with height^2/body resistance ($r = 0.97$, $p < 0.001$). This method may be suitable as it is noninvasive, rapid, and acceptable for children (Davies et al., 1988). However, further cross-validation studies are needed, especially with regard to markedly different body composition in obese children and adolescents.

When bioelectrical resistance was used for the assessment of body composition in children and adolescents, there were doubts about which age-specific equation should be used during growth. The relationship between height^2/resistance and total body water (TBW) is fairly reliable across a wide age range, but with preschool children some validation is necessary. TBW was assessed from $^2H_2$ ^{18}O (DLW) dilution in groups of children aged 4 to 6 years and bioelectrical resistance and reactance were measured in two independent laboratories. No significant differences in the results of TBW measurements were found. Kushner's equation for TBW can be transformed into an equation for FFM using published gender- and age-specific constants for the FFM hydration. The intraclass reliability for estimates of fat mass and FFM using bioelectrical resistance in another independent group of children was > 0.99 for duplicate observations performed two weeks apart (Goran et al., 1993).

The results of measurements using tetrapolar whole-body BIA were compared with the measurements of total body potassium (TBK) using ^{40}K spectrometry and skinfold thickness measurements in subjects aged 3.9 to 19.3 years. A best-fitting equation to predict TBK-derived FFM from BIA and other potential independent predictors was developed and cross-validated in two randomly selected subgroups of growing subjects using stepwise multiple regression analysis.

The technical error associated with BIA measurements was much smaller than that of skinfold measurements; however, the reproducibility of BIA-derived FFM estimates was only slightly better than that of FFM estimates obtained using weight and two skinfold measurements. Best-fitting regression equations for FFM using BIA measurements have been derived (Schaefer et al., 1994). In this study, conventional anthropometry, using published equations for the evaluation of FFM from skinfolds, slightly overestimated TBK-derived

FFM but predicted FFM with a precision similar to the best-fitting equations involving bioelectrical impedance analysis.

Bioelectrical impedance analysis has also been used to study the effect of dietary supplementation in malnourished children. A positive effect was found with a high-protein diet contributing to the acceleration of growth and restoration of body composition (Kabir et al., 1994). Bioelectrical impedance analysis has also been used for the evaluation of body composition in obese children to assess the effect of reduction treatment (Yiannakou et al., 1998).

Marked inconsistencies in body composition evaluation, however, were observed in some studies when using BIA along with other methods (anthropometric measures, four skinfolds) in a field study of children of different ages, gender, and adiposity. Using four different algorithms for the estimation of fat ratio from BIA data, a high intraindividual variance was observed, that is, from 13.8% to 33.4%. The same applied to the prevalence of overweight. When comparing BIA and anthropometric estimation, BIA systematically overestimated fat mass. Considerable inconsistencies were observed especially at low BMI for girls and for small children (Mast et al., 2002). Using the BIA prediction equation derived from the study of Tyrell et al. (2001), correlations between DXA measurements and BIA in the estimation of FFM, fat mass (FM), and percentage of fat mass (PFM) were noted. BIA-FFM underestimated DXA-FFM by a mean of 0.75 kg, BIA-FM overestimated DXA-FM by a mean of 1.02 kg, and BIA-PBF overestimated DXA-PBF by a mean of 2.53%. Further analysis showed, however, that BIA correlated better than anthropometric methods in the estimation of FFM, FM, and PBF, and it was therefore concluded that foot-to-foot BIA is a reliable technique in the measurement of body composition (Tyrell et al., 2001).

The study of Eisenkolbl, Kartasurya, and Widhalm (2001) showed that results of BIA measurements significantly underestimated data ascertained by DXA. However, Sung et al. (2001) in a Hong Kong study of 7- to 16-year-old children concluded that BIA is a valid alternative method to DXA for the measurement of body fat. BIA measurements enabled the evaluation of fat mass index (FM/stature^2 – FMI). The comparison of BMI and FMI showed somewhat higher sensitivity for obesity evaluation of the latter as shown in Japanese children 3 to 5 years old. This conclusion should, however, be further validated in other age groups (Eto et al., 2004).

4.3.1.6 ^{40}K Measurement

^{40}K measurements using whole body counters evaluate body potassium as related to its natural gamma-activity in the human organism. This method was also used for the estimation of body composition in a group of adolescents using hydrostatic weighing and BIA. Estimates of body fat percentage by total body potassium were significantly greater than by either BIA or hydrostatic weighing. When current estimates for the FFM density in children were employed to derive the ^{40}K/FFM, the value for boys was 58.9mEq and for girls 54.2mEq. These data indicate that FFM can be underestimated in growing individuals when using adult-derived values for $^{40}K/FFM$ (Cordain et al., 1989).

4.3.1.7 Total Body Water by Deuterium or Tritium Oxide

Total body water may be measured by isotope dilution by administering a tracer that dilutes equally throughout body water and that can then be measured. Stable, nonradioactive isotopes of water containing deuterium or ^{18}O are used. Deuterium is more often used because it is cheaper; mass spectrometry is then used for analysis. Gas chromatography or infrared absorption can also be used for analysis but requires a greater amount of deuterium. Tritium can also be used as the analysis is cheap and rapid, but it is radioactive and so is not suitable for many individuals, especially younger subjects.

At present, deuterium oxide ($^{2}H_2 O$) is used for measurements of body water and thus also of body composition. Most often it is used as DLW ($^{2}H_2$ ^{18}O), which enables the simultaneous assessment of total energy expenditure (Prentice, 1999).

4.3.1.8 Total Body Electrical Conductivity (TOBEC)

Measurements of body composition by TOBEC are used mainly for the evaluation of hospitalized infants and children for whom permanent monitoring of the nutritional status is indispensable. This approach is considered more suitable for infants and young children because methods using density assume a constant relationship between water and the fat-free component of the body and "adult" composition of lean FFM. The anthropometric assessment of body composition using skinfolds has not been satisfactory in very young children. Methods such as total body potassium, neutron activation, hydrodensitometry, and body volume measurements also require a relatively long confinement within special devices. This is difficult for younger children and completely unrealistic for those who are sick or any children who are shy and afraid of laboratory and clinical procedures.

The TOBEC methodology is one of the most promising body composition techniques, especially for those in the youngest age categories. The technique is safe, quick, totally noninvasive, and more accurate than the majority of other methods (Fiorotto, Cochran, and Klish, 1987). The method is based on the principle that a living organism placed in an electromagnetic field perturbs that field. This perturbation is caused by the electrolyte mass within the organism. Since electrolytes are included in fat-free body mass exclusively, it is possible to accurately separate this tissue from body fat, which is enabled by adequate calibration. The measurement requires one second and is usually repeated three times to achieve a desirable level of accuracy. The pediatric instruments usually give more exact results because they can be calibrated using animal carcasses such as miniature pigs or mature rabbits.

Smaller TOBEC instruments have also been developed and used for infants (Fiorotto, Cochran, and Klish, 1987).

All TOBEC instruments are constructed around a large electromagnetic coil to which sensors are attached. As electromagnetic energy dissipates when a subject enters the coil, more current must be fed into the coil to maintain constant electromagnetic field strength. The amount of current needed for this measurement is directly proportional to the perturbation of the electromagnetic field — that is, to the electrolyte mass of the measured subject. Thus the "TOBEC number" is derived.

For older children and adults, larger TOBEC devices have been developed with motorized carriages in contrast to those for infants. The subject is passed through the instrument at a constant rate and a total of 64 readings are obtained in a sequential fashion. These readings result in a computer-generated curve that is then deconvoluted by Fourier transform. The Fourier-derived constants are used in the calibration equation to assess fat-free body mass (Klish, 1993).

The body composition of obese children and children with Prader-Willi syndrome who also have a high fat content, aged 11.5 ± 3.6 years and 10.1 ± 3.5 years, was assessed. Using TOBEC, the percentage of fat was higher, but the development of lean body mass was significantly lower in children with Prader-Willi syndrome as expressed by an index relating FFM to body height. This latter index improved in some of the patients when treated with growth hormone (Klish, 1993).

4.3.1.9   Magnetic Resonance Imaging (MRI)

The principle of magnetic resonance imaging (MRI) is that certain nuclei with intrinsic magnetic properties range during the transmission of the radio frequency waves in a certain direction of the magnetic field. After the interruption of the transmission of this wave, the nuclei return to their original position and transmit the absorbed energy, which is possible to measure. There is no irradiation in this method and it does not require a high level of cooperation of subjects; however, the measurement setup procedure can take some time. MRI is primarily used for the measurement of visceral fat, although is also used to measure other structures, including thigh and liver (Sohlström, Wahlund, and Forsum, 1993).

In children, this method has been used to assess the thigh muscle and fat tissue in subjects who were treated with growth hormone (GH), children with Turner's syndrome, and those with intrauterine growth retardation (IUGR). Children administered GH were examined before and then at regular intervals during GH treatment. An increase in muscle tissue was identified by MRI as well as a reduction of adipose tissue in the thighs, with a dramatic change in the muscle/adipose tissue cross-sectional area ratio in each period of the treatment. There was a correlation between BMI and muscle and adipose tissue cross-sectional area at each time point ($p < 0.0001$). The muscle cross-sectional area increment also correlated with height velocity

(Leger et al., 1994). MRI could also be used in studies of children treated for various purposes, including obesity, but limited observations have been reported.

4.3.1.10   Computed Tomography (CT)

Whole body scans provide information on the size of individual tissues. However, the organism is subjected to some irradiation, and therefore this method is not recommended for younger children. The measurements are also time consuming and costly. Intraabdominal fat has, however, been measured using CT in some studies (Goran et al., 1993).

4.3.1.11   Ultrasound

High-frequency sound waves pass freely through homogeneous tissues, and part of the emitted energy is reflected at any interface between different tissues — for example, fascia separating muscle and adipose tissue. This reflection is then converted into an electric signal. Correlations with carcass fat measurements are statistically significant, but are not sufficiently high. In adults, the results of this method correlate significantly with measurements of the distance between the tip of the abdomen and L4-5 using a pelvimeter (Kunesová et al., 1995).

4.3.1.12   Whole-Body Air-Displacement Plethysmography (ADP)

The whole-body air-displacement plethysmography (ADP) method has been compared across a wide range of body sizes and showed good precision for body volume and body density measurements in adults and adolescents, provided that aberrant values are rejected. When available, obesity may be defined using this method (Wells and Fuller, 2001), and pair measurements can make the measurements more precise.

4.3.1.13   Comparison of Several Methods: Measuring Children with BIA, TOBEC, and DXA

Ellis (1996) used several methods simultaneously to evaluate body composition in children and young adults. Estimates of the relative and absolute amounts of body fat were highly correlated among several methods: BIA, total body conductivity, and DXA ($r = 0.72 - 0.97$, $p < 0.001$). However, using a Bland and Altman comparison among the estimates revealed significant differences among the methods. The mean differences between methods for body fat ranged from 0.30 ± 6.7 kg to 4.2 ± 2.7 kg while the difference for the percentage of fat ranged from $0.8\% \pm 3.5\%$ to $9.9\% \pm 5.2\%$. Therefore, the classification of fatness into simple categories such as normal, overweight, and obese with regard to the percentage of fat was significantly method-dependent. This important study led to the conclusion that the lack of interchangeability for fatness classification makes it difficult to ensure that similar groups of subjects, homogeneous with regard to fatness, can be accurately selected when different methods are used. This limitation can also restrict the possibility of comparison with the results of various studies, both cross-sectional and longitudinal, that also relates to follow-ups of treatment of obese subjects (Ellis, 1996).

4.3.1.14   Creatinine Excretion

Creatine is the final product of nitrogen metabolism and as such can provide information on the amount of muscle tissue in the body. To obtain sufficiently precise results, it is necessary to collect urine over several days (at least three) and adhere to a certain diet. This is difficult when subjects are not measured in a metabolic unit or hospital (Waterlow, 1994). This method has been used in the past with children.

4.4   Fat Distribution

Another important morphological characteristic of obesity is subcutaneous fat distribution, or fat patterning. Gender differences in the amount and distribution of fat appear at birth. The measurement of ten skinfold thicknesses during the first 48 hours after delivery revealed significant gender differences, especially in the suprailiac skinfold. Generally, there was a trend for higher deposition of fat in all ten skinfolds measured in girls in whom the suprailiac skinfold was significantly greater immediately after birth (Pařízková, 1961, 1963a,b). This gender difference increased during further periods of growth and was largest during puberty.

Fat patterning is evaluated via ratios — for example, between subscapular and triceps skinfold (centrality index), or the sum of skinfolds on the trunk and on the extremities. In later periods of adulthood, when the amount of subcutaneous fat increases even when BMI remains the same, there is less of a gender difference in fat due to an increasing amount in males (Pařízková, 1977). Similar differences have also been found in the total amount of fat as measured by densitometry. Anthropometric indicators enable the evaluation of the fat patterning — for example, *conicity index* (CI), which is associated with a high body weight and centripetal fat distribution (Perez and Landaeta-Jimenez, 2001).

As an individual gets older, an increasing amount of fat is deposited in body cavities, especially in the abdomen. An increased amount of visceral fat is considered the most important health risk with regard to cardiovascular diseases, diabetes, and other metabolic problems. Various methods are used to measure internal fat, most commonly CT scanning. The importance of central adiposity was revealed several decades ago when it was shown that individuals who have a larger deposition of fat on the trunk as compared

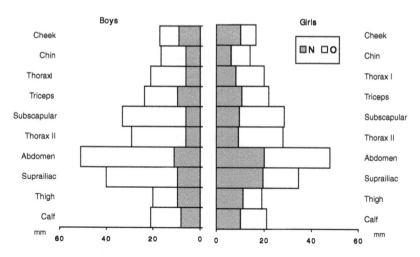

FIGURE 4.7

Comparison of skinfold thickness (mm) distributions in obese (O) and normal-weight (N) boys and girls (12 to 14 years old); centrality index (subscapular/triceps ratio) in obese boys (1.2), in obese girls (1.4); in normal-weight boys (0.8), in normal-weight girls (0.7). (Based on data from Pařízková, 1977, Pařízková, 1972, and Pařízková, 1993.)

to the extremities have a higher risk of pathological features (Daniels et al., 1999; Francis et al., 1999). These include increased blood pressure, diabetes, and dyslipoproteinemia (Vague, 1956; Skamenová and Pařízková, 1963).

More recently a similar situation was described in children. A central pattern of fat distribution in adolescents aged 11.0 to 13.8 years was associated with higher levels of postprandial lipemia after an oral fat load when compared to subjects with a peripheral pattern. These data indicate that the pattern of fat distribution of adipose tissue may be more important than total adipose tissue amount — for example, regarding lipid metabolism (Moreno et al., 2001a). Increased adiposity and the distribution of fat is also related to metabolic and hemostatic parameters (insulin, triglycerides, fibrinogen, plasminogen activator inhibitor: PAI-1, and tissue-type plasminogen activator-antigen [tPA-Ag]). Fibrinogen was mainly associated with upperbody subcutaneous fatness (as measured by an optical device, the Lipometer), which was the main correlate of metabolic and hemostatic parameters. It remains to be investigated whether this type of subcutaneous fat distribution is involved in the expression of metabolic and hemostatic risk factors and if it participates in the dysregulation of the hemostatic system in obese children (Sudi et al., 2001c).

4.4.1 Skinfold Thickness Ratios (Indices)

Figure 4.7 outlines the distribution of subcutaneous fat in normal and obese children at the ages of 12 to 13 years. A comparison of the thickness of the individual skinfolds shows not only markedly higher values but that their mutual relationship is different. The distribution of fat is similarly increased both in obese boys and girls, and the usual gender difference in the amount of total fat and its patterning is lacking. Both obese boys and girls resemble older women as shown by the comparison of the results of measurements in various age groups using the same method (Pařízková, 1963a,b, 1977). Also the relationships between individual skinfolds (for example, using the centrality index: subscapular/triceps skinfold ratio) and relationships between the sums of skinfolds on the trunk and on the extremities were different as compared to normal-weight children (Pařízková, 1963c). In another study in severely obese children aged 10.15 ± 2.01 years the centrality index was positively correlated with TC, LDL-C, TG, and negatively correlated with HDL-C (Marelli et al., 1993).

4.4.2   Waist Circumference, and Waist/Hip and Waist/Height Ratios

Fat distribution has also been evaluated using ratios of various circumference measurements, most often of the waist. In a study using DXA in children 7 to 17 years old, it was demonstrated that waist circumference was the best simple measure of fat distribution, since it was least influenced by gender, race, and overall adiposity (Daniels, Khoury, and Morrison, 2000). Waist circumference (WC) itself was shown, however, to be quite sufficient for the evaluation of intraabdominal fat. In Italian girls, it was revealed that WC was a significant independent risk factor for insulin resistance and blood pressure independently of their age and Tanner stage for puberty (Maffeis et al., 2003).

Indices relating waist-to-hip (W/H; WHR) or waist-to-thigh (W/T; WTR) are also used, and more recently also waist-to-height (W/Ht; WHtR). Gender differences in normal children living in the central part of Spain, aged 4.0 to 14.5 years, were described; the values of the mentioned indices may serve as standard values of fat distribution for clinical practice (Moreno et al., 1997). The indices were validated along with the percentage of overweight; percentage stored fat was validated by significant correlations with triglycerides (TG), alanine aminotransferase (ALT), and insulin in boys, whereas only WHR/Ht showed a close relationship with TG and insulin in girls. Moreover, this index differentiated subjects with abnormal values of TG, insulin, and ALT, especially in girls (Asayama et al., 1998a). In another study of Japanese children, only WHR/Ht – SDS showed enough sensitivity and specificity to predict metabolic derangement in obese girls, and it was therefore recommended that there be a diagnostic criterion that classifies obesity in Japanese adolescent girls into two types according to normal and/or abnormal values of serum triglycerides, alanine aminotransferase, or insulin level (Asayama et al., 2000). Waist/hip ratio was negatively associated with HDL-C and positively associated with TC/HDL-C ratio in pre- and postpubertal girls independent of age and BMI (Guillaume, 1999).

Marelli et al. (1993) found a significant correlation between WHR and TG level. These results confirm that even during childhood, severe obesity is related to blood lipid alterations and at this early stage of life the truncal distribution of adipose tissue is associated with an adverse serum lipid spectrum. Waist/hip ratio/height standard deviation scores (SDS) can serve as an index predicting occurrence of biochemical complications — that is, abnormal values of TG, ALT, and insulin in obese children aged 6 to 15 years (Asayama et al., 1999).

To further validate the abovementioned indices of fat distribution, inter-relationships were examined between BMI, WHR, serum concentration of immunoreactive insulin (IRI), C-peptide, and sex hormone binding globulin (SHBG). In central and gluteal obesity, differentiated by WHR, IRI, C-peptide, and SHBG differed significantly. There was no correlation between WHR and IRI, C-peptide, or SHBG. These results suggest that using WHR for the differentiation of central and gluteal obesity does not help in adolescence, which may be due to morphological changes during puberty (Ilies, Mahunka, and Sari, 1994).

4.4.3   Subcutaneous and Intraabdominal Fat

In a two-decade longitudinal study, the relationships between adiposity on the trunk and on the extremities were followed in French males and females from the age of 1 month to 21 years. The relationship between adult and childhood skinfold ratio measurements was found to be weak in boys and slightly better in girls. From this study and also from previous follow-ups, adiposity measurements in children (which are both associated with metabolic and health problems) could be selected that have the best correlations with the adult values: BMI in both genders, trunk skinfolds in boys, and subscapular/arm skinfold thickness ratio in girls. Consequently, a boy with both a high BMI and trunk skinfold thickness values, or a girl with both high BMI and subscapular/arm ratio skinfold values, are at a greater risk of centralized obesity and accompanying comorbidities later in life (Rolland-Cachera, 1995; Rolland-Cachera et al., 1990b).

Body fat distribution was assessed and quantified using MRI in girls in late puberty. The amounts of subcutaneous and intraabdominal fat were derived from transverse slices at the levels of the waist, hip, and trochanter using magnetic resonance imaging. The results were compared with simple anthropometric measurements. Waist, hip, and trochanter circumferences were highly correlated to the respective related MRI total fat surface area both in early and late pubertal girls ($r = 0.79$ to 0.97), while waist circumference, and waist-hip, waist-thigh, or skinfold ratios were not significantly correlated with intraabdominal fat areas.

Further measurements showed that in late puberty, the MRI-derived amount of subcutaneous fat was significantly larger in the trochanter level compared to that in girls in the early stages of puberty. This was due to a greater deposition of fat in the gluteal area. It could be concluded that circumferences at the trunk are good measures for the related amounts of fat in pubertal girls; this is not true for various ratios of circumferences and/ or skinfold ratios (De Ridder et al., 1992).

The possibility of predicting visceral adiposity from the measurements of waist circumference was further supported by MRI assessments at a level of L4 in subjects with simple obesity aged 8.6 to 15.5 years. Best correlations were found for MRI and waist circumference. In addition, waist/arm, and waist/thigh ratios correlated with visceral fat measured by MRI (Brambilla et al., 1997).

Internal fat was measured in children and adolescents (Goran, Kaskoun, and Shuman, 1995) using CT imaging along with anthropometric methods for the evaluation of intraabdominal adipose tissue (IAAT) in children aged 6.4 ± 1.2 years, weighing 24.8 ± 5.4 kg. Body composition was assessed using BIA and fat distribution evaluated from the individual measurements of eight skinfolds. The ratio of IAAT to subcutaneous adipose tissue (SCAT) was 0.15 ± 0.08, and the ratio of IAAT to total body fat mass was 1.44 ± 0.84 cm^2/kg. IAAT was significantly correlated with body weight (0.54 $p < 0.03$), all skinfold measures ($r = 0.60 \pm 0.78$, $p < 0.02$ to $0\ 0003$) except at the calf, then with fat mass ($r = 0.69$, $p < 0.003$) and the trunk-to-extremity skinfold ratio ($r = 0.78$, $p < 0.0003$). No significant relationship between IAAT and WHR was found in obese children of this age. These preliminary results show the existence of IAAT in young children and also reveal that individual skinfold thicknesses on the trunk and the trunk/extremity skinfold ratio provide a better marker of IAAT than waist/hip ratio (Goran, Kaskoun, and Shuman, 1995).

For the evaluation of IAAT, it is also possible to use another anthropometric approach: the measurement of the distance between L4 and the tip of the abdominal wall. The correlation between these two measurements and the results of ultrasonography in adult obese subjects was significant (Kunesová et al., 1997).

Rolland-Cachera and Deheeger (1998) examined the relationships between waist circumference, WHR, and waist/stature ratio in children. The WHRs were not correlated with either fatness index but the absolute values of waist circumference as well as waist/stature ratio correlated significantly with fatness indices (BMI, triceps, and subscapular skinfolds).

The findings from the Bogalusa Heart Study also emphasized the importance of body fat distribution in children characterized in particular as having a high waist circumference. This parameter may help to identify children likely to have adverse concentrations of insulin and lipids. Compared with a child at the 10th percentile of waist circumference, a child at the 90th percentile was estimated to have, on average, higher concentrations of LDL-C and TG, and lower HDL concentrations. These highly significant differences were independent of weight and height and consistent across race-gender groups (Freedman et al., 1999).

4.4.4 Muscle Arm and Fat Circumferences

Upper-arm fat area (UFE = arm circumference × triceps skinfold/2) was used for the definition of malnutrition and also for the identification of obesity — for example, in Brazilian children aged 1 to 5 years. The prevalence of obesity was analyzed in various regions of the country (De Moura et al., 1998). Rolland-Cachera, Bellisle, and Sempé (1989) and Rolland-Cachera (1995) also used this parameter for the evaluation of obesity in children.

4.5 Striae in Obese Children

Excess fatness can cause striae in obese children and adolescents. Subjects from 3 to 19 years were followed up in a pediatric nutrition clinic. Striae were identified in approximately 40% of patients. Generally, striae were symmetrical on both sides of the body and were most prominent on the thighs, arms, and the abdomen. Less frequently they appeared on the back, buttocks, and over the knees. There was no gender difference in the prevalence of striae but they were more marked in older subjects and after longer periods of obesity (Hsu et al., 1996). Colored striae were also observed in Taiwanese children, most commonly appearing on the thighs, arms, and abdomen (Chen, 1997).

Measurements of type III procollagen propeptide and of adrenal function suggest that striae in the obese children are associated with lower collagen synthesis. As adrenal function was similar in all groups of obese children, those with or without striae, it was supposed that the higher estrogen levels in the obese with striae are due to the aromatase activity of fat tissue (Riganti et al., 1993).

4.6 Growth, Skeletal Age, and Bone Development

As mentioned before, obese children are frequently not only heavier but also taller than their normal-weight or lean peers. In a group of Italian obese children aged 3 to 16 years, percentile distribution of height for age showed that stature was higher in obese children than in normal-weight control children by about 5 to 6 cm. This was the case in both genders until about 11 years in girls and 12 years in boys, which indicates an accelerated growth in obese subjects. After this age, percentile distribution was similar in both obese and normal-weight children. With respect to controls, skeletal age tended to be advanced by about 0.75 year in obese girls at all ages, and about 0.75 to 1.0 year in boys up to 11 years. After this age, the skeletal age of boys

TABLE 4.2

Morphological Characteristics in Normal and Obese Boys and Girls
(Aged 13 to 14 Years)

	BMI	Fat (%)	FFM (kg)	Bi-Iliocristal (cm)	Chest Circumference (cm)	Arm Circumference (cm)
Boys						
Normal ×	19.3	12.5	43.9	22.8	78.6	23.1
SD	2.1	5.9	5.1	1.8	3.3	1.2
Obese ×–	26.6a	29.5a	48.6a	27.7a	88.3a	27.0a
SD	2.9	3.2	5.0	1.0	5.5	2.3
Girls						
Normal ×	20.4	18.1	40.7	26.8	79.2	24.3
SD	3.1	6.0	4.9	2.3	4.2	2.5
Obese ×–	27.8a	31.9a	46.7a	27.4	95.18a	29.6a
SD	4.0	3.7	6.4	1.1	3.8	3.3

[a] Statistically significant differences between groups; bi-iliocristal breadth significantly larger after reduction of suprailiac skinfold thickness.

Based on data from Pařízková, 1972.

was similar to controls and relative to age. Maturation according to skeletal age tended to be earlier as BMI increased and early maturers had higher values of BMI (Vignolo et al., 1998). Similar differences in height were also found in obese Czech children (Figure 4.6) (Pařízková, 1977, 1972, 1995a,b).

Child weight and level of maturity accounted for 54% of the variance in prediction of baseline height percentile. Initial values of height and parental height accounted for only 9% of the variance in changes in height percentile, both adjusted for parental height. Weight change did not correlate with growth adjusted for parental height.

In obese children, bone development is usually advanced as shown in South American or Chinese children (Alcazar, Alvear, and Muzzo, 1984; Xu, 1990). The development of body frame is also different in growing subjects with a longer history of obesity, with some larger measurements in obese adolescents — for example, bi-iliocristal diameter, greater lean body mass (Table 4.2, Pařízková, 1972; 1977) and others. Obese Bulgarian children displayed an accelerated growth and bone maturation varying about ± 1SD over the norm. This was more prominent in girls (Stanimirova, Petrova, and Stanimirov, 1993).

Another study in Italian obese subjects showed that growth charts (referred to 97th, 50th, and 3rd percentile) were superior to those of the normal-weight population up to the age of 13 and 12.5 years for males and females, respectively. Later, growth decreases in both genders. The obese subjects did not differ in height compared to their normal-weight peers at the age of 18 years. Bone age estimated by radiograph of the left hand and wrist using the Tanner-Whitehouse II system was more advanced over chronological age in both genders. The increase of bone age over calendar age did not show a substantial difference during pubertal maturation in boys whereas in girls this difference decreased with advancing sexual maturation (De Simone et al., 1995).

Obese subjects in this study also had significantly higher plasma insulin levels compared to lean controls. A significant positive correlation between plasma insulin levels and height standard deviation score was also found. This study revealed that the growth increase in an obese child starts in the first years of life. This stature advantage is maintained until the beginning of puberty with a growth velocity equal to that of lean subjects.

Skeletal maturation is markedly increased and accelerated in both genders. Bone age in this follow-up remained advanced during the period of pubertal development, and obese subjects showed a less notable growth spurt than normal-weight subjects. The growth advantage gradually decreases and final adult height of obese and normal weight subjects is not different (De Simone et al., 1995).

The excess load from an increased deposition of fat might be one of the reasons for the changes in the bone mineral density of obese children. In a study of obese children aged 11.8 ± 2.7 years, determinations were made at the level of the lumbar spine (L2-4) by a commercial dual-photon absorptiometer (Novolab 22A). Bone mineral density was similar in obese and normal children, and was highly correlated with age ($r = 0.70$), body height ($r = 0.65$), and body weight ($r = 0.55$). The highest values for bone mineral density were found in obese adolescents with the most advanced pubertal status. No gender differences were observed in obese children when pubertal stage was taken into account. Lumbar spine bone mineral density corrected for age was not related to the degree or duration of obesity. No effect of physical activity could be demonstrated in spine mineralization in the obese group (De Schepper, Van den Broeck, and Jonckheer, 1995).

4.7   Lean Body Mass in Obese Children

Increased fat deposition is accompanied by greater development of lean, fat-free body mass (LBM) as shown by hydrodensitometric measurements (Pařízková, 1963c, 1977; Cheek, 1968) and changed bone mineral content. These variables were followed in children aged 7.3 to 16.5 years with mild, moderate, and severe obesity using DXA and by measuring BMC in various parts of the body. No significant differences were revealed in upper or lower trunk or in total BMC and LBM in these three groups of obese growing subjects. Upper and lower fat mass was significantly greater in the severe and moderately obese than in the mildly obese or in normal groups. No differences between moderate and severely obese subjects were observed.

Similar differences were found for trunk and total fat mass. In this study, more marked levels of obesity were thus associated with increased fat mass but not increased BMC and LBM in the obese subjects (Sothern et al., 1998).

In contrast, a DXA study in obese Brazilian children (aged 94.67 ± 10.89 months) showed a significantly greater amount of LBM, higher bone mineral content, higher bone mineral density, and higher total body calcium in the obese compared to normal-weight children of a similar age (Fisberg et al., 1998).

The reported differences of LBM in obese growing subjects in other studies can be explained by variation in the duration, age at the onset of obesity, and degree of obesity, plus different methodologies (Fisberg et al., 1998; Pařízková, 1977).

4.8   Muscle Fibers and Obesity

The relationship between muscle fiber type and body adiposity has also been studied using skeletal muscle biopsies. Such studies have mainly been conducted with adult subjects; however, some information can apply to younger age categories. Findings need to be verified in the future when additional methods suitable for children may be available. The presence of slow fibers in muscle biopsies of the vastus lateralis was inversely related to body fatness in adult subjects. Metabolic evidence evaluated using the respiratory exchange ratio (RER) indicated that fatter men with a lower proportion of slow muscle fibers used less fat during exercise on a bicycle ergometer at a workload of 100W than lean men (those with high proportion of slow fibers) (Wade, Marbut, and Round, 1990).

This evidence supports the hypothesis that muscle fiber type is an etiological factor in the development of obesity and that the processes concerning the metabolism of lipids during work are related to the proportion of various types of fibers in skeletal muscles. These mechanisms can apply at earlier periods of life as a certain ratio of slow-to-fast twitch muscle fibers are present at birth (Åstrand and Rodahl, 1977).

Decreased activity of fat-oxidizing enzymes in biopsies from the vastus lateralis muscle was shown in obesity-prone adult subjects, but a similar study was not executed in children for obvious reasons. No differences in fiber type composition but a smaller area of type I and 2B fibers was found in postobese women compared to controls. Significantly lower values for hydroxyacyl-coenzyme-A-dehydrogenase (HADH), a key enzyme in b-oxidation of fatty acids, and of citrate-synthetase, a rate-limiting enzyme in the Kreb's cycle, were revealed in the postobese women. These findings were matched with a trend for lower aerobic power (VO$_2$ max) and lower food and fat intake. As shown in other studies, a high level of aerobic power facilitates the utilization of lipid metabolites and contributes to a reduction and/or maintenance of a low amount of stored fat (Pařízková, 1977). RMR and RER did not differ but tended to be lower in the postobese women. This could explain the lower fat oxidation previously found in postobese subjects; however, when adjusting data for age and VO_2 max, the differences in enzyme activities were no more significant among postobese and control subjects (Raben et al., 1997). As mentioned earlier, a high level of aerobic power output corresponds with a higher utilization of lipid metabolites.

4.9 Summary

The estimation of body composition — the absolute and relative amounts of adipose tissue and lean, fat-free body mass — is one of the most important factors in the diagnosis of obesity. As most of the approaches are more complicated and demanding than the simple evaluation of basic anthropometric characteristics — that is, height and weight of the organism — the BMI has commonly been used. For children, due to changes in body proportionality, special growth grids have been created. Cutoff points indicating special percentiles as criteria for overweight and obesity have been established by the International Obesity Task Force (IOTF) of the World Health Organization. However, these vary slightly for individual child populations, especially for those whose data were not used for the generation of the definition of the criteria. Therefore, some researchers have suggested that population-specific criteria be developed. Of considerable potential importance is the so-called adiposity rebound (AR) of BMI phenomenon, which occurs approximately after the sixth year. This follows a temporary decrease in BMI following the first year of life, with BMI increasing from the 6th to about the 18th year. The timing of the AR may be important from the point of view of obesity later in life, which develops more often when AR of BMI appears earlier than in the standard population. Crossing over percentiles is a further important indicator of obesity development. BMI correlates most significantly with the percentage of stored fat, but in cases of morbid obesity the results could be spurious.

For the assessment of body composition, the most traditional methods are densitometric — for example, underwater weighing, which is best with simultaneous measurement of the air in the lungs and respiratory passages. Total body composition measurements using deuterium (or tritium) for body water, ^{40}K measurements, ultrasound, and creatinine excretion have also been widely used for a long time. More recent body composition measures developed include dual-energy x-ray absorptiometry (DXA), bioelectrical impedance analysis (BIA), total body electrical conductivity (TOBEC), computer-assisted tomography analysis (CT), and magnetic resonance imaging (MRI). The latter methods are mostly used in clinics or scientific institutions, and are more expensive and demanding for both researchers and their subjects.

Anthropometric methods such as circumference measures or skinfold thickness measurement are recommended given their greater simplicity, low cost, and the potential to use them under field conditions. They correlate well with more sophisticated methods, which in some cases were only recently considered suitable for children (e.g., CT measurement involves exposure to a small amount of radiation). The results of all of the methods mentioned correlate mutually but do not give identical results.

The use of various methods of body composition assessment in obese children enables not only more exact diagnoses of obesity and its degree, but they also evaluate in greater detail the changes after reduction treatment during growth and development. Fat distribution over body surfaces (trunk, extremities; comparing circumferences, skinfolds) or assessing fat deposited intraabdominally and subcutaneously is another essential characteristic that correlates significantly with clinical symptoms and health risks.

5

Energy Expenditure and Physical Activity

Energy expenditure — along with energy intake and the resulting energy balance and turnover — plays an essential role in the deposition of fat in the human organism and in the development of obesity. Physical activity is the main variable that can change energy expenditure at all ages. A reduction in physical activity due to sedentary behaviors during leisure time can have a negative effect on energy balance, and unfortunately our understanding of nondetectable, low-level activity in children is limited (Dietz, 1991).

The numerous gaps in our understanding of energy expenditure in a range of contexts, particularly in children, include the inability to collect exact measurements of energy expenditure over extended periods of time. The same is true at the other extreme. We have a poor understanding of the contribution of small amounts of nonweight-bearing physical activities such as fidgeting while sitting. Some suggest that in children, such activities may account for more energy output than once thought (Dietz, 1991).

More longitudinal studies are necessary as the short-term measurements of energy expenditure in children who are already obese do not always reveal the true relationship between total energy expenditure (TEE) and activity energy expenditure (AEE) and adiposity during growth. Possible differences between obese and lean individuals may also not be revealed. As mentioned previously, the level of physical activity in children and youth today is generally quite low and in many places may still be decreasing, regardless of the individual's level of adiposity. This situation appears to exist both in the industrially developed countries and in Third World countries where the economic and social situation has changed very rapidly in the recent past.

Obesity does not develop overnight. The condition is the result of long-term metabolic, hormonal, functional, and psychological adjustments related to a different energy balance and turnover in the organism, influenced substantially by the environment and also based on one's genetic background. Therefore, ad hoc short-term measurements cannot provide a true picture of any parameter, including the history of the level of physical activity and TEE during earlier periods of growth. To understand the causes of obesity in a comprehensive manner, including the contribution of energy expenditure, would require measurements over a long period starting with the very beginning of any increase in weight and deposition of excess fat. Potentially, one might need to consider the period preceding the development of overweight. With respect to physical activity and energy expenditure in childhood, parent-child relationships and physical activity patterns are also important (Fogelholm et al., 1999).

5.1   Components of Energy Expenditure

Energy expenditure is composed of a number of components. TEE includes the following:

Basal metabolic rate (BMR): The minimal rate of energy expenditure compatible with life (under conditions of quiet sleep).

Resting metabolic rate (RMR): The rate of energy expenditure usually measured under resting conditions, as described below. RMR is the most commonly used measure as BMR is more difficult to ascertain.

Thermic effect of food (TEF) or the thermic effect of a meal (TEM) also known as diet-induced thermogenesis (DIT): Energy used in digesting, absorbing, storing, and disposing of ingested nutrients (James and Schofield, 1990). The thermic effect of food is usually estimated as 10% of total energy expenditure.

Activity energy expenditure (AEE): Energy expended in physical activity. Physical activity provides the greatest potential to vary total energy expenditure (Figure 5.1).

Measurement of BMR is usually undertaken by indirect calorimetry under basal conditions, which in practice means that the measurements are taken during sleep or just after waking. It is also recommended that the individual fasts overnight and avoids intense physical activity the preceding day. This methodology is not feasible in subjects living under normal home conditions and therefore is usually reserved for laboratory or clinic settings.

A number of regression equations for the estimation of BMR have been developed. The FAO/WHO/UNU Expert Consultation (Rome, 1981; World Health Organization, Geneva, 1985) suggested new equations for children and adolescents that were published in a WHO document (1985) and further developed by James and Schofield (1990) (Table 5.1). For this estimation of both weight and height, only weight is used for the calculations. The values of BMR are also used for the calculation of TEE by multiplying the time spent in various activities by the respective "energy cost" calculated based on a BMR multiple (Table 5.2 and Table 5.3).

Resting energy expenditure (REE) is usually evaluated on the basis of the uptake of oxygen (by indirect calorimetry) under resting conditions in a

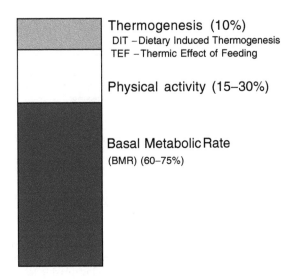

FIGURE 5.1
Components of daily energy expenditure in normal subjects.

TABLE 5.1

Equations for Predicting Basal Metabolic Rate from Body Weight (W) in Children and Adolescents

Age Range (years)	Kcal.day^{-1}	r	SD[a]	MJ.day^{-1}	r	SD[a]
Males						
0–3	60.9 W – 54	0.97	53	0.255 W – 0.226	0.97	0.222
3–10	22.7 W + 495	0.86	62	0.0949 W + 2.07	0.86	0.259
10–18	17.5 W + 651	0.90	100	0.0732 W + 2.72	0.90	0.418
Females						
0–3	61.0 W – 51	0.97	61	0.255 W – 0.214	0.97	0.255
3–10	22.5 W – 499	0.85	63	0.0941 W + 2.09	0.85	0.264
10–18	12.2 W + 746	0.75	117	0.0510 W + 3.12	0.75	0.489

[a] SD, standard deviation of differences between the actual and predicted estimates.

Based on data from WHO, 1985.

comfortable environment and ambient temperature and after at least 30 minutes repose.

TEE during one or more days can also be measured by direct and/or indirect calorimetry in special calorimetry chambers. Obese adult subjects have been studied under such conditions, but confinement in an isolated chamber for a long period of time is not acceptable for younger children. TEE can also be measured under normal free-living conditions using doubly

TABLE 5.2

Physical Activity Ratios (PAR) of Selected Activities

PAR	Value Range	Activity
1.2	(1.0–1.4)	Lying at rest, sitting or standing quietly
1.6	(1.4–1.8)	Washing, dressing
1.4	Sitting, playing	
2.5	Strolling around	
2.8	(2.4–3.3)	Walking on level, speed 3–4 km.hr–1
3.2	Walking at a normal pace	
4.7	Walking uphill slowly	
5.7	Walking uphill at normal pace	
7.5	Walking uphill fast	
2.8	(2.4–3.3)	Walking downhill
3.8	Cycling, gymnastics	
5.1	Dancing, swimming	
6.7	(5.9–7.9)	Walking, speed 6–7 km.hr–1, football, running, cross-country walking, paddling, etc.
9.0	(7.9–10.5)	Aerobic dancing, playing tennis competitively

Based on data from WHO, 1985 and James and Schofield, 1990.

TABLE 5.3

Examples of the Calculation Used to Derive Energy
Expenditure in a 10-Year-Old Girl (Body Weight 33.8 kg)

Activity	Hours	kcal	kJ
Sleep at $1.0 \times$ BMR	9	435	1820
School at $1.5 \times$ BMR	4	290	1210
Light activity at $1.5 \times$ BMR	4	290	1210
Moderate activity	6.5	690	2890
High activity at $6.0 \times$ BMR	0.5	145	610
Total expenditure		1850	7740
Growth		65	270
Total requirement per 24 hours $1.65 \times$ BMR		1915	8010

Based on data from WHO, 1985.

labeled water (DLW) (Prentice, 1999), a technique that has often been used in studies of obese children (Maffeis et al., 1996; Molnar et al., 1995; Maffeis, Schutz, and Pinelli, 1992a). AEE can be evaluated as the difference between TEE and (REE + TEF).

Physical activity (PA): Any bodily movement produced by skeletal muscles that results in an increase in energy expenditure.

Physical activity level (PAL): Expresses the ratio between BMR and TEE. PAL = TEE during 24 hr/BMR during 24 hours.

Physical activity ratio (PAR): A similar index relating the values per minute: PAR = TEE min^{-1}/BMR min^{-1}.

Exercise (E): A subcategory of physical activity that is structured, repetitive, and purposeful in the sense that improvement or maintenance of physical fitness is often an objective (Nieman, 2003). AEE can be evaluated by direct measurement (calorimetry) or by a procedure suggested by the WHO (1985) and James and Schofield (1990). The calculation of BMR and the use of multiples of BMR (METs) (Table 5.2) for individual physical activities are in widespread use. An example for a normal child is provided in Table 5.3. Individual evaluation encompasses the ability to consider the time and intensity of workload in activity and/or exercise.

5.2 Resting Metabolic Rate (RMR) and Resting Energy Expenditure (REE)

Resting metabolic rate (RMR) is most often ascertained by measuring subjects under quiet resting (nonsleeping) conditions. RMR can be assessed directly or by using prediction equations. When it is measured directly, the individual must rest for a minimum of 30 minutes in an ambient temperature before the measurement is taken. As mentioned previously, this parameter usually replaces the measurement of BMR due to its relative ease of measurement. However, RMR can be calculated using the regression equations recommended by the WHO (1985) and James and Schofield (1990). As these equations were derived mainly on the basis of measurements in normal-weight children, results must be evaluated with caution when applied to obese children.

The measurements of Kaplan et al. (1995) provide some useful working examples. The assessment of REE in pediatric practice using various prediction equations does not readily apply to obese children. REE was measured by indirect calorimetry and compared with the results of the following prediction equations: FAO/WHO/UNU (WHO, 1985), the Harris-Benedict (H-B) equation, and two equations of Schofield, one using weight (Scho-WT) and the other using weight and height (Scho-HT/WT). The results of the study in children and adolescents (aged 0.2 to 20.5 years) showed that the Schofield HT/WT equation predicts REE in children with clinical nutritional problems better than the equations that use weight alone (Kaplan et al., 1995). However, in view of the wide variability in REE measurements in children of various levels of fatness, it is preferable not to predict REE in obese children but to measure it directly whenever possible.

Other measurements in a sample of prepubertal and pubertal children aged 10 to 16 years showed that the indirect calorimetry method (using the ventilatory hood system) did not agree with the results of the calculations using five regression equations. All equations overestimated RMR in obese subjects by 7.5 to 18.1%. Additional regression equations have been derived

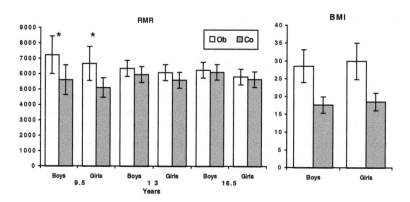

FIGURE 5.2
Comparison of body mass index (BMI) and resting metabolic rate (RMR) in obese (Ob) and normal-weight (Co) boys and girls aged 9.5 to 16.5 years. * indicates ($p < 0.05$). (Based on data from Molnar and Schutz, 1997.)

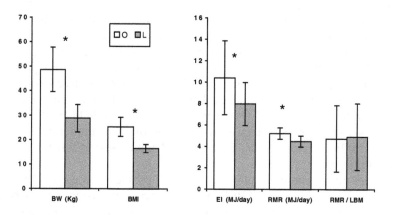

FIGURE 5.3
Comparison of morphological characteristics (body weight, body mass index), energy intake (EI), resting metabolic rate (RMR, MJ per 24 hours) in obese (O) and normal-weight (L) boys and girls. * indicates ($p < 0.05$). (Based on data from Maffeis, Schutz, and Pinelli, 1992.)

on the basis of measurements of a further cohort of obese children and adolescents and provided reliable results compared to direct measurements (Molnar et al., 1995). Figure 5.2 shows the comparison of RMR and BMI in normal and obese children.

The study of Tounian et al. (2003) showed that RER in obese children was higher than in constitutionally lean children. There was an association between RER and fat-free, lean body mass (LBM), which is usually larger in obese than in normal-weight children. Fat mass was correlated with the rate of fat oxidation. In another study, RMR, BMI, and food intake were higher in obese than normal-weight children (Figure 5.3) (Maffeis, Schutz, and Pinelli, 1992a). When adjusted for fat-free mass, RMR did not vary. The energy intake was the same in both obese and normal-weight children. The main determinant of RMR was thus fat-free LBM. However, the gender difference remained significant after fat-free mass (FFM) adjustment. The adjusted values of RMR decreased slightly but significantly between the ages of 10 to 16 years (Molnar and Schutz, 1997).

Nonresting energy expenditure has been reported to be significantly lower among pubertal than prepubertal girls. After adjustment for age and body composition, it was noted that RMR, nonresting energy expenditure, and TEE were all significantly lower among black girls than among white girls. Differences in RMR and TEE among premenarcheal girls were associated with parental weight status and girls' race-ethnicity, whereas differences in nonresting energy expenditure were associated with pubertal stage and race-ethnicity (Bandini et al., 2002).

Other studies have also confirmed higher resting energy metabolism (expenditure) in obese than in nonobese children and adolescents, but the REE related to fat-free mass was not significantly different. Fat-free LBM explained 73.1% of the variability in REE; gender, age, and surface area added little to this (2.6 to 3.8%). Fat-free mass was the most important predictor of REE, followed by waist circumference and age. Differences in REE between the obese and nonobese subjects do not seem to justify the maintenance of obesity (Rodriguez et al., 2002). When body composition is accounted for, RMR does not differ significantly between obese and normal-weight Chinese boys (Stensel, Lin, and Nevill, 2001).

African-Americans may have lower resting energy expenditures than whites. Body composition measured by DXA in 5- to 17-year-old subjects showed that when trunk FFM was included in the model in place of whole-body FFM, the ethnic differences in REE decreased. Trunk fat-free, lean mass partially explained the lower REE found in obese African-American children and adolescents. The lower REE of girls and of African-Americans may contribute to the difficulty in weight management in these groups, as a different approach has to be used (Tershakovec et al., 2002a).

Body fatness can be affected through EE by genetic factors. An association of the mitochondrial protein 2 (UCP-2) gene and obesity in children has been analyzed because it was suspected that UCP-2 may have an influence on energy expenditure. The research showed that the UCP-2 genotype was related to body composition and REE in children aged 6 to 10 years. Overweight children and nonoverweight children of overweight parents were genotyped for a 45-base pair deletion/insertion (del/ins) in 3'-untranslated region of exon 8 and for exon 4 C to T transition. Greater BMI in del/ins children was independent of race and gender. Body composition was also different according to UCP-2 genotype. All body circumferences and skinfold thickness examined were significantly greater in del/ins than in del/del children. Body fat mass as determined by DXA was also greater in del/ins than in del/del children. In children genotyped at axon 4, no significant differences in BMI or body composition were found among the 3 exon 4 genotypes. Neither REE nor RQ was different according to UCP-2 exon 4 or exon 8 genotype. The exon 8 ins/del polymorphism of UCP-2 appears to be associated with childhood-onset obesity. The UCP-2/UCP-3 genetic locus may also play a role in body weight development during childhood (Yanovski et al., 2000).

5.3   Thermic Effect of Food (Diet-Induced Thermogenesis)

Excess fatness may have an effect not only on RMR but also on the thermic effect of food (TEF, or diet-induced thermogenesis [DIT]). This phenomenon was studied in a group of obese and normal-weight children aged 8.8 ± 0.3 years. RMR was higher in obese than in normal-weight children, and when RMR was adjusted for fat-free mass, values were no longer significantly different. The thermic response to a liquid-mixed meal, expressed as a percentage of the energy content of the meal, was significantly lower in obese than in normal-weight children (Figure 5.4) (Maffeis et al., 1993d). These data indicate that the defect in thermogenesis reported in obese adults originates earlier in life than was previously assumed. A meal high in fat was considered a risk for weight gain based on meal-induced thermogenesis (Maffeis et al., 2001).

The relationships between REE, DIT (assessed by indirect calorimetry), and body fat distribution were analyzed in normal-weight and obese children distributed in groups of abdominal (WHR > 0.9) and gluteal-femoral obese (WHR < 0.8). No differences in REE and DIT were seen among children with different types of obesity. Therefore, it was concluded that body fat

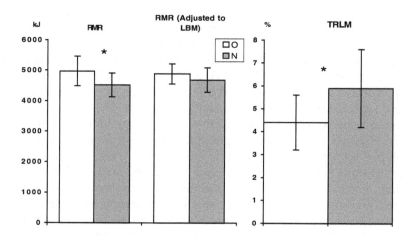

FIGURE 5.4

The comparison of resting metabolic rate (RMR) and the thermic effect of mixed liquid meal (TRLM) in prepubertal obese (O) and nonobese control (N) children. * indicates (p < 0.05). (Based on data from Maffeis et al., 1993.)

distribution in obese and normal-weight adolescents has no influence on REE and TEF (Zwiauer et al., 1993).

5.4 Total Energy Expenditure and Physical Activity

There is considerable evidence to suggest that participation in physical activity as a youngster has a bearing on functional status as an adult. Similarly, it may be contended that the physical activity experiences of children and adolescents play a major role in the development of appropriate lifestyle behaviors in the adult years. Tracking of physical activity behaviors across the growing years and into adulthood is central to understanding the persistence of benefits of physical activity being maintained. One of the limiting factors in our understanding of a range of health issues is the need for valid and reliable measures of physical activity.

Studies of TEE, including the energy spent on physical activity (AEE) in children can be quite difficult. Due to the excessive cost it is unusual to use more sophisticated and costly methods such as the DLW technique for the measurements of TEE on a routine basis, along with measurements of BMR and/or RMR. However, DLW ($^2H_2\ ^{18}O$) has been more widely used during the last decade (Davies et al., 1998; Prentice, 1999).

5.4.1 Methods

A number of methods have been used to measure the physical activity status of children and adolescents. Westerterp (1999) grouped the available techniques into five general categories: behavioral observation; questionnaires (including diaries, recall questionnaires, and interviews); physiological markers such as heart rate; calorimetry; and motion sensors.

Methods vary in sophistication from the relatively simple and easy-to-administer self-report and monitoring methods to the more costly laboratory-based procedures. The laboratory-based methods are more precise but are not suited to large numbers of individuals while the reverse is true for the field methods such as self-report and monitoring procedures. Readers are encouraged to access a number of reviews devoted to physical activity assessment in children and adolescents (Heath, Pate, and Pratt, 1993; Melanson and Freedson, 1996; Montoye et al., 1996; Pate, 1993; Sallis, 1991; Simons-Morton et al., 1990). In addition, a review of the assessment of physical activity level in relation to obesity provides a useful summary (Westerterp, 1999).

There are numerous considerations regarding the choice of a measure of physical activity, including the reliability, validity, and efficacy of the instrument (Hills, Byrne, and Pařízková, 1998). Reliability is the extent to which a method produces similar values on two or more occasions (Baranowski et al., 1990). Precision and accuracy relate to the ability of a measurement technique to achieve the right answer. Validity in turn refers to the extent to which the method is a true indication of the variable (in this case physical activity) being assessed (Hills, Byrne, and Pařízková, 1998).

The energy cost of PA and TEE can be expressed by multiples of BMR and MET values. This characterizes the intensity of workload related to BMR and, therefore, the energy expended. MET values have been derived mostly on the basis of measurements in adults but have also been used for children (WHO, 1985). Using this procedure, TEE per day can be calculated. However, during the same physically defined workload (for example, two watts per kg of body weight on a bicycle ergometer), 12-year-old children increased their energy expenditure related to BMR by approximately 29% less than 18-year-old individuals and adults (Pařízková, 1985).

The multiples of BMR that characterize the intensity of a workload for adults are higher due to the reduction of BMR with aging. Therefore, their use can be misleading when using the WHO procedures for children, especially at younger ages. This phenomenon can partly explain the trend for a higher physical activity level (PAL) in children, especially of preschool age. The transition from resting to active conditions in a young individual is a relatively smaller change than in an older person. However, this principle applies to normal-weight children and less to the overweight and/or obese.

Bigger, fatter individuals, as a function of their weight, BMI, body composition, and spontaneous physical activity, are more akin to a much older individual. The BMR to characterize estimation of energy expenditure using the above-mentioned procedure should be supplemented by the measurement of young individuals during standardized workloads and deriving more exact multiples of the intensity of each workload. The example given in Table 5.3 shows how such evaluations are made, and as a crude approximation of TEE, this can still be quite useful.

The DLW method provides a measurement of total daily energy expenditure over a time frame of one to three weeks (Schoeller and Hnilicka, 1996). PAL can be calculated by expressing the average daily metabolic rate (ADMR) from DLW as a multiple of BMR (PAL = ADMR/BMR).

The main advantage of DLW is that it provides a noninvasive method for the assessment of TEE under conditions of normal living, and in spite of both advantages and disadvantages of the technique (Prentice, 1999), it has been used in both adults and children. The principle involves the oral application of a mixture of ^2H_2O and $H_2\,^{18}O$ to enrich the body's water pool with ^2H and ^{18}O. The plateau concentration of the isotopes measured three to four hours after dosage enables the estimation of the water pool, which is used for both DLW calculation and for the estimation of fat mass to lean body mass ratio. The ^2H equilibrates with body water, and the rate constant for its disappearance is proportional to water turnover. The ^{18}O equilibrates with both water and the bicarbonate pool that is generated from the carbon dioxide appearing as the end product of oxidative metabolism. Their rapid equilibrium is due to the carbonic anhydrase reaction, and the rate constant for [18]O disappearance is proportional to the sum of water and bicarbonate turnover. The difference between the two rate constants gives a measure of carbon dioxide production from which energy expenditure can be evaluated using classical indirect calorimetric equations (Prentice, 1999).

The DLW technique is considered the criterion measure or gold standard for TEE measurement. Like all measures the technique has inherent strengths and weaknesses. The major advantage of the technique is its precision, but this needs to be weighed against the substantial cost. As a laboratory-based procedure (at least for assessment of samples), the technique is prohibitive for any large-scale, population-based assessment of energy expenditure. Further, the technique provides a gross measure of energy expenditure and is unable to define the nature of the activity or types of activity the individual has been involved in.

A study by Goran et al. (1993) using the DLW technique with 4- to 6-year-old children quantified associations between energy expenditure, heart rate, resting energy expenditure, and body composition. Findings included a significant association between resting heart rate and energy expenditure. Measures of heart rate and other parameters such as body composition have been considered legitimate options for the measurement of energy expenditure in a larger number of subjects.

Heart rate (HR) monitors and derivatives are in widespread use, commonly in conjunction with training programs. Monitors are able to capture heart rate data over an extended time frame. This may include the registration of the number of beats in certain bands of heart rate across the measurement period, commonly during the waking hours of the day. The results of these HR measurements form the basis of the estimation of energy expenditure. When HR is correlated with oxygen uptake (by indirect calorimetry) under rest conditions and/or at various levels of workload, an assessment of energy output using individual regression equations of the relationship between HR and O_2 uptake is possible.

Other forms of monitoring devices, including mechanical and electronic derivatives, include a wide range of uniaxial and triaxial accelerometers or movement registration systems (Westerterp, 1999). Numerous concerns have been raised regarding the reliability of energy cost measurement of various physical activities using accelerometers — for example, when walking uphill or downhill, the incline must be taken into consideration or estimates may be inaccurate (Terrier, Aminian, and Schutz, 1999). For validation purposes, physical activity of children was measured simultaneously by DLW and accelerometers (Hoos et al., 2003).

The use of the Tritrac accelerometer (and deriving METs), along with self-reported physical activity, has enabled physical activity determinants to be derived in obese children. There is a moderate correlation between these two parameters of physical activity ($r = 0.46$). The difference between the measurements using Tritrac is 1.6 METs and using self-reported activity, 2.3

METs. In the prediction of activity, variance has been considered according to factors in a hierarchical analysis (socioeconomic level, body composition, fitness, hedonics of child and adult activity behaviors) (Epstein et al., 1996).

The evaluation of physical activity level using the Tritrac yielded more reliable estimates of the physical activity level in obese children aged 8 to 15 years than a self-reported measure. Correlations between the values of energy output by accelerometer (expressed in METs) and adjusted heart rates ($r = 0.71$) were significantly higher than correlations between adjusted heart rates and self-reported METs ($r = 0.36$). Self-reported METs had higher mean standard errors in estimating heart rates, were significantly greater than accelerometer METs, and systematically overestimated accelerometer METs (Coleman et al., 1997). This means that the information on physical activity levels in obese children using questionnaires may not be objective.

Accelerometers have revealed a fivefold variation in physical activity among healthy 5-year-old children. Girls displayed lower activity than boys at this age both at school and during weekends, and measurements using accelerometers may be able to help identify children at risk for obesity development (Metcalf, Voss, and Wilkin, 2002).

AEE (measured by DLW and indirect calorimetry) and energy expenditure assessed physical activity from 7-day recall (PAR) in U.S. prepubertal and pubertal boys were inversely related to adiposity. Abdominal visceral fat and subcutaneous fat were not related to AEE of activity hours after partial correlation with fat mass, maturation, and age. Fat mass is more closely related to AEE than the time spent in activity as identified by physical activity recalls (Roemmich et al., 2000).

A longitudinal study of physical activity (measured by Caltrac activity monitors, diary, and a questionnaire) showed that in the biracial U.S. cohort of the NHLBI Growth and Health Study (NGHS), there was a dramatic decrease of overall physical activity during the transition from childhood to adolescence (Kimm et al., 2000). The number (not duration) of moderate to vigorous physical activity exercise bouts in children was related to the relative reinforcing values of physical activity (RRVPA) measured in the laboratory, which can contribute to the prediction of physical activity level along with obesity. This indicated that RRVPA is a determinant of physical activity level and that it may be more reinforcing for children to engage in multiple, short exercise bouts than fewer, more extended bouts (Epstein et al., 1999). Results using the triaxial accelerometer (Tracmor 2) were compared with the DLW method ($^2H_2$ ^{18}H) measurements in 6.2-year-old children (± 2.2 y), and it was again shown that this method is a valid instrument for the measurement of physical activity in children (Hoos et al., 2003).

A number of self-report measures are available but they vary substantially. These questionnaires usually describe the type, duration, and frequency of daily physical activities that are not always possible to obtain from the assessments of TEE or sums of HR over longer time periods. This is essential for evaluations as only a relevant intensity and type of exercise can result in significant changes to morphological and functional variables.

Therefore, an effort has been made to create and validate questionnaires and also to evaluate children's activity. Questionnaires may be used simultaneously with the other approaches of energy expenditure measurements. The self-report questionnaires represent the most commonly employed methods of physical activity assessment. Generally, instruments of this type are suitable for individuals over 10 years of age. Assistance is essential from teachers and parents when working with younger children.

The Children's Activity Rating Scale (CARS) with five levels made possible the categorization and discrimination of eight physical activities, and therefore children's level of energy expenditure. Observers were trained to follow young children under field conditions, and there was a satisfactory agreement of the results of observations gained by individual examiners. These data demonstrate that CARS can encompass a wide variety of physical activity and levels of energy expenditure. Mean values of energy expenditure for eight activities representing the five levels of CARS were pretested by measuring VO_2 and heart rates in 5- to 6-year-old children. These values ranged from 1 to 5.2 METs, that is, 14.5 to 80.6% of VO_2 max, and heart rate from 89 to 183 beats.min^{-1} (Puhl et al., 1990). This type of assessment may enable the evaluation of energy expenditure when more sophisticated and expensive methods are not available (DuRant et al., 1993).

5.5 Physical Activity and Energy Expenditure as Related to Fatness

Physical activity level generally fluctuates and decreases with age (Roemmich et al., 2000; Reilly et al., 2004). The exact evaluation of physical activity level in individual subjects during growth and living under normal conditions is difficult. Precise and accurate methods such as the DLW technique are too expensive and not available to all researchers. Physical activity epidemiology is essential for the evaluation of the effect of physical activity levels on a child's development and also on the prevalence of obesity. Physical activity level generally fluctuates and decreases with age (Roemmich et al., 2000; Reilly et al., 2004).

To date, many samples have not been adequately described and/or the statistical procedures employed were not satisfactory. As a result of the studies that have been conducted there are varying opinions regarding the relationships between physical activity and fatness, including significant differences in reported physical activity levels in lean and obese children. In relation to childhood obesity, the influence of TEE is also somewhat unclear as some studies report a reduced TEE (Griffiths, Rivers, and Payne, 1987; Roberts et al., 1988) and others do not (DeLany et al., 1995; Treuth et al., 1998). An improvement in the existing methods of physical activity epidemiology is necessary (Caspersen, Nixon, and DuRant, 1998).

As mentioned previously, only certain levels of intensity, duration and type of physical activity, and exercise can stimulate changes in body adiposity through increased energy expenditure (see Chapter 4). Few individuals display a consistent regulation of energy balance and size of body fat stores. There is evidence that a low energy output is not counterbalanced with a decreased hunger and amended satiety mechanisms in individuals with a genetically determined susceptibility to weight gain and obesity. About 80% of the variance between subjects' RMR can be explained by the amount of lean, fat-free body mass, and a further 10% is accounted for by fat mass, plasma T3, and noradrenaline levels (Astrup, 1998).

When evaluating the increasing prevalence of obesity, many studies, such as in U.S. or Canadian child populations, reveal that reduced physical activity may be the main causal factor (Dowda et al., 2001; Goran and Treuth, 2001; Tremblay and Willms, 2003). Poor urban planning may be a contributing factor as there are not enough suitable spaces for many young people to participate in physical activity and exercise. In 5- to 7-year-old German children, overweight was associated with physical inactivity, unsuitable eating habits, and low SES (Muller et al., 1999). Reducing sedentary activities may therefore be another good approach in the prevention and treatment of obesity in children (Robinson, 1999).

Obese Australian children exhibited significantly lower daily accumulation of total counts by accelerometer, less medium and vigorous physical activity (MPA and VPA, as evaluated by METs), as well as significantly fewer 5-, 10-, and 20-minute bouts of both medium and vigorous physical activity. The obese children also reported significantly lower levels of physical activity self-efficacy, were involved in significantly fewer community organizations promoting physical activity, and were significantly less likely to report their father or male guardian as physically active (Wake, Hesketh, and Waters, 2003).

The same conclusions were derived for a population in the West Indies where a stronger impact of inactivity in childhood than later in adolescence was considered (Caius and Benefice, 2002). A significant relationship was found between childhood obesity and computer usage, TV watching, total hours in sedentary behavior, and maternal BMI. An indirect significant relationship with childhood obesity was shown if a parent was home when the child got home, and if a father participated in exercise with his child. Caloric intake, total time in physical activity, demographic variables, and father's BMI showed no significant relationship with children's BMI (Arluk et al., 2003). In the United States, only a small part of the variance in a child's BMI was related to TV viewing, but not video games (Geiss, Parhofer, and Schwandt, 2001).

In a study in children aged 4.1 to 13.6 years, it was reported that REE was higher in the obese than in normal-weight children, which was apparent after adjustment for fat-free, lean body mass. Obese children also had a higher percentage of fat oxidation, lower carbohydrate oxidation, and a lower respiratory quotient (Paz-Cerezo et al., 2003).

A decline in physical activity during adolescence was observed in both white and black girls followed from 9 to 10 until 18 to 19 years (National Heart, Lung, and Blood Institute Growth and Health Study). Lower levels of parental education were associated with a greater decline in activity for white girls, both younger and older; for black girls, this association was only revealed at an older age. Pregnancy was associated with a decline in activity in black girls, but not among white girls in whom activity declined along with smoking. A higher BMI was associated with a greater decline in activity in both white and black girls (Kimm et al., 2002). The role of sedentarism is considered a most important factor that needs to be evaluated more carefully (Reilly et al., 2003), for example following TV and video viewing as a marker of inactivity (Proctor et al., 2003; Vandewater, Shim, and Caplowitz, 2004). The effect of physical activity on the autonomic nervous system has also been compared in obese and nonobese, lean children (Nagai and Moritani, 2004).

One of the recent studies to consider level of physical activity in relation to time spent watching TV and participating in video games found that increased TV viewing did not reflect reduced 24-hour energy expenditure as assessed by heart rate monitoring. TV viewing was also not related to submaximal VO_2 results, muscle strength, or poor dietary intake. As is the case in other studies, children of low SES spent more time watching TV (Grund et al., 2001b). For a more complete picture of children's physical activity in relation to time devoted to TV viewing, it would be prudent to assess both time spent watching TV and the frequency, intensity, time, and type of other physical activities subjects participated in during the remainder of their time. This information would be useful to identify whether the time spent watching TV is compensated for by more intense activity at other times. It is important to note that in the studies mentioned in this area, confounding factors such as diet, genetics, and many others were mostly not controlled.

5.5.1 Genetic Factors

Some studies suggest that there is also a significant genetic component that predisposes both a low level of spontaneous physical activity and an increased deposition of fat. Infants of obese mothers have low energy expenditures, which is associated with obesity, whereas no such finding was observed in infants with nonobese mothers (Davies, Day, and Lucas, 1991; Roberts et al., 1988). In another study, RMR was 6% lower in children with one obese parent than in other children studied (Goran et al., 1995). Family membership accounted for 57% of the variance in spontaneous physical activity, indicating that a genetic predisposition is involved (Zurlo, Ferraro, and Fontvieille, 1992). Familial clustering of obesity is a common phenomenon — for example, obesity in twins.

Berkowitz et al. (1985) found that neonatal adiposity was not significantly associated with parental adiposity and gender and did not predict adiposity later in childhood. However, in a stepwise multiple regression analysis, the daily physical activity level in children and parental adiposity were significantly associated with childhood adiposity. The age or gender of the child did not significantly correlate with childhood adiposity. The increase in parental adiposity or the decrease of daily physical activity level was likely to increase the adiposity in 4- to 8-year-old children.

Genetic factors are assumed to play an important role in RMR and thermic effect of feeding. Measurements in prepubertal children subdivided according to family history showed that average RMR was similar in obese children with or without a family history of obesity, but were higher than in the normal-weight control children. Adjusted for FFM, average RMRs were comparable in all three groups of children. The thermic effect of feeding calculated as a percentage of RMR was lower in the obese than in control children. These measurements failed to support the view that family history of obesity can significantly influence the RMR and TEF of obese children with obese parents (Maffeis et al., 1993e).

In another study of obese children, resting metabolic rate (RMR) was studied as a function of body weight, and higher values were found in obese than in lean children. Child weight accounted for 72 to 78% of the variance in RMR. When parental weight was included, the prediction of RMR did not improve. After six months of treatment obese children decreased their percentage of overweight but RMR remained unchanged. These data indicate that the RMR does not change when the percent of overweight results from the increase of height and no change in weight (Epstein et al., 1989a).

RMR is a familial trait, but its effect can be attributed mainly to the familial resemblance of body size and composition, that is, FFM and fat mass. A low level of RMR for a given FFM is a risk factor for increased weight gain and obesity. Based on a meta-analysis, weight-normalized formerly obese subjects have a fivefold greater chance of having a very low RMR when adjusted for body size and composition than matched control subjects who were never obese (Astrup, 1998).

Obese and lean adolescent siblings were compared for RMR (indirect calorimetry), aerobic power (VO_2 max in absolute and relative values), and body composition. Obese siblings had an increased amount of stored fat, and similar lean, fat-free mass. RMR did not differ among obese and lean siblings. Aerobic power was greater in obese siblings, but it was the same when adjusted for fat-free mass (Elliot et al., 1989).

Energy balance, of which AEE has a large effect, plays an important role in the development of obesity during childhood (Roberts, 1995). Results of studies reveal significant relationships between the degree of physical activity and the percentage of fat (Davies, Day, and Lucas, 1991; Pařízková, 1977, 1996). However, some results are controversial and do not confirm these relationships. Measurements of TEE and AEE have shown higher or similar values in obese than nonobese children, although obese children were usually more sedentary. Obese children spend less time participating in moderate and more vigorous physical activities than lean children (Maffeis, 1998), and their higher energy expenditure is due to a higher energy cost of every-day activities resulting from carrying the extra load of excess fat.

5.5.2 Physical Activity and Adiposity in Early Life

The effect of physical activity on adiposity in children has been studied often since birth and in relation to parents' adiposity. Physical activity measures were not associated with neonatal adiposity, nor was neonatal activity significantly correlated with adiposity in later childhood. Two groups of young children at a low- (group N) and high-risk of developing obesity (group O), judged by parental obesity, were studied in relation to energy intake. Energy intake was 16% lower in group O. Total energy expenditure was determined by the heart rate method (Griffiths, Rivers, and Payne, 1987).

In many studies no significant differences in physical activity levels related to overweight have been found. Reduced energy expenditure in early infancy has been associated with the later development of obesity in children born to overweight mothers, and physical activity level is already associated with risk factors for cardiovascular diseases in childhood (Eisenmann, 2003). The Longitudinal Framingham Heart Study supported the hypothesis that a higher level of physical activity during early childhood results in a reduced deposition of fat (Moore et al., 2003). This study also showed that children who spent most of their time watching television during childhood had the greatest increase in stored fat over time (Proctor et al., 2003). A key factor in overweight children may be a more marked risk for further increase of adiposity due to low levels of physical activity during the preschool period (Trost et al., 2003).

The relationship between energy expenditure and later body composition has been studied in healthy children aged 6.67 ± 0.81 years with body composition evaluated using a standard deuterium oxide dilution technique. Total energy expenditure was measured at the age of 12 weeks using the DLW technique, and there was a wide variation in total energy expenditure, 71.2 ± 20.0 kcal.kg^{-1} body weight, and 91.4 ± 25.0 kcal.kg^{-1} of fat-free mass. However, the correlation between energy expenditure at the age of 12 weeks and body fatness was not significant. In addition, the energy expenditure of infants who at any time in later childhood became overweight was not significantly different from the rest of the group. It was not possible to prove any relationship between early total energy expenditure and body fatness at the age of 6.67 years (Davies, Connolly, and Day, 1993).

Observations in 18-month-old children have shown significant correlations between physical activity levels and caloric intake. Children with a higher caloric intake tended to have lower activity levels. This finding suggests that these two risk factors influencing the development of obesity are likely to occur together in young children (Vara and Agras, 1989). At the preschool age, very active children tended to have a higher food intake than inactive children (Pařízková, 1977, 1991).

Physical activity during growth varies according to age and gender. The level of physical activity is high when BMI decreases during the preschool period and decreases along with the age of adiposity rebound. It may be that all these characteristics are signs of a certain level of maturity for entering primary school. Usually physical activity decreases with increasing age, most commonly after entering primary school. This decrease in activity relates not only to the time spent at school but also during leisure time and weekends, and during and after puberty (Pařízková and Hainer, 1989). Activity was lower in young females compared to males in a group of African-American freshmen as reflected in the Lipid Research Clinic's physical activity questionnaires (Kelley, 1995). There appears to be similar trends in physical activity during adolescence.

A significant association between body weight and physical activity (r = 0.63) was found in 5- to 6-year-old German children; however, the association between fatness and physical activity was weak in preschool children (r = 0.29) (Kortzinger and Mast, 1997). Another study (Klesges, Haddock, and Eck, 1990) of preschool children used direct observation, motion sensor evaluation, and parental reports; no marked associations between physical activity and weight status, and no cardiovascular risks such as blood pressure, were found. As mentioned earlier, this was not true in a study by Davies, Connolly, and Day (1993), who found a significant correlation between the level of physical activity and adiposity in preschool children. However, differences in the results of the above-mentioned studies may be explained by the varying frequency, intensity, duration, and mode of physical activity, and also other factors that were not checked in all of the groups compared.

In a study following TEE (using DLW) in groups of children aged 6 to 8 years with a high and low risk for obesity (with obese or nonobese parents), no significant differences were found (Greene et al., 1998). Regression analysis showed that lean FFM, BMR, body weight, and the percentage of stored fat were better predictors of TEE in high-risk children than parental BMI. A trend to greater adiposity characterized the high-risk group, suggesting that these children may be particularly susceptible to the development of obesity later in life. The time spent in active and sedentary activities was assessed by questionnaire (7-day leisure diary) in two groups of normal-weight children aged 6 to 8 years. These children were either at a high (parental BMI > 29.5 kg/m^2) or low risk of obesity (parental BMI < 28.2 kg/m^2). High-risk children spent significantly more time in active pursuits overall, but were more sedentary on weekends. This may be due to lesser parental encouragement for sports, resulting in a lack of sufficiently intensive exercise to influence the somatic and functional development of children.

Studies in different countries showed that most children, especially those who are obese, spend several hours per day in sedentary activities. Spanish children aged 2 to 5 years of age watched TV for 9 hours per week, those aged 6 to 9 years watched 12.5 hours, and those aged 10 to 13 years watched for 14.6 hours per week. The presence of a TV set, computer, or video games in the child's room increased with age and was in the order of 15%, 9%, and 10%, respectively. Many children also watched TV during breakfast or dinner (Bercedo-Sanz et al., 2001). There appears to be a positive relationship between TV viewing and fatness, that is, children who spend more time with TV watching have increased body weight, BMI, skinfolds, fat mass, and a prevalence of overweight. Similar results were found in U.S. children aged 9 to 12 years (Huston et al., 1992; Vandewater, Shim, Caplowitz, 2004).

Preschool children's TV viewing time depends on the mother's status: those mothers who are in a low-income group, and who have depressive symptoms or are obese, have children who spend three or more hours watching TV per day. The attention and effort to reduce time spent in sedentary activities with the TV set should therefore also be aimed at mothers and their personal situations (Burdette et al., 2003). Accelerometry was used as an objective method for the evaluation of sedentary behavior in young children 3 to 4 years old, with the application of special cutoffs for accelerometry output, which enabled higher sensitivity of activity and/or inactivity evaluation (Reilly et al., 2003). Median time spent in moderate to vigorous physical activity represented only 2% of monitored hours at age 3 years and 4% at age 5 years in Scottish children (mixed longitudinal study), indicating a high level of inactivity from an early age (Reilly et al., 2004). In Australian children aged 5 to 11 years a significant inverse association was found between PAL (evaluated by DLW and BMR; PAL= TEE/BMR), BMI, and body fat. Vigorous physical activity measured by the Tritrac-R3D method correlated significantly and negatively with body fat (Abbott and Davies, 2004).

5.5.3 Physical Activity and Adiposity in School-Aged Children and Adolescents

Numerous studies have considered the relationship between energy intake, physical activity, and body fat. White and black girls aged 9 to 11 years enrolled in the National Heart, Lung, and Blood Institute Growth and Health Study provide some indicative information. Multivariate regression analyses showed that age, the number of hours of television and video watched, the percent of energy from saturated fatty acids, and the activity-patterns score best explained the variation in BMI and the sum of three skinfold measurements in black girls. In white girls, the best model included age, the number of hours of television and video watched, and the percent of energy from total fat (Obarzanek et al., 1994). This study indicates that the percentage of stored fat is related to energy intake and expenditure in both black and white girls.

Parameters of body fatness, food intake, and its composition and the level of physical activity were also specified as the most important factors of obesity in Mexican-American girls (Calderon et al., 1996). These data indicate that the association between activity and fatness only appears at a later age.

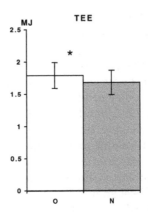

FIGURE 5.5

Comparison of total energy expenditure (TEE) in obese (O) and nonobese (N) adolescents. * indicates (p < 0.05). (Based on data from Bandini, Schoeller, and Dietz, 1990.)

The reported relationship between level of physical activity and body fat varies in some studies with respect to gender. In Swedish adolescents aged 14 to 15 years, a significant relationship was found in boys between physical activity level (PAL = TEE/RMR), TEE evaluated by the minute-to-minute monitoring method, RMR by indirect calorimetry, and body composition (evaluated by skinfolds). The same result was not seen in girls (Ekelund, Yngve, and Sjostrom, 1998).

The etiology of the so-called low RMR syndrome is probably heterogenous, but low plasma T3 and catecholamine levels and Trp64Arg polymorphism of the β_3-adrenergic receptor may be responsible in some cases. Obese subjects with a low value for energy expenditure over 24 hours achieve a smaller weight loss during dietary treatment than subjects with a high value of 24-hour energy expenditure. However, it was assumed that the present lifestyle with physical inactivity might only influence those subjects who are predisposed psychologically and metabolically to reduced activity, and therefore are also susceptible to weight gain and obesity (Astrup, 1998).

Autonomic nervous system function is associated with fatness and activity. Results of a study in Japanese children showed that obese children have reduced sympathetic and parasympathetic nervous activity as compared to lean children who have similar physical activity levels. This autonomic reduction, which is associated with fat deposits in the inactive state, might be an etiological factor in the onset or development of obesity in childhood (Nagai and Moritani, 2004).

Total energy expenditure (measured by DLW) was significantly greater in a group of obese than nonobese 12- to 18-year-old adolescents (Figure 5.5) (Bandini, Schoeller, and Dietz, 1990). Basal metabolic rates determined using indirect calorimetry were highly correlated with FFM in both obese and nonobese groups (r = 0.77, and 0.94, respectively). The basal metabolic rate adjusted for FFM was significantly higher in males than females and in the

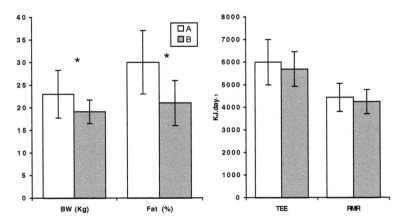

FIGURE 5.6
Differences in body weight (BW kg), percentage of stored fat (fat %), total energy expenditure
(TEE), and resting metabolic rate (RMR) between Pima Indian (A) and white (B) children aged
5 years. * indicates (p < 0.05). (Based on data from Salbe et al., 1997.)

obese subjects. The ratios of total TEE/BMR were not significantly different
in obese and nonobese groups. These results indicate that BMR and TEE are
not reduced in adolescents who are already obese (Bandini, Schoeller, and
Dietz, 1990). However, any difference in both TEE and BMR that may have
preceded the full development of obesity may be a factor. This can be elucidated only by a longitudinal prospective study.

Physical activity levels have also been compared in two populations that
vary markedly in the prevalence of obesity: Pima Indian children and white
children aged 5 years. Total energy expenditure and RMR were measured
by the DLW method and indirect calorimetry. Different indices of physical
activity level were then calculated, including AEE = TEE – (RMR + 0.1 × TEE)
and physical activity level PAL = TEE/RMR. Pima children were significantly heavier than their white peers of the same age and were also fatter.
Total energy expenditure and RMR were similar in both groups (Figure 5.6)
in both absolute values and after adjustment for body weight, FFM, FM, and
gender. Both Pima and white children had PAL levels 20 to 30% lower
(1.35 ± 0.13) than currently recommended by the World Health Organization
(1.7 to 2.0). However, the calculated indices of physical activity were comparable in these two racial groups. Therefore, the differences in physical
activity could hardly be the cause of obesity in Pima Indian children at the
age of 5 years (Salbe et al., 1997a,b).

Some more profound metabolic differences genetically established in Pima
Indians may be the cause, along with a suggested higher food intake in this
obesity-prone population. Important information for the ever-decreasing
physical activity levels in both groups serves as a warning signal for improving the preventive measures for childhood obesity. The time spent in sedentary activities, especially in television viewing in Pima Indian children aged

9.7 ± 2.1 years, predicted weight gain 8 years later at the age of 17.1 ± 1.2 years (Salbe et al., 1998).

The relationships between the level of physical activity and obesity in older Pima Indian and Caucasian children aged 9.9 and 9.7 years, respectively, were also assessed. Pima Indian children were taller, heavier, and fatter. Girls reported significantly lower past-year and past-week sport leisure activities than Caucasian girls and also spent more time watching television. Pima boys also reported lower past-week, sport leisure activity than Caucasian boys. In Pima Indian boys, past-year sport leisure activities correlated negatively with BMI (r = -0.49) and percentage of stored fat (r = -0.56). No similar correlations were found in Pima Indian girls, which was similar to the above-mentioned study (Fontvieille, Kriska, and Ravussin, 1993).

Children of obese Pima Indian parents were significantly heavier and tended to be fatter with a higher absolute fat mass when compared with offspring of thin, lean parents. During both normal and overfeeding conditions, the larger part of variance in 24-hour energy expenditure in a respiratory chamber was accounted for by differences in FFM (54 and 68%, respectively). The differences in the level of spontaneous physical activity accounted for approximately another 19% and 21 percent (Freymond et al., 1989).

In Pima Indian children, decreasing physical activity from 5 to 10 years of age is accompanied by an increase in weight and adiposity, which is further associated with decreases in insulin sensitivity (ISI). In children whose decrease in activity was smaller, the decrease of ISI was also smaller, which was independent of the changes of weight and adiposity. The establishment and maintenance of an increased level of physical activity can be relevant not only from the point of view of obesity epidemiology but also from the point of view of increasing prevalence of type 2 diabetes in children (Bunt et al., 2003). Physical activity correlated significantly negatively with sum of skinfolds in Hong Kong boys, but not in girls (Rowlands et al., 2002).

In a study by Schutz (1989), measurements of energy expenditure by indirect calorimetry showed a linear relationship between body weight and 24-hour activity energy expenditure. The absolute rate of energy expenditure, especially during weight-bearing activities, is not lower in the obese compared to lean subjects since the hypoactivity does not fully compensate for the greater gross energy cost of a given activity. Similar conclusions have been reported by other researchers (Maffeis et al., 1996; Maffeis, Zaffanello, and Schutz, 1997). However, when discriminating TEE and AEE, the results revealed that in spite of comparable TEE in both obese and normal-weight subjects, the level of activity and energy expended from activity was lower in obese children (Figures 5.7 and 5.8).

The measurement of total daily energy expenditure (TDEE) in free-living conditions (assessed by heart rate using individually determined regression lines at various levels of activity) in obese and nonobese children, aged 9.1 ± 1.6 years and 9.2 ± 0.4 years, respectively, showed higher values of TDEE in obese children. However, the time spent in physical activity was lower in the obese than in the nonobese. This result seemed to be compensated by a

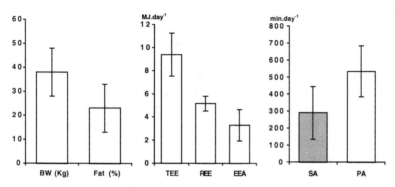

FIGURE 5.7
Body weight, percentage of stored fat (fat %), total and resting energy expenditure (TEE, REE), and energy expenditure for activity (EEA), for both sedentary (SA) and nonsedentary physical activities (PA) in 9-year-old boys with broad range of characteristics. Relationship of SA and % fat, r = 0.46 (p < 0.05). (Based on data from Maffeis, Zaffanello, and Schutz, 1997.)

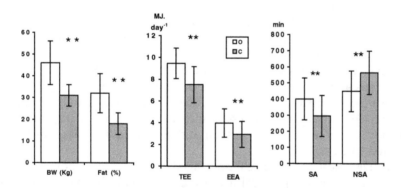

FIGURE 5.8
Comparison of body weight (BW), percentage of stored fat (fat %), total energy expenditure (TEE), energy expenditure for activity (EEA, MJ/day), and duration of sedentary (SA) and nonsedentary activities (NSA) in obese (O) and nonobese (C) 8- to 10-year-old children. ** indicates (p < 0.01). (Based on data from Maffeis et al., 1996.)

higher energy cost of activity due to higher body weight. In addition, under sedentary conditions obese children expend more energy than control children. Energy intake was comparable in both groups, but this lack of difference may be due to underreporting by obese subjects (Maffeis, Zafanello, Schutz, 1997). Time devoted to sedentary activities was directly proportional to fat mass percentage (r = 0.46, p < 0.05), which suggests the importance of the role of muscular activities in the prevention of the deposition of excess fat. Total energy expenditure was significantly higher in the obese group than in the nonobese group, and the energy expenditure for physical activity together with thermogenesis was significantly higher in obese children (Maffeis et al., 1996).

Higher energy expenditure in obese subjects during laboratory functional testing such as walking and running on a treadmill was found in a group of prepubertal children (Maffeis et al., 1993b). At the same speed of exercise during the test the energy expenditure was significantly greater in the obese than in control children. Energy expenditure per kg of total and/or FFM was comparable for both groups. Obese children had a significantly larger pulmonary ventilatory response to this workload than did normal-weight control children. Heart rate was comparable in boys and girls combined but significantly higher in obese subjects. These data indicate that walking and running are energetically more demanding for the obese than for normal-weight subjects. Similar results were gained during functional testing in other groups of obese children (see Chapter 12) (Pařízková, 1977). This also helps to explain why obese individuals spontaneously reduce their physical activity levels, especially weight-bearing activities such as running and walking.

In a group of obese and nonobese prepubertal children, TEE was significantly higher than energy intake in the obese children, but comparable to total energy expenditure in the nonobese children. This discrepancy may also be explained by the underreporting of food intake in the obese children, an invalid method in this age group (Maffeis et al., 1994a).

A study by Almeida, Fox, and Boutcher (1998) reported on the measurement of physical activity level using the Tritrac accelerometer during two weekdays and two weekend days. In addition, an estimation of body fat from triceps and subscapular skinfolds in adolescent girls (14.9 ± 0.6 years) and boys (15.2 ± 0.8 years) was made. Results revealed significant correlations between activity and fatness in girls ($r = -0.438$, $p < 0.05$), but not in boys. Boys were more active in total and had a limited range of fatness compared to girls.

A further study of Italian children aged 6 to 14 years showed a poor response to voluntary physical activity and exercise during leisure time, along with incorrect nutritional habits, which also concerned subjects enrolled in sport activities (Caldarone et al., 1995). Clearly, an inadequate lifestyle can be a concern for children from an early age when desirable physical activity and dietary habits and a necessary fitness level should be established. To neglect this critical period would mean the correction later may be more and more difficult as it is hard to persuade children to take part in activities that are perceived as too difficult and thus unpleasant for them (Borra et al., 1995).

Some studies have not shown the expected effect of physical activity. For example, a study in a multiethnic sample did not show any differences in physical activity between obese and nonobese girls in grades 5 through to 12. Hispanics and Asians reported lower activity levels than other racial groups. Only 36% of the entire sample and less than one-fifth of either Asians or Hispanics met the year 2000 goal for strenuous physical activity, which decreased with age (Wolf et al., 1993). The time spent participating in games in obese and nonobese Italian children was not different, and the type of game, that is, sedentary or active, was not associated with body mass index (Chiloiro et al., 1998).

Another study of obese and normal-weight children did not show any between-group differences in daily activities (using a questionnaire). However, the sport grades at school were lower and the participation in the training teams of sport clubs less frequent among obese than normal-weight children. Obese children were also less fit as judged from the pedaling time in an exercise test on a bicycle ergometer and from the maximum oxygen uptake (VO_2 max) related to lean body mass (Huttunen, Knip, and Paavilainen, 1986).

Measurements lasting two days did not reveal any differences between obese and nonobese boys and girls' physical activity levels, or their total attitude toward physical activity. There were no significant relationships between child and maternal activity level, attitude toward physical activity, and adipose level. Obese and nonobese children showed similar levels of physical activity and attitude toward activity, which was unrelated to maternal factors measured. However, the levels of physical activity were generally low in both obese and nonobese subjects and did not seem to have an important role in their weight control (Romanella et al., 1991). Unfortunately, measurement was undertaken across a very short period of time.

Comparisons between other groups of obese and nonobese adolescents have confirmed the lack of differences in TDEE, measured by DLW. This applied to the period of weight maintenance (intake $1.61 \times BMR$), and also to the period of carbohydrate overloading ($2.45 \times BMR$) (Bandini et al., 1989). BMR measured by indirect calorimetry increased comparably in both obese and nonobese adolescents under such conditions.

In a study of French adolescents aged 12 to 16 years, the relationships between daily energy expenditure (DEE) evaluated from a long-term measurement of heart rate and whole body indirect calorimetry, body composition (skinfolds and BIA), and physical activity were examined. Individual relationships between energy expenditure and heart rate were computed and regression equations derived, enabling the evaluation of energy expenditure under free conditions over five days, including the weekend. Intra-group variability in DEE, adjusted for differences in FFM, increased during weekends, especially in males. These results were related to the level of physical activity. Nineteen percent of males and 43% of females had a decrease in energy expenditure during weekends compared with school days without any physical training (Vermorel et al., 1998). This indicates the passive character of leisure time in adolescent subjects.

Groups of fifth graders, subdivided according to the level of obesity, were examined for TDEE using DLW, RMR, and body composition measures (tertiles of subscapular plus triceps skinfolds). No differences in FFM between the groups were revealed, while the highest tertile group weighed 14 Kg more than the lowest. Mean energy expenditure using either day was nearly identical (Figure 5.9). No differences in RMR, energy expended in activity, or TDEE were observed between the three groups. A reduction in

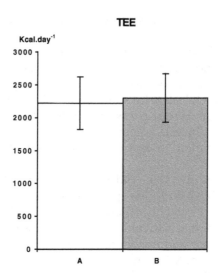

FIGURE 5.9
Daily total energy expenditure (TEE) in groups of obese prepubertal children from highest (A) and lowest (B) tertiles of body weight and fatness. (Based on data from DeLany et al., 1995.)

RMR or TDEE could not explain differences in obesity in these prepubertal children. However, the fact that the heaviest children expended the same amount of energy in activity and had the same TDEE as the leanest while weighing 14 Kg more indicates that the obese children had a reduced activity level (DeLany et al., 1995). This could be explained by the greater energy demands for the same movement due to an excess fat load interfering especially during dynamic, weight-bearing activities.

Studies using DLW have shown that as a group, obese children consume more energy and have a higher TEE than lean children. In many follow-ups, energy intake has been reported as the same and sometimes lower in obese children. Therefore, it was assumed that energy imbalance is particularly due to a decreased TEE and cannot explain the deposition of excess fat. However, underreporting of food intake in the obese and higher energy efficiency in subjects predisposed and developing obesity was also considered. This question requires further research focused on complex longitudinal studies evaluating simultaneous and repeated energy intake and output along with BMI and body composition changes, at least from the beginning of an increased deposition of fat.

Additional results have also shown comparable energy expenditure in obese and normal-weight children after adjustment for body size. Therefore, at least on a group basis, there does not appear to be any defects in energy metabolism that would predispose obesity (DeLany, 1998; DeLany et al., 1995, 1998). However, a low level of physical activity is associated with increased body fatness in some cross-sectional studies, and more importantly, in some longitudinal studies in both normal-weight and obese children. These findings indicate that a low level of physical activity is important in the development of pediatric obesity and that intervention programs with increased exercise are essential for its rectification, especially in subjects with low physical activity levels.

5.5.4 Longitudinal Studies of Physical Activity, Fatness, and Cardiovascular Risks

The Amsterdam Growth and Health Longitudinal Study (AGAHLS) showed that the development of fat is fairly predictable, especially on the basis of the repeated assessments of the level of physical activity. This study is the longest study executed repeatedly on the same subjects, from 13 to 27 years of age. The protocol includes measurement of four skinfolds, dietary intake (cross-check dietary history interview in a time frame of the last three months), and physical activity level (standardized activity interview based on a questionnaire, retrospective over the previous three months).

The results showed a steep decrease in energy expenditure from the age of 13 years from about 4500 METS per week to 3000 METS at the age of 27 years. Data on dietary intake confirmed the decrease of energy per Kg of body weight from about 225 kJ per day at the age of 13 years to about 155 kJ at the age of 27 years. The energy turnover was higher in males than in females during adolescence, with energy intake 15% and energy output 20% higher in boys. At the age of 23 years, the gender difference in energy intake was reduced to 10%, and the difference in energy output disappeared.

Low stability coefficients were found for physical activity (0.34: 0.19–0.49), but higher coefficients were revealed for dietary intake (0.55: 0.45–0.64) and fat mass (0.63: 0.56–0.71). Somewhat surprisingly, fat mass was negatively related with daily energy intake. The longitudinal relationship between fat mass and physical activity corrected for dietary intake between the ages of 13 and 27 years showed a significant negative relationship when fat mass was estimated from the sum of four skinfolds but not when estimated from the values of BMI (Kemper et al., 1999). Therefore, this unique longitudinal study involving the same subjects provides much more reliable results and also reinforces the effect of physical activity and exercise on body adiposity.

With regard to risk, injuries must be considered when recommending increased physical activity and exercise. Obese children may be more threatened than nonobese children (see Chapter 6), especially during certain sport activities. A well-planned program with sound equipment and supervision can help to avoid accidents (Flynn, Lou, and Ganley, 2002).

5.6 Social Class, Fatness, and Physical Activity

Social class affects the prevalence of obesity and participation in regular exercise. In low socioeconomic districts, the rate of overweight and obese children was up to 23% higher and the enrollment in sports activity was low. In contrast, in high social class districts, the rate of overweight and obese children was lower and the rate of sporting children higher (Petersen, 1998).

Observations in preschool children from low-income families showed that during free play periods 58% of time was devoted to sedentary activities, and only 11% to vigorous physical activities. Children's BMI, teacher-rated type A behavior, parent-reported mother and father BMI, parents' vigorous activities, and family history of cardiovascular diseases (CVD) risks were the independent variables studied. The multiple regression of moderate-intensity activity was significant; family cardiovascular risk, parent vigorous activity, and father's BMI accounted for a significant amount of variance. The results indicate that the parental role in modeling physical activity for their young children may extend beyond the confines of their home (Sallis et al., 1988).

5.7 Summary

Energy expenditure as related to energy intake is one of the most important determinants of body adiposity. Individual components such as basal metabolic rate (BMR), resting metabolic rate (RMR), and thermic effect of food (TEF, or diet-induced thermogenesis [DIT]) were followed in obese and normal-weight children, and differences were found in relation to age, gender, duration, and degree of obesity. RMR and BMR were mostly higher in obese subjects, but when related to lean, fat-free body mass, the differences between obese and normal-weight children were commonly not apparent. Thermic effect of food expressed as a percentage of the energy content of a meal was lower in the obese. Findings on the activity energy expenditure (AEE) as a part of total energy expenditure (TEE) were mostly lower in the obese, but previous results have been contradictory, possibly due to methodological problems. Total energy expenditure was not always lower in the obese and in some studies was found to be higher. This is due to the additional burden of fat, which for the same physically defined task demands greater strain and energy output (especially of dynamic, aerobic character when lifting one's own body weight). However, when considering the nature of different activities, reduced activity was most common in the obese and was often characterized by TV viewing — a key marker of sedentarism. Familial clustering of not only obesity but also physical activity habits and lifestyle often showed the effect of genetic, hereditary factors.

Most studies revealed that physical activity levels have been decreasing during recent decades in all groups of individuals. Therefore, it might be concluded that at present, both obese and nonobese children display low levels of physical activity. As the average BMI of the adult population has been increasing, it could be suggested that even growing subjects who are lean at present may become overweight or obese in adulthood, provided poor lifestyle behaviors are maintained. This concerns children in all countries including those of the Third World, where social, economic, and lifestyle habits including diet and physical activity level and workload have changed markedly and rather rapidly.

The results of studies to date indicate that children — particularly those of obese parents and those with low levels of physical activity — are predisposed to obesity, especially when an inadequate diet is also present. The classic adage of the multifactorial origin of childhood obesity, including physical inactivity, seems to be valid in spite of contradictions regarding the relationship between activity and fatness presented in some studies.

Carrying an excess load of stored fat increases the energy cost of the same dynamic activity. For example, running on a treadmill with a load (James and Schofield, 1990) results in a higher energy cost than without a load when completing the same exercise. The higher energy cost of dynamic activities and lower mechanical efficiency in the obese increases the strain and discomfort of any physical activity. This is the most common reason for the spontaneous reduction of such activities when measured repeatedly during prolonged periods of time (Kemper et al., 1990, 1999) and, as such, is recognized as one of the most important causes of the globally increasing obesity found in children and adolescents. An increase in energy expenditure is fundamental to the successful reduction of adiposity. This can best be achieved with a stepwise exposure to dynamic aerobic exercise that is progressively prescribed at an individualized intensity to maximize energy expenditure in a given period of time and according to individual management of obesity.

6

Evaluation of Functional Status

The level of physical fitness and physical performance is among the most important characteristics of the human organism. There are different indicators of functional capacity, the most important being cardiorespiratory fitness and endurance, motor and sensorimotor development, muscular strength, motor skill and coordination. Psychological factors also play a significant role in functional performance.

An appropriate level of physical fitness and performance are essential ingredients not only for a meaningful standard of participation in sport and athletic activities but as an essential ingredient of the functional status of all individuals. For example, a particular standing in cardiorespiratory fitness and skill would concern everybody. Functional characteristics and capacity to perform daily living tasks with ease may be far more important criteria than body size and other capacities usually assessed.

The evaluation of functional status in marginally malnourished children from some developing countries has demonstrated that in certain functional characteristics, especially those concerning the cardiovascular and respiratory systems, such individuals were on a higher level than normally fed children from industrially developed countries. Obese children may also have a range of suboptimal functional characteristics. Workload testing is a valid means of evaluating the functional status of obese children (Owens et al., 1999) and has enabled the definition of a particular treatment approach and its consequences.

Physical fitness has been defined as an ability to carry out daily tasks with vigor and alertness without undue fatigue, with ample energy to enjoy leisure time pursuits, and to meet unforeseen emergencies (Nieman, 2003). Numerous other definitions of fitness exist but all largely express the same views. Physical fitness is partly conditioned genetically and is also related to health status. Fitness can be increased significantly by the process of adaptation to various types of physical activity and exercise that stimulate the individual systems related to physical performance (Åstrand and Rodahl, 1977; Niemann, 2003).

Physical fitness is comprised of numerous components. An adequate level on one of the components of fitness does not necessarily mean a corresponding adequacy in another item. This is particularly the case in obese children.

Excess fat does not always interfere with individual functional characteristics in the same manner so the level of physical performance and fitness in the young obese individual is modified in a characteristic way, not always negatively. This chapter outlines some of the more important issues in relation to functional status of an individual and considers both the development and the evaluation of these items.

Physical and motor-related components of fitness that may have some bearing on locomotor ability and movement characteristics of children include indices of cardiorespiratory function, flexibility, muscular strength and endurance, and agility. Cardiorespiratory capacity is most frequently linked with general health maintenance and is an important limiting factor in the performance of all aerobic tasks in both weight-supported tasks such as riding a bicycle ergometer and activities such as walking and running.

Observations in obese children have revealed a less efficient cardiopulmonary response. Heart rate, systolic blood pressure, and forced vital capacity are significantly different in this population during and after exercise. A significant positive correlation has been reported between heart rate and biceps skinfold thickness (Tang et al., 2002).

6.1 Cardiorespiratory Function

6.1.1 Criteria and Methods

Cardiorespiratory function can be evaluated by different tests. It is commonly assessed through measurements of aerobic power expressed as the oxygen uptake during a maximal or peak workload (VO_2 max) on a treadmill or bicycle ergometer. Functional capacity can be expressed in the absolute ($ml.O_2^{-1}.min^{-1}$) and relative values, that is, values related to total and/or lean, fat-free body mass ($ml.O_2^{-1}.min^{-1}.kg$ BW^{-1} and/or LBW^{-1}). The capacity to transfer oxygen to the working tissues, mainly skeletal muscles, depends on the efficiency of the heart muscle, and vascular and respiratory systems. Therefore, the peak value of oxygen uptake during a defined period of time (commonly one minute) of workload gives the best information on the level of aerobic power and cardiorespiratory efficiency of the individual. Key elements are the duration of the increasing workload and the final value of peak or max O_2 uptake.

The evaluation of aerobic fitness using absolute values of maximal oxygen uptake (VO_2 max) can be misleading as it can be quite high even in obese subjects, and not always reveal the "true" level of physical fitness. As this test measures O_2 during a dynamic, weight-bearing workload, it is necessary to consider body weight, especially its total value, including stored fat. VO_2 max is therefore related to total and/or lean body mass. However, relating O_2 to lean, fat-free body mass is also not logical as it is not possible to execute the workload without an individual's own weight of fat, and the work performance must be realized with the simultaneous loading by an excess inert mass. A similar parallel may be to exercise with a suitcase or a knapsack equivalent to the excess weight.

The level of performance achieved must also be taken into account. When evaluating aerobic power, it is desirable to consider the conditions during which it was achieved, for example, the distance covered and speed or the slope of the treadmill. During the bicycle ergometer test, the level of performance can also be expressed in physical terms (Watts.min^{-1}). Real performance is more important in everyday life than a theoretical value of the consumed O_2.

Simultaneously, other variables such as CO_2 output, the respiratory quotient (RQ), ventilation (in absolute values and related to total and lean, FFM), breathing frequency, and blood pressure are usually assessed. Individual parameters are commonly expressed over one minute. More recent studies with newer technology enable the breath-by-breath analysis of all the parameters mentioned.

Functional capacity of the cardiorespiratory system is often evaluated during other types of workload — for example, during a standard workload (equal to various proportions of VO_2 max such as one-third, one-sixth, and so on), or at the level of PWC_{170} (the physical working capacity at the level of 170 beats per minute).

DuRant, Dover, and Alpert (1983) assessed indices of working capacity in children and found that PWC_{170} discriminated between underweight, normal-weight, and overweight children. This finding is indicative of overweight and obese children scoring lower on PWC than normal-weight children. In contrast, the results from other indices tended to overestimate the capacity of overweight children equating them with normal-weight children. The submaximal PWC_{170} is an appropriate regimen for the assessment of aerobic capacity.

Some contention surrounds the choice of the most suitable ergometer procedure to employ in PWC_{170} estimation. These concerns have related to the initial loading, load increments, number of workloads, and duration and frequency of pedalling. Cognizant of these concerns, the authors have used the following protocol. Physical working capacity (PWC_{170}) can be ascertained following heart rate response to exercise at three successive workloads on a mechanically braked Monark cycle ergometer following an appropriate warm-up and familiarization with equipment. Three workloads are suggested with an initial load of 1 watt per kilogram of body weight (1 W.kg^{-1}) and the further two increments of 0.5 or 1 watt depending on the heart rate reached, with each load lasting two minutes. Subjects pedal at a rate of 60rpm (range 58 to 62). The seat of the cycle ergometer should be adjusted to the position of maximum comfort for each subject. Data on the above-mentioned workloads are used to ascertain both PWC_{170} (kpm.min^{-1} and Watts^{-1}) and PWC_{170} (kpm.kg.$^{-1}$min^{-1} and Watts.kg^{-1}). A similar procedure was also used in the earlier International Biological Programme (IBP) for the evaluation of physical fitness, body composition, and motor abilities of a representative sample of 2471 Czech subjects 12 to 55 years old (Seliger et al., 1978).

Aerobic power is differentiated from anaerobic power (the capacity to work involves a period under anaerobic conditions), and therefore is an important factor in cardiorespiratory fitness. Ventilatory threshold (VT, or anaerobic threshold AT or VT), is defined as the greatest oxygen uptake at which pulmonary ventilation stops to increase linearly with increasing exercise intensity, and starts to take a steeper slope. This measure is also used for the evaluation of the efficiency of the cardiorespiratory system and the overall level of physical fitness and performance. A detailed description of these functional measurements is provided in a number of textbooks on exercise physiology (Åstrand and Rodahl, 1977; McArdle, Katch, and Katch, 1991). In many studies, approaches are used simultaneously to provide a more accurate characterization of different aspects of cardiorespiratory fitness.

6.1.2 The Effect of Age, Gender, and Body Composition in Normal and Obese Children

Reviews of the epidemiological studies on physical fitness and physical activity in normal-weight children show significant developmental trends and gender differences. Some comparisons show that aerobic power (VO_2 max) related to body mass remains stable from 6 to 16 years in boys. However, when comparing different groups in individual age categories, some developmental trends might be obscured because of the lack of homogeneity of subjects in these groups. Longitudinal studies in which repeated measurements of individual characteristics with increasing age are taken show the developmental trends. Such studies are rare due to the difficulty in preserving the same groups over a number of years. A longitudinal study on adolescent boys (from 10.8 to 17.8 years of age) showed an increase in aerobic power (VO_2 max.min^{-1}.kg body weight^{-1} and/or kg lean body mass^{-1}) until 14 to 15 years and then a decline. The decline is less or not apparent in trained subjects enrolled in regular sport training (Pařízková, 1977).

Meaningful comparisons between different studies can be limited, even when considering a single parameter such as cardiorespiratory function. Groups of children tested using different protocols and procedures and at various chronological and maturational age and degrees of obesity make comparisons awkward. For example, treadmill protocols may use different speeds and workloads and may or may not use a slope. Moreover, these procedures are not always described in detail in the literature. Therefore, it is only possible to consider the conclusions. To directly compare the individual values is difficult due to the methodological differences mentioned and may give spurious conclusions. Therefore, wherever possible a more detailed description of individual studies is given in this volume.

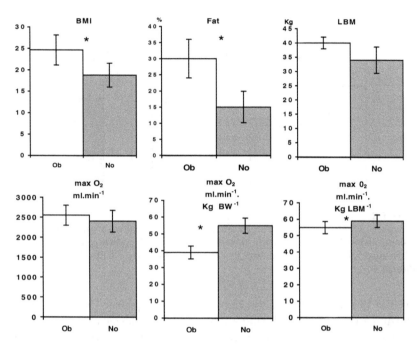

FIGURE 6.1

Comparison of body mass index (BMI), percentage of stored fat (%), lean fat-free body mass (LBM, kg), aerobic power expressed as oxygen uptake during maximal workload on a treadmill in absolute values as related to total and/or lean, fat-free body mass in obese (Ob) and normal-weight (No) boys. * indicates ($p < 0.05$). (Based on data from Pařízková, 1977, Pařízková, 1968a, 1998.)

Normal-weight girls have lower aerobic power than boys by approximately 25%, which usually decreases during prepubertal and pubertal periods. Reports on physical activity have shown that boys are about 15 to 25% more active than females (Sallis, 1993). This review indicated that older youth and especially girls are at an increased risk of obesity, mainly due to a sedentary lifestyle.

6.1.3 The Effect of Obesity

Figure 6.1 shows a comparison of body composition and aerobic power of normal-weight and obese boys at the age of 11.7 years. Obese boys of the same age were slightly taller and heavier in total, lean, and fat body mass. The absolute values of VO_2 max.min^{-1} were the same in both groups (Pařízková, 1977). This result was also found in other studies (Elliot et al., 1989; Maffeis et al., 1994a). However, when maximal oxygen was related to total and/or lean body mass, the values were significantly lower in the obese. The peak level of maximal oxygen uptake was achieved in obese boys after a shorter period of running on a treadmill at a lower speed, with the performance achieved being worse in the obese children.

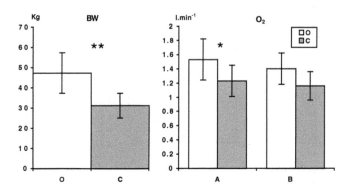

FIGURE 6.2

Comparison of body weight and oxygen uptake during maximal workload on a (A) treadmill (2% slope) and a (B) stationary bicycle in obese (O) and control, normal-weight (C) prepubertal children aged 9.5 ± 0.8 years. * indicates (p < 0.05); ** indicates (p < 0.01). (Based on data from Maffeis et al., 1994b.)

Similar measurements of the maximal aerobic power (VO_2 max) (Figure 6.2) using an open circuit during a workload on a bicycle ergometer showed higher absolute values in obese children aged 9.5 ± 0.8 years compared to normal-weight control children of the same age. When expressed per kilogram of fat-free mass, the differences disappeared (Maffeis et al., 1994b). Results related to total body mass were not given in this study.

Measurements in obese Tunisian girls showed lower values of maximal oxygen uptake per kilogram of body weight along with a lower BMR, energy expenditure, and physical activity level (Figure 6.3), along with a markedly increased energy intake (Pařízková et al., 1995a).

Performance characterized by the oxygen uptake evaluated during a standard workload on a bicycle ergometer was also significantly different in normal-weight and obese boys. During the same workload, the oxygen uptake and heart rate were significantly higher in the obese; therefore the same performance was executed under conditions of a higher energy output (see Chapter 12) (Pařízková, 1977).

It is rare in the literature to find international comparisons between studies with a consistent protocol, but this was possible in the 1960s in the framework of the International Biological Program (IBP) (see Pařízková, 1985; Seliger et al., 1978). This large international study followed somatic, body composition, cardiorespiratory, and motor development of a sample of 2471 subjects aged 12 to 55 years; unfortunately, this study was not repeated with a comparatively complex program.

Obese children 6 to 17 years old had higher absolute oxygen uptakes during a treadmill exercise test, which, however, were decreased significantly when related to body mass or body surface area. The ventilatory efficiency as a slope or as a simple ratio of anaerobic threshold did not differ between obese and normal-weight children. The absolute metabolic cost of exercise was higher

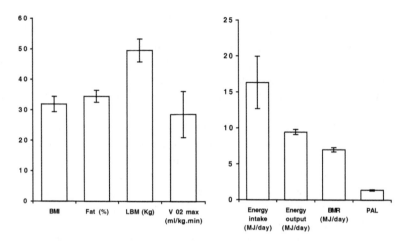

FIGURE 6.3

Body mass index (BMI), percentage of stored fat (% fat), lean body mass (LBM, kg) aerobic power (oxygen uptake during maximal workload related to body weight, VO_2 max.kg^{-1}), energy intake and output, basal metabolic rate (BMR), and physical activity level (PAL = 1.35) in obese Tunisian adolescent girls. (Based on data from Pařízková et al., 1995.)

in the obese children, who also rated perceived exertion during test to be substantially higher (Marinov, Kostianev, and Turnovska, 2002).

Aerobic power was evaluated in another study during an incremental treadmill test in obese and nonobese prepubescent girls aged 7 to 12 years. Open circuit calorimetry was used and maximal oxygen uptake (VO_2 max.kg body weight^{-1}) was significantly lower in obese subjects (23.0 ± 3.9 ml.kg^{-1}.min^{-1}) compared to normal-weight controls (36.0 ± 0.9 ml.kg^{-1}.min^{-1}). Exercise tolerance was also longer in nonobese girls, although this result was not statistically significant. These data also indicate that excess body weight, due to increased fatness, diminishes cardiopulmonary performance and attenuates exercise tolerance in prepubescent obese females similar to other subjects (DeMeersman et al., 1985).

Similar observations were found in other groups of obese children aged 9 to 14 years, in which gas exchange was assessed during exercise. Maximal oxygen uptake (VO_2 max) as related to total body weight was significantly lower in obese subjects than in normal-weight children. Ventilatory anaerobic threshold (VAT) as a percentage of VO_2 max was similar in both groups. A significant correlation was found between VAT and VO_2 max in both obese and normal-weight children. The habitual level of physical activity was lower in the obese subjects compared to controls. These results show that the level of physical fitness is reduced in obese children. Fitness can be assessed by the measurements of VAT, which does not require a maximal workload and is therefore suitable for the evaluation of subjects with exercise intolerance (Zanconato et al., 1989).

Other measurements also revealed lower aerobic power (VO_2 max.ml^{-1}.min^{-1}, VO_2 max.ml^{-1}.kg^{-1} body weight) and reduced physical working capacity

(PWC$_{170}$). Both of these parameters were significantly lower than in normal-weight children (Tamiya, 1991). Measurements in Russian children showed that those with moderate, average, or slightly higher body mass had the highest level of physical working capacity PWC$_{170}$.kg body weight^{-1}. With increasing weight, a decrease in working capacity was apparent, and this was most pronounced in obese subjects (Malova, Simonova, and Fetisov, 1993).

The relationship between the content of stored fat, ranging from normal to gross obesity, was assessed in adolescent females. Skinfold thickness correlated significantly with the absolute values of maximal oxygen uptake. That is, the higher the body weight and fatness, the higher the maximal oxygen uptake in absolute values, but correlated significantly negatively with oxygen uptake per kilogram of body weight and treadmill endurance time ($r = 0.49$ and 0.42, respectively).

Obesity did not affect submaximal walking economy (Rowland, 1991). These results indicate that increased fat levels increase oxygen uptake during a workload but functional fitness — that is, the performance achieved declines because of the inert load created by excess stored fat.

In another study of obese girls aged 7 to 11 years, no relationship was proved for VO$_2$ max (assessed on a bicycle ergometer test) and the percentage of stored fat (DXA). Significant correlations were found for VO$_2$ max and leg lean mass and/or total lean body mass. These data suggest that aerobic power is mainly dependent on lean, fat-free body mass when not using weight-bearing exercise on a treadmill (Fernandez et al., 1998a). However, in other studies, a significant negative relationship between VO$_2$ max and body fatness was found (see Pařízková, 1977). Such relationships, however, appear to be most significant when the range of the assessed values is sufficiently large. In homogeneous groups they may not be apparent at all.

Obese children often display abnormal reactions to exercise, but their real lack of fitness is also sometimes questioned. In obese subjects aged 9 to 17 years, size-independent measures of exercise — that is, the ratio of O$_2$ uptake (VO$_2$) to work rate during progressive workload and the temporal response VO$_2$, carbon dioxide output (VCO$_2$) and minute ventilation (VE) at the onset of exercise — were used. The ability to perform external mechanical work was corrected for VO$_2$ max at unloaded pedaling (change in VO$_2$ max, that is, delta VO$_2$ max) and in anaerobic threshold (delta AT). On average, children's responses were in the normal range. However, in one-third of the obese children tested, values of delta VO$_2$ max or delta AT of more than 2SD below normal were found. With increasing age, no increase of delta VO$_2$ max, or delta AT, was found in obese children and adolescents, which is usual in normal-weight children. Although the response time of VO$_2$ max was normal (with regard to predicted values) those for both VCO$_2$ and VE were prolonged (Cooper et al., 1990). These results indicate that not every obese child is unfit and that testing cardiorespiratory response is indispensable for the selection of subjects with more serious functional impairment.

The effect of excess fat on functional capacity seems to be dependent on the nature of the individual at the onset of obesity.

Thai children aged 9.2 years with differing degrees of adiposity were evaluated using the following tests: evaluation of maximal oxygen uptake (VO_2 max during a submaximal bicycle ergometer testing); vital capacity; 50-meter run; flexibility (sit-and-reach); and abdominal strength and endurance (30-sec sit-ups). The usual gender differences were seen, that is, better results in boys except for flexibility. However, gender differences in fitness levels were not apparent in obese groups, unlike in normal-weight children. The performance levels varied significantly according to the degree of obesity, especially in the VO_2 max test (Pongprapai, Mo-suwan, and Leelasamran, 1994).

Oxygen uptake and energy output measured by open circuit spirometry during walking at four different speeds was assessed in obese boys and girls. Energy output was related to total and lean, FFM (measured by hydrodensitometry). ANOVA analysis revealed significant differences in the energy output between the speed conditions. There was no significant difference between genders such as in the amount and distribution of fat (see Chapter 4) (Pařízková, 1977).

A nonlinear increase in energy output with increasing speed indicated a decreasing efficiency with increasing speed of walking. Biomechanical factors may be important in this respect. These factors include the extra energy output needed to accelerate the extremities and trunk, increased energy output due to increased inertia, and increased upper-body forward lean to maintain balance at faster speeds of movement. An increased load in the form of excess fat may be responsible for this lower efficiency (Katch et al., 1988b).

The level of cardiovascular fitness was evaluated in groups of children aged 8 to 13 years with high and low adiposity (evaluated by three skinfolds: triceps, subscapular, and suprailiac). Physical working capacity (PWC_{170}) was used for the evaluations. The most important predictor of cardiovascular fitness in high-adiposity children was the physical activity score computed for each child from a two-day observation period. Thirty-eight percent of the variance in PWC_{170} was accounted for by age, BMI, and physical activity scores (Taylor and Baranowski, 1991).

Measurements of VAT in children aged 4 to 16 years on a treadmill showed significantly lower values in obese compared to normal-weight peers. The habitual level of physical activity assessed by questionnaires was 27% ($p < 0.01$) lower in the obese compared to healthy controls. Strikingly lower ventilatory thresholds in the obese children may cause those children to avoid moderate or strenuous exercise because of the higher degree of effort needed. This mechanism is also assumed as essential for the maintenance of obesity during childhood (Reybrouck et al., 1987, 1997).

Oxygen uptake (VO_2 max) and carbon dioxide output (VCO_2) were measured in obese children aged 11 ± 3.8 years during a workload on a treadmill.

The analysis of respiratory gas exchange was measured breath by breath. The BMI of the obese children was 25.0 ± 0.20. To eliminate the effect of body weight, the slope of VO_2 versus VCO_2 was evaluated. This slope was calculated below the ventilatory threshold (S1) and above the ventilatory threshold (S3). The comparison of the results showed that S3 was significantly steeper in the obese compared to normal-weight children in a comparable age range (10.8 ± 2.2 years). The steepest values for S3 were found in the subjects with the highest degree of obesity. This approach has limitations since in a large proportion of subjects (48%) the VT could not be achieved.

However, these measurements again demonstrated that cardiorespiratory exercise function in obese children is reduced, especially during dynamic, weight-bearing exercise (Reybrouck et al., 1997). From these results, it follows that obesity interferes with athletic activities, mainly those with a dynamic performance component and of an aerobic nature, such as running or cycling.

In studies undertaken by the author (Hills and Parker, 1988, 1990) obese subjects were grossly disadvantaged in some movement tasks recording lower scores on PWC_{170} than normal-weight subjects, even following correction for body weight. Obese subjects also scored appreciably higher 600-meter run times than lighter counterparts, and ability to balance in the stork stand test was inferior. The relatively short duration tasks of standing broad jump and shuttle run were less of a problem for obese subjects. Significant positive correlations were found between both height and sitting height and standing broad jump indicative of the advantage gained via body dimensions favoring linearity. Significant negative correlations were found between body weight and PWC_{170} ($kpm.kg^{-1}.min^{-1}$), the sum of three circumferences and PWC_{170}, and the sum of four skinfolds and PWC_{170}. In the obese group only a limited number of high correlations between physical and motor fitness variables were found compared to the lighter group. Both groups showed a strong association between grip strength and most measures, but correlations were stronger in the normal-weight group. The most significant relationship was between the strength measure and body mass (0.662 versus 0.864). Similar findings were seen for all other measures in the normal-weight group except PWC_{170} ($kpm.kg^{-1}.min^{-1}$). The relationship between cardiorespiratory working capacity and many anthropometric and body composition measures was pronounced in this group.

The results of this study indicate the greater working capacity of normal-weight prepubertal children compared with obese children and support the evidence derived from similar studies of older children. Obese children, due to their greater fat content, showed an operational disadvantage in PWC_{170} $kpm.kg^{-1}.min^{-1}$ and negative correlations between PWC_{170} and body weight. The results have implications for the involvement of obese children in aerobic physical activity by adding objective evidence in contrast to the many generalized claims made by other studies regarding movement capacity and quality of movement in this population (Hills and Parker, 1988).

The results of a fitness test on a treadmill (PWC_{170}) correlated negatively with C-reactive protein (CRP); this relationship was more pronounced in boys than in girls (Isasi et al., 2003). Thoren et al. (1973) postulated that the additional weight carried by children at the lower levels of obesity may be sufficient to provide a training effect that could enhance their physical fitness status but such a benefit would be possible only through regular physical activity. The possible training effect would relate to the slight overload stress provided by the additional adipose tissue being transported. As will become evident in following sections of this volume, training with appropriate exercise prescription can provide significant positive effects on movement capability.

Ward and Bar-Or (1986) have described the lack of habitual physical activity that too often characterizes the obese individual as "secondary inactivity." Unfortunately, this level of inactivity contributes to a withdrawal from the physical activity setting, which, if left unchecked, can lead to further inactivity. It is this cycle of inactivity and increased adiposity that is recognized as the major factor in the registration of subnormal physical working capacity. As the level of obesity increases, mobility of the obese child is made more difficult and compounds the already vulnerable physical condition of the individual. With further worsening, any advantages gained via fat-free weight increase would be outweighed by the increased inactivity.

When evaluating the results of performance tests, for example, on a treadmill it is necessary to take into account the effect of environment and other factors. For instance, obese youngsters ran significantly longer during distraction (music) than without it (De Bourdeaudhuij et al., 2002); therefore, attention-distraction had a positive effect on perseverance, which might influence the evaluation of the level of physical fitness ascertained.

Physical activity is important during childhood for the adequate development of the functional capacity of the cardiopulmonary system, and the progressive but slight reductions in level of activity in the obese means that they are predisposed to inappropriate development of this system.

6.2 Lung Function Measurements

The development of obesity leads to deterioration in a number of indices of lung function, including vital capacity and maximum ventilatory volume (MVV). Obese individuals frequently complain of breathlessness on mild exertion and are more susceptible to respiratory infections with the heavier chest wall serving to impede normal respiratory movements. An improvement in exercise tolerance and a feeling of well-being can be gained via weight reduction.

Some studies, for example, in Taiwanese children, did not show differences among obese and normal-weight children with regard to some lung function tests (forced expiratory volume in the first second, peak expiration flow rate, forced vital capacity, Tang et al., 2001), in spite of differences in triceps skinfold thickness, which correlated with body mass index. It seems that tests performed under rest conditions, that is, without workloads, are less or not at all influenced by excess fat.

Lung function can be evaluated in greater detail by the measurements of forced expiratory flow and MVV. These values are, in some studies, often reduced by obesity to between 60 and 70% of predicted normal values. In Singapore, more obese children had significantly lower values for each test of lung function. The results seem to indicate a narrowing of small airways and increased respiratory inertia possibly due to excessive accumulation of fat in the chest wall and abdomen leading to respiratory limitation (Ho et al., 1989).

Comparisons with predicted normal values for height, gender, and body surface area (BSA) revealed significantly reduced values (mean % predicted) in the obese with respect to a range of values. Residual volume (RV), total lung capacity (TLC), minute ventilation (VE), and resting energy expenditure (REE) were increased. These results show altered pulmonary function due to obesity during growth, characterized by a reduction in diffusing capacity, ventilatory muscle endurance, and airway narrowing. The changes may reflect extrinsic mechanical compression on the lung and thorax, and/or intrinsic alterations within the lung (Inselma, Milanese, and Deurloo, 1993).

Spirometry was performed on a group of obese children before and every 3 minutes after a workload on a treadmill. The majority of obese children had at least a 15% fall in at least one of the three monitored pulmonary function parameters. The same result was observed in less than a half of the normal-weight children. The mean percentage falls in forced expiratory volume (FEV) and forced expiratory flow ($FEF_{25-75\%}$) were significantly greater in obese children than in the controls. The pattern of bronchospasm, which appeared soon after workload, was consistent with that found in the asthmatic population. The degree of fall in $FEF_{15-75\%}$ significantly correlated negatively with triceps skinfold thickness. These results reveal that bronchospasm of the smaller airways occurs more frequently in obese children and is related to subcutaneous fat. This might contribute to the avoidance of exercise and increased workloads in obese subjects due to bronchial hyper-reactivity; however, this finding requires further research (Kaplan and Montana, 1993).

In children with mild obesity, pulmonary volumes are within the normal range. In severe obesity, the main factor is the decreased distensibility of the chest wall, which becomes worse over time and is the cause of the alteration in ventilatory volume, flow, and transfer factors (Bosisio et al., 1984).

Expiratory reserve volume (ERV) of the lungs and its relation to vital capacity (ERV/VC) was examined in a group of prepubertal boys and girls. The relationship of these respiratory parameters to the percentage of body fat was assessed using regression analysis. The regression for preadolescent boys and for adult men was similar, but this was not so for girls. In this group, the expiratory reserve volume increased with increasing fatness:

(ERV/VC) × 100 = 29.3. + 0.19 fat%, r = 0.48, p < 0.03). In all groups there was no correlation with age or height. In contrast to adults in whom body weight correlates significantly with the above-mentioned parameter, no such relationship was seen in younger subjects (Barlett, Kenney, and Buskirk, 1992). Spirometric data showed positive dependence of lung function on BMI in girls with increasing BMI values. This was not the case in boys (Fung et al., 1990).

Reduction in functional residual capacity (FRC) and diffusion impairment were the most usual abnormalities found in a study of obese children (Li et al., 2003). Standardized pulmonary function tests (spirometry, lung volumes, and single-bit diffusion capacity for carbon monoxide) and DXA measurements were used, and it was found that a reduction of static lung volume correlated with the degree of obesity.

Pulmonary function tests, polysomnography, and multiple sleep latency tests also showed abnormal results in obese children. Forty-six percent of obese subjects had abnormal polysomnograms, and there was a positive correlation between the degree of obesity and the apnea index, as well as an inverse correlation between the degree of obesity and the degree of sleepiness on multiple sleep latency tests. These results reveal that obese adolescents have a high prevalence of mild sleep-disordered breathing. Obstructive sleep apnea syndrome improved after tonsillectomy and adenoidectomy (Marcus et al., 1996).

Another study of adolescents aged 10.3 ± 4.4 years, with a history of morbid obesity and breathing difficulty during sleep, showed that 37% of the group had marked abnormalities (apnea, hypopnea, excessive arousal levels, or abnormalities in gas exchange). A sleep history questionnaire showed that all patients snored. Pulmonary tests indicated that 28.5% of subjects had a restrictive defect and 47% of subjects possessed obstructive changes. Multiple regression analysis revealed a significant association between weight, age, or gender and any physiological measure on the polysomnogram. Most of the abnormal polysomnograms were only mildly abnormal during adolescence, but in two cases the abnormalities were so severe that they required clinical intervention (Mallory, Fiser, and Jackson, 1989).

6.3 Blood Pressure, Cardiac and Aortal Function, and Obesity

In high-income countries, the decline in blood pressure in 5- to 34-year-olds of both sexes and from a range of ethnic groups for at least the last 50 years indicates that exposures (e.g., diet) acting in early life are significant determinants of blood pressure. However, the prevalence of cardiovascular diseases is still high in both developed and developing countries along with increasing childhood obesity; there is a possibility that favorable blood pressure trends may be plateauing. This indicates the necessity of interventions

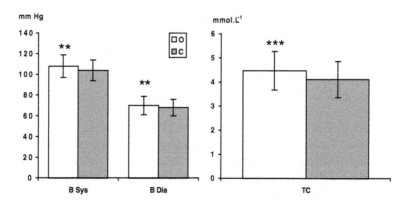

FIGURE 6.4

Comparison of systolic and diastolic blood pressure (B Sys, B Dia), and total cholesterol (TC) in obese (O) and control, normal-weight (C) children. ** indicates (p < 0.01); *** (p < 0.001). (Based on data from McMurray et al., 1995.)

in early life to prevent an increase in blood pressure in adulthood, which includes childhood obesity prevention (McCarron, Smith, and Okasha, 2002).

The Amsterdam Growth and Health Study revealed that longitudinal measurements of body fat percentage in the early teenage years seems to be the most important cardiovascular disease indicator in predicting risk levels in young adults. The amount of physical activity measured in young adulthood is the only behavioral parameter to show a significant interrelationship with other cardiovascular disease risks (Kemper et al., 1990, 1999).

Systolic and diastolic blood pressure was significantly elevated in the obese compared to the normal-weight control children (Figure 6.4) (McMurray et al., 1995). Another study in Italian children aged 6.6 to 14.4 years with a wider range of BMI followed weight, height, waist and hip circumferences, and blood pressure. Insulin sensitivity was evaluated by an Insulin Tolerance Test (ITT). The results of this study suggested that blood pressure in children is more closely related to body fat distribution and insulin resistance than to excess weight (Salvatoni et al., 1997).

Blood pressure in healthy boys and girls aged 4 to 18 years increased regularly with advancing years and was always more closely correlated with height and total body weight than with age. This association became much stronger during puberty in males. Correlation with body height was not found after puberty, but the correlation with body weight remained and increased. In children whose weight in relation to height was greater by 20% or more, the risk of an increased blood pressure was a multiple of 2.5 in boys and 2.0 in girls. However, the extent to which the increase in blood pressure is due solely to excess weight and fatness, and to other possible factors such as the level of maturity and early development of other tissues (muscle, bone), needs to be studied in greater detail (Andre, Deschamps, and Gueguen, 1982).

In adults, significant correlations between blood pressure and the level of obesity have been reported. In childhood, some studies reveal the same findings; however, exploratory analysis indicates an occasionally strong but quite variable relationship between blood pressure and BMI, which differs by age, gender, and the particular blood pressure measure under consideration (Labarthe, Mueller, and Eisser, 1991).

A 3-year longitudinal study followed self-reported behavior, height, weight, skinfold, blood pressure, and BMI in a sample of matched cases. Data were analyzed according to ethnicity, age, and gender, and a greater proportion of females were obese as seniors. Overweight trends for each of the four groups by ethnicity and gender were stable over the period of the study. Later, a marked increase in obesity among black females was found. Blood pressure correlated significantly with percent of ideal body weight, skinfold thickness, and BMI, indicating that increasing obesity is associated with an increase in blood pressure in both black and white subjects (Adeyanju et al., 1987). The positive relationship between fatness and blood pressure becomes more apparent when obesity has been established for a long period of time. The hypothesis that the early onset of obesity is associated with obesity later in adolescence is supported by these results and is indicative of a persistent health risk.

The effect of obesity on echocardiographic parameters (the thickness of the interventricular septum and of the posterior wall, end diastolic left ventricular internal dimension, and left ventricular mass) was studied in groups of Japanese children aged 6, 12, and 15 years. Left ventricular parameters were normalized for height. Significant correlations between the indices of obesity and left ventricular internal dimension or left ventricular mass were revealed. The obesity index was more strongly correlated than BMI with posterior wall thickness and left ventricular internal dimension. The most important finding concerned the significant effect of obesity on left ventricular parameters as early as 6 years of age (Kohno, Tanaka, and Honda, 1994).

In obese children in China, blood pressure was higher and significantly related to BMI values. An increase of one BMI unit was associated with, on average, an increase of 0.56mm Hg and 0.54mm Hg in systolic (SBP) and diastolic blood pressure (DBP), respectively. In normal-weight children, the increase in SBP and DBP was 1.22 and 1.20mm Hg, respectively. An increase of BMI is conclusively associated with elevated SBP and DBP in nonobese children; an increase in the adjusted BMI was associated with an increase in SBP and DBP in both obese and nonobese children (He et al., 2000).

Obesity, which significantly increases blood pressure, can also result in left atrial enlargement (Daniels et al., 2002). General and visceral adiposity have been associated with an increased left ventricle mass (Humphries et al., 2002). Left ventricular diastolic filling as related to adiposity was also studied. Left ventricular diastolic function, flow velocity patterns of the pulmonary vein, and the mitral valve were measured by pulse Doppler echocardiography in asymptomatic obese children. All obese subjects had abnormal pulmonary venous flow velocity patterns. The mitral flow velocity pattern in the obese was also characterized by a decrease in early diastolic filling. These indices, however, did not correlate with an increase in BMI percentage. This study suggests that BMI can predict the abnormality of left ventricular diastolic filling (Harada, Orino, and Takada, 2001).

The stiffness of the abdominal aorta using transthoracic echocardiography in both normotensive and hypertensive obese children, compared to controls, was measured. Aortic strain (S) and pressure strain elastic modulus measurements differed significantly in the hypertensive obese group, along with increased cholesterol levels and higher body mass index (Levent et al., 2002).

No correlation was found between the length of QT interval and obesity; however, the prevalence of a long QT interval in children generally is greater than previously considered (Fukushige et al., 2002).

The variability of heart rate in children is influenced by age, but the physique had no significant effect in normotensive healthy children. The effect of fat load can appear only when its amount is increasing during a longer period of growth, especially when achieving excess values.

There is a contraversion on the autonomic control of cardiac function involvement. A study using power spectral analysis of heart rate variability showed an increase in sympathetic tone coupled with a reduction in vagal tone. This finding makes way for the hypothesis that autonomic nervous system changes depend on the time course of obesity development (Riva et al., 2001). Noninvasive autonomic nervous system function tests were evaluated in obese and control children. The results of Valsalva ratio, 30/15 ratio, and heart rate responses to deep breathing significantly differed in the obese children; orthostatic test differed insignificantly. Ophtalmic examinations were normal in both groups. The results indicate normal activity of sympathetic and hypoactivity of the parasympathetic nervous system, implying parasympathetic nervous system dysfunction as a risk factor in childhood obesity (Yakinci et al., 2000).

An increased heart rate and higher blood pressure were found in obese normotensive children that were associated with parasympathetic heart rate control decrease. These children had higher casual and ambulatory blood pressure, and higher fasting glucose, insulin, and triglyceride levels. Overall heart rate variability values were not significantly lower in the obese subjects (Martini et al., 2001).

The above-mentioned research findings confirm that cardiac function is significantly influenced by excess weight and fatness, especially when initiated at an early age. In growing overweight individuals, the increased insulin levels may be a risk factor for the accumulation of increased left ventricular mass after correction for growth, which is not dependent on obesity level, blood pressure, or insulin (Urbina et al., 1999).

Microvascular function is also negatively associated with obesity. Skin microvascular response (measured using Doppler imaging), to iontophoresis of acetylcholine (Ach) and sodium nitroprusside (SNP), was significantly negatively correlated with percentage of body fat. In addition, subjects stratified in the upper quintile based on two-hour postfeeding glucose levels showed significantly lower vasodilatation to both Ach and SNP. A clustering of high postfeeding glucose, impaired microvascular function, increased insulin resistance, and higher central fat distribution (higher waist-to-hip ratio) was found. These observations reveal that risk factors for adult cardiovascular disease begin to cluster in normal children, which might have marked effects with regard to atherosclerosis later in life (Khan et al., 2003).

Mechanical properties of the common carotic artery (CCA) and endothelial function of the brachial artery were studied in a group of obese children (mean age 12 years), who had a vascular high resolution echographical analysis. Cross-sectional compliance (CSC), cross-sectional distensibility (CSD), and incremental elastic modulus (Einc) were analyzed at the CCA site. The brachial artery dilation (FMD) was measured after hyperhemia (with stimuli for endothelial dependent and independent function). Fat mass was ascertained by DXA, along with insulin resistance and glucose tolerance test. The obese children had significantly lower CSC, CSD, and FMD, as well as higher values of Einc. The CCA stiffness was related to the amount of stored fat and overweight, and also to insulin resistance. The android fat distribution was related to endothelial dysfunction (Aggoun et al., 2002). Endothelial dysfunction was associated with low plasma apolipoprotein A-I and with insulin resistance. These changes may, along with android fat distribution, be the main risk factors of the arterial changes in severe obesity — that is, arterial wall stiffness and endothelial dysfunction — and thus are of considerable concern as possible early events in the genesis of atheroma (Tounian et al., 2001).

6.4 Hematological Parameters

Plasma hemostatic measures, D-dimer, fibrinogen, and plasminogen activator inhibitor-1 (PAI-1) were evaluated in obese boys aged 7 to 11 years. Boys had significantly greater fibrinogen and D-dimer concentrations than girls; additionally, black children had significantly greater fibrinogen and D-dimer concentrations than whites. Fibrinogen was positively associated with the percentage of stored fat ($r = 0.40$, $p < 0.01$), subcutaneous abdominal tissue ($r = 0.40$, $p < 0.01$), total fat mass ($r = 0.42$, $p < 0.01$), and BMI ($r = 0.41$, $p < 0.01$). PAI-1 was positively associated with visceral adipose tissue ($r = 0.49$, $p < 0.01$), subcutaneous abdominal adipose tissue ($r = 0.32$, $p < 0.01$), FFM ($r = 0.50$, $p < 0.01$), and insulin ($r = 0.61$, $p < 0.01$). D-dimer was positively associated with the percentage of stored fat ($r = 0.40$, $p < 0.01$), subcutaneous abdominal adipose tissue ($r = 0.37$, $p < 0.05$), total amount of stored fat ($r = 0.40$, $p < 0.01$), and BMI ($r = 0.43$, $p < 0.010$). Multiple regression analysis revealed that for fibrinogen, gender and the higher percentage of stored fat explained significant independent portions of the variance.

Significant predictors for PAI-1 were higher amounts of visceral adipose tissue and fat-free mass. The significant predictor for D-dimer was ethnicity. General adiposity and visceral adipose tissue may play a role in regulating plasma hemostatic factors in obese children. Increased fatness of the individual is associated with unfavorable concentrations of hemostatic factors that in turn are implicated with cardiovascular morbidity and mortality later in life (Ferguson et al., 1998).

In healthy adults, a positive correlation of white blood cells (WBC), the percentage of stored fat, and leptin was reported. This relationship was also analyzed in children aged 10.3 ± 3.2 years. BMI, sum of skinfolds, percent of ideal body weight, arm fat area, and body fat measured with BIA were correlated with WBC, lymphocytes (L), and neutrophils (N). Spearman rank correlation coefficient and stepwise variable selection analysis were performed. Simple linear regression analysis showed an inverse correlation of WBC with age, and a direct correlation for percent of body weight and body mass index. Neutrophils correlated significantly with body weight, percent of ideal body weight, sum of skinfolds, arm fat area, body fat mass, and body mass index. Using stepwise variable selection analysis, WBC correlated with percent of ideal body weight and N with BMI alone. These results agree with those found for the adults. It is possible that the relationship between WBC and percent of body fat may be mediated in part through the effect of leptin, which is directly involved in proliferation of hemopoietic stem cells (Perrone et al., 1998b).

6.5 Physical Performance and Motor Abilities

A number of studies have found that increased body fatness has a negative influence on children's physical performance, particularly in activities requiring the body to be projected through space as in jumping. Earlier studies of the performance of adults have also highlighted the inverse relationship between body fat and the ability to move total body weight. Åstrand and Rodahl (1977) maintained that such a relationship is due to the fact that body fat adds to the mass of the body without making a contribution to force-generating capacity, subsequently becoming additional weight to be moved during tasks that involve weight bearing. Although the disadvantages of the condition have often been mentioned, much of the evidence has not been quantified and has resulted in considerable subjective reporting of movement capacity.

6.5.1 Motor Skill

For the most part, motor skills are age and gender dependent, with the efficiency of movement progressively improving throughout childhood and

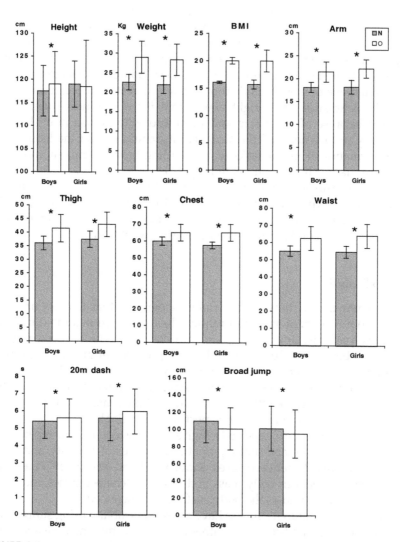

FIGURE 6.5

Comparison of morphological characteristics (height, weight, BMI, arm, thigh, chest, waist circumferences, (cm)) and motor performance (20-m dash, broad jump), in normal-weight (N) and overweight (O) 6.4-year-old children. * indicates (p < 0.05). (Based on data from Pařízková, 1998, Pařízková, 1996a.)

into early adolescence. Motor skill development is also highly influenced by environmental influences. Risk factors that negatively impact on performance levels include previous injury, decreased endurance fitness, and level of adiposity (Birrer and Levine, 1987). In preschool children, the performance level of jumping on the spot and in the 20-m dash was significantly worse in overweight compared to normal-weight peers (Figure 6.5) (Pařízková, 1996a).

Motor skills consist of a number of specific but interrelated components that include agility, flexibility, and speed, each of which has a bearing on the performance of physical activity tasks. Generally, the efficacy of movement progressively improves during the childhood years, with development highly dependent on environmental influences. Some of the factors affecting motor skill development include motivation, interest, practice, training, and body characteristics. One might expect that the obese individual, who is ridiculed because of body size and form and who is also more likely to voluntarily reduce habitual physical activity, could exhibit inadequacies in the performance of motor tasks (e.g., standing broad jump, sit-and-reach, flexed arm hang, shuttle run, plate tapping).

Motor performance involving individual limbs and/or smaller muscle groups, and all types of performance that do not require the manipulation of an individual's own weight in space, are influenced much less in the obese than other modes of dynamic, weight-bearing workloads.

6.5.2　Flexibility

Gender comparisons have traditionally recognized that females are more flexible from 5 years of age to adulthood. Reasons cited include differences in activity patterns, limb length, and muscle mass. The reduced physical activity of obese individuals, as well as the presence of greater amounts of adipose tissue, has contributed to suggestions that the obese have reduced joint flexibility. Borms (1986) has suggested that a limited range of motion can result in lower work efficiency and limited movement and that quality and aesthetics of movement is an aspect often overlooked.

Docherty and Bell (1985) reported a high and consistent relationship between measures of flexibility and anthropometric measures of linearity and found mostly similar results between sexes. Krahenbuhl and Martin (1977) assessed the relationship between body mass and flexibility characteristics and found that flexibility decreased as the body surface area increased.

Most studies of children's fitness have assessed flexibility using simple measures such as the sit-and-reach test rather than more comprehensive and objective analyses of the range of motion of major joints. Further, only a limited number of studies have considered the effect of body fat on flexibility, and the results of these studies are inconsistent. Therefore, the utilization of a comprehensive flexibility protocol with obese prepubertal children, along with a test of agility, a component of fitness that relies partly on flexibility, is warranted.

6.5.3　Strength

Strength is related to parameters of body size such as height and weight. Watson and O'Donovan (1977) reported that many human performance variables are more highly related to the cube of height than to body weight.

In growing children, the relationship between size and muscular strength is so great that it probably obscures other, more subtle influences, such as those differences due to variation in body shape. Obese children are superior to nonobese children in measures of back and grip strength. Grip strength serves as a good indicator of absolute strength, and it increases monotonically with body weight and percent of body fat. However, excess fat does not appear to negatively influence this strength indicator (McLeod, Hunter, and Etchison, 1983).

Laubach and McConville (1969) showed that strength was negatively related to skinfold thickness, while Lamphiear and Montoye (1976) found strength more highly related to biacromial diameter, upper arm circumference, and triceps skinfold thickness than other measures.

Back strength is one of the few items that is superior in obese children (Kim, Matsuura, and Inagaki, 1993; Suzuki and Tatsumi, 1993). This is logical as muscle strength is related to muscle and lean body mass of the individual. A static workload not requiring weight bearing over a distance is not influenced by an excess load of stored fat and may be even higher due to greater lean body mass in the obese (Pařízková, 1977).

The obese group was also inferior to the normal group in stepping up and down on a stool where body weight produces a considerable overload on the cardiorespiratory system. Wear (1962) suggested that the relationships found may be due partly to indirect factors other than excess weight itself, such as lack of physical activity, which may affect performance. In studying children, Palgi et al. (1984) and Gutin et al. (1978) found a significant relationship between percent of body fat and slower run times over 1 to 2 km, results that support the disadvantage of transporting additional body fat in running tasks.

6.6 The Effect of Obesity on Motor Performance at Different Ages

Motor abilities can be influenced by excess weight from a very early age. Groups of normal-weight and obese babies were compared, and a delayed gross motor development was found in the obese. A significant correlation was found between excessive weight and gross motor delay. Over the following year, both weight and motor development reverted to normal in the majority of infants (Jaffe and Kosakov, 1982). It was suggested that a comprehensive evaluation of the motor-delayed overweight infant be performed before concluding that the delay in motor development might be caused by other factors, not just an increased body weight and fatness.

The potential deteriorating effect of excess fat on dynamic performance increases with age and the longer the duration of obesity. In preschool children, the effect of increased weight and BMI is only apparent in some areas, such as broad jump and the 20-m dash (Figure 6.5) (Pařízková, 1996a), and much less so in other measured variables. The significant effect of increased weight and fat is most marked during puberty.

Sawada (1978) found inferior performances in the 50-m dash, running and jumping, repeated side-step jumping, and vertical jumping. Sawada also noted that half of the obese group experienced difficulty in chin-ups, results that were similar to those reported in an earlier study by Wear (1962).

Obese boys aged 12 to 14 years were tested in 19 physical fitness and motor ability items, and body fatness was evaluated by 6 skinfolds and bioelectrical impedance analysis. Obese boys had significantly poorer results in the 1500-m run, 5-minute run, 50-m run, running long jump, and many other variables. Obese boys were superior in back strength only. These data confirm previous studies on the differentiated effect of excess fatness on physical performance (Pařízková, 1977), which has the most negative influence during dynamic workloads of aerobic, weight-bearing activity.

The association between fitness and fatness was examined in girls aged 7 to 17 years. The measurements included 5 skinfolds, the sit-and-reach test, sit-ups, flexed arm hang, and motor performance items such as standing broad jump and vertical jump, arm pull strength, flamingo stance, shuttle run, the plate tapping step test, and also PWC_{170}. Age-specific partial correlations between fatness and each fitness item, controlling for stature and weight, showed that subcutaneous fat accounted for health-related fitness of the variance in each of the items. The most important items for health-related fitness were the step test and PWC_{170}. The fattest girls had generally poorer levels of physical fitness compared to lean girls (Malina et al., 1995).

Gender differences in fitness levels were not apparent among obese boys and girls; neither was the amount of fat and its distribution (Pařízková, 1977). This might be one of the reasons for the undifferentiated physical performance levels between genders. The performance level varied significantly according to the degree of obesity, especially in VO_2 max tests, the 50-m run, and sit-up test (Pongprapai, Mo-suwan, and Leelasamran, 1994).

A balance test (Bruininks-Oseretsky) and two computerized posturography tests were used for the evaluation of the effect of an increased body weight. The results of the balance tests correlated negatively with body weight, BMI, percentage of fat, and total fat mass. Overweight subjects had lower scores than normal-weight ones, supporting the view that overweight adolescents have poorer balance (Goulding et al., 2003b).

The level of motor ability and coordination of an individual influences physical activity level. Similarly, difficulty in visual coordination is also considered as a possible cause of the problems during exercise in obese children that may result in the preference for sedentary behaviors (Petrolini, Iughetti, and Bernasconi, 1995).

6.7 Summary

Functional capacity and the level of physical fitness are significantly altered by excess fat. Various components of them are influenced in a different way; two of the most important and essential for health, cardiorespiratory efficiency and aerobic fitness, belong to those mostly deteriorated. Skill tasks that do not require lifting of an individual's own weight are affected less, or not at all. Muscle strength, which depends significantly on fat-free, mostly muscle mass, can even be increased. Numerous tests and methods are used; for aerobic fitness the measurements on the treadmill, bicycle ergometer, and/or using step-test, etc. are used, either during maximal or standard workload defined specifically. As indicators, the oxygen uptake, carbon dioxide output, respiratory quotient (RQ), and ventilation are mosty often evaluated either in absolute and/or relative values (per kg total body, or lean, fat-free body mass) along with the assessment of the physical working capacity ($PWC_{170,\ i.e.,}$ at the level of heart rate of 170 beats per minute) and anaerobic threshold (AV). Results of all these tests characterizing dynamic working capacity are more or less changed by excess fatness, especially when relative values of these parameters are used (especially per kg body weight, the most valid indicator). This was demonstrated in a number of studies in groups of obese subjects of different age and gender, revealing deteriorated fitness of dynamic, aerobic performance tasks requiring the transfer of an individual's own body weight along the distance which gave corresponding results. Functional and fitness parameters correlated significantly with a number of anthropometric indicators, especially those characterizing body composition and the degree of adiposity. Also, further lung function measurements, such as vital capacity and forced volume, were negatively influenced by excess fatness. Blood pressure at rest and during workload was increased in the obese, especially in those with visceral adiposity. Increased left ventricle mass and further deviations may predict abnormalities of left ventricular filling in the obese. Stiffness of abdominal aorta, parasympathetic nervous system dysfunction, microvascular and endothelial dysfunction, and unfavorable concentrations of hemostatic factors indicating increased functional and health risks were also revealed, and were associated with further body composition, metabolic, biochemical, and hormonal deviations. Motor skills such as agility, flexibility, speed, and balance tests are also significantly changed, along with visual coordination of movement. Handicaps appear in special tests early in life already, and mostly develop undesirably further with increasing duration and degree of obesity.

According to the increasing interest in prescribing improved physical activity regimes and exercise for weight reduction, the evaluation of the above-mentioned parameters at any age and stage of obesity must be the focus of attention.

7

Food Intake

Increased energy intake has long been considered the single most important item in the pathogenesis of obesity. Energy excess that is ingested or "economized" during the metabolic processes in the organism due to individual hormonal and biochemical characteristics, or which is simply not used, contributes to the enhanced deposition of fat. The composition of food and the relationship between the individual components of food items also have an important role in an increased adiposity level.

However, many studies in both adults and children have not shown any significant differences between the food intake of obese and normal-weight subjects. Similar to studies on physical activity status or energy expenditure (EE), food intake research has commonly been undertaken with individuals who are already obese and often in a maintenance period of obesity rather than during a dynamic phase. Further, observation periods in such studies are generally very short, rarely lasting longer than one week. Like normal-weight subjects, obese subjects display a "nutritional individuality" (Widdowson, 1962), from the point of view of energy intake, output, and overall food behavior and choice.

Parental attitudes and beliefs regarding obesity proneness in children are important in relation to the development of the child's eating behavior (Hood et al., 2000). The Special Child Feeding questionnaire can be used to assess aspects of child-feeding perceptions, attitudes, and practices and their relationships to the child's developing food-acceptance patterns, the control of food intake, and obesity development (Birch et al., 2001). For long-term control, educational strategies should focus on the consumption of a varied and balanced diet. They should also provide orientation and reassurance with regard to desirable, healthy body weight and shapes, and the social meaning and importance of eating (Westenhoefer, 2002).

Increased intake of food in obese children does not seem to be caused by a lack of nutritional knowledge, which depends on age and type of school education. Nutritional knowledge can also vary in obese and nonobese children (Reinehr et al., 2003). A study of English children showed some of the psychological features associated with the development of eating disorders, including a link between concerns and self-esteem based on physical appearance. This may help to explain why childhood obesity may enhance the risk of developing eating disorders later in life (Burrows and Cooper, 2002). At present, food advertisements, especially in TV programming, can alter food consumption not only in the obese but also in normal-weight children (Halford et al., 2004b). Motivation for eating as a potential factor in obesity development has been analyzed by cross-sectional analysis (Hawks et al., 2003).

Food and portion sizes have been compared in the United States between 1989 and 1995 (Smiciklas-Wright et al., 2003). Concern with respect to increased prevalence of obesity was raised with changes in childhood food consumption patterns (St.-Onge, Keller, and Heymsfield, 2003). The Z-score for BMI in girls may be predicted by examining food purchased away from home (Thompson et al., 2004). "Couch potatoes and French fries" have been considered as characteristics of present physical activity, sedentary, and dietary behaviors and BMI in adolescents (Utter et al., 2003).

7.1   Methods

Food intake can be evaluated using a number of procedures, such as direct weighing, but this is only possible under special conditions (in a metabolic unit, in a hospital, or when funding permits an appropriate number of dietitians). The use of questionnaires, food diaries (inventory method), interviews, and/or a combination of these methods are more common. The nature and comprehensiveness of questionnaires and the duration of the analysis period can vary. Most common time periods for evaluation are 1 week or a representative 3- to 4-day block of time including at least 1 weekend day. Telephone interviews have also been used, for example to gain information on the last day of a study. A comprehensive description of methods is not the function of this volume but is available in numerous textbooks on nutrition (e.g., Dwyer, 1994; Hunt and Groff, 1990).

7.2   Development of Food Behavior in Early Life

As early as the 1930s, it was demonstrated that when given choices of nutrients children select an adequate diet without adult supervision. Children grew well and were healthy despite patterns of intake at individual meals that were not predictable and were also highly variable. A later study in young children from 2 to 5 years of age in which 24-hour food intake was measured on 6 days also showed great variability in energy intake at each of the 5 daily meals. However, the total daily energy intake was relatively constant for each child. The mean coefficient of variation for each child's energy intake for individual meals was 33.6%, but for total daily energy intake it was 10.4%. In most cases, a meal high in energy was followed by a meal of lower energy, or vice versa (Birch et al., 1991).

These findings point to the existence of satisfactory mechanisms to preserve an adequate energy balance. However, this might only apply when food intake is well balanced in macro- and micronutrients and only when satiety mechanisms with regard to energy balance in the individual are involved. When highly attractive foodstuffs with a high energy density are available, this ability can be compromised and an inadequate food intake can occur. Over time this could result in obesity. The effect of the family and the whole environment of the child, including mass media and television, can also play a significant role.

The early periods of growth are particularly important in the development of appropriate eating habits. Eating behavior has to be viewed as a complex phenomenon involving the coordination of cognitive, social, motor, and emotional development, which are under the regulation of both central and peripheral factors (Hammer, 1992). Besides providing necessary biological substrates for growth, development, and maturation processes, food intake and eating habits are also important for social interactions. For example, the formation of the mother–infant relationship plays an essential role at the beginning of an individual's life.

In the United States, dietary patterns changed in children aged 2 to 10 years during the period 1978 to 1988. Intake of macronutrients remained fairly stable during this period and exceeded the RDAs while daily vitamin and mineral intake was lower in 1988 for the majority of subjects studied (Alberton et al., 1992). A further study of U.S. children (Kennedy and Goldberg, 1995) confirmed the change in food consumption patterns. These trends have been linked with the increasing prevalence of obesity. The ratio of obese children and adolescents consuming unhealthy foods appears to be increasing.

A number of factors can modify food behavior in early childhood. In a group of healthy infants, suckling was measured twice in a laboratory during the first month and its effect on the development of early adiposity was followed. Multiple regression analysis revealed that parental education and a measure of feeding behavior, that is, the interval between the bursts of suckling, accounted for 18% of the variance in triceps skinfold measures at one year of age. A lower level of education of the parents and shorter intervals between the bursts were associated with greater adiposity. Other feeding variables, such as the pressure of suckling and the number of reported feeds per day, accounted for 21.5% of the variance in skinfold thickness at 2 years of age. Fewer but larger feeds and a higher suckling pressure were associated with greater adiposity. These data indicate that greater adiposity in early age is related to a vigorous infant-feeding style. That is, suckling more rapidly at a higher pressure, with a longer suck and burst duration and a shorter interval between bursts of suckling, causes a higher energy intake. The differences in feeding style could also be genetically endowed. In this study, breastfeeding protected children against early adiposity only to the age of 6 months (Agras et al., 1987).

Body size and food ingestion behavior are related in infants with different risks of obesity that is, obese and lean mothers (Berkowitz et al., 1995). Of all the risk factors for development of obesity, including maternal and paternal BMI, gender, feeding mode (breast, bottle, or a combination), 3-day food intake, nutritive suckling behavior during laboratory test feeding. and parental education, along with the interactions between them, nutritive suckling behavior was higher in the high-risk group with obese mothers at the age of 3 months. In this sample, infant food intake and nutritive sucking behavior at 3 months of age contributed to measures of body size at 12 and 24 months (Berkowitz et al., 1998).

As mentioned in Chapter 4, the effect of the early diet on the development of BMI is undisputed. A follow-up study of nutrition and growth from 10 months to 8 years of age in French children showed a positive correlation of BMI at the age of 8 years with energy intake at the age of 2 years. However, this correlation became insignificant when adjusting BMI at 2 years. As mentioned in Chapters 3 and 4, the percentage of energy as protein ingested at the age of 2 years correlated positively with BMI and subscapular skinfold at the age of 8 years, after adjustment for energy intake and parental BMI. The percentage of energy contributed from protein at the age of 2 years was also negatively associated with the age of adiposity rebound.

Therefore, the higher the protein intake at 2 years of age, the earlier the adiposity rebound and the higher the subsequent BMI level. Protein at the age of 2 years was the only nutrient intake associated with the fatness development pattern in following years. The association between protein intake and obesity is also consistent with the increased values of body height and generally accelerated growth of the obese children; this might also be related to the role of IGF-1 and other hormones (Rolland-Cachera et al., 1995). Some studies have confirmed this finding (Scaglioni et al., 2000), but others have not (Hainer et al., 1999; Hoppe, Molgaard, and Michaelsen, 2000).

A high-fat, low-protein diet such as human milk is adapted to a high-energy demand for growth in early childhood that may not always be the case with bottle-feeding. Bottle-fed children more often become obese in later years than breast-fed children. A high-protein diet in early childhood could therefore increase the risk of obesity along with other co-morbidities later in life (Rolland-Cachera et al., 1995; Rolland-Cachera, 1995). A comparison of the age of adiposity rebound and BMI related to diet in countries with different nutritional habits and RDAs could also contribute to these conclusions (Gillman et al., 2001; Pařízková and Rolland-Cachera, 1997); which are still under discussion (Butte, 2001).

7.3   Food Intake and Obesity

As indicated earlier, there is some confusion about the evidence that the obese overeat. This parallels the limited evidence that the obese are more

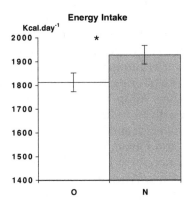

FIGURE 7.1

Comparison of energy intake in obese (O) and normal-weight (N) children. * indicates (p < 0.05). (Based on data from Greco et al, 1990.)

sedentary. Some studies show a decreased energy intake in the obese when compared to normal-weight children. Understanding of the biological basis of obesity has grown rapidly during the last decade, and this work has particularly concerned the identification of a novel endocrine pathway involving the adipose tissue secreted hormone leptin and the leptin receptor in the hypothalamus. Plasma leptin levels are regulated inter alia by feeding and fasting (Schonfeld-Warden and Warden, 1997) and may play an important role, not only in food intake, but also in the utilization of energy and deposition of fat in the body (see Chapter 9).

Food intake has been assessed in obese and normal-weight children aged 7 to 11 years. An interview and a food diary were used during the 2 days prior to the study, and the questionnaire was administered over 1 week. Food intake in obese children did not exceed that of children with normal body weight rather, it was lower (Figure 7.1) (Greco et al., 1990). The group consumed approximately 15% of energy as proteins, 35% as fats, and 50% carbohydrates. No difference was noted between obese and normal-weight children. The percentage of carbohydrates was lower and the percentage of proteins and fats was higher than RDAs. A significant increase with age was noted for protein and fat intakes, along with a considerable reduction of carbohydrates. These deviations involved the majority of both obese (70%) and normal-weight children (80%).

In a group of white and Mohawk children aged 4.2 to 6.9 years, TEE was measured using the DLW method. In addition, mothers completed the Willet-food-frequency questionnaire to report the usual dietary intake of children. Total energy intake assessed by the food-frequency questionnaire was significantly higher than total energy expenditure. Over- and underestimation of energy intake were not related to gender or body composition of children. It was concluded that use of such questionnaires significantly overestimates energy intake of children (Kaskoun, Johnson, and Goran, 1994).

This study also confirms the methodological problems seen in food intake analysis in young children (see Chapters 1 and 3).

Energy intake in two groups of young children with a low (Group N) and high risk of obesity (Group O) as judged from parental obesity was assessed. Energy intake was 16% lower in Group O as assessed by dietary record along with TEE, ascertained by monitoring heart rate. The energy intakes of all children together, and also in Group N, showed the usual wide variability and absence of correlation with body size; however, in group O, a significant relationship between body weight and height with energy intake was found ($r = 0.5$) (Griffiths, Rivers, and Payne, 1987).

In a group of obese and nonobese Italian children aged 10.1 ± 2.1 years, the energy intake was the same. When expressed in relation to total and/or FFM, the energy intake was lower in the obese than in the nonobese children (189.5 ± 74.5 versus 292.0 ± 109.2 kJ.kg body weight^{-1}.day^{-1}, $p < 0.001$, or 251.9 ± 91.2 versus 333.0 ± 122.6 kJ.kg fat-free body mass^{-1}.day^{-1}). The composition of the diet was comparable for both groups; however, obese children ate more protein than controls, in particular, from animal origin (14.6 ± 3.7 versus $13.6 \pm 3.0\%$ of energy). The animal/plant ratio was 2.4 ± 1.7 versus 2.1 ± 1.1, $p < 0.05$. The intake of saturated fats and cholesterol was comparable in both groups. No correlation was found for the intake of nutrients and the percentage of body fatness at the age of 10 years.

A cross-sectional study of overweight and nonoverweight schoolchildren (aged 11 years) showed, however, that the overweight ate significantly less (8948.7 vs. 9590.1 kJ/day, $p < 0.01$). Carbohydrate intake was significantly lower in the overweight group compared to nonoverweight children (250.9 ± 58.8 vs. 222.1 ± 77.4 g/day). These data indicate that the excess fatness in overweight children is not due to an increased food intake in this case but to a decreased energy output (Rocandio, Antosegui, and Arroyo, 2001). Further study showed that obese children were also significantly less active than controls, but no difference was found in obese versus nonobese children in relation to the time spent in sport activities, both at school and during leisure time (Maffeis et al., 1993b). These differences in physical activity may explain, at least partly, the differences in body fatness.

However, along with elevated fat mass and serum lipid levels, an increased energy intake (2 to 3 times) compared to normal-weight children was found by Lahlou et al. (1997). Another study in obese 4- to 16-year-old children showed that they eat significantly more total energy, total fat, and saturated fatty acids (g) than nonobese subjects. Step-wise multiple regression showed greater total energy intake (when controlled for physical activity), but not of fat and saturated fatty acids, which had the strongest relationship to the percentage of body fat (Gillis et al., 2002). These children were younger than the other groups of the obese. Greater intake of energy from fat was found in children with high risk of obesity, and there was a significant linear trend toward increasing fat intake (% energy) with increasing risk of obesity and enhanced body fatness (McGloin et al., 2002).

A 6-month investigation on food consumption and habits showed that children with excess weight had an energy intake that was approximately 20% higher than the recommendation for normal-weight subjects. With regard to RDAs, the highest intake was that of protein, the second being carbohydrates. Clearly, morbidly obese teenagers exhibited definitely higher energy intake than normal subjects (Jerk and Widhalm, 2000). A study of Appalachian children indicated a pattern of food consumption that was high in fatty and sugary food and low in fruit and vegetable consumption. Analysis of physical activity showed that overweight children reported more episodes of video/computer play compared to nonoverweight children, especially boys (Crooks, 2000). At 1 year of age, the protein intake was higher in obese than in nonoverweight children; a follow-up was done at the age of 5 years. Children of overweight parents were also heavier. Multiple logistic analysis confirmed that protein intake at 1 year of age was associated with overweight at 5 years. In children from overweight mothers, prevalence of overweight at 5 years tended to be higher in bottle-fed than in breast-fed ones (Scaglioni et al., 2000). Parental overweight was a major risk for children's overweight, but early high protein intake was considered to influence the development of adiposity as indicated by Rolland-Cachera et al. (1995).

A longitudinal study with children aged 2 and 15 years followed the effect of energy and macronutrient intake and BMI, triceps (TC), and subscapular skinfold (SS) thickness. Across this period, energy-adjusted fat and carbohydrate intake were inversely related to SS measures, but not to either BMI or triceps skinfold. The best predictor of fatness was previous adiposity, which had the effect of strengthening as the age interval shortened. Parental BMI, maternal SS, and paternal TC contributed to the variance of the corresponding measure at some, but not all ages (Magarey et al., 2001a, 2003).

Eating style and its relationship to children's adiposity were examined in children aged 3 to 5 years who attended a university preschool setting. Children completed controlled, two-part meals, reflecting children's precise ability to adjust food intake in response to changes in energy density of the diet. An eating index, reflecting this ability to regulate energy intake, was correlated with morphological characteristics of children. These correlations showed the association between fat stores and responsiveness to energy density cues. Pearson's correlation coefficients revealed that children with greater body fat stores were less able to regulate energy intake accurately.

The most important predictor of children's ability to regulate energy intake was parental control in the feeding situation. Mothers who were more active in controlling their children's food intake had children who showed less ability to self-regulate energy intake ($r = -0.67$, $p < 0.0001$). This suggests that the optimal environment for children's development of self-control of energy intake is not when healthy food choices are provided but when children are allowed to assume their own control of how much they consume (Johnson and Birch, 1994). This might also contribute to the prevention of development of increased body adiposity in early life.

Measurements in a study by Forbes and Brown (1989) showed that energy required for weight maintenance in a group of adolescent and adult subjects of widely varying body size was directly proportional to body weight (r = 0.92). A greater lean body mass and greater energy demands for carrying an increased load of excess fat explained the increased energy requirement in the obese.

With regard to micronutrients, zinc concentration in plasma and erythrocytes were significantly lower in obese children. The higher urinary zinc excretion in the obese means that zinc nutritional status is altered (Da Nascimento-Marreiro, Fisberg, and Franciscato-Cozzolino, 2002).

At present, there is an unsatisfactory consensus on food intake in the obese; the varying designs and methodologies of individual studies make comparisons difficult. Conclusions are contradictory, which may be due to subject differences, particularly in duration, degree, and the stage of obesity and other factors, such as the intensity of physical activity, which was commonly not controlled.

7.4 The Effect of the Composition of the Diet and Eating Behavior

The composition of the diet, especially fat, is particularly important in early childhood. Essential fatty acids provide the substrates for arachidonic acid, docosahexaenoid acid, and their metabolites, which are essential for an adequate maturation of the central nervous system, visual development, and intelligence (Hardy and Kleinman, 1994).

There is still only limited evidence on the relationship between the composition of a child's early diet and the development of chronic diseases, including obesity, later in life. However, the essential role of the individual nutrients in particular periods of growth and development has been more frequently documented in recent studies and analyses (Barker, 1990, 1994, 1995; Pařízková, 1996; Prentice and Jebb, 1995; Prentice et al., 1988).

The effect of protein in early life on adiposity development was mentioned in Chapters 3 and 4, and will be also considered in Chapter 8. Composition of the diet was compared in obese and lean subjects in a group of 8- to 12-year-old children (Valoski and Epstein, 1990). There were no differences in energy, fat, calcium, iron, Vitamin A and C, thiamin, and riboflavin intakes between groups. A study of Spanish obese and nonobese adolescents showed no difference in energy intake of adolescents. However, obese subjects derived a greater proportion of their energy from protein (19.8% vs. 16.4%) than did nonobese controls. The proportion of energy from fats was also higher in the obese (45.4%) than in the nonobese (38.7%), and the obese also consumed greater amounts of cholesterol (Ortega et al., 1995). This study also confirmed that it is necessary to check and manage the diet for both total amount of energy and composition of various macrocomponents.

The dietary intake of children 7 to 14 years of age in a small Italian community also showed a higher intake of protein (up to 15.8% of energy) with an increased animal/vegetable protein ratio (1.5 to 2.1). The intake of fats was higher than 35.9% of daily energy and the polyunsaturated/saturated fatty acid ratio was low, ranging from 0.3 to 0.5. The intake of cholesterol exceeded the recommended level (231 to 347 mg per day) and the daily intake of total carbohydrates was also low (45.3 to 48.5% per day). Crude fiber intake increased with age from 2.8 g to 4.5 g per day. However, the comparison did not reveal any significant differences (Pantano et al., 1992).

The effect of fat intake on fat mass was studied in a longitudinal study (Magarey et al., 2001a) and also in white and Mohawk children 4 to 7 years of age. Body composition (via BIA, skinfolds) and energy expenditure based on physical activity level were also assessed. Before statistical analysis, FM was adjusted for FFM and the intake of fat was adjusted for nonfat food intake. No influence of gender or ethnicity on fat intake was found, and there was no influence of ethnicity on the relationship between fat intake and fat mass. Adjusted mean intakes for the groups of children based on parental obesity status are presented in Figure 7.2. The fatty acid composition

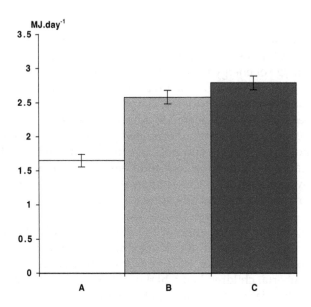

FIGURE 7.2
Adjusted mean values (x ± SE) of fat intake for nonfat intake in children with a nonobese father and mother (A), obese father and nonobese mother (B), and obese father and mother (C). A significant relationship between fat mass and fat intake, r = 0.48, p < 0.01, was revealed. (Based on data from Nguyen et al, 1996.)

of fat (Ailhaud and Guesnet, 2004) was also considered to be an early determinant of childhood obesity.

Nguyen et al. (1996) reported on the influence of maternal obesity on
dietary fat intake of children. They found a significant correlation between
fat mass and fat intake in boys, but not in girls, when adjusted for physical
activity and energy expenditure. Therefore, mothers may contribute to the
development of obesity in their children by influencing the dietary fat content of boys. Dietary fat intake contributed to obesity independent of physical
activity and energy expenditure.

Imbalances in the contribution of macronutrients to the total energy intake
also appear more marked in overweight and obese Spanish adolescents. In
this study, a greater proportion of their energy intake came from fats and a
lower percentage from carbohydrates; however, no differences in total
energy intake were found. Obese subjects also had significantly larger intakes
of cholesterol. The situation was more pronounced in females, who consumed 50% of their energy from fat, 21.9% from protein, and only 27.5%
from carbohydrate. The most significant result of this study is the confirmation that the diet composition, rather than energy consumption, was the
main factor responsible for obesity in both young women and men (Ortega
et al., 1996). There are also significant associations between diet and certain
hormones with a high-fat and low-carbohydrate diet associated with leptin
levels (Park et al., 1998).

A study by Tucker, Seljaas, and Hager (1997) showed that the percentage
of body fat in children aged 9.8 ± 0.5 years varied according to their diet
composition. Children's energy intake was positively related to their adiposity; the percentage of energy from fat was also positively related to adiposity
before and after controlling for potential confounders (fatness, fitness, physical activity, and parental body mass). The percentage of energy derived from
carbohydrates was inversely related to adiposity under the same conditions.

The percentage of body fat also correlated positively with intakes of total,
saturated, monounsaturated, and polyunsaturated fat, and correlated negatively with carbohydrate intake and total energy intake adjusted for body
weight in boys and girls aged 9 to 11 years (Gazzaniga and Burns, 1993). All
associations remained after an adjustment for energy intake, resting energy
expenditure (REE), and physical activity. These results provide further
confirmation that the composition of the diet, particularly the ratio of fats,
may play an important role in the development of children's obesity, independent of total energy intake, REE, and physical activity.

Obese prepubertal children had a higher relative fat intake than nonobese
children, and their fat mass was associated with this factor. The low postabsorptive RQ in obese children may indicate a compensatory mechanism by
increased fat oxidation (Maffeis, Pinelli, and Schutz, 1995). A fat meal (48%
fat) was a risk for fat gain as it reduced thermogenesis and resulted in a
higher fat balance than an isocaloric and isoproteic low-fat meal (Maffeis et
al., 2001).

Further studies have shown that total energy intake and diet composition (especially saturated fats) are positively associated with the development of obesity. Many studies have reported an intake of fats exceeding 30% of energy intake and therefore recommend a lower proportion in the diet. However, this mainly concerns children over 2 to 3 years of age. In infants and younger children, fats are an indispensable part of their high-energy needs and limited dietary capacity. The proportion of fats in the diet is thus dependent on the age of the child and should not be severely decreased at an early age. Reduced-fat diets in very young children are problematic. Children placed on a very low-energy and low-fat diet due to hypercholesterolemia have shown marked problems with growth and development (Lifshitz and Moses, 1989; Widhalm, 1996). Mindful of proper development of the child, the diet should contain no more than 30% of total energy intake from fat, less than 10% from saturated fat, and less than 300 mg of cholesterol per day (Widhalm, 1996). Therefore, the definition of appropriate fat intake for any child must be made with great care.

Measurements of dietary intake and composition in obese children showed that the percentage of dietary lipids correlated directly with serum level of triglycerides (TG) and inversely correlated with HDL-C. The percentage of dietary carbohydrates was inversely correlated to TG and ApoB/A1 and directly correlated to basal insulin. The prevalence of dyslipoproteinemia and hypertension was significantly higher in the families who showed hyperinsulinemia. The patients who reported a dietary animal/plant lipid ratio of greater than 1.0 also showed a significantly higher prevalence of cardiovascular disease in their families. Again, the composition of the diet seems to be more important than excessive energy intake with regard to dyslipoproteinemia, which along with excess weight plays the main role in obesity-related diseases (Riganti et al., 1993).

Experimental evidence supports polyunsaturated fatty acids of the omega-6 series as potent promoters of adipogenesis *in vitro* and adipose tissue development *in vivo* during the gestation/lactation period. This was also confirmed by epidemiological studies in infants as well as by the assessment of the fatty acid composition of mature breast milk and formula milk. Smaller unnoticed changes in fatty acid composition of ingested fats over the decades might be important determinants of the increasing prevalence of obesity in children (Ailhaud and Guesnet, 2004).

A further study of Italian children and youth has confirmed the inadequacies of energy intake macronutrient distribution and preference for inadequate foodstuffs in youth. More than two-thirds of children consumed more than 70 g of soluble sugars per day and 10% exceeded 150 g per day. Snacks accounted for 34% of the total daily energy intake and an imbalance in energy distribution of macronutrients. Only 62% of adolescents were able to correctly match the perception of their body weight with the actual measurement. The majority of youth consumed a regular breakfast but it was rarely nutritionally adequate. Obesity prevalence reached almost 30% (Ferrante et al., 1995).

The consumption of sugar-sweetened drinks is directly associated with obesity in children. With each additional serving of drink, both BMI and frequency of obesity increased after adjustment for anthropometric, demographic, dietary, and lifestyle variables (Ludwig, Peterson, and Gortmaker, 2001). Similarly, excessive fruit juice consumption could have an impact on obesity; however, it had no effect on anthropometric indices in German children (Alexy, 1999). The trend to increased consumption of fruit juices and their contribution to an excess of energy intake in some children may be due to a preference for foods with a sweet taste (Dennison, 1996). Further, children who ate quick-service food twice a week or more at baseline through adolescence had the greatest mean increase in BMI compared to those who ate it only once a week or not at all (Thompson et al., 2004).

7.5   Eating Behavior and Food Preferences

Food preferences in 3- to 5-year-old children were related to parents' weight status and skinfold thickness; children who preferred fat had heavier parents. Fat preferences were significantly related to triceps skinfold measurement ($r = 0.61$, $p < 0.01$). In contrast, epidemiological studies provide evidence that sugar consumption as well as total carbohydrate consumption is associated with leanness (Anderson, 1995).

The most marked relative changes in the composition of diet and nutritional patterns have occurred in the countries of the Third World. For example, in southern Africa, urban black 5-year-old children consumed a low-fat (30% of energy), high-carbohydrate (61% of energy) diet in 1984, but they consumed a typical Westernized diet in 1995 (fat 41% and carbohydrate 52% of total energy) (MacKeown et al., 1998).

As mentioned in Chapter 3, a high-fat diet accompanying acculturation is assumed to be one of the causes of the increasing prevalence of obesity in many populations. Similar changes in fat ingestion (but also of sugar) were found in Canadian Inuits (Shephard, 1991, in Papua New Guinea, and in Samoa (Chapter 2), and were connected with an increasing prevalence of obesity, diabetes, and cardiovascular diseases. In addition to dietary changes, the reduction in physical activity and workload that impact on energy balance together with energy intake must be considered, as was the case in the United States (St.-Onge and Heymsfield, 2003).

Another interesting scenario relates to the increased susceptibility of immigrant groups coming to northern Europe and experiencing changes in food intake, diet composition, and patterns of eating. As mentioned in Chapters 2 and 3, diseases related to overnutrition, such as obesity, cardiovascular diseases, and diabetes, are most often considered in this respect (Wandel, 1993).

An evaluation of eating behavior in obese Italian prepubertal and adolescent girls aged 9.9 ± 0.88 and 15.56 ± 1.61 years showed an increased food intake in both groups. Compared to RDAs, energy intake was higher in 36% of girls in the younger group and in 46% in the older group. Protein intake was increased in 78% of the younger and 66% of the older girls. A decreased calcium intake was found in the majority of girls, and total cholesterol was increased in 33% of the younger and 23% of the older obese girls (Bianco et al., 1993).

Morbid obesity, defined as body weight exceeding 100% of reference weight, has been reported in the United States and European countries, including Austria. Twenty-two Austrian adolescents with a BMI of 32.5 ± 3.9kg/m^2 were divided based on age of onset of obesity, that is, subjects who became obese between the 9th and 11th year (group 1) and those who were already considered obese as infants (group 2). In group 1, insulin, total cholesterol (TC), LDL-C, and triglyceride levels were higher than in group 2. The majority of these adolescents had an energy intake 20% higher than normal-weight children; ate more restaurant meals such as pizzas, noodles, and pasta; and ate fewer vegetables and fruit. Family doctors and pediatricians, and/or parents and caregivers, never tried to rectify the preferences of these children (Widhalm, 1999).

Eating in the absence of hunger may represent a stable phenotypic behavior in overweight girls aged 5 to 7 years (Fisher and Birch, 2002). Binge eating was revealed as a prevalent problem among obese children and adolescents who sought help for their obesity. There are marked differences in self-esteem and a range of eating-related characteristics in children with and without binge eating. No differences were found in the degree of obesity and depression. There is an urgent need to pay particular attention to disordered eating including binge eating in adolescents (Decaluwe and Braet, 2003).

7.6 Thermic Effect of Food (Diet-Induced Thermogenesis) and Obesity

The thermic effect of food (TEF, or diet-induced thermogenesis [DIT]) was similar and did not significantly change in groups of obese and normal-weight children during overfeeding (Bandini et al., 1989). However, insulin and 3.5.3-triiodothyronin levels did increase significantly but did not differ between the groups. Plasma norepinephrine (NE) and urinary excretion of 4-hydroxy-3 methoxymandelic acid (VMA) did not increase during overfeeding. The TEF did not appear to be reduced in obese adolescents; therefore facultative TEF does not appear to be a significant factor in weight maintenance during adolescence.

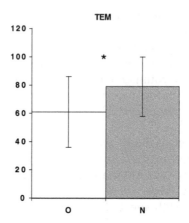

FIGURE 7.3
Comparison of the thermic effect of mixed liquid meal (TEM kj.3hr^{-1}) in prepubertal obese (O) and control, nonobese (N) children. * indicates (p < 0.05). (Based on data from Maffeis, Schutz, and Pinelli, 1992b.)

In contrast, Maffeis, Schutz, and Pinelli (1992b) showed that the thermic effect of a mixed liquid meal (at an energy level corresponding to 30% of the 24-hour pre-meal resting metabolic rate) was significantly lower in obese compared to control children (Figure 7.3). This was true despite the higher energy content of the test meal in the obese. Another study (Maffeis et al., 2001) showed that in obese 10-year-old girls a high-fat meal is able to induce lower thermogenesis and a higher positive balance than an isocaloric and isoproteic low-fat meal. This again indicates the importance of diet composition.

Measurements executed under resting conditions and after exercise also showed that thermogenesis was significantly greater in a lean relative to an obese group. The percentage of fat mass was the best predictor of TEF at rest and during postexercise recovery. Absolute basal energy expenditure was higher in the obese than in lean adolescents, and no significant differences were observed between groups in relation to basal energy expenditure per kg of FFM. Therefore, even when lean and obese adolescents are comparable with respect to FFM, thermogenesis is blunted in obese subjects (Figure 7.4) (Salas-Salvado et al., 1993).

Post-meal (chocolate milkshake) energy expenditure (TEM) was compared in normal (BMI = 17.8kg/m^2) and obese (BMI = 35.9kg/m^2) adolescent girls. Cumulative TEM was calculated as the integrated area under the TEM curve with RMR at baseline. The meals resulted in a greater rise in insulin and glucose for the obese compared to nonobese subjects and a significant increase of TEM for both groups. The cumulative TEM was 61.9% greater for the nonobese when expressed relative to body mass, and 33.2% for the nonobese when expressed relative to the fat-free body mass. Expressed relative to the meal, the TEM was 25.5% less for the obese. These observations support an energy conservation hypothesis for obese female adolescents (Katch et al., 1992).

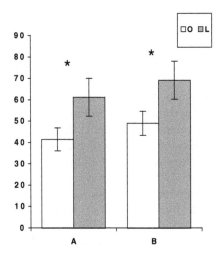

FIGURE 7.4
Comparison of thermogenesis after a test meal in obese (O) and lean, normal-weight (L) 15-year-old subjects under rest (A, kcal.3 hours[-1]) and postexercise (B) conditions. * indicates (p < 0.05). (Based on data from Salas-Salvado et al., 1993.)

7.7 The Role of Food Consumption Patterns in the Development of Obesity

The role of metabolic and/or behavioral daily rhythms with regard to food intake was studied in obese children (Bellisle et al., 1988). Daily energy consumption and the distribution of intake over the waking hours were studied in a group of children aged 7 to 12 years, divided into 5 fatness categories. No difference in the estimated daily energy intake was observed between groups; however, the distribution of intake during the waking hours was different. Obese and fatter children ate less at breakfast and more at dinner than their lean peers; lunch and dinner represented a higher ratio of daily intake. The energy value of breakfast and afternoon snacks was inversely related to the degree of fatness of children. These observations did not exclude hyperphagia during other periods, but a possible contribution of disturbed metabolic and/or behavioral cycles in the development of over-weight was suggested (Bellisle et al., 1988). These results confirm the old adage that to prevent obesity breakfast should be eaten and a greater pro-portion of daily intake ingested during the first half of the waking hours. Correspondingly one should eat more modestly at the end of the day, with an early dinner.

The role of diet composition was not significant when parental obesity (BMI) was taken into account; however, the percentage distribution of the intake of energy among the different meals, particularly dinner, explained the inter-individual variance of fatness in children of both genders (Maffeis et al., 2000). Maffeis et al. (1999b) used a multiple regression analysis in Italian schoolchildren with relative weight as the dependent variable, and the percentage of the energy intake ingested at breakfast, morning snack, lunch, afternoon snack, dinner, postdinner snack, and age as independent variables. Overweight was positively correlated with food intake at dinner and negatively correlated with an afternoon meal.

In another study of obese and overweight children more of an imbalance was noted in energy profiles of the obese compared to normal-weight subjects. A significant difference was found between the amounts of energy supplied by carbohydrates. Obese children had less satisfactory breakfast habits, which may contribute to poorer food choices over the rest of the day, and in the long term, to an increased risk of obesity (Ortega et al., 1998).

In a study of preschool children (24 to 36 months), overweight subjects had a lower consumption at lunch than normal-weight children when high carbohydrate pre-loads (fruit juice and banana, 30 min before lunch) were tested. A high-protein pre-load (chicken meat) had no effect on lunch consumption. When energy intake derived from food consumption was analyzed, the same tendency for food consumption was revealed (Araya et al., 1995).

Italian adolescents often show disorders of dietary behavior, predisposing them to obesity and to anorexia nervosa. Recommendations for improvement dietary improvement include promoting a regular breakfast and a balanced intake of animal and vegetable foods with an increased calcium intake to maximize bone density (Agostoni et al., 1994). Later development of osteoporosis, especially in women, is related to early intake of calcium and balanced food intake (U.S. RDAs, 1989). Dairy products, vegetables, and especially enriched cereals form the basis for an adequate diet during this period of development.

In Czech children who also have increased obesity prevalence, the omission of breakfast was found in approximately 54.1% of cases, especially in larger cities. The majority of children had a mid-morning snack and a school lunch. In villages where obesity prevalence was greater, the number of children who had a school lunch was smaller (Kovářová et al., 2002). Omitting breakfast was also a common finding in obese Spanish children (Aguirre and Ruiz-Vadillo, 2002).

In Japan, the undesirable effects of a Westernized lifestyle have negatively influenced eating habits, caused irregular food intake patterns and a reduction in physical activity. Unfortunately, an increasing number of working mothers also promote the eating of processed food and thus increase energy intake from fat (Murata, 1992). Education systems trying to promote optimal nutrition and lifestyle practices are often overwhelmed by the effect of the mass media. Most commercials for fast-food products do not consider health promotion but rather promote the ready availability and easy preparation of attractively packaged foods for the whole family.

Eating behavior, including the rate of consumption of food, was measured during two lunch meals in obese and normal-weight children aged 11 years. Obese children ate faster and did not slow down their eating rate toward the end of the meal as much as normal-weight children. The obese also indicated they had less motivation to eat before lunch than normal-weight children. A deficient satiety signal or an impaired response to such signals in obese growing subjects could possibly explain these differences (Berkeling, Ekman, and Rössner, 1992).

Eating behavior has also been compared in obese and normal-weight adolescents using several tests with vanilla drinks. No significant differences were found with respect to the absolute amount of the drink and/or energy intake consumed. However, differences were found in the amounts prior to and after the tests. Results indicated a greater sensitivity and higher responsiveness to external stimuli in the obese (Widhalm, Zwiauer, and Eckharter, 1990).

Food intake can influence gastric electrical activity as measured by electrogastrography (EGG) as well as being related to nutritional status and adiposity. The electrogastrographic power normally increases postprandially. However, when normal-weight and obese children aged 6 to 12 years were assessed, the response to a mixed meal was not affected by BMI values. Gastric electrical rhythm and rate and gastric power were also not influenced by age and gender (Riezzo, Chiloiro, and Guerra, 1998).

Another factor often cited for its contribution to the development of childhood obesity is between-meal snacking. A study in Antigua (Bartkiw, 1993) indicated that children consume significant amounts of food between meals. Whilst some of the components of snacks had an adequate nutritional value, most were undesirable. This could play a major role in the deterioration of health.

Behaviors and concerns related to weight were measured by questionnaire in fourth-grade children attending a rural school in central Iowa. Weight-related behaviors and concerns rose with increasing weight-for-age and BMI, and were more prevalent among girls than boys. The frequency of drinking diet soft drinks was positively correlated with weight-for-age and BMI, and tended to climb with an increase in weight-related behaviors and concerns. Girls were more likely than boys to report a desire to be thinner, whereas boys were more likely than girls to want to be taller. The desire for less body fat was significantly associated with an increase in the frequency of weight-related behaviors and concerns than with the frequency of drinking diet soft drink, weight-for-age, and BMI (Gustafson-Larson and Terry, 1992).

Resting energy expenditure, RQ, plasma glucose, and insulin concentrations were studied in obese children with respect to the effect of different kinds of meals. These parameters increased sooner, steeper, and higher with the liquid meal (LM) than with the three consecutive small meals (SM) in obese boys and girls aged 12.7 ± 0.6 years. The magnitude of TEF was greater after the LM than with the SM. These results indicate that the frequency of

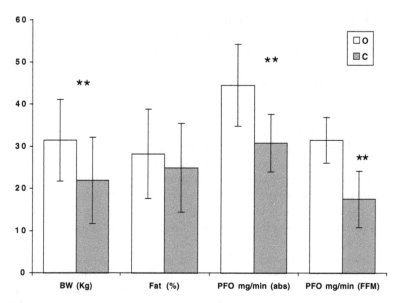

FIGURE 7.5

Comparison of morphological characteristics and postabsorptive fat oxidation (PFM mg.min^{-1}) in absolute values and as related to fat-free, lean body mass (FFM) of obese (O) and normal-weight (C) prepubertal children. * indicates ($p < 0.05$); ** ($p < 0.01$). (Based on data from Maffeis, Pinelli, and Schutz, 1995.)

food consumption influences the immediate thermogenic response as well as changes in the respiratory quotient, glycemia, and insulinemia followed simultaneously (Molnar, 1992). This may also be related to the development of adiposity.

7.8   Utilization and Oxidation of Macronutrients

Fat may not be metabolized in the same way in prepubertal normal-weight and obese children. Postabsorptive fat oxidation expressed in absolute values was significantly higher in obese than in nonobese children, but not when adjusted by analysis of covariance with fat-free mass as the covariate (Figure 7.5). In obese children and in the whole group, fat mass and fat oxidation were significantly correlated ($r = 0.65$; $p < 0.001$). The slope of the relationship indicated that for each 10 kg of additional fat mass, resting fat oxidation increased by 18 g per day. The higher postabsorptive rate of fat oxidation in obese children as compared to onobese subjects may favor the achievement of a new equilibrium in fat balance opposing further increases of the adipose tissue (Maffeis, Pinelli, and Schutz, 1995).

The oxidation of the individual items of fat, that is, of exogenous (meal intake) and endogenous fat (lipolysis) and their ratios, were considered in children with a wide range of BMIs (Maffeis et al., 1998a). The relationship between adiposity and fat oxidation during the postprandial period after a mixed meal was also examined. The use of stable isotope (^{13}C) enriched fatty acids added to a mixed meal and indirect calorimetry enabled the differentiation between exogenous and endogenous sources of fat oxidation. During the 9-hour postprandial period, children oxidized an amount of fat comparable to that ingested in the meal. Exogenous fat represented the average 10.8% (0.9%) of total fat oxidation.

Endogenous fat calculated as the difference between total fat oxidation and exogenous oxidation represented 88.2% (0.9%). Endogenous fat oxidation as well as exogenous fat oxidation were highly correlated with total fat oxidation (r = 0.83, p < 0.001, r = 0.84, p < 0.001, respectively). Exogenous fat oxidation when expressed as a proportion of total fat oxidation correlated directly with fat mass, while endogenous fat oxidation as a proportion of total fat oxidation was inversely related to it. As mentioned earlier, the enhanced exogenous fat oxidation may be considered as a mechanism to prevent further increase in adiposity, and hence to maintain fat oxidation at a sufficient rate under conditions of the exposure to exogenous fat in a meal (Maffeis et al., 1998a; Maffeis et al., 1999a). Similar results were found in a study of Hungarian children with higher oxidation rates of fat in obese as compared to normal-weight peers. Both fat-free, lean body mass and fat mass were important determinants of the rate of fat oxidation (Molnar and Schutz, 1998).

The effect of obesity on carbohydrate oxidation (exogenous compared with endogenous carbohydrate) after the consumption of a mixed meal was studied in obese and normal prepubertal children aged 8 years (Rueda-Maza et al., 1996). Total carbohydrate oxidation was calculated by indirect calorimetry (hood system) whereas endogenous carbohydrate oxidation was estimated from carbon dioxide production (VCO_2), the isotopic enrichment of breath $^{13}CO_2$, and the abundance of ^{13}C carbohydrate in the meal ingested. The time course of ^{13}C in breath was measured over 570 minutes and followed a similar pattern in both groups. Although total carbohydrate oxidation was not significantly different among both groups, exogenous carbohydrate utilization was significantly greater and endogenous carbohydrate oxidation was significantly lower in obese compared with normal-weight children. The rate of carbohydrate oxidation was positively related to the body fat (r = 0.65, p < 0.01). This study suggests that in the postprandial phase, a smaller proportion of carbohydrate oxidation is accounted for by glycogen breakdown in obese children. The sparing of endogenous glycogen may result from decreased glycogen turnover already present at prepubertal age (Rueda-Maza et al., 1996).

Energy expenditure measured by indirect calorimetry was also followed at rest and after an oral sucrose load of three grams per kg of body weight in overweight girls aged 14.54 ± 0.38 years. The thermic effect of eating was evaluated by computing the area under the curve of the EE response and above resting EE during the first 3 hours after the sucrose load. REE (kcal.day^{-1}) was higher in the overweight subjects and when REE was related to FFM the values were lower in the obese than in the normal-weight children. As mentioned in Chapter 5, a linear correlation between REE and FFM was found in both control and overweight subjects (r = 0.78 and 0.68, respectively; p < 0.05 and 0.001). Actual REE in the obese children was significantly lower than the values predicted from regression equations of REE on FFM in controls to the actual FFM in obese children. The thermic effect of eating was identical in overweight and normal-weight subjects regardless of whether it was expressed as an absolute value, a percentage of energy intake, or standardized by FFM (Tounian et al., 1993).

7.9 Summary

Findings in relation to food intake in the obese compared to normal-weight individuals are not homogeneous. Some recent data suggest an increased energy intake in long-term studies, but other studies have shown the same or even lower energy intake in the obese. This is particularly the case when measurements were undertaken over shorter periods. Food intake and behavior are dependent on early influences during infancy and the family situation (obese or normal-weight parents) and nutritional habits. The changes in dietary intake that have occurred during the last decades and relate more to the composition (more fat and sugar) than the amount of food are reflected in obesity prevalence during growth. Children of obese parents have higher fat intake than the recommended 30% of energy intake, which also contributes to higher weight. An increased protein intake early in life can result in earlier adiposity rebound (AR, which can also result in later obesity; however, this was not confirmed in other studies. Consumption of total carbohydrates is usually lower in the obese but sugar intake is higher, including an increased intake of snacks and soft drinks. Additionally, the overconsumption of fruit juices can contribute to obesity development. Studies of food behavior and the distribution of food intake of the obese during the day frequently showed the omission of breakfast and increased eating during the afternoon and evening. Eating in the absence of hunger and later development of binge eating have also been reported. In addition, the obese eat faster and do not slow down toward the end of the meal. There is little evidence to support a change in gastric electrical activity in the obese. Findings on thermic effect of food are inconsistent, especially when adjusted to fat-free mass. Thermogenesis after a meal was mostly higher in lean than in obese subjects, but when related to FFM, differences were generally not apparent. Exogenous and endogenous fat may not be handled in the same way in normal-weight and obese subjects. Postabsorptive fat oxidation is generally higher in the obese and correlated with adiposity; however, it was generally not different when related to fat-free mass. Fat mass and fat oxidation are correlated, which has been proposed as a protective mechanism to prevent further fattening.

8

Biochemical Characteristics

8.1 Serum Lipids, Lipolysis, and Body Adiposity

Nutritional status and adiposity are significantly associated with a number of biochemical parameters, including serum lipids and lipoproteinemia (Anavian et al., 2001). Commonly, total cholesterol (TC), high-density lipoprotein (HDL-C) and low-density lipoprotein cholesterol (LDL-C), and triglycerides are assessed (Lai et al., 2001). Apolipoprotein A1, B, and E have been analyzed in studies of obese children and youth less frequently. The results concerning the changes in lipid metabolism, one of the most regular phenomena accompanying obesity, are also mentioned in other chapters, along with the assessments of other parameters.

In the Bogalusa Heart Study, 3311 children and young adults, grouped according to gender, age, and race from a biracial community, were examined. A significant positive relationship between ponderosity and LDL-C was found in older age groups (22 years) but was absent in the younger age groups. It may be speculated that such relationships might appear later in life after a longer period of increased weight and fatness. A significant negative association was found between ponderosity and HDL-C, which was particularly apparent in males at the age of 22 years.

As a measure of central obesity, subscapular skinfold thickness correlated similarly with serum lipoproteins. This enabled the development of a regression model using the subscapular skinfold to predict serum lipids (Wattigney et al., 1991). Similar relationships between serum lipid level and obesity were found in Japanese children (Yamamoto et al., 1988).

In another study a positive relationship between serum lipids and fatness was found in preschool children. The percentage of fat correlated significantly with the serum levels of total cholesterol (TC) and triglycerides (TG) in children aged 4.7 years, indicating the importance of adiposity and dislipoproteinemia at an early age (Pařízková, 1996b; Pařízková et al., 1986). DuRant et al. (1993) also showed that more favorable serum lipid and lipoprotein levels were associated with lower levels of fatness and higher levels of cardiovascular fitness in children aged 4 to 5 years. Physical activity appeared to have an indirect association with serum lipid and lipoprotein values through its relationship with higher fitness levels and lower body adiposity. Similar relationships were reported by Gutin (1998).

Correlates of the serum level of HDL-C were examined in black and white girls aged 9 to 10 years in the framework of the NHLBI Growth and Health Study. Each 10mm increase in the sum of 10 skinfolds was associated with a decrease of 1.4 mg.dL^{-1} of HDL-C, and each unit increase in the triceps/ subscapular skinfold ratio was associated with an increase of 2 mg.dL^{-1} LDL-C. In addition, each 10% increase in polyunsaturated fat intake was associated with an increase of 3.4 mg.dL^{-1} HDL-C. The associations of sedentary activity and sexual maturation with HDL-C were mediated by the differences in adiposity. HDL-C serum levels were, on average, 3.6 mg.dL^{-1} higher in black compared to white girls (Simon et al., 1995).

Aerobic conditioning is effective in the modification of dyslipoproteinemia and the health risks of atherosclerosis and without a reduction in excess fat, health cannot be effectively promoted (Fripp et al., 1985). Obesity among Greek adolescents was associated with unfavorable lipid profiles, similar to findings in other countries. Adolescents living in urban areas had a significantly higher level of total and LDL-C, but this was more consistent with lower socioeconomic status. There was evidence that TC, LDL-C, and HDL-C levels were significantly affected by qualitative aspects of diet evaluated using a food frequency questionnaire. The results of this study provides further support for the protective effect of a traditional Mediterranean pattern of living and eating in the rural areas of Greece. A more favorable lipid profile was found in adolescents, and this may partly explain the very low incidence of coronary heart diseases (CHD) in this part of Europe (Petridou et al., 1995).

The serum lipid level of children in Milan, Italy, was also comparable to other Western European data but higher than in southern Italy, where dietary intake and body fatness is generally lower. This difference is also related to a lower socioeconomic level. In obese children, higher levels of ApoB, triglycerides, total cholesterol (TC), and LDL-C and lower levels of HDL-C were seen, with higher values in obese boys than girls. An assessment of dietary intake showed the significant effect of nutritional factors. A higher TC/HDL-C ratio was found in children of the lower quartile for polyunsaturated fatty acid intake (Giovannini et al., 1992).

The increased prevalence of risk factors, as characterized by an unfavorable profile of serum lipids for later atherosclerosis, has also been reported in other child populations with increased obesity, including in Poland (Malecka-Tendera et al., 1997, 1998; Obuchowitz and Szczepanski, 1986) and the Czech Republic (Lísková, Hosek, and Stozicky, 1998; Šonka et al., 1993). Significantly lower serum HDL-C levels were found in the obese compared with normal-weight boys (Figure 8.1) (Ferrer-Gonzales et al., 1998).

A study of Polish children revealed a significant association between BMI and atherogenic lipid profile in boys, that is, positive correlations of BMI with TC, LDL-C, TG and a significant negative correlation with HDL-C. In

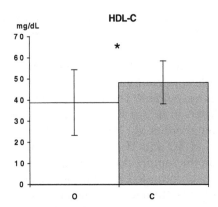

FIGURE 8.1
Comparison of serum level of HDL-C (mg/dL) in obese (O) and control, normal-weight (N) boys 5.3 to 9.9 years old. * indicates ($p < 0.05$). (Based on data from Ferrer-Gonzales et al., 1998.)

girls, a significant negative correlation was found for BMI and HDL-C (Malecka-Tendera et al., 1997). Another study in obese children aged 10 to 11 years showed higher values of Apo B and a lower Apo A-1/B ratio. Significant correlations were found between Apo A-1 and physical fitness, triceps skinfold thickness, birth weight, physical fitness, and triceps skinfold, and between Apo A-1/B ratio and triceps skinfold thickness. When both obese and normal-weight children were grouped together, a correlation was found between BMI and TC, Apo B, and the Apo A-1/B ratio. Multiple regression equation analyses indicated a significant positive contribution to the Apo A-1 level by HDL-C and physical fitness, and a negative contribution by birth weight (Sveger et al., 1989).

In a group of mildly obese children 9 to 12 years old, the level of LDL-C, TG, and the atherogenic index were significantly higher and the HDL–C significantly lower than in the normal-weight group. These results indicate that the fat percentage evaluation is suitable for the differentiation of mildly obese children in two distinct subtypes based on serum lipid profiles, and that the excess fat percentage can predict future development of atherogenesis (Tamura, Mori, and Komiyama, 2000).

The prevalence of obesity in Austrian children is 19% at the age of 7 to 9 years and 29% in 15- to 19-year-old boys. There is a decrease in prevalence in girls from 16 to 13% in the same age intervals. Levels of TG were within the normal values in both obese and normal-weight children; however, in the nonobese, TG serum level was significantly lower. No significant differences were found in TC, HDL-C, and LDL-C between obese and nonobese children and adolescents, although a higher TC/HDL-C ratio was found in the obese subjects (Elmadfa et al., 1994).

A further study (Lecerf, Labrunie, and Charles, 1998) of obese children aged up to 17 years reported the relationship between serum lipids, level of obesity, and waist-to-hip ratio. In boys, TG increased and LpA1 (a lipoprotein particle containing only Apo A-1) decreased with overall obesity. In obese girls, TG and insulin increased, and LpA1 decreased with upper body fat distribution; however, following multivariate analysis, these correlations were only found in boys.

An Italian study showed that 23% of the obese primary schoolchildren studied were hypercholesterolemic and 21% had hypertriglyceridemia; however, hypertension was not evident. This high percentage of obese and hyperlipidemic young children indicates a serious health risk and the need for early intervention (Menghetti et al., 1995). In Belgian children aged 6 to 12 years, increased levels of TC and TG were also seen, along with a marked prevalence of obesity in the sample studied. In girls, TC correlated positively with the energy density of saturated fat, cholesterol, and protein intake, and negatively with the polyunsaturated/saturated ratio of fat intake and energy density of carbohydrate intake. No such relationships were observed in boys. In addition, no relationships between TG and nutritional factors were observed in both genders. In boys, TC and TG correlated positively with BMI while, in girls, this relationship was observed for TG and BMI. It was concluded that environmental and family factors have a different effect with regard to gender, being more pronounced in girls (Guillaume, 1998).

Concentrations of TG and HDL in preschool children are correlated with central obesity (evaluated by the waist:arm ratio), and this result is independent of current height and BMI. Increasing birth weight was not associated with more a favorable blood lipid profile at the age of 31 and 43 months (Cowin and Emmett, 2000). Overweight was associated with a low level of HDL, along with hypertriglyceridemia and a high level of LDL in Taiwanese children 7.27 ± 0.46 years old (Lai et al., 2001). Higher serum glucose, insulin, cholesterol, and triglycerides than the nonobese children of the same age was also shown in obese Taiwanese children aged 11.3 ± 2.4 years (Hwang et al., 2001).

The effect of obesity and fat patterning on lipoproteinemia has been studied in Japanese children and youth (Asayama et al., 1995). In boys, anthropometric indices of obesity correlated with risk factors of atherosclerosis and strong correlations were observed among the indices of overweight, adiposity, and body fat distribution. In contrast, only the indices of body fat distribution, but not those of overweight or adiposity, were correlated with serum biochemical indices in the obese girls. This study indicated that body fat distribution is significantly related to certain biochemical complications of childhood obesity, and the androgenic fat patterns induce metabolic derangements during growth and development.

When an oral tolerance test was administered in obese and nonobese adolescents, a significant increase in triglyceride (TG) serum concentration after 2 and 4 hours was found in both groups. In a comparison of pastprandial lipemia in adolescents with a central versus peripheral pattern of fat distribution, higher variables were found in those with a central pattern of fat distribution (Moreno et al., 2001a). Another study in obese adolescents aged 11.0 to 13.8 years related to serum lipids and fat distribution characterized by the waist-to-hip ratio and triceps/subscapular ratio also used a fat tolerance test. The results were also evaluated according to the type of obesity and peripheral and/or central fat distribution. Postprandial lipemia did not differ between obese and nonobese adolescents, but a higher post-prandial lipemia concentration was also observed in subjects with a central pattern of fat distribution. These data also confirm that lipid metabolism disturbances may occur during growth depending more on the type of fat distribution than on its total amount in the organism (Moreno et al., 1998).

Body mass index increased more in hypercholesterolemic girls during the 6-year longitudinal Bogalusa Heart Study but was not different after 6 years in hypercholesterolemic and nonhypersterolemic boys. The association between BMI and blood lipids became stronger with increasing age along with the same insulin and blood pressure (Tershakovec et al., 2002a).

8.2   Lipid Metabolism in Adipose and Muscle Tissue

Lipolytic activity of the adipose tissue of obese children is decreased. *In vivo* lipolysis that reflects the mobilization of lipid stores from the subcutaneous adipose tissue shows decreased sensitivity to epinephrine in childhood-onset obesity. As an *in vivo* index of lipolysis, glycerol flux was measured using a nonradioactive tracer dilution approach and plasma-free fatty acids (FFA) concentration. At the basal state, obese children had a 30% lower rate of glycerol release per unit of fat mass than control children. To study lipolysis regulation, epinephrine was infused stepwise at fixed doses. In lean children, glycerol and FFA increased +249–246% of basal values but in the obese only increased +55–77%. The resistance of lipolysis to epinephrine did not show any relationship with the Arg64 polymorphism of the beta-(3)-adrenorecep-tor gene (Bougnères et al., 1997). In obese children, plasma apoA-I and HDL-C are independent predictors of leptin concentration during weight loss (Holub et al., 1999).

Lower rates of lipolysis contribute to a racial disparity between African-American (AA) and white-American (WA) children. The former are hyper-insulinemic and the rates of type 2 diabetes and obesity are also higher. Body lipolysis was measured in both groups with ^{2}H (5) glycerol after an overnight fasting and was approximately 40% lower in AA than WA children. Fasting insulin levels were higher in AA children; lipolysis correlated positively with fat mass, percent body fat, and abdominal fat mass. In multiregression anal-ysis models after controlling for insulin and body composition, race remained a significant contributor to the variance in lipolysis. An early metabolic phenotype may mediate fat trapping and susceptibility to the development of obesity in AA children (Danadian et al., 2001).

There is limited information about intramuscular lipid stores in children due to the invasive character of muscle biopsies. The development of nuclear mag-netic resonance spectroscopy enabled determination of intramyocellular trig-lyceride stores (ICML), accessible energy that may decrease skeletal muscle glucose utilization in obese and nonobese adolescents (11 to 16 years). Both intra- and extracellular content were significantly greater in the soleus muscle of the obese (BMI = 35 ± 1.5kg/m^2) than in control subjects (BMI = 21kg/m^2). A strong inverse correlation was found between IMCL and insulin sensitivity. This persisted and became even stronger after controlling for percent body fat and abdominal subcutaneous fat, but not when adjusting for visceral fat. In obese adolescents increases in total body fat and central adiposity were accompanied by higher ICML and ECML lipid stores (Sinha et al., 2002).

Skeletal muscle energetics was measured *in vivo* by nuclear magnetic resonance spectroscopy during a plantar flexion exercise in girls (8.6 ± 0.3 years, BMI 22.6 ± 4.2kg/m^2), subdivided further according to parents' leanness or obesity. Skeletal muscle energetics, specifically inorganic intracellular phosphate (P$_1$), phosphocreatine (PCr), and PH measured during plantar flexion, did not differ in both groups of girls with or without predisposition to familial obesity (Treuth, Butte, and Herrick, 2001).

In obese children, the concentrations of alanin-aminotransferase (ALT), cholinesterase (ChE), gamma-glutamyltransferase (GT), and ALT/AST index were significantly higher. Concentrations of ALT and ChE were positively correlated with insulin and the insulin/glucose index, BMI, and waist/hip ratio. These results indicate that biochemical parameters such as ALT and ChE may be useful as indirect measures of fat deposits in obese children (Martos-Estepa et al., 2000).

8.3   Protein Metabolism and Uricemia in Obesity

In prepubertal children, obesity is associated with an absolute increase in whole-body protein turnover that is related to an increased lean fat-free mass. Both factors contribute to the explanation of the higher resting energy expenditure (REE) in the obese compared to nonobese children (Chapter 5). A significant relationship was found between protein synthesis and FFM (R = 0.83, $p < 0.001$) and protein synthesis and REE (r = 0.79, $p < 0.005$) (Kiortsis, Darach, and Turpin, 1999).

The relationship between uricemia and adiposity was examined in adolescent girls. Both dietary factors and clearance of uric acid (CIU, which was not influenced by an increased intake of water) appears to be responsible for hyperuricemia in young obese subjects (Grugni et al., 1998).

A significant positive relationship between adiposity and C-reactive protein (CRP) has also been shown. Obese children tended to have high CRP levels and elevated blood pressure, along with slight dislipidemia. These results indicate that CRP is one of the useful indices of childhood obesity, a major contributor to the development of atherosclerosis (Hiura et al., 2003).

Plasma homocysteine levels are associated with the indices of obesity and insulin resistance in obese children and adolescents, and change along with weight and body composition due to reduction treatment (Gallistl et al., 2001b).

8.4 Mineral Metabolism

Mineral metabolism may also be altered in obese children. During an oral glucose tolerance test (OGTT), serum calcium and phosphate decreased, and serum parathyroid hormone (PTH) and calcitonin (CT) increased less in obese than in nonobese children. When obese children received a high carbohydrate content diet, changes in mineral metabolism occurred that were characterized by a secondary increase of PTH and 1,25(OH)2D3. Calcium decreased and PTH and CT increased less markedly during OGTT. Bone mineral content (BMC) measured by a photon absorptiometer and BMC/bone width ratio were lower in obese than in nonobese children (Zamboni et al., 1988).

Along with other biochemical variables, the parameters concerning mineral metabolism and some hormones were changed in a group of 8- to 11-year-old obese children (who were on a diet rich in energy and carbohydrates). In basal conditions alkaline-phosphatase (AP), osteocalcin (CT), parathyroid hormone (PTH), calcitonin (CT), and 1,25 dihydroxyvitamin D3 (1,25 (OH) 2D3) levels were significantly higher, along with increased levels of glucose immuno-reactive insulin (IRI). Levels of 25-hydroxyvitamin D3 (25OHD3) were lower in obese children compared to controls. Urinary excretion of calcium (Ca/Cr) and phosphate (TmP/GFR) were lower in obese than in nonobese children, and hydroxyproline (OH-P/Cr) and cyclic AMP (cAMP/GF) were higher in obese children (Zamboni et al., 1988).

8.5 Total Antioxidant Capacity and Lipid Soluble Antioxidant Vitamins

Total antioxidant capacity (TAC) is decreased in obese children. Reduced plasma levels of lipid soluble antioxidant vitamins (α-tocopherol and β-carotene) were also found in obese children compared to controls (Molnar et al., 1998). The differences remained significant after correction for lipemia. Reduced plasma concentrations of the main lipid-soluble antioxidants may increase the risk of cardiovascular diseases in obese children and youth. Reduced serum levels of fat-soluble antioxidants were also confirmed in obese children in the NHANES-III study (Strauss, 1999). Serum levels of β-carotene were also significantly lower in obese children than in normal-weight children. After adjustment for serum TG and TC levels, α-tocopherol was also lower in the obese but no significant differences were observed in the intake of β-karotene, α-tocopherol, fruit, or vegetables between obese and nonobese children (Strauss, 1999).

The antioxidative Cu/Zn-SOD (superoxide dismutase) response to obesity-related stress in obese and normal-weight children was followed, and the antioxidant response as Cu/Zn-SOD was significantly higher in obese children (Erdeve et al., 2004).

8.6   Summary

Serum lipids, namely total cholesterol (TC), LDL-C cholesterol, TG, Apo-B, TC/HDL, atherogenic index in absolute values and/or as related to BMI, total and central adiposity, and waist/hip ratio were increased in the obese in most studies. These results have been consistent for many years. HDL-C and ApoA-1/B ratio were reduced, and were negatively associated with body fatness. Plasma Apo A-1 and HDL-C are also independent predictors of leptin concentration during weight loss. The association of serum lipids with BMI becomes stronger with age, along with the same insulin level and blood pressure. Lipolytic activity of the adipose tissue is reduced in obese children, and the mobilization of lipid stores from subcutaneous fat tissue showed decreased sensitivity to epinephrine. Obese children also have a lower level of glycerol release per unit of fat mass than normal-weight children. Reduced mobilization of TG may contribute to the increased accumulation of fat, which is also obviously related to reduced physical activity. Lower rates of lipolysis vary in different ethnic groups: white-American had higher rates than obese African-American subjects. Lipolysis correlated with fat mass, percentage fat, and abdominal fat mass. Both intra- (IMCL) and extracellular (EMCL) TG stores in the soleus muscle were higher in the obese. A negative correlation was found between IMCL and insulin sensitivity, which remained or became even stronger after adjustment for body fat percentage and abdominal subcutaneous fat. ALT, ChE, and GT, ALT/AST were significantly higher in the obese, and the concentration of ALT and ChE was positively correlated with BMI, W/H ratio, insulin, and insulin/glucose index. Whole body protein turnover is increased in the obese and protein synthesis correlated with FFM and REE. Hyperuricemia was also found in the obese.

C-reactive protein (CRP) also correlated with adiposity; plasma homocysteine levels were associated with indices of obesity and insulin resistance, and their changes along with weight loss after reduction treatment. Mineral metabolism may also be altered as shown by changes in its parameters during an oral glucose tolerance test (OGTT). Total antioxidant capacity is decreased; reduced levels of β-carotene and α-tocopherol were found in the obese, even when no differences in their intake were revealed.

9

Hormonal Characteristics

Hormonal activities are essential for the maintenance of normal body composition. Disturbances in hormonal secretion and clearance have often been considered as the main causes of increased body fatness, particularly in those who are very obese. However, primary hormonal abnormalities such as Cushing syndrome are very rare. Many studies in growing children with very different approaches have simultaneously monitored hormonal levels, metabolic parameters, and their mutual associations with obesity characteristics. Most of the features that characterize obesity and relate to hormonal function are considered to be secondary and may have resulted from a change in overall metabolic status of an obese individual. Comparative studies involving children are difficult to interpret as mentioned previously. This difficulty is further compounded by the differentials in level of sexual maturation (often not assessed) in the young people being studied. In summary, efforts to compare and generalize the results from individual studies, often conducted under completely different sets of conditions, could result in spurious conclusions.

Obese children as a group are characteristically taller than children who have a normal body weight. In most cases these differences are only temporary and the normal-weight children usually catch up to their obese peers with increasing age and maturity. A number of hormones and their interactions are changed by increased adiposity and are also related to the temporarily accelerated growth of the obese.

9.1 Insulin-Like Growth Factor (IGF)

IGF displays a wide range of metabolic effects. The prevailing component of IGF in the plasma is bound to a specific binding protein (BP). It is presumed that BP modulates the biological activities of IGF. BP3 is regulated by growth hormone (GH) and has a high affinity for IGF. The GH-independent BP1 and BP2 show lower affinities.

Increased linear growth with a normal or high insulin-like growth factor (IGF-1) level is apparent in spite of low growth hormone (GH) secretion during the prepubertal period. In a study of children with simple obesity and normal children with shorter stature, it was revealed that peak levels of GH in the growth hormone releasing factor (GHRF) test were significantly lower in children with simple obesity. There was also a significant positive correlation with sigma IGFBP-1. With pubertal stage matching, serum GHBP and IGF-1 levels were significantly higher in children with obesity than in the other group of normal-weight children. The results of this study lead to the hypothesis that increased dietary intake and hypernutrition during growth cause hyperinsulinemia that increases GH receptor and IGF-1 secretion despite low GH secretion. Hyperinsulinemia may also increase free IGF-1 by lowering IGFBP-1. These two mechanisms are supposed to be nutrition-related hormonal changes and can explain the temporary accelerated growth of obese children. The increased IGF-1 may contribute to the decreased GH secretion due to negative feedback in simple obesity during childhood (Yasunaga et al., 1998).

The study by Bideci et al., (1997) showed significantly increased values of IGF-1 in obese children, but IGFBP-3 levels did not differ from the control group. IGF-1 and IGFBP-3 levels were significantly higher in the obese pubertal as opposed to prepubertal children. A positive linear correlation was found between BMI and IGF-1 levels ($r = 0.51$, $p < 0.05$); therefore Bideci et al., (1997) suggested that obesity had a considerable effect on IGF-1 levels during growth. The results of another study suggest that in prepubertal and early pubertal girls, IGF-1 concentration in blood is related to overall body size. Along with sexual maturation, this relationship between IGF-1 and somatic size diminishes, and relationships between IGF-1 and both fatness and physical fitness start to appear (Beckett, Wong, and Copeland, 1998).

In obese girls aged 15.0 ± 1.0 years, with a mean BMI of 31.1 ± 3.8 kg.m², the following associations using Spearman's correlation coefficients adjusted for age were revealed. IGF-1 correlated with body height, fasting insulin, and BP3 levels. In contrast with recent data on adults, no relationship was found with BMI, waist-to-hip ratio, and blood lipids. IGF-2 was correlated with insulin and BP3 levels. BP1 and BP2 were negatively correlated with BMI and insulin, and positively correlated with SHBG levels. The ratio BP1/BP2 was related to TC and LDL-C. Furthermore, BP2 showed a negative correlation with waist-to-hip ratio, TG, and uric acid levels (Wabitsch et al., 1997b). This study provided a new insight into the physiological role of IGF; BP, BP1, and BP2 seem to be insulin-regulated. They are associated with several metabolic parameters, possibly due to their modulation of IGF-1 metabolic actions. High BP1 and low BP2 levels appear to reflect a higher atherogenic risk, which is increased in obese subjects.

Free forms of IGF-1 in circulation are normal in children with simple obesity (Hasegawa et al., 1998). Increased values of IGFBP-3 along with increased insulin were found in obese children in which IGF-1, free IGF-1, free IGF-1/IGF-1. and IGFBP-1 levels were not significantly different from nonobese children. A negative correlation of IGFBP-1 and insulin level in obese children was also found. This study indicated that normal growth in obese children might be maintained due to normal IGF-1 and increased IGFBP-3 levels, which are stimulated by increased insulin levels or nutritional factors, or by an increased responsiveness to GH (Park et al., 1999).

Fasting serum levels of IGF-1, IGF binding protein-3, and type 1 procollagen C-terminal peptide (PICP) were assessed in groups of obese children and adolescents at different stages of puberty. The effect of insulin, GH, and weight loss was also studied. The growth velocity (GV) was greater in obese boys and girls than in controls during the prepubertal phase, and puberty development had a significant effect. Fasting insulin values correlated with IGFBP-3 in the obese, accounting for 24.8% of variation in prepubertal subjects and 17.1% in pubertal subjects. In normal-weight subjects, no relationship was revealed. In prepubertal control subjects with normal weight, PICP and standard deviation score (SDS) of BMI correlated with IGF-1, accounting for 12.9% of the variation, and the SDS of BMI correlated with IGFBP-3, explaining 27.8% of the variation (Falorni et al., 1997b).

In obese pubertal subjects, no significant correlations were revealed, but PICP and SDS of BMI accounted for 14.3% of the variation in the IGF-1/IGFBP-3 molar ratio. These results demonstrate that IGF-1 and IGFBP-3 are influenced by age, gender, sexual development, and nutritional status. An influence of insulin on IGFBP-3 serum levels was observed in the obese. The relationship of IGF-1 to PICP in normal-weight subjects, and the IGF-1/IGFBP-3 molar ratio to PICP in the obese, supports the concept that IGF-1 influences skeletal growth. The increased IGFBP-3 serum values in the obese suggest a possible role in controlling the growth stimulus induced by the nutritional status (Falorni et al., 1997b).

IGFBP-1 was strongly associated with insulin sensitivity and fatness in early prepubertal children aged 9.8 to 14.6 years. Insulin sensitivity, IGF-1, and obesity are important predictors of IGFBP-1 levels in pubertal children. IGFBP-1, which is suppressed by insulin, may increase free IGF-1 levels and thus contribute to somatic growth in obese children. Similar mechanisms may appear in pubertal children where growth acceleration and insulin resistance occurs simultaneously (Travers et al., 1998).

Both total and phosphorylated IGFBP-1 concentrations were decreased in obese children, and the increased IGF-1 level in obese children was related to the reduced total IGFBP-1 level but not to the change in the IGFBP-1 phosphorylation status (Kamoda et al., 1999). A study by Saito et al. (1998) showed that the fasting IGFBP-1 level was suppressed in prepubertal obese children (22.1 ± 18.4 mu.g.l^{-1}, $p < 0.001$) compared to control children (76.0 ± 62.9 mu.g.l^{-1}). However, obese children had normal insulin levels. The IGFBP-1 level may be a useful predictor for the early identification of the development of insulin resistance in prepubertal obese children. The results of the study by Attia et al. (1998) suggest that the compensatory hyperinsulinemia that characterizes adolescent obesity chronically suppresses levels of IGFBP-1. Low IGFBP-1 concentrations may serve to increase the bioavailability of free IGF-1, which may then contribute to low circulating GH, total IGF-1, and IGFBP-3.

Significant positive relationships were found between BMI and somatomedine-C/insulin-like growth factor-1 (SM-C/IGF-1), between IRI and SM-C/IGF-1, and also between BMI and immunoreactive insulin (IRI). These data seem to indicate that SM-C/IGF-1 in obese children is regulated by IRI dependent on BMI; this regulating effect of insulin may be important in obesity since human growth hormone production to stimulating factors is reduced.

9.2   Growth Hormone (GH)

Obesity is associated with a decrease in growth hormone (GH) synthesis and excretion and an increased GH clearance, along with high insulin and IGF-1 levels, which may interfere in the complex interactions of various hormones (Vanderschueren-Lodeweyck, 1993). GH secretion is impaired, which is considered a consequence rather than a cause of obesity. GH also regulates the synthesis of IGF-I in adipocytes. Increased amounts of IGF-I and GH-binding protein could be secreted from an enlarged amount of adipose tissue in the obese in spite of GH hyposecretion and a decrease in the generation of IGF-I in each adipocyte. This may contribute to the normal or increased IGF-I and GH-binding protein levels in obese subjects (Su-Youn-Nam and Marcus, 2000).

Previous studies have also shown an exponential decline in the calculated daily secretion rate of GH as a function of age in healthy men. There is also a significant negative correlation between the daily GH secretion rate and indices of obesity, for example, BMI. For each increase in BMI of 1.5 kg/m^{-2} there is a 50% decrease in the amount of GH secreted per day. At puberty and throughout adulthood, gonadal steroid hormone concentrations in blood positively determine GH release.

As shown in a study on prepubertal children with exogenous obesity, the GH-IGF axis is significantly altered even when most changes in the peripheral IGF system appeared to be independent of the modifications in GH secretion (Argente et al., 1997b). Serum concentration of the high-affinity growth hormone binding protein (GHBP) was increased in obese children and adolescents. GHBP correlated significantly with percent of body fat, waist and hip circumferences, body weight, and waist-to-hip ratio, as well as with serum leptin concentration, uric acid, insulin, total cholesterol (TC), LDL-C, LDL-C/TC ratio, triglycerides, and height standard deviation scores (SDS). Age, gender, and stage of puberty had no effect on GHBP. Multiple regression analysis using age, gender, anthropometric variables, fat percentage, and waist circumference as independent variables revealed significant associations between GHBP and leptin, triglycerides, TC, LDL-C, LDL-C:HDL-C ratio (Kratzsch et al., 1997). Waist circumference, an indicator of abdominal body fat mass, is a major determinant of GHBP levels during childhood, while leptin may be one candidate for a signal linking adipocytes to the growth hormone receptor–related GHBP release. Increased serum GHBP levels may further reflect metabolic abnormalities in obese children and adolescents. An increase in 24-hour growth hormone level concentration can result from an incomplete modified fast in obese early pubertal girls (Kasa-Vubu et al., 2002). Circulating leptin levels decreased during a treatment program, which resulted in a reduced body weight in a study by Kratzsch et al. (1997). A comparison between groups of normal-weight and obese children showed a similar response of GH to GH-releasing factor. The neuroregulation of GH release appears to be similar in normal-weight and obese peripubertal children (Volta et al., 1995).

GH-secretory bursts and mean serum GH concentrations are proportional to serum estradiol and testosterone. Body composition and especially visceral adiposity appear to be dominant negative determinants of GH production since the relationships between GH secretion and age, testosterone, or sleep are all attenuated or abolished by adiposity (Vedhuis and Iranmanesh, 1996).

9.3 Insulin

Insulin resistance and hyperinsulinemia coexist in preadolescent boys and girls with moderate and severe obesity (Caprio et al., 1996a). A study of obese adolescents by Rocchini et al. (1987) showed consistently a significantly elevated fasting insulin concentration and abnormal insulin response to an oral glucose tolerance test, along with significantly higher systolic and diastolic blood pressure and elevated 24-hour urinary sodium excretion. Significant correlations were also found among fasting insulin, body weight, blood pressure, waist circumference, and BMI (Bedogni et al., 2002).

Increases in insulin resistance at puberty were mostly related to fat mass. Increased abdominal, visceral, subcutaneous, and muscular compartments may increase insulin resistance at puberty beyond that due to total body fat. Serum concentrations of leptin and IGF-1 may further modulate homeostasis model (HOMA) beyond the influence of fatness and of its distribution (Roemmich et al., 2002). However, these conclusions are limited according to cross-sectional design and use of HOMA.

As ascertained by ultrasonography, hyperinsulinemia is associated with visceral fat accumulation, which may be the most sensitive method of predicting insulin resistance associated with metabolic derangements in children (Tamura, Mori, and Komiyama, 2000). Hyperinsulinemia can be predicted by subnormal sex hormone binding globulin concentration in prepubertal obese children (Galloway, Donaldson, and Wallace, 2001) and there is an early relationship between fasting insulin and insulin resistance, independent of body fat, with resulting health risk factors (Sinaiko et al., 2001).

Insulin-stimulated glucose uptake measured at two physiological levels of hyperinsulinemia was reduced in obese subjects compared to nonobese subjects. Defects in oxidative and nonoxidative glucose metabolism were revealed in all obese preadolescents at the higher infusion rate using a euglycemic hyperinsulinemic clamp. The ability of insulin to inhibit lipid oxidation was impaired in obese subjects at two levels of hyperinsulinemia (180 and 480 mmol). Increases in basal and glucose-stimulated insulin levels during the hyperglycaemic clamp reflected the reductions in glucose uptake during the insulin clamp in obese preadolescents. Along with an increase of BMI, a decrease of insulin sensitivity correlated significantly and inversely with increases of blood pressure, triglycerides (TG), subcutaneous fat, the percentage of total body fat, and the stage of sexual maturation. Findings in overweight/obese African-American girls aged 5 to 10 years related to hyperinsulinemia in response to glucose load suggested that the early stages of metabolic decompensation, which can result in type 2 diabetes, may occur already during growth (Young-Hyman et al., 2001).

Fasting, circulating insulin was assessed in white and black adolescents aged 11 to 18 years, along with C-peptide as a noninvasive measure of insulin secretion by beta cells (Jiang, Srinivasa, and Berenson, 1996). The C-peptide:insulin ratio served as an indicator of hepatic insulin extraction, and the insulin-to-glucose ratio as a measure of insulin sensitivity. BMI was positively related to insulin and C-peptide, and inversely with a C-peptide-to-insulin ratio in both ethnic groups of adolescents in this study. Both increased insulin secretion and decreased insulin clearance contributed to hyperinsulinemia in obese adolescents.

In prepubertal obese children, both immunoreactive and bioactive GH concentrations were low. Therefore, nutritional factors and insulin may contribute to sustain normal growth by modulating several components of the IGF-IGFBP system (Radetti et al., 1998a). Another study hypothesized that overnutrition causes hyperinsulinemia, which increases growth hormone (GH) receptors and IGF-1 secretion despite low GH secretion. Hyperinsulinemia may also increase free IGF-1 by lowering IGFBP-1. As mentioned earlier, these two mechanisms are supposed to be the hormonal changes related to nutrition in children with simple obesity and can also explain the growth of children with simple obesity. The increased IGF-1 may contribute, due to negative feedback, to reduced GH secretion in obese children (Yasunaga et al., 1998).

The development of hyperinsulinemia and insulin resistance was examined in children, with obesity lasting various periods of time and with continuous weight gain, compared to normal-weight children. Early in the evolution of obesity, insulin and C-peptide responses to a normal meal were increased by 76 and 80%, respectively. The first insulin peak was higher and occurred later in the obese subjects than in normal-weight children. The obese children had more insulin peaks within the 6-hour period after the lunch than normal-weight children. In contrast, fasting plasma insulin and C-peptide levels remained normal during the initial years of obesity, then increased progressively and

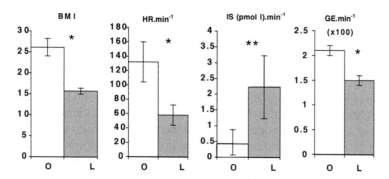

FIGURE 9.1

Comparison of BMI, hepatic insulin resistance (HIR), insulin sensitivity (IS), and glucose effectiveness (GE) in obese (O) and lean (L) pre-pubertal children. * indicates (p < 0.05) ** (p < 0.01). (Based on data from Hoffman and Armstrong, 1996.)

significantly with the duration and degree of obesity (Le Stunff and Bougnères, 1994).

Insulin sensitivity, evaluated as the rate of glucose uptake during a three-step hyperinsulinemic euglycemic clamp, was comparable in obese and normal children. Initially higher than normal in obese children, the maximal rate of glucose uptake decreased with both obesity duration and age of children, indicating the progressive development of insulin resistance (Le Stunff and Bougnères, 1994).

Insulin sensitivity was markedly lower in the obese prepubertal children compared to a lean group of peers, whereas glucose effectiveness was higher in a study by Hoffman and Armstrong (1996). Hepatic insulin resistance was also higher in the obese, with an increased insulin secretion over the first 19 minutes following glucose, although plasma glucose levels were higher (Figure 9.1). Results show that obese prepubertal children have peripheral and hepatic insulin resistance. The increases in glucose effectiveness and insulin secretion may be compensatory responses to these defects in insulin secretion.

Gonzales Moran et al. (1989) studied circadian rhythms of insulin and cortisol in obese and nonobese children. Hyperinsulinemia was confirmed in the group of obese children, and the plasma cortisol levels were higher in male obese and control children. No correlation was found between body fat and cortisol and/or insulin levels. Both normal-weight and obese children showed circadian rhythms. The rhythm for cortisol was similar in both normal and obese children; however, the insulin rhythm was disturbed in the obese. The acrophase was delayed 2 hours when values for both genders were evaluated together but only by 1 hour when girls were evaluated separately. The acrophase of cortisol and insulin rhythms in both obese and control groups is not interdependent. The alterations cited were not related to the duration of obesity in children. Radetti et al. (1998b) found that insulin secretion in obese children is pulsatile as in adults, and its secretion pattern is related to body weight.

Increased values of insulin also appear in the saliva of obese compared to normal-weight children. Insulin was investigated along with glucose, total protein, and amylase activity in the saliva of normal and obese children following a meal. Considerable variability in the values of these parameters was found in different subjects, and all values were higher in obese children than in normal-weight children. The concentration of insulin and the other parameters was on average higher than the maximum insulin level in normal children, and in some of the obese children, the concentration was more than four times higher. The progressive hypersecretion of insulin may thus promote an increased predisposition to type II diabetes mellitus at a later age (Kamarýt et al., 1989). Sex-hormone-binding globulin (SHGB) concentration can serve as a marker for hyperinsulinemia during prepuberty (Galloway, Donaldson, and Wallace, 2001).

In Pima Indian children the insulin sensitivity index decreased from 5 to 10 years of age, and increases in body weight and adiposity were associated with decreases of insulin sensitivity and physical activity (Bunt et al., 2003). In Pima Indian children, all health risk factors were increased; for example, insulin resistance syndrome (IRS) was associated with an increased body weight. After adjustment for current weight, age, and sex, lower birth weight was associated with higher systolic blood pressure, fasting plasma insulin and 32–33 split pro-insulin concentrations, glucose and insulin concentrations 30 minutes post-glucose, subscapular/triceps skinfold ratio, and plasma total and LDL cholesterol concentrations. Lower birth weight was associated with increased calculated insulin resistance. The highest levels of IRS variables and total and LDL cholesterol were found in children of low birth weight, but high fat mass was identified at 8 years. Taller height at this age predicted higher fasting plasma insulin concentrations, insulin resistance, and plasma total and LDL-cholesterol concentrations. The most insulin-resistant children were those who had short parents but had themselves grown tall (Bavdekar et al., 1999).

The results of the study of Gascón et al. (2000) in children 6 to 9 years old revealed a strong relationship between insulin and SHGB, which was shown as a marker for hyperinsulinemia and/or insulin resistance. The changes in SHGB levels in the obese did not affect free androgen index (FAI) and thus did not cause the changes of the androgenic status. Insulin has an important role in the regulation of SHGB levels.

Impaired glucose tolerance, hyperinsulinemia, and insulin resistance are the most important metabolic complications of obesity. These characteristics can eventually result in noninsulin-dependent diabetes (NIDDM) (Olefski, Kolterman, and Scarlett, 1982). Even if values are within the normal range, a relatively increased glycemia and high insulinemia may be considered in untreated obese children as a metabolic adjustment to insulin resistance and to intracellular glycopenia. Type 2 diabetes mellitus can develop later in life more frequently in the obese, especially those who have been overweight since childhood. In young patients with type 1 diabetes, growth was also increased before diagnosis, and the pubertal growth spurt was reduced.

Adolescent overweight was overrepresented; it was related in females with diabetes to poor metabolic control but showed no further acceleration in early adulthood (Domargard et al., 1999).

9.4 Steroid Hormones, Sexual Maturation

Altered steroid metabolism has also been found in obese children when compared to their normal-weight peers (Juricskay and Molnar, 1988a,b). There was a trend for a higher secretion of steroids in obese children than in nonobese children, but the differences were greatly reduced when the excretion rate was related to total body weight. Correlations were sought between body weight and the excretion of certain steroid groups, such as C2105 corticoid metabolites and compounds representing the androgen line, androsterone, then ethiocholanolon and dehydroepiandrosteron. In normal-weight children, the correlations between these parameters were significant.

The study of Chalew et al. (1997) showed that the integrated concentration of cortisol was reduced in obese children. However, the study by Juricskay and Molnar (1988a,b) indicated that the excretion of cortisol metabolites was increased along with the increased excretion of androgen metabolites and pregnenediol, a metabolite of pregnanolon. There was a trend for increased excretion of all steroid groups, which in certain cases was significant. Wide variability was also observed in the steroid excretion in obese children. In about one-third of the obese children studied, there was a hypersecretion of some components of the steroid spectrum. This phenomenon was frequent in boys (Juricskay and Molnar, 1988b).

Hyperphagia and obesity are the characteristics of hypercortisolism. A single-dose dexamethasone suppression test was performed in obese children to rule out hypercortisolism. A single dose of dexamethasone significantly increased the high leptin levels in obese children. Therefore, it was hypothesized that glucocorticosteroids up-regulate leptin levels in human subjects (Kiess et al., 1996).

Klein et al. (1998) showed that in the prepubertal or early pubertal stages of growth and development, obese children had similar estradiol levels and equivalent bone ages at a younger chronological age than nonobese children. Leptin levels did not correlate with estradiol level or bone age.

Menarche is related *inter alia* and also to a certain level of fat deposition during puberty in girls. The changes in circulating concentrations of leptin could be a hormonal signal that influences gonadotrophin secretion. A study in adolescents and young adults aged 13 to 19 years with significant variability in the level of fatness showed that in perimenarcheal and young adult girls, LH and FSH responses to GnRH were negatively correlated with BMI and circulating leptin. Decreased LH and FSH responses to GnRH were associated with increased adiposity and hyperleptinemia. These data are consistent with a direct neuro-endocrine negative effect of excess leptin on the central reproductive system in obese girls. In boys of comparable adiposity, no influence of BMI or leptin on gonadotrophin concentrations was revealed. This is another aspect of the sexual dimorphism characterizing human leptin physiology (Bouvattier et al., 1998).

Menarche is a key biological marker of maturity in girls. In a study by Stanimirova, Petrova, and Stanimirov (1993), menarche occurred in Bulgarian obese girls at the age of 12.1 ± 1.30 years of age, with height of 154.5 ± 5.35cm, body weight of 57.20 ± 5.00 kg, and total body fat of 32.27 ± 2.12%. Menarche occurred approximately 7 months earlier than in nonobese girls. These results provide further confirmation of the link between obesity development and physiologically mediated parameters of growth. The evaluation of pubertal stage is difficult in normal-weight children and more in the obese; self-assessment was not sufficiently reliable (Bonat et al., 2002).

Precocious puberty in obese children may be related to excess weight, and bone age may often be advanced along with the accelerated growth. A group of obese children was studied when undergoing an ACTH stimulation test during which they received an intravenous bolus of 250 micrograms of Cortrosyn. Blood samples were then taken at 0 and 6 min for 17-OHprogesterone, 17-OHpregnenolone, dehydroepiandrosterone, androstenedione, and cortisol levels. In two of the overweight children, there was a suspicion of congenital adrenal hyperplasia, but these subjects did not differ from the other obese subjects with regard to linear growth rate and degree of skeletal maturation. Normal-weight children displayed all measured values within reference ranges (Jabbar et al., 1991).

Hyperandrogenemia and hyperinsulinemia were found in girls with precocious menarche and central distribution of fat (larger waist circumference, waist-to-hip ratio, greater absolute and relative fat mass vs. controls in each pubertal stage). Fasting insulin levels, free androgen index, and blood lipid levels were more closely related to central fat than to total fat mass (Ibanez et al., 2003).

9.5   Beta-Endorphins and Somatostatin

The relationships between plasma beta-endorphin, insulin concentration, body fat, nutritional parameters, diet history for energy and macronutrient intake of overweight or obese prepubertal children aged 5.8 to 9.6 years have also been investigated. Obese children were characterized by significantly higher average concentrations of beta-endorphins along with increased insulin compared to normal-weight children. An analysis of concentrations in relation to the percentage of body fat revealed that beta-endorphin concentrations increased more with increasing fatness than insulin concentrations. A significant positive correlation between beta-endorphin and insulin levels was noted only in the obese subjects. In addition, there was a significant positive correlation between beta-endorphin levels and energy and macro-nutrient intake in this group. In both groups, the percentage of energy from fat correlated positively with beta-endorphin concentrations.

Energy and fat intake also showed a significant positive correlation with insulin levels in both groups. These results indicate that the level of beta-endorphins may be useful as an indicator of appetite in overweight and obese prepubertal children whose food intake has not yet been restricted (Obuchowitz and Obuchowitz, 1997).

There is relatively little information on somatostatin concentrations in obese children and their response to a meal. Following ingestion of a mixed meal, the reaction of somatostatin was the same as in normal-weight, control children. Although integrated insulin response over 180 min was higher in the obese group, the integrated somatostatin response did not differ from controls. After an oral glucose load, no change in circulating somatostatin concentrations was found (Rosskamp, Becker, and Zallet, 1986).

9.6   Leptin

The role of leptin in childhood obesity and specifically during puberty and adolescence, has received considerable attention in the recent past (Apter, 1997; Frelut, 1997; Moran and Phillip, 2003). Leptin, a recently defined hormone (Ma et al., 1996; Zhang et al., 1994), is the product of the adipose tissue-specific ob gene and is involved in the regulation of metabolic processes and the deposition of fat. Leptin provides information to the central nervous system on the energy stored in the body deposits of fat and appears to function as a link between adiposity, satiety, and physical activity. Leptin therefore appears to have a range of roles, such as a growth factor in a range of cell types, a mediator of energy expenditure, a permissive factor for puberty, a signal of metabolic status, and a modulator between the fetus and the maternal metabolism. It also interacts with other hormonal mediators and regulators of energy status and metabolism such as insulin, glucagon, the insulin-like growth factor, growth hormone, and glucocorticoids. Leptin also appears to act as an endocrine and paracrine factor and perhaps also as an autocrine factor (Margetic et al., 2002). Many of the interactions of leptin with the periphery appear to be direct; however, many are also centrally mediated under different physiological states.

The identification of the ob gene and its adipocyte-specific protein leptin has provided the first physiological links to the regulatory system controlling body weight. In experimental animals, specifically the (ob/ob) mouse, extreme obesity is attributed to mutation in the gene-encoding leptin that has profound effects on appetite and energy expenditure. Until recently, however, there was not enough equivalent evidence on the role of leptin in the control of stored fat in humans. A longitudinal study showed that plasma leptin is important for the prediction of weight gain in obese children (Savoye et al., 2002).

Present knowledge reveals that the leptin system is highly complex. As mentioned earlier, leptin is involved in a range of physiological processes in a manner far transcending the initial lipostatic content. Leptin is produced in white adipose tissue and also brown fat, the placenta, and fetal tissues (heart, bone, and cartilage). Leptin is still widely described as a satiety factor but also has a stimulatory effect on energy expenditure (Stehling et al., 1997). Therefore, leptin interacts with both components of energy balance.

Caprio et al. (1996b) found a significant correlation between serum leptin levels and subcutaneous fat deposits in children and adults. Surprisingly, a weaker correlation was found with visceral fat mass. In this study, leptin levels remained unchanged under both euglycemic and hyperglycemic hyperinsulinemic conditions in both obese and nonobese subjects. Early in the development of juvenile obesity, leptin levels are increased and more closely related to subcutaneous fat mass. Acute elevations of insulin concentrations do not affect circulating leptin levels.

The relationship of leptin and body fat mass (BFM), subcutaneous adipose tissue (SAT) levels (15 sites by Lipometer optical device), and waist-to-hip ratio (WHR) was followed in obese children and adolescents, along with leptin and insulin. In a body fat distribution model, WHR with the 4 SAT-layers of 4 upper-back and 2-triceps explained 75% of the variation in leptin. These results suggest that SAT-layers and their topography are main determinants for leptin in obese children. Maturity in the obese is associated with higher values of upper-body SAT-layers and lower values of abdominal and lower extremity SAT-layers (Sudi et al., 2000d). Regarding different ethnicity, leptin (which was higher in obese females than males) correlated well with anthropometric measurements (body weight, BMI, skinfolds) and with the grades of obesity in children in the United Arab Emirates (Adeyemi and Abdulle, 2000).

Physiological factors that influence leptin include fasting, exercise, and exposure to the cold, each of which causes a fall in ob gene expression and a corresponding reduction in the circulating level of leptin. However, the nature of the leptin complex may reduce its potential as a target in the treatment of obesity. The administration of human recombinant leptin seems to provide only limited effects (Van Gaal et al., 1999).

Leptin is known to decrease food intake and increase energy expenditure in ob/ob mice. Variants of the ob gene were not found in humans, and relatively little is known about the action of leptin on food intake and energy expenditure in humans, although circulating leptin concentrations are positively correlated to body fat stores (Van Gaal et al., 1999). Leptin exerts its central effects through several neuroendocrine systems, including neuropeptide Y, glucagon-like peptide-1, melanocortin, corticotrophin-releasing hormone (CRH), and cocaine and amphetamine-regulated transcript (CART). In obese children leptin was related to adiposity and also to plasminogen activator inhibitor 1-antigen (Sudi et al., 2000e).

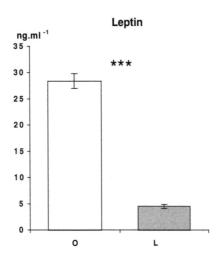

FIGURE 9.2
Leptin levels in obese (O) and normal-weight (L) children (ng.ml^{-1}). *** indicates (p < 0.001). (Based on data from Lahlou et al., 1997.)

Obese subjects have significantly higher serum leptin concentrations than normal or lean individuals (Figure 9.2) (Lahlou et al., 1997). Body fat mass correlates significantly with serum leptin concentrations in newborns, children, and adults. Females who are characterized by an increased percentage of stored fat also have higher serum levels of leptin. Circulating leptin concentrations change under conditions of extreme variations in energy intake such as fasting or overfeeding.

Measurements in white and black children and adolescents (aged 9 to 20.5 years) showed significant sex-by-race interaction on serum leptin levels, adjusted for subscapular skinfold thickness and age. Girls had serum leptin levels that were on average 2.15 times those of boys. There was an age-by-sex interaction, with serum leptin concentrations decreasing with age in boys but not in girls. A strong inverse relationship between serum testosterone levels and serum leptin levels in boys appeared to explain the effect of age (Ambrosius et al., 1998).

Newborns with intrauterine growth retardation have significantly lower serum leptin levels than those with normal growth, and leptin levels were only positively correlated with BMI in a study by Jacquet et al. (1998). These data indicate that the development of adipose tissue and the accumulation of stored fat are the major determinants of fetal and neonatal serum leptin levels. Sexual dimorphism was evident in utero. In female fetuses, higher levels of leptin were found during the last weeks of gestation, and this was consistent regardless of growth status at birth. At this time, subcutaneous fat is already deposited in significant amounts and can vary according to the term, gender, or metabolic status of the mother (Pařízková, 1993b, 1977).

In a study by Hassink et al., (1997), leptin was also present in all newborns (mean concentration 8.8 ng.mL^{-1}, SD = 9.6). In this study, serum concentration also correlated significantly with newborn weight and arm fat. Comparisons with older children indicated that leptin levels in newborns cannot be explained by adiposity alone. For example, there was no correlation between leptin and insulin. Leptin was also present in all mothers (mean value 28.8 ng.mL^{-1}, SD = 22.2 ng.mL^{-1}). Leptin concentration correlated with pre-pregnancy BMI, BMI at the time of delivery, and arm fat. In addition, maternal leptin correlated with serum insulin, but there was no correlation between maternal and newborn leptin concentrations.

A number of newborns (13%) had higher levels of leptin than their mothers. These results seem to indicate that leptin plays an important role in the intrauterine and neonatal development and that the placenta provides a source of leptin for a growing fetus (Hassink et al., 1997).

In other studies birth weight correlated with cord leptin levels. Gender differences in plasma leptin concentration were present at birth in umbilical cord blood, then at the age of four weeks. Plasma leptin levels at 4 and 14 weeks were lower than leptin concentrations observed in umbilical cord plasma, and an increase of its values was observed during this period of growth (Helland et al., 1998). Maffeis et al. (1998b) confirmed that female newborns have significantly higher serum leptin levels than males in cord blood. IGF-1 was significantly lower in newborn males compared to females while insulin and cortisol did not differ. Also in this study, birth weight correlated with leptin concentration in newborns (r = 0.56, p < 0.001). When gender was taken into account in the statistical analysis, the concentration of circulating hormones (insulin, cortisol, IGF-1, S-HBG) did not independently affect leptin inter-individual variability (Maffeis et al., 1998a).

At the beginning of life, leptin correlates with the indicators of body mass and neonatal cord leptin concentrations correlate significantly with birth weight and body mass index. In this study, gender differences were absent with regard to cord blood leptin. Maternal obesity had no effect on cord leptin, whereas exogenous maternal steroids increased neonatal leptin concentrations (Shekhavat et al., 1998). These findings indicate the importance of the fetal and neonatal periods for the development of leptin levels along with BMI. Leptin concentrations in human milk do not differ in the mothers of obese and nonobese infants. These results suggest that milk-borne leptin has no significant influence on adiposity during infancy (Uysal et al., 2002).

Significantly higher serum leptin concentrations were also found in obese Finnish children when compared to normal-weight children during the first five years of life, but serum concentrations of leptin did not show any significant relationship to dietary parameters or serum lipids in normal-weight children of the same age. The results also suggested that serum leptin concentration expresses more the amount of body fat as it may also play a role as a predictive factor for childhood adiposity (Hakanen et al., 1998).

A longitudinal study of plasma leptin levels has been executed in Australian children who were assessed at the age of 12 and 18 months, and for a proportion of the group at the age of 10.1 ± 1.6 years. The results showed that the baseline leptin continued to predict greater values of BMI percentile change over time and remained a potentially useful indicator of an increasing weight gain (Steinbeck et al., 1998).

The results of an ongoing prospective study on characteristics of leptin after long-term storage describe its relationship to body weight from birth to old age in a population-based sample of Swedish women. The group was first examined at the ages of 38 to 60 years and reexamined 24 years later. Low values of self-reported birth weight were related to higher leptin levels in adulthood ($p < 0.01$), after controlling for age and adult weight. This might be related to the findings of Barker (1998) and others who have indicated low birth weight as a risk for the later development of diseases, including obesity. Prospective analyses also showed that high leptin levels in 38- to 46-year-olds predicted subsequent long-term weight gain ($p = 0.003$), although the opposite (but nonsignificant trend) was seen in women initially aged 50 and older. This study indicated that leptin values from frozen serum could serve to predict the risk of an increased weight gain later in life in women aged 38 to 46 years. The retrospective analysis on birth weight values also suggested that leptin resistance in adulthood might have a fetal origin (Lissner et al., 1998).

Serum leptin levels were higher in diabetic than in healthy children; these differences cannot be explained by age, adiposity, or stage of pubertal development. They can be elucidated as conditioned by metabolic perturbation intrinsic to the diabetic state, or chronic hyperinsulinemia (Luna et al., 1999).

Leptin levels were significantly higher in children in prepuberty and at early stages of puberty and did not correlate with estradiol levels or bone age (Klein et al., 1998). The relationship between serum leptin levels and energy expenditure was also studied in Pima Indian children aged 5 years. Body composition was assessed by isotopic water dilution, total energy expenditure (TEE), and resting metabolic rate (RMR) using doubly labeled water (DLW) and indirect calorimetry. Total physical activity was evaluated as the ratio of TEE/RMR. Serum leptin levels correlated significantly with TEE, both in absolute values and when adjusted for body size and with physical activity level. Significant and positive correlations were found for serum leptin level and the percentage of stored fat, and these correlations were similar after adjusting for the percentage of body fat in both genders (Salbe, Nicolson, and Ravussin, 1997b).

As shown in experimental models with laboratory rodents, defects in leptin or its receptor in the hypothalamus result in obesity development. Leptin administration can cause weight loss in both ob/ob mice and in normal-weight control animals. However, this has not yet been replicated in humans. These observations suggest that humans may be resistant to endogenous leptin levels (Considine, 1997). However, some results have been achieved with subcutaneous injections of leptin in obese children (O'Rahilly et al., 2003).

The measurements of serum leptin concentrations in obese children aged 14.5 ± 1.2 years showed mean values of 21.1 ± 12.1 ng.ml^{-1}. At a given BMI level, a one to fourfold range of leptin plasma levels was noticed. Seventy-five percent of these values were out of the range of mean $\pm$ 2 SEM. Age,

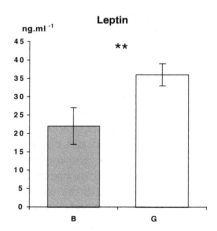

FIGURE 9.3
Leptin levels in obese boys (B) and girls (G). ** indicates (p < 0.01). (Based on data from Lahlou et al., 1997.)

gender, and/or gender maturity stage did not appear to explain these marked differences. BMI correlated significantly with leptin levels (r = 0.79; p < 0.001). These data suggest that the biological background as reflected by low or increased leptin concentrations in severely obese children is heterogeneous (Frelut et al., 1997) and cannot be explained by single-factor analysis.

Serum leptin levels increase during growth and development, and this increase continues in girls during sexual maturation, along with fattening, but decreases in boys. Suppression of testosterone increased leptin levels in boys, and the resumption of puberty was associated with decreased leptin levels. In girls, serum leptin levels did not change with the alteration of the pituitary-ovarian axis and were permanently higher than in boys. Serum leptin levels were also significantly higher during the night (Palmert, Radovick, and Beopple, 1998). There is a hypothesis that leptin could contribute to the regulation of GH secretion (Coutant et al., 1998). Forward stepwise regression analysis selected the change in total body fat in young females over a 6-month period as the most powerful determinant of the percentage of increase in the nocturnal leptin concentration (Matkovic et al., 1997).

Measurements in girls showed higher serum levels of leptin (Figure 9.3) (Lahlou et al., 1997). This applies even after correction for the differences in body fat mass. In a multiple regression analysis with age and body mass index (percent of body fat) as fixed variables, testosterone had a potent negative effect on serum leptin levels in boys, but not in girls. Argente et al. (1997a) also found a marked variation of serum leptin levels in boys and girls, which significantly depended on the maturational stage. Along with progressing puberty, leptin increased permanently in girls and decreased in boys. In obese children, leptin levels were markedly increased, and a significant correlation of leptin and BMI was again found in this study.

Overweight children, especially girls, tend to mature earlier than leaner children. It was also found that menstruation starts at a certain level of adiposity and body weight, which led to a hypothesis that the degree of body fatness can trigger the neuroendocrine events that lead to the onset of puberty; leptin levels are higher in obese children. Leptin receptors were identified in the hypothalamus, gonadotrope cells of the anterior pituitary, and ovarian follicular cells, and also in Leydig cells. Leptin accelerates gonadotropin-releasing hormone (GnRH) pulsatility in hypothalamic neurons, and also has an influence on the anterior pituitary. However, a high level can have also inhibitory effects on the gonads. Obese children also have increased adrenal androgen levels, which may be involved in the accelerated growth in height of the obese before puberty, in spite of lower GH levels. It was revealed recently that leptin also has a specific role in stimulating the activity of enzymes for the synthesis of adrenal androgens.

In vitro experiments using newly developed human adipocytes in primary culture showed that both testosterone and its biologically active metabolite dihydrotestosterone are able to reduce leptin secretion into the culture medium up to 62%. Using the semi-quantitative reverse transcriptase-PCR method, testosterone was found to suppress leptin mRNA to a similar extent. These results indicate that apart from the differences in body fat mass, the higher androgen concentrations in obese boys are responsible for the low leptin serum concentration when compared with obese girls (Wabitsch et al., 1997a). A critical leptin level is obviously needed to maintain menstruation (Kopp et al., 1997).

In another study, Ellis and Nicholson (1997) confirmed a significant positive relationship for serum leptin and body mass index. The percentage of fat and fat mass was gender dependent and not influenced by ethnicity. At each degree of sexual maturation, females had higher levels of leptin than males. This difference remained significant when leptin was normalized for fat mass. In boys and girls, the mean leptin/fat mass ratios were relatively invariant during sexual maturation, and no differences were observed between the oldest children with the highest degree of sexual maturation and in young adults. The finding of a higher average serum leptin and leptin/fat mass ratio at prepubertal ages may suggest that there are gender differences in leptin synthesis, clearance rates, bioactivity, and/or leptin transport.

Along with the elevated serum leptin levels and increased fat mass, the follow-up of obese children revealed an increased intake of energy (two to three times) compared to normal, lean children (Lahlou et al., 1997). Obese children had higher leptin levels even when they were normalized with fat mass. Gender differences, that is, higher serum levels of leptin in girls and a significant correlation between leptin and fat, were also seen in this study. It appears that serum leptin reflects but does not halt fat storage in obese children. When serum levels of leptin were normalized to body adiposity, leptin in females was found to be increased independently by obese status, sexual maturation, and being female.

Leptin was also positively associated with percentage of fat intake and negatively associated with percentage of carbohydrate intake. These results show that a high-fat, low-carbohydrate diet was related to leptin levels (Park et al., 1998). Correlations between serum leptin levels, BMI, and percentage of fat were also found in diabetic children, but insulin-dependent diabetes was not associated with higher leptin concentrations (Verrotti et al., 1998).

Other studies have confirmed significant relationships between leptin and age, gender, level of pubertal development, BMI, and insulin (Hassink et al., 1997). Serum leptin levels were 4 to 5 times higher in obese children and adolescents compared to normal-weight children of the same age (Falorni et al., 1997a). Using partial correlation analysis in subjects subdivided according to gender and pubertal stages, log values of serum leptin and fasting insulin values, adjusted by age and standard deviation scores for BMI, correlated significantly, with a weaker correlation in boys than in girls. In obese children, leptin concentrations correlated better with total insulin area (TIA) under the curve during a glucose tolerance test (evaluated before the therapeutic program started) than with fasting insulin level.

Total adiposity but not insulin or insulin resistance index is the main determinant of leptin in obese children. In contrast to obese girls, the FFM and TG contribute significantly to the variation in leptin in obese boys (Sudi et al., 2000a). In obese children, there is no inverse association between leptin and cortisol, found usually in adults, but there is a significant relationship between insulin and cortisol (Sudi et al., 2000c).

The leptin receptor itself may not be specifically involved in the control of leptin secretion, and supports the concept of relative resistance to leptin in common obesity (Lahlou et al., 2000). Leptin circulates in serum bound to high molecular weight proteins, which can be hypothesized to regulate its functional efficiency. Leptin-binding activity (LBA) was found to reflect circulating leptin levels, as well as body composition and hormonal milieu. Leptin binding, in addition to leptin, may play an important role in the regulation of appetite and in the "leptin resistance" in obese youth (Diamond et al., 2000).

Two very severely obese children who were members of the same pedigree had very low leptin levels in spite of markedly increased stored fat. In both, a homozygous frame-shift mutation involving the deletion of a single guanidine nucleotide in codon 133 of the gene for leptin was found. The severe obesity in these congenitally deficient children provides the first genetic evidence that leptin is an important regulator of energy balance in humans (Montague et al., 1997). Another study of extremely obese German children, however, did not show leptin deficiency mutation (Hinney et al., 1997).

As shown in an experimental model (mice), leptin acts as a skeletal growth factor, with the direct effect on skeletal growth centers (Shalitin and Phillip, 2003). For physical maturity, the timing of AR is an indicator rather than a certain level of adiposity (Williams and Dickson, 2002).

The hypothesis was tested that juvenile obesity in humans may be caused by leptin resistance mediated through genetic variations in isoforms of the hypothalamic leptin receptor. Obese Danish men with a history of juvenile onset obesity were followed, and the results of this study showed that it is unlikely that mutations in the coding region of the long isoform of the leptin receptor are a common cause of juvenile-onset obesity (Echwald et al., 1997).

Increased adiposity contributes to higher levels of PAI-1-Ag, which was associated with leptin and insulin, but not after adjustment for fatness. BMI was the main determinant for the variation of leptin, which does not seem to be independently linked with fibrinolytic parameter. However, an unfavorable metabolic and fibrinolytic risk profile may begin to act from puberty in the obese (Sudi et al., 2000e). Further data of Sudi et al. (2000b) do not support that leptin alone serves as an independent predictor of blood pressure in obese children and adolescents.

Restrained eating and leptin levels showed a significant inverse association in obese girls aged 8 to 12 years, which remained significant after adjustment for fat mass, and which is the most important biological predictor of leptin levels. In the case when lower leptin levels caused reduced energy expenditure, restrained eating might be responsible for weight gain in obese subjects because of a positive energy balance (Laessle, Wurmser, and Pirke, 2000).

Human leptin and leptin receptor genes and their mutations were followed as models of serum leptin receptor regulation. It was revealed that leptin is not needed for ObR gene expression. It was suggested that leptin plays a role in receptor down-regulation because soluble Ob receptor (sObR) levels are negatively correlated with leptin levels and BMI in control subjects, whereas sObR levels are not depressed in obese leptin-deficient, or leptin-receptor-deficient individuals (Lahlou et al., 2002). Before the beginning of gonadal activity in obese and control children, dehydroepiandrosteron sulfate (DHEAS) levels are explained partly by leptin and BMI. In addition to BMI, IGF-1 in part accounts for androstenedione (AD) levels. Increased androgen secretion in children with premature adrenarche may be explained by parameters other than leptin or BMI (L'Allemand et al., 2002).

9.7 Ghrelin, Adiponectin, Thyroid Hormones, Tumor Necrosis Factor Alpha, Gastric Inhibitory Peptide

Ghrelin is a new gut-brain, growth-releasing peptide isolated from human and rat stomach — gastric mucosa that induces weight gain and increases appetite and food intake. This reduces fat utilization and facilitates fat storage. It may interact with glucose metabolism. Circulating levels of ghrelin as a function of gender, adiposity, and pubertal status were followed in a study by Bellone et al. (2002). In human obesity, ghrelin seems to be down-regulated. Fasting plasma ghrelin levels in Japanese children and adolescents (mean age 10.2 ± 2.8 years, BMI $28.0 \pm 4.5 \text{kg/m}^2$) were negatively correlated with BMI and waist circumference, but not with percent of overweight or percent of fat, whereas fasting leptin levels were positively correlated with all of the following parameters: BMI, waist circumference, percent of overweight, and percent of body fat. Further, plasma ghrelin levels were negatively correlated with fasting immunoreactive insulin, homeostasis model assessment insulin resistance index, and quantitative insulin sensitivity check index values. There was no association between plasma ghrelin and leptin, but ghrelin correlated with PAI-1 concentrations. These observations suggest that the down-regulation of ghrelin secretion may be a consequence of higher insulin resistance associated with visceral fat distribution and elevated PAI-1 concentrations, but not the consequence of total body fat accumulation related to leptin (Ikezaki et al., 2002).

In a sample of children (mean age 9.4 years), 10 single-nucleotide polymorphisms were found. One common polymorphism of the ghrelin gene, which corresponds to an amino acid change in the tail of the prepro-ghrelin molecule, was significantly associated in children with a higher BMI and with lower insulin secretion during the first part of an oral glucose tolerance test, although no difference in glucose level was observed. These observations suggest that variations in the ghrelin gene contribute to obesity in children and may modulate glucose-induced insulin secretion (Karbonits et al., 2002).

Molecular screening of the ghrelin gene showed the association of Leu77Met variant with earlier onset of obesity (Miraglia-del-Giudice et al., 2004). A study in Italian children showed that the Leu77Met polymorphism of the ghrelin gene seems to play a role in anticipating the onset of obesity in children, suggesting that ghrelin may be involved in the pathophysiology of childhood obesity (Miraglia-del-Giudice et al., 2004).

Gastric inhibitory polypetide (GIP) and glucagon-like peptide-1 potentiate glucose-induced insulin secretion. Their abnormal secretion may be involved in the pathogenesis of the insulinemia in obese children. Using a hyperglycemic clamp with a small oral glucose load, it was possible to assess GIP response in obese and lean prepubertal children and adolescents. Basal insulin and C-peptide concentrations and insulin secretion rates were significantly greater in obese subjects. Under conditions of stable hyperglycemia, the ingestion of a small amount of glucose resulted in similar GIP responses in both lean and obese subjects. Therefore, in juvenile obesity, excessive alimentary beta-cell stimulation may be independent of the release of GIP (Heptulla et al., 2000).

Adiponectin is a new adipokine with anti-inflammatory and insulin-sensitizing properties; it was also found to have independent negative associations with obesity and hyperinsulinemia/insulin resistance in adults. In a study with Pima Indian children, plasma adiponectin concentrations were negatively correlated with percentage of body fat and fasting plasma insulin concentrations cross-sectionally both at 5 and at 10 years of age. At age 10, percentage of body fat but not fasting plasma insulin was independently associated with fasting plasma adiponectin concentrations. Longitudinally, plasma adiponectin concentrations decreased with increasing adiposity. These results confirm similar results gained in adults of an inverse relationship between plasma adiponectin concentrations and adiposity in children.

It seems that hypoadiponectinemia is a consequence of the development of obesity in childhood (Stefan et al., 2002).

TSH, T3, and T4 were significantly higher in the obese compared to normal-weight children aged 4.5 to 16 years. Twelve percent of the obese children had TSH, 15% had T3, and 11% had T4 concentrations above the twofold standard deviation of normal-weight children. The degree of overweight was associated with T3, T4 and TSH. Thyroid hormones did not correlate significantly with leptin (Reinehr and Andler, 2002).

Another study in obese and normal-weight children also showed increased levels of TSH and T3 in the obese. In most subjects, however, these increases were not accounted for by thyroid autoimmunity or iodine deficiency. TSH elevations with normal thyroid hormone levels in obese children do not need any thyroxic treatment, provided that thyroid disorders are excluded (Stichel, L'Allemand, and Gruters, 2000).

In obese children TSH was not related to hemostatic markers — that is, factor VII coagulant activity (VIIc) and factor VIII coagulant activity (VIIIc), tissue type plasminogen activator antigen (tPA-Ag), and plasminogen activator inhibitor-1 antigen (PAI-1-Ag) — as markers of cardiovascular risk. An inverse association between fT4, factor VIIc, and fibrinogen was found, which remained significant after adjustment for body fat mass. These findings demonstrate a close relationship between thyroid function and hemostatic markers of cardiovascular risk in obese children and adolescents, and suggest that thyroid dysfunction is associated with an unfavorable hemostatic status already during growth (Gallistl et al., 2000c).

Tumor necrosis factor-alpha (TNF-alpha), a polypeptide cytokine produced primarily by mononuclear phagocytes, plays a key role in the initiation of the inflammatory response, but has a multitude of effects in many tissues. A multivariate regression analysis of the interactions between TNF-alpha and insulin on circulating leptin levels among normal and overweight children showed that plasma insulin levels had a significant positive association with leptin levels even after adjusting for BMI in normal-weight children only. Plasma TNF-alpha levels were positively associated with leptin levels even after adjusting for BMI in girls only. This study showed that plasma insulin plays certain role in leptin expression among normal-weight children. However, it was shown that TNF-alpha plays a more significant role in leptin expression among girls only (Chu et al., 2002).

In contrast to adult subjects, prepubertal obese subjects show intact adrenomedullary responses to caffeine (Bondi et al., 1999).

9.8 Summary

As primary hormonal disturbances causing greater adiposity are quite rare, some hormonal deviations in obese children are mostly considered secondary and resulting from a changed metabolic status. However, an increasing number of studies do not always report corresponding findings. Obese children are usually temporarily taller in spite of a decrease in growth hormone (GH) synthesis and increased GH clearance. Urinary GH excretion is reduced before and after puberty in spite of comparable height, and GH increases during puberty are less in the obese. Blunted GH response to provocative stimuli was also found. Affinity of GHBP is increased in the obese and in some studies was associated with percentage of fat, waist and hip circumferences and ratio, body weight, serum leptin, uric acid, insulin, TC, LDL-C, LDL-C/TC, TG, and height standard deviation scores (SDS).

IGF-1 levels are increased in the obese, and this has many metabolic effects. The greatest component of IGF-1 is bound to specific protein (BP), presumed to modulate its biological activities. IGF-1 correlates with height, overall body size, fasting insulin, and BP 3 levels. The association diminishes with increasing age, and the relationship of IGF-1 to fatness and fitness starts to appear. Some studies lead to the hypothesis that increased dietary intake during growth causes hyperinsulinemia, increased GH receptor, and IGF-1 secretion, despite low GH secretion. GH also regulates the synthesis of IGF-1 in adipocytes, the increased amounts of which (and of GHBP) could be secreted from large amounts of adipose tissue in spite of GH hyposecretion.

Pro-collagen C-terminal peptide (PICP) increases during puberty with a more rapid decrease in girls and in normal-weight subjects (NWS). PICP association to IGF-1 in normal-weight children and the PICP to IGF-1/IGF-1BP molar ratio in the obese supports the concept that IGF-1 influences skeletal growth. IGF BP-1, which supports growth, is associated with insulin sensitivity and fatness in the obese during early puberty. Body mass index and immunoreactive insulin, which are interrelated, are also significantly associated with somatomedin-c/IGF-1.

Hyperinsulinemia and an abnormal response to an oral glucose tolerance test (OGTT) exist in the obese along with increased blood pressure and Na secretion. Increased insulin resistance (IR) was found to be related to fat mass, mostly visceral; the latter is the predictor of insulin resistance. The ability to inhibit lipolysis by insulin is impaired. Along with increased BMI, insulin sensitivity correlates significantly with blood pressure, TG, subcutaneous fat, percentage of FM, and stage of sexual maturation, as found in, for example, African-American girls 5 to 10 years old. Type 2 diabetes mellitus can occur in early growth. Circadian rhythms of insulin showed impairment. Increased values of insulin were also found in saliva. In Pima Indians, insulin sensitivity decreased from 5 to 10 years, which was associated with an increase of body weight, adiposity, and health risks, and a decrease in physical activity.

A trend for a higher secretion of steroid hormones in the obese was found; in normal-weight children steroids correlate with body weight, but not in the obese. In one-third of the obese, hypersecretion of some components of the steroid spectrum was found, especially in boys. Hyperphagia and obesity are characteristics of hypercortisolism. Obese children had similar estradiol levels and equivalent bone age at a younger chronological age than normal-weight children. Leptin did not correlate with estradiol levels and bone age. Menarche can occur earlier in obese girls and precocious puberty may be related to body weight. LH and FSH responses to GnRH were negatively correlated with BMI and circulating leptin.

Decreased LH and FSH responses to GnRH were associated with increased adiposity and leptin. A direct neuroendocrine negative effect of excess leptin on the central reproductive system exists in obese girls. Hyperandronemia and hyperinsulinemia were also found in girls with precocious menarche and central fat distribution. β-endorphins and somatomedin increase more along with adiposity than insulin. β-endorphin is also an indicator of appetite.

Leptin produced in, for example, white and brown adipose tissue and fetal tissues, has a number of roles in energy regulation. Leptin correlates with adiposity, and decreases more with aging in boys; an inverse relationship between serum testosterone and leptin levels was found in boys. In girls, leptin levels are higher, and this sexual dimorphism exists from the fetal period; newborns with intrauterine growth retardation (IUGR) have lower leptin levels. Birth weight, BMI, and arm fat correlate positively with leptin. No correlation between maternal and newborn leptin levels were found, and maternal obesity had no effect on cord blood leptin. Prospective analyses show that adult leptin levels can predict long-term weight gain. Leptin levels are also higher in diabetic children. There is also a positive correlation between leptin and percentage fat intake; total adiposity, not insulin and IR, is the main determinant of leptin in obese children. The leptin receptor itself may not be specifically involved in the control of leptin secretion, and supports the concept of relative resistance to leptin in common obesity. Leptin binding activity (LBA) reflects circulating leptin levels and body composition. Increased adiposity contributes to an increased level of PAI-1-Ag, which is associated with leptin and insulin, but not after adjustment for fatness. Body mass index is the main determinant for variability of leptin, which does not seem to be independently linked with fibrinolytic parameters characterizing health risks.

Ghrelin seems to be down-regulated in the obese, which may be a consequence of increased IR associated with visceral fat accumulation and increased PAI-1 concentration. Fasting values of ghrelin negatively correlate with BMI and waist circumference, not with percentage of overweight or of fat, whereas leptin positively correlates with BMI, waist circumference, percentage of overweight, and percentage of fat. Plasma ghrelin concentration negatively correlates with fasting immunoreactive insulin (IRI), and correlates positively with PAI-1 concentrations. Ghrelin gene variation can contribute to obesity in children.

Abnormal secretion of gastric inhibitory polypeptide (GIP) and glucagon-like peptide-1 may be involved in the pathogenesis of hyperinsulinemia in obese children. Adiponectin, which longitudinally decreased with increasing body fat, negatively correlated with percentage fat and fasting plasma insulin concentration in Pima Indian children 5 to 10 years old. TSH, T3, and T4 were increased in the obese 4.5 to 16 years old, and were associated with the degree of overweight; no correlation with leptin was found. TSH was not related to hemostatic markers. Thyroid dysfunction may be associated with an unfavorable hemostatic status already during growth.

A multivariate regression analysis of the interactions between tumor necrosis factor α (TNFα) and insulin on circulating leptin levels among normal-weight and obese children showed that plasma insulin levels were significantly positively associated with leptin levels even after adjustment for BMI in normal-weight children only. In girls only, plasma TNFα levels were positively associated with leptin levels, even after adjusting for BMI.

10

Psychosocial Aspects of Obesity

10.1 Psychosocial Determinants of Obesity

A wide range of psychosocial determinants of the overweight or obese condition has been cited, but most are poorly understood. There is less of an understanding and certainly little consensus regarding the aetiology of these factors. For example, we do not know how widespread these determinants are and whether they are genetically mediated, triggered by the environment, or potentially, a mix of both. For instance, how pervasive are the social pressures on young children to be thin? What are the psychosocial pressures associated with the use of restricted dietary practices in this population (Garrow, 1999)?

Some prominent American researchers, e.g. Dietz (1992) have claimed that psychosocial problems are the most prevalent consequence of childhood obesity. There are widespread examples of discrimination against fat people of all ages, and the most vulnerable are young people. Therefore, the most potentially damaging consequence of childhood obesity for many youngsters may be the detriment to psychological well-being. Obese children are consistently rated by their peers as lazy, dirty, and ugly, along with being cheats and liars (Wadden and Stunkard, 1985). Adiposity and psychopathology were associated with loss of control over eating (Morgan et al., 2002). Eating disordered behaviors and psychopathology can vary in obese and normal-weight children, along with fatness (Tanoffsky-Kraff et al., 2004).

Numerous studies have considered the attitudes and preferences for particular features in others; among these studies was an exploration of various forms of disability, including obesity. Results have consistently demonstrated that individuals of all ages rate the obese lowest. The most common explanation for this phenomenon is that generally, children with other disabilities are considered unfortunate victims of the environment whereas the obese are deemed to be somewhat responsible for their plight. The reason many obese adults may dislike drawings of obese children is that the images remind them of their own situation.

The social stigma and marginalization (Strauss and Pollack, 2003) associated with the ungainly appearance of many obese individuals is generally poorly understood. In fact this issue may not even be acknowledged by less empathetic normal-weight individuals. In countries where the favored body size and shape for a male is tall and lean with an athletic body build, those who do not match up, including obese individuals, may be ridiculed and also made to feel like social outcasts. Present society views the obese with much more disdain than decades ago.

This phenomenon is also particularly commonplace in childhood and adolescence where young people can be malicious and vindictive to those who are different. Psychiatric aspects of obese children and adolescents have been examined in the past 10 years (Zametkin et al., 2004). This area is of great importance for further research, as we have a poor understanding of the impact of an increasingly heavier and fatter population on size acceptance.

In addition to the social stigma, obese individuals commonly report a fear of participating in social activities, including sport and recreation. Many obese individuals dread being on view in public places and wearing swimsuits or sporting clothes. The obese child is potentially more sensitive and therefore vulnerable to the comments of his or her peers, and this may be the main reason many avoid physical activity settings and normal social contacts. The need for a degree of self-esteem and self-worth is critical to a well-balanced individual. If these traits are damaged or missing, the obese individual may consider him- or herself ugly and unattractive to the people around, which can lead to unhappiness and depression. This scenario may perpetuate a vicious cycle in which misery and discontent with physical appearance can precipitate the use of food as solace and a corresponding increase in weight and potentially further discontent. Coincidentally, physical activity level may decrease and inactive behaviors predominate.

A good example of social discrimination was provided in the findings of a study by Gortmaker et al. (1993), who obtained follow-up data on a nationally representative sample of men and women who were 16 to 24 years old at baseline. Seven years later, women whose BMI was greater than the 95th percentile had completed fewer years at school, had higher rates of poverty, and were less likely to be married than those who had been normal weight at baseline. The work of Lissau and Sorensen (1994) found that the strongest predictors of the development of later obesity were indices of parental neglect rather than the level of education or parents' occupation.

As early as the 1970s Bruch (1974) contended that social attitudes toward the body, a preoccupation with physical appearance, and an overwhelming emphasis on beauty (which means thinness) in our society were contributing factors in mild forms of body image distortion in nonobese individuals during growth. These factors may be the basis of the early and subsequent widespread condemnation of overweight and obesity as undesirable and ugly. The strength of such community beliefs is a powerful illustration of the psychological and social context in which young people with a weight problem find themselves.

Stunkard (1989) was also an early proponent of the thesis that obesity can be triggered by psychological problems, a particular concern for the childhood and adolescent years. For example, the tendency to overeat and satisfaction gained from eating highly processed foods containing a high proportion of fat and/or sugar can originate from stress at school or in the family. The stressor or prompt to overeat may be the separation or divorce of parents, stress of exams or a disruptive time with peers. In addition, Bruch (1974) identified the difficulties faced by obese children who have overprotective parents with such parents being more likely to use food as a comfort rather than in response to hunger. In contrast, Wadden et al. (1989) found no association between measures of anxiety or depression and weight category in high school girls (mean age of 15.8 years). However, Hills and Byrne (1998) found that overweight girls were significantly more dissatisfied with their size and shape and consequently more of them were attempting to lose weight.

The effect of child and adolescent obesity on immediate mental health and long-term medical complications has become a focus of attention due to their increasing prevalence. Recent advances in neuroscience and genetics are important tools for mental health professionals who can contribute to the reduction of the consequences of childhood obesity; even modest weight-loss goals correlate with significant health benefits (Zametkin et al., 2004).

The psychological ramifications of the above-mentioned issues are too often not considered in the prevention, treatment, and management of obesity. Therefore, a psychological evaluation of the obese child or adolescent may be an appropriate suggestion as a standard measure for use in clinical practice. There is little doubt that the use of a psychosocial approach as an adjunct to the treatment of an obese child would be valuable, and it may be one of the more important keys to a successful and lasting result.

Many overweight children have symptoms of depression. Erikson et al. (2000) have reported on a relationship between depressive symptoms and BMI in preadolescent girls, but not in boys of the same stage of development. Observations of obese children and particularly adolescents in many countries underline their marginalization. Such a situation may further aggravate the social and emotional consequences of an increased weight and fatness and accompanying health problems (Strauss and Pollack, 2003). This scenario can also manifest itself in older age groups, and mental health may be threatened in more sensitive individuals. A dose-response relationship between the number of episodes of depression during adolescence and the risk of adult obesity has also been observed, especially in female subjects. This relationship was differentiated according to age with no association seen in late adolescent boys and similarly, early adolescents boys and girls (Richardson et al., 2003). However, only chronic obesity in children aged 9 to 16 years of age was associated with psychiatric disorders, such as oppositional defiant disorder in both genders and depressive disorders in boys. When this sample of obese youth was followed longitudinally, chronic obesity was associated with psychopathology (Mustillo et al., 2003). The evaluation of the quality of life in obese children underlined the necessity of understanding what life is like for such children in order for their treatment and rehabilitation programs to be more effective (Ravens-Sieberer, Redegeld, and Bullinger, 2001).

Recent research also indicates that the adult preoccupation with weight, restrictive dietary practices, and other harmful methods of weight regulation is also common in the childhood and adolescent years (Drummer et al., 1987; Hills and Byrne, 1998; Smolak, Levine, and Gralen, 1993; Stein and Reichert, 1990; Wertheim et al., 1992). To prevent distorted attitudes about food, weight, and exercise, there is a need to determine what motivates these attitudes, when they first begin to emerge, how they evolve over time, and which individuals are most vulnerable (Killen et al., 1993). Extensive research has assessed body image and weight-control practices of different populations, but, like many other areas of study, there has been considerable variability in the assessment protocols employed. Therefore, the interpretation of results in many instances reflects the assessment methodology utilized as much as the data collected or the varying statistical procedures utilized to interpret the data. As a result, to adequately assess psychological characteristics such as body image and weight-control practices, the efficacy of the assessment protocols used must be considered.

Binge eating symptoms have commonly been reported in severely obese adolescents seeking weight-reduction treatment, and symptoms were strongly related to the results of testing of psychopathological traits (Decaluwe, Braet, and Fairburn, 2003; Isnard et al., 2003). Overweight appeared to precede the appearance of binge eating symptoms (Decaluwe and Braet, 2003). Overweight girls more commonly report concerns about weight, shape, and eating and attempted dietary restraint. This group also displayed more negative self-esteem related to their athletic competence, physical appearance, and global self-worth and also displayed more symptoms of depression (Burrows and Cooper, 2002).

Obesity in children can also be related to the loss of control of eating. which may cause more severe cases of obesity along with greater psychological distress (Morgan et al., 2002). The same study also showed a dose-response relationship between reduced sleeping hours and obesity in children. Short sleeping hours may contribute to obesity through increased sympathetic activity, elevated cortisol secretion, and decreased glucose tolerance. Parental obesity or lifestyle factors like long hours of television watching (a potential contributor to reduced sleeping) and physical inactivity were also significantly associated with obesity in Japanese children aged 6 to 7 years (Sekine et al., 2002). The restraint score for eating was significantly negatively associated with leptin levels in obese girls aged 8 to 12 years (Laessle, Wurmser, and Pirke, 2000).

Research associated with analyses of weight- and eating-related issues has largely concentrated on female populations (Brodie and Slade, 1988; Bruce and Agras, 1992; Cash and Green, 1986; Dennison, 1996; Littrell, Damhorst, and Littrell, 1990) and to a lesser degree on gender differences in early adulthood (Andersen and DiDomenico, 1992; Altabe and Thompson, 1992a). Considerably less work has involved adolescents and younger children, and very few studies have focused on differences between subjects categorized on the basis of body composition or satisfaction with physical appearance (Byrne and Hills, 1993, 1995, 1997; Hills and Byrne, 1998).

10.2 Definition of Body Image

Body image is the picture one has of his or her body (Schilder, 1950). It is a self-concept construct that has been conceptualized in various ways, and as a result, a range of related terms with differing connotations have evolved. These include body percept, body concept, body-ego, body ideal (Kolb, 1975), body schema (Schontz, 1969), body boundary (Fisher and Cleveland, 1968), body awareness, body identity, body structure, body self, and social body concept (Bruch, 1974). While the term "body image" is recognized as a generic label, its interpretation has been dependent on the individual researcher's definition (Thompson, Penner, and Altabe, 1990).

Body image is acknowledged as a complex, dynamic, and multidimensional aspect of the personality (Koff, Rierdan, and Stubbs, 1990). The lack of agreement in defining the concept and the resultant rival approaches in methodology has contributed to difficulties in measuring body image (Burns, 1979). This remains the most criticized feature of body image research (Altabe and Thompson, 1992b; Offman and Bradley, 1992).

Fisher (1990) categorized research dealing with body image issues into nine primary focal areas, including the perception and evaluation of body appearance; accuracy of perception of body size, body sensations, spatial position, and body boundaries; distortions associated with psychopathology and brain damage; responses to body damage; cosmetic alterations; and sexual identity of one's body. The most pertinent of these to overweight, obesity, and weight-control practices are perception and evaluation of physical appearance and accuracy of perceptions of body size.

Obese children are significantly more likely to engage in dieting behaviors to express concern about their weight, to restrain their eating, and to exhibit more dissatisfaction with their body image than average-weight children, especially in girls (Vander-Wal and Thelen, 2000). However, do all obese individuals have a body image disturbance? Some might contend that this is true, but it is not the case, and dissatisfaction with the body is not always a central factor. Some obese individuals (more particularly adults) are able to look at their bodies in a realistic manner and recognize the need to diet and exercise without a significant emotional involvement. Others do not regard their extra body fat as undesirable, either for cultural or personal reasons.

10.3 Appearance-Related Body Image

Body image has both self-perceptual and subjective (attitudinal and affective) components (Garfinkel et al., 1992). Body dissatisfaction and self-esteem are associated with various problematic eating attitudes and behavior patterns (Israel and Ivanova, 2002). Garner and Garfinkel (1981) proposed that body image could be separated into two elements: body image distortion and body dissatisfaction. Body image distortion was considered indicative of perceptual feelings about the body, while body dissatisfaction results from a disturbance in thoughts and is associated with a desire to alter physical appearance (Brownell, 1991; Brownell, Rodin, and Wilmore, 1992; Danforth and Sims, 1992; Garfinkel et al., 1992). Williamson (1990) added an alternative conceptualization of body size dissatisfaction composed of two parts: body size distortion and preference for thinness. Thus, body image disturbance could result from a cognitive inability to assess body appearance (body image distortion) or body size (body size distortion) accurately. Alternatively, disturbance could result from a subjective evaluation that the body does not meet the ideal (body dissatisfaction) and in particular the lean ideal (preference for thinness).

10.3.1 Body Size Distortion

Body size distortion involves a perceptual disturbance in which individuals seem unable to assess their body size accurately. Body size distortion was first studied by Slade and Russell (1973) who noted a greater body size overestimation in anorexic subjects compared to controls. Others have suggested that size overestimation is not specific to eating disordered populations (Thompson, 1986; Thompson and Thompson, 1986). However, it has been suggested that a cognitive inability to accurately assess body size may be an important diagnostic criterion in discriminating between excessive dieting and disordered eating practices (Garfinkel et al., 1992).

10.3.2 Body Dissatisfaction

Body dissatisfaction represents an attitudinal or affective dimension in which one expresses a certain level of satisfaction with the body or specific body parts (Garner and Garfinkel, 1981). Body dissatisfaction is associated with various problematic eating attitudes and behavior patterns, including dietary restraint, weight preoccupation, binge eating, and the risk of developing eating disorders (Rosen, 1990).

In the assessment of disordered eating behaviors, body dissatisfaction is the best predictor of dietary restraint (Gralen et al., 1990). Streigel-Moore et al. (1989) noted that body dissatisfaction more accurately predicted students whose eating symptoms worsened during their first year of studies than perceived stress, ineffectiveness, perfectionism, and competitiveness. Cognizant of research concerning attitudes toward exercise, body dissatisfaction may also influence motivations for exercise, with individuals dissatisfied with physical appearance more likely to exercise for weight control and to improve muscle tone (Byrne and Hills, 1995; McDonald and Thompson, 1992).

Body dissatisfaction and weight concerns appear from very early in life, at the age of 5 years. No direct relationships have been found between girls' weight and weight concerns. However, girls' body dissatisfaction and mothers' weight concerns were independently and positively associated with higher weight concerns among girls (Davison, Markey, and Birch, 2000).

10.3.3 Preference for Thinness

The third type of body image disturbance proposed by Williamson et al. (1989) is indicative of an individual's "ideal body size," or a body size that is used as a standard for judging satisfaction with current body size. Research suggests that individuals who intensely fear weight gain prefer a body size that is significantly thinner than those who do not have such fears (Williamson et al., 1985; Williamson et al., 1989).

10.3.4 Body Size Dissatisfaction

Dissatisfaction with body size may be the strongest predictor of overall body dissatisfaction (Cash and Green, 1986) and associated weight-modifying behaviors (Gustafson-Larson and Terry, 1992). A lower self-concept has been noted in girls with higher body weight from 5 years of age (Davison and Birch, 2001b). Both the negative self-evaluation of these subjects and concern of their parents about their weight status appeared related to self-restriction of food to control weight. Parents therefore have a significant effect in this respect; family environment influences the development of behavioral controls of food intake in overweight children, and family members should be involved in their child's treatment (Birch and Davison, 2001).

Delineation of the body size dissatisfaction concept into separate components has enabled research in appearance-related body image to assess perception of, and attitudes toward, physical appearance in different populations. However, there has been a bias in the research toward the assessment of certain populations. Females of all ages have been more commonly studied than males, and adults and college students have been more regularly assessed than children and adolescents. Consequently, there is a paucity of data considering gender differences across the childhood and adolescent years. Because adolescence is a period commonly associated with the emergence of disordered behavioral patterns such as anorexia and bulimia nervosa (and obesity) (Attie and Brooks-Gunn, 1989) an understanding of age and gender differences in the appearance-related body image of children and adolescents is important.

An example of a study that highlights the aforementioned gender differences is that of Israel and Ivanova (2002), which found that girls with higher degrees of obesity reported lower physical self-esteem than girls who were moderately overweight. For boys, however, the opposite pattern was shown. Nevertheless for both genders, cognitive and social self-esteem predicted general self-esteem, whereas physical self-esteem did not. Fat phobia belongs to pathological traits of obese youth, and should be defined when following obese subjects (Bacon, Scheltema, and Robinson 2001).

Many areas need to be understood in relation to the antecedents of dissatisfaction of body weight. For instance, the Kids' Eating Disorder Survey (KEDS) and Binge Eating Scale followed psychological problems in obese children, and documented an improvement in child behavior problems and competence, but no change in symptoms of disordered eating as a result of a standardized behavioral weight control program (Epstein et al., 2001). Additionally, a study of Australian youths showed the effect of SES on self-esteem; it was lowest in overweight girls of middle/upper SES, and greatest among boys of low SES, despite the latter being more likely to be overweight (O'Dea and Caputi, 2001). The researchers concluded that being overweight did not appear to adversely affect the physical self-esteem of low-SES children, particularly boys.

10.4 Relevance of Psychological Accompaniments of Physical Growth during Childhood and Adolescence

During childhood, physical growth changes are characteristically slow and gradual. The small changes in appearance and increases in height do not generally require wholesale revisions to the image a child has of his or her own body. Similarly, through most other stages of life the body changes imperceptibly and so does one's body image.

In contrast, the more rapid changes during the adolescent period, such as increase in size, changes in body proportions, primary and secondary sex characteristics and facial appearance, mean that minor adjustments in body image are not sufficient for some individuals. It is important to mention that while adjustment and coping with changes in body image are important for many young people, body image is not of uniform importance and significance to adolescents across the entire period of growth. Adolescence is a period when self-awareness of appearance and body shape becomes more important. However, this self-awareness can appear much earlier, for example, at the beginning of the school years, and may result in a deterioration of food habits and or physical activity participation.

The hormonal activity that occurs during puberty contributes to observable bodily changes, the most obvious being those of secondary sexual characteristics. Despite the commonality of physical changes, there are individual differences in the onset and rate of change during this period. Social comparison during puberty (Thornton and Ryckman, 1991) is particularly relevant in young people, so the timing of puberty may be a more important aspect of pubertal development than actual pubertal status (Simmons, Blyth, and McKinney, 1983).

Pubertal timing is usually defined as a measure of an individual's relative development in comparison with the maturation status of the reference group (Alsaker, 1992). Richards, Regina, and Larson (1990) also reported that behavior patterns are influenced more by "social age" than chronological age. Thus, for school children, the reference group would most likely be other students within the same grade.

Early researchers postulated that personality adaptation is affected by body shape, which influences the impression a person makes on others and how one views oneself (Schonfeld, 1966). Bernstein (1990) suggested that the "bio-psychosocial phenomenon" of body image is an individual's view of him- or herself not only physically, but also physiologically, sociologically, and psychologically. Thus, it has been argued that during late childhood and early adolescence, self-awareness is particularly intensified due to the complexity of changes. These include physical changes, the increase of introspection, the importance assigned to physical traits by the peer group, and the increased tendency to compare oneself with culturally determined standards (Littrell Damhorst, and Littrell, 1990; Thornton and Ryckman, 1991).

Statistical analysis of school performance of obese children in Spain showed that obese children of both genders had significantly better results than normal-weight children. This observation may be explained by the additional time spent in academic pursuits compared with being physically active. It is also possible that obese children attend school more diligently in order to be better accepted by their peers and to counterbalance their negative body image (Zoppi et al., 1995).

In a group of black, inner-city school children, 35% were obese according to triceps skinfold thickness criteria. Behavioral characteristics were assessed using the Child Behavior Checklist (CBCL) and the hyperactivity subscale of the Connor's Parent's Questionnaire. Obese children were more likely to have abnormal scores. Referring to CBCL subscale scores, a higher "sex problem" score was noted in obese girls. There was a significant trend for obese boys and girls to have higher CBCL subscale scores. These data supplement the limited information on obese children and are consistent with previous findings suggesting subtle behavior differences in obese children. Also the proportion of obese children placed in special education or remedial class settings was twice that for children with normal body weight (Tershakovec, Weller, and Gallagher, 1994).

Psychological functioning and its association with the changes in BMI during 1 year were evaluated in boys and girls aged 9 years of age. Increases of BMI were significantly associated with unfavorable changes in physical activity attitudes, activity preferences, perceived physical activity competence, self-concept, and body image. There was limited support for the hypothesis that overweight children are more sensitive to changes in body shape than children with normal weight. These data illustrate that growing obese subjects may be overly concerned with body weight and shape (Kolody and Sallis, 1995).

Personality and intelligence were followed up in obese Chinese children aged 9.8 years (Li, 1995). While the prevalence of childhood obesity in China has been low, it has increased significantly in recent years, with the increase representing a large absolute number of the population (see Chapter 2). The system of one child per family may be contributing to this problem as single children might be spoiled more frequently. Li (1995) also found that children with severe obesity had significantly lower performance on a score of IQ (Wechsler Intelligence Score) than control children with normal weight. Simultaneously, a significantly higher EPQ psychoticism score (Eysenck Personality Questionnaire) was found in severely obese children, which indicates that obesity has more serious consequences in a population less adapted to hyperalimentation and obesity than in the other populations. It should be noted, however, that these results were not found in children with a milder degree of obesity (Li, 1995). Another Chinese study confirmed other abnormalities in the obese, including an increased baseline secretion of insulin and C-polypeptide. Total IQ, speech IQ, and operational IQ along with thyroid function were relatively lower in the obese than in controls, and gonad development and maturity took place earlier in the obese (Zhang and Li, 1996). It may be speculated that in this particular Chinese cohort their obesity pathogenesis was caused, at least in part, by an endocrinological deviation. Similar findings in other child populations have not been replicated.

Simple obesity has also been linked with other metabolic disturbances. For example, Obrebowski, Obrebowska-Karsznia, and Gawlinski (2000) noted significantly reduced odor-detection thresholds in children with simple obesity. Smell and taste were assessed and in 77% of cases electrogustometric thresholds were below the normal range.

In a study by Mills and Adrianopoulos (1993), it was revealed that patients with the early onset of obesity demonstrated a greater frequency and higher levels of emotional distress and psychiatric symptomatology than those with late onset of obesity. These findings support the belief that obesity is associated with greater internal psychological conflicts. Therefore, childhood obesity can also serve as a predictor variable for possible psychological problems and disturbances in obese populations in later life.

Therefore, in addition to the biological changes that characterize the adjustment at puberty, psychological adjustments occur in relation to physical changes. At the perceptual level, individuals and their peers react to bodily changes that are observable and make comparisons based on these observations. Due to individual variability in biological maturation, there are common changes noticed in all young people but at the same time there are extensive differences related to the rate of change and to genetic diversity. Each individual alters his or her mental image of their body form as it changes and, in a similar way, responds to social reactions that these bodily changes elicit. Social responses will also have a great bearing on one's psychological state. This will depend on where in the range one is perceived, from approval to disapproval, admiration to ridicule, acceptance or rejection.

Adolescence is a period of physical and psychosocial change that for many involves a stressful reevaluation of self-concept and interpersonal relationships (Emmons, 1992). Well before the onset of puberty, in fact during the younger elementary school years, individuals understand that thinness in women and athletic leanness in men are considered physically attractive and socially acceptable (Davies and Furnham, 1986). There is also evidence that body dissatisfaction and dieting increases at the time of puberty (Smolak et al., 1993). Early maturing females display these attitudes and behaviors before others (Gralen et al., 1990).

Of added interest, Strauss and Mir (2001) found a twofold increase in smoking among normal-weight adolescent girls who reported trying to lose weight. In contrast, prevalence of smoking was similar among overweight adolescent girls who tried to lose weight compared to those who did not, with similar trends reported in boys. Tobacco use is common among normal-weight adolescents trying to lose weight, and its use is also associated with a cluster of other unhealthy dietary practices.

10.5 Sociocultural Influences

Body image is influenced by culturally defined standards of physical attractiveness. Fallon and Rozin (1985) suggested that body image includes the perception of cultural standards, perception of the extent to which one matches the standard, and the perception of the relative importance that members of the cultural group and the individual place on the match.

Physical appearance is emphatic because it determines a large extent of the initial attraction to others and is a key factor in how individuals are judged. Although the physically attractive "ideal" may vary across cultures, physical appearance is of importance to most cultures (Furnham and Baguma, 1994). Individuals are more satisfied if they meet the idealized standards of attractiveness (Cok, 1990). Information that explains the obese condition has a minimal effect on children's attitude and their behavioral intentions toward peers presented as obese (Bell and Morgan, 2000). In order to assess appearance-related body image, it is necessary to define the yardstick against which physical attractiveness is judged and the ramifications of meeting or failing to meet the level of physical appearance deemed "ideal." This has changed profoundly not only during recent decades (e.g., when comparing beauty queens, the most famous movie stars, and subjects presented in commercials for different items, etc.), but also across many centuries when comparing the idols presented in ancient pictures and sculptures.

10.6 Physical Appearance

Spring et al. (1994) proposed that across all societies the most valued body shape is that which is associated with health and prosperity. While the lean physique is considered ideal in Western societies, to ready them for marriage, young Nigerian females from affluent families spend up to two years in "fattening huts" in order to achieve the desired endomorphic physique. Likewise, men from Cameroon enter fattening huts to emerge appearing fat and prosperous and demonstrating prestige (Pasquet et al., 1992).

In general, the body type considered physically attractive depends on gender, social status, and sociocultural context. Western society lauds physical attractiveness, and having the "perfect" body symbolizes self-control, mastery, and acceptance (Brownell, Rodin, and Wilmore, 1992). Some in modern society strive for physical perfection and reward those thought to embody the "ideal" (Rodin and Larson, 1992). Attempts to attain the physical ideal are based on the belief that the body is malleable using diet and exercise (Brownell, 1991). The value placed on physical attractiveness is very evident in the fashion, fitness, diet, and cosmetic industries (Rodin and Larson, 1992). In a less obvious way, the value placed on physical attractiveness is reflected in body image disturbances and the related pathogenic weight-control practices (Wertheim et al., 1992; Wiseman et al., 1992).

As a self-concept construct, body image is greatly influenced by an individual's perception of physical attractiveness. Numerous studies have shown that perceptions of physical attractiveness are positively correlated with an individual's self-concept, self-esteem, personal judgment, depression, and emotional disturbance (Koff and Rierdan, 1991; Rosen, Gross, and Vara, 1987). An individual's objective level of physical attractiveness can influence psychological experiences and development. While the cumulative effects of unattractiveness can negatively influence mental health, an individual's self-perceptions of physical appearance can differ considerably from reliable objective perceptions of physical attractiveness (Butters and Cash, 1987). Thus, self-perceptions can have more salient implications for mental health than objective evaluations. These findings have important implications for the support of obese children and adolescents. Making access to sedentary activities contingent on the completion of some level of physical activity may help to reinforce activity in obese children. Changes in physical activity level depend in part on the targeted physical activity goal (Goldfield et al., 2000), and there is clearly the need to address the seriousness of the level of adiposity with a reinforcement of one's self-concept and body image.

10.7 The "Ideal" Body Shape

Despite the cultural valuation of body shape in relation to health and prosperity, the shape differs in relation to a society's degree of industrialization

(Spring et al., 1993). In affluent cultures characterized by an abundance of processed foods and convenient lifestyles, it is easy and unhealthy to become overweight and difficult to remain thin. Thus, it could be argued that in industrialized societies where the dominant causes of morbidity and mortality are chronic diseases associated with obesity, the ideal body type for both sexes is one that is predominantly lean and thin.

The body shape considered "ideal" is not necessarily the one that is biologically determined and for many is not biologically attainable (Olmstead et al., 1985). Attitudes toward what constitutes a socially desirable body shape are learned early in life (Cash, 1990). What is not learned, however, is that due to biological differences very few individuals will meet societal expectations. If body size and weight are normally distributed only a minority of individuals can be expected to match "naturally" the ectomorphic, almost prepubertal female ideal (Rodin and Larson, 1992), or the male body ideal of "muscular mesomorphy" (Loosemore and Moriarty, 1990).

As the average weight of many populations is increasing, the "real–ideal" difference is also increasing. Fallon and Rozin (1985) concluded that a woman's perception of the ideal female body shape is a thin one, most likely thinner than the average weight of the population. Studies on female adolescents reflect weight concerns comparable to those evidenced in women. Fisher et al. (1991) reported that almost two-thirds of the adolescent females tested described themselves as overweight, three-quarters believed they were above the healthiest weight for age and height, and four-fifths were above the weight deemed to make them most happy. Another study of adolescents found that whereas girls were more likely than boys to report a desire to be thinner (60.3 versus 34.8%), boys were more likely to want to be taller (67.2 versus 49.1%) (Gustafson-Larson and Terry, 1992).

10.8 Body Weight or Body Fatness — The Real Issue?

Body weight and fatness are fundamental elements by which people everywhere are judged (Spring et al., 1994). The stigma attached to being overweight or obese in Western cultures has implications for individuals of all ages. In Western society the sexes appear to differ in the perception and appraisal of total body weight. The term "weight" appears to have a different meaning for males and females (Silberstein et al., 1988), and weight is an issue of central importance to women. Females are faced with the paradox of a hormone-induced increase in body fat at puberty and a socioculturally driven desire to be thin (Wilmore, 1991). Further, for females the term "weight" may relate closely to perception of personal body size. Females may equate underweight with thinness, low adiposity, and an ectomorphic body type, all of which are viewed as favorable. In contrast, males may equate underweight as ectomorphy, and overweight as endomorphy, both of which are viewed as unfavorable.

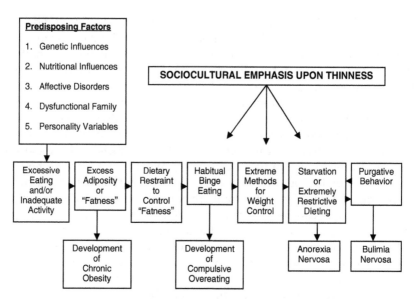

FIGURE 10.1
An etiological model for eating disorders. (Based on data from Williamson, 1990.)

Williamson (1990) devised a theoretical model, illustrated in Figure 10.1, which delineated how body-image distortion, preference for thinness, and body size dissatisfaction interact with fear of fatness to produce a static and dynamic disturbance of appearance-related body image. It is evident from the model that a multidimensional approach incorporating measurements of each component of body image disturbance must be employed if a comprehensive assessment of appearance-related body image is to be achieved.

Due to the varied approaches to defining body image (Sturmey and Slade, 1988), the number of appearance-related body image assessment procedures has proliferated, with the majority focusing on the perceptual and subjective components. Figure 10.2 illustrates the categorization of these measurement procedures.

10.9 Summary

The intensity of body image disturbances fluctuates widely even over short periods of time. When things are going well and a person with a body image disturbance is in good spirits, he or she may not be troubled by the disability although it may never be far from one's awareness. In contrast, in esteem-lowering experiences and a depressive mood state, the unpleasant aspects of life may become focused on his or her obesity and the body becomes the explanation and symbol of unhappiness.

PHYSICAL APPEARANCE-RELATED BODY IMAGE ASSESSMENT

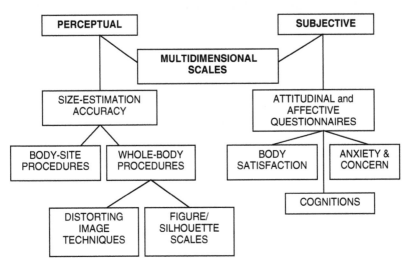

FIGURE 10.2
Categorization of appearance-related body image assessment measures. (Based on data from Byrne and Hills, 1993.)

Despite such short-term fluctuations in intensity, body image disturbances persist with remarkably little change over long periods of time and in concert with considerable variation in life circumstances. For example, weight reduction can have little influence for some individuals, much to their surprise and dismay.

A number of factors may predispose an obese person to a disturbed body image. These include the age of onset of obesity, presence of emotional disturbances, and negative evaluation of obesity by others during the formative years. Disturbances in adulthood are often commonplace in those who became obese during childhood or adolescence. While relative indifference to the condition may characterize much of childhood, adolescence is the most common period where a disturbed body image is likely to begin.

With the level of devaluation of obesity in society, it may appear redundant to mention negative evaluations as a cause. Obese individuals who have a body image disturbance are often preoccupied with obesity, irrespective of their social status and intelligence. Body weight is the overriding concern, and the individual sees the world in terms of body weight. The individual may envy those who are thinner and feel contempt for those who are fatter.

Nevertheless, it is a mistake to assume that all obese individuals are psychologically or emotionally disturbed. There are no more anxious or depressed people among the obese than in the general population. Therefore, psychological problems do not occur in all obese individuals.

Irrespective of the mix of contributing factors to one's overweight or obese state, it is highly likely that psychosocial factors will be important in most cases. Some may argue that such factors are not as important as the physiological or metabolic; however, such factors may hold the key to treatment and management of the condition at all ages for many individuals.

11

Health Problems

Obesity in childhood is associated with numerous medical problems related to physiological, metabolic, and structural changes (Gunnell et al., 1998; Kiess et al., 2001; Zwiauer et al., 2002). Health problems in the obese very often include hyperlipidemia, increased total cholesterol (TC), and triglycerides (TG), along with decreased HDL-C and increased LDL-C (see Chapter 8), as well as coronary heart disease, elevated blood pressure, hyperinsulinemia, carbohydrate intolerance, diabetes mellitus, impaired heat tolerance, deterioration in hormonal release, and others. Additional complications include sleep apnea, osteoarthritis, orthopedic and respiratory problems, gall bladder disease, and many others. This profile of health problems is not confined to the industrially developed countries but is a result of the rapid "Westernization" of other countries. For example, increased blood TC levels in children have also been found in other countries, with accompanying health risks (Couch et al., 2000).

Nevertheless, it is important to understand that obesity has not been conclusively earmarked as a primary independent risk factor for these problems. Parent-reported health status of overweight and obese Australian primary school children showed that parental concern about their child's weight was strongly associated with the child's actual BMI. Despite this, most parents of overweight and obese children did not report poor health; a high proportion did not report any concern. This may well be a problem from the point of view of early identification and diagnosis of obesity in children and a timely intervention (Wake et al., 2002).

Many pediatricians and general practitioners perceive obesity in childhood as a serious problem that should be treated as early as possible, particularly as childhood obesity contributes to approximately 30% of adult obesity (Greecher, 1993; Davis et al., 1993a,b). Few longitudinal studies have considered the delayed, long-term effects of childhood obesity with respect to adult disease. Approximately one-half of adolescents with more severe obesity, that is, with a BMI at or above the 95th percentile, become obese adults (Dietz, 1998c).

Moreover, there is some evidence that obesity that develops during childhood and persists until adolescence can increase adult morbidity and mortality. As the severity of obesity can predict morbidity, the persistence of childhood obesity may be expected to account for a disproportionate share of the consequences in the adult years. In men who were obese during adolescence, all-cause mortality, and especially the mortality from cardiovascular diseases and colon cancer, was higher. In both genders early obesity increased the prevalence of cardiovascular diseases and diabetes in adulthood. This may be related to the amount and distribution of fat. Various adverse psychosocial consequences were also more frequent in females who were obese in childhood. This included completion of fewer years of education, higher rates of poverty, and lower rates of marriage and household income. The same result has not been found in males (Dietz, 1998b). Increased adiposity, eating disorders, and psychopathology are already significantly associated in childhood (Tanoffsky-Kraff et al., 2004).

11.1 Dyslipidemia, Hemostatic Factors, and Cardiovascular Risks

Vanhala et al. (1998) suggests that adult obesity developed from childhood may be more problematic than adult-onset obesity due to an increased risk of the metabolic syndrome. Some authors suggest that irrespective of adult body mass, adolescent obesity is associated with elevated health risks, dyslipidemia, increased blood pressure (Mijailovic, Micic, and Mijailovic, 2001), and higher adult mortality (Must et al., 1992). A specific role of intra-abdominal adipose tissue on morbidity risk in adulthood was suggested to exist in childhood (Morrison et al., 1999) that was independent of total body fat. This has not been definitively demonstrated but may direct the effort for effective prevention and treatment of childhood obesity (Maffeis and Tato, 2001). Percent of body fat and fat mass evaluated by DXA in Pima Indian children (from 5 to 19 years of age) correlated significantly with BMI, and were significantly related to metabolic measures (fasting and 2-hour plasma glucose, systolic and diastolic blood pressure, TC, HDL, fasting insulin, and TG). Body mass index was strongly associated with measures of adiposity by DXA, and these measures showed a similar association with cardiovascular risk factors (Lindsay et al., 2001).

In the Bogalusa Heart Study, subjects were partially examined at the age of 2 to 17 years and were reexamined at ages 18 to 37 years (mean follow-up at 17 years). Child overweight was related to adverse risk factors among adults, but associations were weak and were attributable to the strong persistence of weight status between childhood and adulthood. Although obese adults had adverse levels of lipids, insulin, and blood pressure, the level of these risk factors did not vary with childhood weight status or with the age of obesity onset. Results of this important longitudinal study indicate the need for additional research data; however, both primary and secondary prevention of obesity in childhood is emphasized (Freedman et al., 2001b).

This especially concerns children with a family history of cardiovascular diseases as shown in African-American and European-American subjects (Dekkers et al., 2004).

Further results of the Bogalusa Heart Study with subjects (black and white) followed from 8.1 and 14.4 years to 22.5 and 30.9 years indicated that increases in adiposity, regardless of initial status of body fatness, alter cardiovascular risk variables toward increased risk beginning in childhood. Body mass index, skinfolds, SBP, DBP, LDL, HDL, TG, insulin, and glucose were evaluated. Females, particularly blacks, displayed a greater rate of increase in adiposity than males. In a multivariate analysis, the rate of increase in adiposity was related independently to baseline age and the rate of baseline adiposity was related to adverse changes in measured cardiovascular risk variables, except glucose. The changes in BP, LDL-C, and HDL-C were greater in whites, while the rate of increase in insulin was greater in blacks. Females displayed greater changes in BP, HDL-C, and insulin; males displayed greater changes of TG (Srinivasan, Mayers, and Berenson, 2001).

Other studies have revealed that overweight in adolescence can predict a broad range of adverse health effects that are independent of adult weight after 55 years of follow-up. Morbidity and mortality of obese adolescents aged 13 to 18 years, characterized by a BMI higher than the 75th percentile for age in a large national survey, was assessed in the Harvard Growth Study and compared to their lean peers (BMI 25 to 50th percentiles). Subjects who were still alive were interviewed about their medical history, weight, functional capacity, and risk factors. Cause of death was assessed from death certificates. The analysis revealed that obesity during adolescence was associated with an increased risk of mortality from all causes and disease-specific mortality among men, but not among women. The relative risks among men were 1.8 for mortality from all causes and 2.3 for mortality from coronary heart disease. The risk of morbidity from coronary heart disease and atherosclerosis was increased among men and women who had been overweight in adolescence. The risk of colorectal cancer and gout was increased among men and the risk of arthritis was increased among women who had been overweight during adolescence. Overweight during adolescence was a more powerful predictor of these risks than overweight in adulthood (Dietz, 1998a; Must et al., 1992).

A 50-year longitudinal study of a group of obese adolescents demonstrated that the mortality and morbidity from cardiovascular diseases were significantly increased compared with a group of subjects who were lean during adolescence. In addition, the influence of adolescent obesity on adult morbidity and mortality appeared independent of the effects of adolescent obesity on adult weight status. A more marked deposition of fat on the trunk starts to appear during adolescence (Pařízková, 1977). Therefore, adolescent-onset obesity may be the forerunner to adult obesity as well as influencing mortality and morbidity in its own right (Dietz, 1993). This is one of the most important reasons why obesity should be managed as early as possible, at the latest during adolescence (Csabi et al., 2000). This concerns not only appropriate diet but also the level of physical activity, which was shown to be too low not only in countries like Canada (Tremblay and Willms, 2003), but also China (Tudor-Locke, Ainsworth, and Adair, 2003).

Risk factors for coronary heart disease are present in obese adolescents, including an increased level of serum lipids with lower HDL-C, increased blood pressure, and a reduced fitness level (Berenson et al., 1993). These problems occur more frequently in children from families with an increased prevalence of these problems (Becque et al., 1988). It is even more important to intervene when individuals are further handicapped by their family history. However, with regard to adult health risk (according to blood pressure, carotic artery intima-media thickness, fibrinogen concentration, TC, LDL-C, HDL-C, TG, fasting insulin, 2-hour glucose concentration, BMI, percentage of body fat) in a prospective familial cohort study in Newcastle upon Tyne, little tracking from childhood overweight to adulthood obesity was found when using a measure of fatness independent of body build. Only children who were obese at the age of 13 years showed an increased risk of obesity as adults (50 years). No excess adult health risk from childhood or teenage overweight was found. Being thin in childhood offered no protection against adult increased adiposity, and the thinnest children were found to have highest adult risk at every level of adult obesity (Wright et al., 2001). The members of this cohort were born in 1947; the results could be different in subjects born recently and under a different set of life conditions.

The evaluation of other long-term data on the health status of obese children showed that 28% had hyperlipidemia, 25% had an elevated blood pressure, and 30% also had asthma. Sixty-three percent of these children had obese mothers, 31% had obese fathers, and 50% had one or more obese siblings (Unger, Kreeger, and Christoffel, 1990). In relation to risk factors for atherosclerosis in obese children, the following anthropometric parameters were suitable predictors: body mass index in subjects below 9 years of age, BMI and waist circumference in males over 9 years, and BMI and waist/hip/height ratio in females aged over 9 years (Perrone et al., 1998a).

The effect of early obesity and the delayed consequences were followed in a study by Guo et al. (1998). Mathematical models were fitted to individual semiannual BMI values from 2 to 18 years of age and then at 2-year intervals from 18 to 25 years. Analyses showed that the higher the peak velocity and the BMI values at peak velocity and at maximum, the more likely adulthood obesity would develop. Birth weight also had an important role: the lower the birth weight, the more likely the development of obesity in adulthood. In addition, the later the peak velocity and maximum BMI, the higher the TG, and the higher the BMI at maximum velocity, the lower the HDL-C.

A 40-year weight history and adult morbidity and mortality was described in a cohort of Swedish subjects followed in Stockholm between 1921 and 1947 (DiPietro, Mossberg, and Stunkard, 1994). The sample of overweight children remained overweight as adults. After the age of 55 years, BMI values started to decrease in both males and females. From postpuberty onward, female subjects were heavier than males. Subjects who died during the 40-year study and those reporting cardiovascular diseases were significantly heavier at puberty and adulthood than were subjects who remained healthy. There was a marked increase in BMI between the postpubertal period and age 25 among those who subsequently died, those who developed cardiovascular disease, and particularly those who developed diabetes. In contrast, those reporting cancer had a lower BMI throughout. This study provides further evidence that overweight and obesity in adolescence may continue until adulthood and may be associated with serious health risks and increased morbidity and mortality later in life. However, it is necessary to also consider the effect of range of fatness then and recently, and the additional effect of further factors on delayed consequences of early obesity that were not controlled. This needs to be analyzed in future studies.

The association between risk factors for coronary heart disease including obesity in 15- to 16-year-old schoolboys and adult mortality rates was examined in localities characterized by a fourfold difference in adult mortality from coronary heart disease. Increased body fat, smoking, poor diet, and physical inactivity were found in pupils from a school in a high-risk area compared with those in a low-risk area. Lipids, maximum oxygen uptake, and hypertension were similar in children from both schools. The risk of coronary heart disease seems to reflect the adult mortality rates in the area (Freeman et al., 1990). The reduction of obesity prevalence in childhood is therefore one of the important tools available to reduce coronary heart disease later in life (Freedman, 2002).

Measurements in lean, fit children showed lower total cholesterol (TC), low-density lipoprotein cholesterol (LDL-C), and triglyceride levels (TG), and higher high-density lipoprotein cholesterol (HDL-C) levels than in unfit children, except after adjustment for body fat and/or abdominal fat. Unfit children appear to be at an increased risk of unhealthy levels of serum lipids due primarily to increased body fatness.

Cardiovascular risks were associated with leptin levels and nutrition in Korean girls aged 15.4 ± 1.5 years compared to normal-weight girls of a comparable age. Circulating leptin levels were significantly higher in obese girls and were significantly correlated not only with body weight and body fat but also with systolic blood pressure, fasting blood sugar, TC, TG, and LDL-C. After correction for BMI, leptin was significantly correlated with percent of body fat, TC, and LDL-C. Several cardiovascular risk factors were positively associated with circulating leptin, which in turn was positively correlated with percent of fat intake and negatively with percent of carbohydrate intake. These results show that a high-fat, low-carbohydrate diet was related with leptin levels, and simultaneously with several cardiovascular risks (Park et al., 1998).

Another study showed that the dietary intake of energy, fat, fiber, and cholesterol was similar among groups of children at high risk for cardiovascular disease based on family history but who varied in blood TC (Kelley et al., 2004).

Assessments of lipid profile have commonly been studied with hematological and hormonal characteristics in relation to the health risks in childhood obesity.

This particularly relates to studies undertaken more recently as the interrelationships between all factors mentioned have a significant effect on present or later morbidity. In German obese children and adolescents, for example, increased cholesterol was significantly associated with P-selectin and D-dimer as markers of platelet activation, endothelial cell dysfunction, and activation of the coagulation system. These results suggest an unfavorable intercorrelation between metabolic and hemostatic risk factors for coronary heart disease in childhood obesity (Gallistl et al., 2000b).

A number of possible interrelationships have been suggested between metabolic and hemostatic parameters resulting from increased fatness. Sudi et al. (2001a) assessed TG, insulin, glucose, fibrinogen, plasminogen activator-inhibitor (PAI-1), tissue type plasminogen-activator-antigen (tPA-Ag), and body composition in children. Waist and hip circumference was measured, and subcutaneous adipose tissue layers (SAT-layers) at 15 sites were assessed using an optical device, the Lipometer. Fat distribution was evaluated using factor analysis, and upper-body subcutaneous fatness was mainly associated with fibrinogen. In girls, significant correlations between most measures of adiposity, including waist circumference, were also associated with hemostatic parameters. PAI-1, TG, and age were the main determinants for tPA-Ag, together with glucose, fibrinogen, and percentage of body fat mass, which contributed to PAI-1. Another study showed that in the obese subjects, insulin, PAI-1, and fragment 1+2 of pro-thrombin (F1+2) were positively correlated with BMI (Valle et al., 2000).

Obese children (with normal or increased blood pressure) had a significantly higher concentration of TC and TG and lower HDL-C levels. There was also an increase in platelet aggregation and a decrease in nitric oxide (NO) production in hypertensive children (both obese and normal weight), reflecting a significant negative correlation. A significant positive correlation was observed between platelet aggregation and BMI; an increased lipid peroxidation and higher blood and plasma viscosity were also noted but only in obese hypertensive children. Multivariate analysis showed significant interactions between the effects of obesity and hypertension on platelet aggregation and thiol oxidation. This indicates that an increased platelet aggregation and oxidative insult contribute to the development of hypertension and the promotion of vascular damage (Haszon et al., 2003).

A study of children in the United Kingdom revealed that fibrinogen and factor VII levels are associated with fatness but did not support the concept that these indicators are related to fetal growth or social class in England and Wales (Cook et al., 1999).

Apo-E polymorphism seems to influence some lipid profile abnormalities associated with obesity in children; however, clustering of risk factors and insulin resistance seem not to be dependent on ApoE polymorphism (Guerra et al., 2003). Obese, hypertensive, and diabetic children originate from families with cardiovascular disease and higher BMI. Their lipoprotein-A and B may be predictive of future cardiovascular diseases (Glowinska, Urban, and Koput, 2002).

During the six years of longitudinal observations in the Bogalusa Heart Study, BMI was increased more in hypercholesterolemic than in nonhypercholesterolemic 5- to 12-year-old girls but not boys. The association between BMI and blood lipids as well as insulin and blood pressure has become stronger with increasing age, especially in girls (Tershakovec et al., 2002a).

C-reactive protein concentration in children was correlated with several cardiovascular risks, but only fibrinogen, HDL-C, heart rate, and systolic blood pressure remained statistically significant after adjustment for ponderal index (Cook et al., 2000).

11.2 Blood Pressure and Cardiovascular Disorders

Once considered rare, primary hypertension in children has become increasingly common in association with obesity and other risk factors (Burke et al., 2004). These factors include family history of hypertension and ethnic predisposition for hypertensive disease. Obese children have approximately a threefold increased risk for hypertension compared to their normal-weight peers. The risk of hypertension in children increases across the entire range of BMI with no well-defined threshold effect. As is the case in adults, a combination of factors, including overactivity of the sympathetic nervous system, insulin resistance, and abnormalities in vascular structure and function, may contribute to obesity-related hypertension in children (Sorof and Daniels, 2002). New standards for BMI in childhood with regard to blood pressure criteria were recently established in Australian youth (Burke et al., 2004). Leptin was not found to be an independent associate of blood pressure in obese individuals during growth according to Sudi et al. (2004).

Large increases in BMI during adolescence may have a detrimental effect on systolic blood pressure (SBP) in middle life, as shown by a longitudinal study from birth to 43 years in U.K. subjects. Birth weight was determined from maternal health information and related to SES (Hardy et al., 2004).

The results of the FRESH Study showed that in 9- to 11-year-old children the level of physical fitness assessed using a treadmill test was usually higher in boys and fatness and TG serum levels were higher in girls. Systolic blood pressure correlated positively with fatness in girls, but in boys there was only a trend toward a similar relationship. LDL-C in boys correlated positively with fatness and negatively with the level of physical fitness. Using multivariate analysis, physical fitness was the primary correlate of total and LDL-C. In girls, fitness correlated positively with total and LDL-C, but this finding was reversed in boys. Fatness correlated negatively with HDL-C only in boys. Evidently, boys were more physically active, fitter, and carried less body fat. The level of physical fitness in boys was also positively associated with more favorable serum lipid levels. Along with other studies, these data suggest that consistent relationships among fitness, activity, fatness, blood pressure, and lipids are likely to emerge as children approach adolescence (Stewart et al., 1995).

Results of studies from the National Heart, Lung, and Blood Institute (NHLBI) have confirmed that both obesity and high blood cholesterol levels in U.S. children are higher than optimal. A study by Ernst and Obarzanek (1994) suggested that the benefit of reducing the prevalence of these conditions in children and adolescents would be revealed later in life. Research has focused on the predictors of the transition to the obese state, the feasibility, efficacy, and safety of long-term dietary intervention during growth, and the effects of school-based programs that include various systems of positive interventions with respect to obesity.

Another study confirmed some of the previous observations, including that the level of actual physical activity does not vary among obese and nonobese children. Correlations of physical activity and total cholesterol were low and not significant. However, both systolic and diastolic blood pressure and total cholesterol were higher in obese children. These observations indicate that obesity is associated with higher blood pressure and total cholesterol regardless of the actual level of physical activity of children (McMurray et al., 1995). Generally, activity levels are low with a narrow range in all that might make any relationships less marked and significant.

Increased blood pressure is manifested in the obese under resting conditions and during physical activity. Comparisons of hypertensive obese and nonobese adolescents before and during a treadmill test revealed no differences under resting conditions, but during moderate exercise (stage II Bruce test), the differences became significant. The same was found during maximal exercise. Heart rate response to exercise was also greater in normotensive obese than in nonobese adolescents. These data show that obese hypertensive adolescents have higher blood pressure during exercise than lean, nonobese hypertensive adolescents. During exercise testing on a treadmill, it is possible to identify hypertensive adolescents and also to identify different mechanisms from those at rest that induce blood pressure elevation during exercise (Tulio, Egle, and Greilly, 1995). Under these conditions, an increased percentage of stored fat is a functional as well as a health handicap. Another study of 14- to 15-year-old obese boys and girls showed 2 or more risk factors for cardiovascular diseases in 25% of subjects, especially increased values of TC (Anding et al., 1996) and a lower score of cardiorespiratory fitness.

In a 3-year longitudinal study of anthropometric parameters and blood pressure in adolescents, there was a relatively greater proportion of female to male students who were overfat as seniors. Overweight trends for each of the four groups (that is, black and white boys and girls) were stable over the study period. A sharp increase in obesity occurred among black females. A significant association was found between percent of ideal weight, skinfold thickness, BMI, and blood pressure among females of both ethnic groups. These observations add support to the hypothesis that the early onset of obesity is an indicator of obesity in the later years of adolescence with many of the accompanying health risks including hypertension (Adeyanju et al., 1987).

Measurements in obese Czech children aged 9 to 16 years admitted to a sanatorium for the treatment of obesity showed percent of body fat from 29 to 44% (derived from skinfold measurements and using regression equations for Czech children) (Pařízková, 1977). Fat distribution was evaluated using the waist-to-hip ratio and in addition, blood pressure, lipoproteins, apolipoproteins, OGIT, and IRI were evaluated. The level of physical fitness was assessed by a treadmill test. Paired tests and multiple regression analyses showed that fatness, diastolic blood pressure, and TG are independent factors for metabolic syndrome in obese children. These results provide further evidence that in this age range, body fatness is related to risk factors for cardiovascular disease and diabetes (Lísková, Hosek, and Stozicky, 1998).

In children with simple obesity an increased systolic blood pressure was associated with hypersinulinemia, hyperleptinemia, and visceral accumulation regardless of family history of hypertension during growth and also later in adulthood (Nishina et al., 2003). In girls, waist circumference was also independently associated with cardiovascular risk factors, especially with diastolic blood pressure (DBP) and insulin resistance, and also independently of age and Tanner's stage of sexual maturation (Maffeis et al., 2003). The dietary intake of children with a high risk of cardiovascular diseases has been followed and analyzed (Kelley et al., 2004).

Obese hypertensive students had a higher heart rate at rest than nonobese normotensive subjects. Variability of blood pressure, both systolic and diastolic, and during daytime and sleep periods was higher in obese than in nonobese. Findings of increased heart rate and blood pressure variability in obese children with isolated systolic hypertension suggest that sympathetic nervous system hyperactivity may contribute to its pathogenesis (Sorof et al., 2002). An increased excretion of cortisol metabolites in hypertensive obese children compared to obese and normal-weight children with normal blood pressure has also been found (Csabi, Juricsay, and Molnar, 2000).

Arterial stiffness may be an indicator of early vascular changes related to the development of cardiovascular disease. Stiffness of the abdominal aorta using transthoracic echocardiography in normotensive and hypertensive obese children compared to controls was measured. Aortic strain and pressure strain elastic modulus measurements were significantly different in the obese hypertensive group, in which BMI and TC were also higher (Levent et al., 2002). Changes of BMI from adolescence to young adulthood are related to intima-media thickness at 28 years and atherosclerosis risk (Oren et al., 2003). Carotid intima-media thickness (IMT) was related to obesity throughout life as revealed in the Bogalusa Heart Study between the ages of 4 and 45 years. The cumulative effects of childhood-onset obesity (BMI 95 percentile) that persists into adulthood were therefore proven. IMT values were not increased in subjects who were obese only during childhood, or in thin subjects who became obese as adults (Freedman et al., 2004).

BMI can predict left ventricular diastolic filling in asymptomatic obese children and cell adhesion molecules (sICAM-1) may be a useful marker of endothelial dysfunction and early atherosclerosis. A significant correlation was found between endothelial dysfunction markers and obesity as well as TG level in subjects 5 to 19 years old (Glowinska et al., 2001).

11.3 Insulin Resistance and Diabetes Mellitus

A study in Finland revealed that obesity is also associated with an increased risk of insulin-dependent diabetes mellitus (IDDM, type 1 diabetes mellitus) in children (Freedman, 2002). The prevalence of obesity in children affected by IDDM was on average twofold from the age of 2 years onward compared to control children. In logistic regression analysis, the development of obesity 1 to 4 years before the diagnosis of IDDM was associated with an increased risk of disease in boys as well as in girls. This also held true after adjustment for maternal education and place of residence (Hypponen et al., 1998). Obesity and diabetes in association with leptin were reviewed (Moran and Philip, 2003). Relationships among serum insulin, leptin, blood pressure, and visceral fat accumulation in obese children were also evaluated (Nishina et al., 2003).

Insulinemia of the mother can also influence the body fat of her children. A follow-up study in women with past gestational diabetes showed that the incidence of obesity in their offspring might have been reduced by antenatal insulin therapy (Simmons and Robertson, 1997). However, prenatal exposure to the metabolic effects of mild, diet-treated gestational diabetes mellitus (GDM) does not increase the risk of childhood obesity. Obesity prevalence in the offspring of mothers either with or without GDM showed a slightly higher prevalence in the offspring of mothers without GDM. There was also no difference in mean BMI adjusted for age and gender in these two groups of offspring (Whitaker et al., 1998). Offspring of the mothers with uncompensated diabetes mellitus had significantly thicker skinfolds at birth when compared to the offspring of normal, healthy mothers (Pařízková, 1963a). Changes of BMI during childhood show the association between thinness in infancy and the presence of impaired glucose tolerance or diabetes in young adulthood. An increase in BMI after two years of age is also associated with these disorders (Bhargava et al., 2004). Increased insulin resistance and type 2 diabetes has increased in India, especially in urban areas, and is associated with prenatal and postnatal factors. Accelerated growth is a risk for increased adiposity and insulin resistance, especially in children born small. Urban lifestyles with poor diets and sedentarism are further promoting factors for obesity and type 2 diabetes similarly as in other populations (Yajnik, 2004).

Observations in Pima Indian children show that there has been an increase in type 2 diabetes, which is attributed to the diabetic intrauterine environment. There are, of course, also interactions between the effect of genetic and factors acting during pregnancy (Dabeleaand Pettitt, 2001). The relative weight and 2-hour fasting plasma glucose were the variables most predictive of type 2 diabetes in Pima Indians aged 5 to 19 years who participated in a longitudinal population-based study and were characterized by normal glucose tolerance. Fasting insulin was a significant predictor of diabetes but did not add to the predictive value of relative weight. Against a background of parental diabetes, high-fasting insulin concentrations predict diabetes, which is compatible with the hypothesis that insulin resistance is an early metabolic abnormality leading to type 2 diabetes. However, in this particular study, its predictive value did not add significantly to that of relative weight, which is also an indicator of body adiposity and with which fasting insulin is correlated (McCance et al., 1994). Impaired glucose tolerance in young adulthood is related to serial changes of BMI during childhood (Bhargava et al., 2004).

Pima Indians may have an increased parasympathetic drive to the pancreas, which could result in a primary hypersecretion of insulin and contribute to their increased prevalence for obesity and diabetes. Both insulin and pancreatic polypeptide (PP), surrogate markers of pancreatic vagal tone, were measured in lean and obese Pima Indian and Caucasian children. Pima Indian subjects had a higher fasting insulin and PP (Weyer et al., 2001).

Insulin resistance with respect to glucose metabolism has been shown in obese adolescents. However, the urinary sodium excretion and the pressor system remain insulin-sensitive. The sensitivity of the sodium retaining action to hyperinsulinemia has been reported as higher in obese subjects when compared to nonobese. For this reason, when the compensatory endogenous hyperinsulinemia is raised by insulin resistance, these factors may result in chronic sodium retention and pressor system stimulation and subsequent hypertension in the obese (Miyzaki et al., 1996).

The incidence of type 2 diabetes is also dependent on adiposity rebound (AR). The condition decreased progressively from 8.6% in subjects whose adiposity rebound occurred before the age of 5 years to 1.8% in those in whom it occurred after 7 years. Early AR was preceded by low weight gain between birth and 1 year. These results indicate that large differences in the incidence of type 2 diabetes are associated with growth rates *in utero*, weight gain in infancy, and age at AR (Eriksson et al., 2003a). The Bogalusa Heart Study showed that family situation influences insulinemia in children: offspring with a high risk for coronary artery disease develop excess fatness beginning in childhood and then later manifest hyperinsulinemia in young adulthood (Yussef et al., 2002).

Insulin sensitivity has correlated inversely with intramyocellular (IMCL) triglyceride stores even when adjusted for percent of body fat and abdominal subcutaneous fat mass. Extramyocellular lipid contents were also strongly related to insulin sensitivity (Sinha et al., 2002).

There were established threshold values for visceral abdominal tissue (VAT), VAT/SAT (subcutaneous AT), and sagittal abdominal diameter as a risk for metabolic derangement (of insulin level, TG, and alanin aminotransferase) in obese adults. Waist girth, sagittal diameter by CT, and waist/hip ratio were evaluated as anthropometric surrogates of VAT. However, these values were lower with regard to biochemical complications in Japanese obese boys aged 6 to 14 years. These values can be used for classifying obese boys into two types: those with medical problems and those without (Asayama et al., 2002).

Multiple regression of the data from a 14-year longitudinal study in Italian children showed that relative BMI and insulin resistance at childhood were independent predictors of adult BMI in girls. A multivariate logistic regression analysis showed that high relative BMI and low insulin resistance index at baseline predicted obesity in adulthood for girls, no matter their age, stage for sexual maturation, and parents' BMI. In boys, insulin resistance was not a significant predictor of adult obesity. These data indicate that obesity in childhood tracks into adulthood; in obese girls, insulin resistance during childhood appears to oppose the risk of adult obesity (Maffeis et al., 2002).

11.4   Multimetabolic Syndrome (MMS)

The increasing prevalence of insulin resistance syndrome (syndrome X, metabolic syndrome) with further above-mentioned health problems in various child populations has been the focus of attention from both genetic and environmental points of view (Weiss et al., 2004; Ten and Maclaren, 2004). There are secular trends in variables associated with the metabolic syndrome of children and adolescents in North America (Eisenmann, 2003).

The prevalence of multimetabolic syndrome (MMS) documented in obese adults has also been examined in obese children aged 12.3 ± 2.2 years (Molnar, Decsi, and Csabi, 1997), from the point of view of hypertension, hyperinsulinemia, hypercholesterolemia, hypertriglyceridemia, low HDL-C, and impaired glucose tolerance. In a subgroup, physical fitness and fat-soluble natural antioxidants were also studied. Multimetabolic syndrome was documented in 16 to 20% of obese children. Resting tachycardia, low physical fitness, and reduced a-tocopherol plasma concentration were also part of MMS in obese children (Molnar, Decsi, and Csabi, 1997). The evaluation of exercise tolerance (exercise duration, PWC_{170}, and VO_2 max) in obese children with MMS showed a low level of fitness in children with multiple cardiovascular risk factors (Torok and Molnar, 1999).

A longitudinal study of Australian children aged 7.4 to 8.9 years has also confirmed that syndrome X variables clustered among children who had a tendency to deposit more fat on the trunk. In this sample, there was no evidence that infant size predicted development of the insulin resistance or dyslipoproteinemia of the syndrome at the age of 8 years (Dwyer et al., 2002).

Different homeostatic control of metabolic syndrome characteristics exists in obese and nonobese children. This influences hyperinsulinemia and dyslipoproteinemia, including high TG and low HDL, impaired glucose tolerance, hypertension, and/or type 2 diabetes. BMI, waist circumference, trunk-to-total skinfolds, systolic blood pressure, glucose, uric acid, fasting insulin, TG, and HDL were also identified in this study. Leptin also seems to play a key underlying role in metabolic syndrome, especially in obese children (Moreno et al., 2002), and Eisenmann (2004) has also reported secular trends in variables associated with the metabolic syndrome in children and adolescents in North America.

The relationship between morbidity and extreme values of BMI was evaluated in a group of 17-year-old Israeli adolescents. Functional limitations prevailed at both extremes of BMI distribution. Overweight was associated with hypertension and joint disorders in the hip, knee, and ankle (Lusky et al., 1996).

11.5 Hepatic Problems

In obese children and adolescents, hyperinsulinemia is an important contributor to the development of a fatty liver, apparently more so than overweight and increased fatness, blood glucose, or serum lipids. This was the finding in a study of Japanese children where the prevalence of fatty liver was 24.1% (Kawasaki et al., 1997). The results of a study in Italian children aged 4.3 to 20 years also confirmed the importance of hepatic damage due to obesity during growth and its relationship with metabolic alterations. Steatosis was found in 55.4% and hyperaminotransferasemia in 20.3%, and both these conditions together were found in 15.4% of children. In patients with an ultrasonographic pattern of steatosis of the liver, there were significantly higher levels of liver enzymes (ALT, AST, gGT), triglycerides, and insulinemia. The degree of insulinemia correlated significantly with the presence or absence of steatosis (Bergoni et al., 1998).

Nonalcoholic steatohepatitis, in which fatty change and inflammation in the liver occurs, also appears increasingly in obese children (Chitturi, Farell, and George, 2004). In a 10-year-old and a 14-year-old boy, cirrhosis from nonalcoholic statohepatitis was observed, with one boy progressing to cirrhosis with symptomatic portal hypertension within a 2-year period (Molleston et al., 2002). The significance of obesity as a risk factor for cholecystolithiasis in children and adolescents was not proved (Kachele et al., 2000).

11.6 Respiratory Diseases, Asthma

Respiratory symptoms were reported as worse in the obese during growth as the result of measurements in 7800 English and Scottish children aged 5 to 11 years. Logistic regression analysis showed an increased liability to some respiratory symptoms in subjects with the highest weight and triceps skin-fold thickness. Positive associations were found between weight for height and the prevalence of bronchitis, with comments such as "chest being wheezy" and "colds usually going to the chest." These data indicate that some respiratory illnesses can be reduced by preventing overweight or obesity in children (Somerville, Rona, and Chinn, 1984), and this seems to be related to some respiratory problems often found in obese children (see Chapter 6). In severely obese boys, a fall in pulmonary function was observed in measures of the ratio of forced expiratory volume in one second (FEV_1) to forced vital capacity (FVC), and respiratory rates at 5 and 15 minutes after the exercise on a bicycle ergometer. Significant negative correlations between pulmonary function changes after exercise with BMI and skinfolds were also found in obese youngsters (Gokbel and Atas, 1999) and in another study, obesity was considered as a risk for asthma in children (Von Kries et al., 2001).

In adults, a positive association between asthma and obesity has been reported. Levels of obesity were associated with asthma symptoms in 4- to 11-year-old English children regardless of ethnicity. This association was more consistent for BMI than for sum of skinfolds, partly because obese children were more advanced in their maturation than other children. The association was also stronger in girls than in boys but only in a multiethnic inner-city sample (Figueroa-Munoz, Chinn, and Rona, 2001). In a general population sample where prevalence of obesity and asthma (lung function, bronchodilator responsiveness, and daily peak flow variability) were found, the following results emerged. Girls rather boys who were obese at 11 years of age were more likely to have current wheezing at ages 11 and 13 but not at ages 6 or 8 years. Girls who became overweight or obese between 6 and 11 years of age were 7 times more likely to develop new asthma symptoms at 11 or 13 years. At age 11 their peak flow variability and bronchodilator responsiveness were significantly more likely to be increased (Castro-Rodriguez et al., 2001).

The Children's Health Study (Southern California) showed that the risk of new-onset asthma was higher in children who were overweight, especially in boys. The effect of being overweight was higher in nonallergic children than in allergic children; therefore, it was concluded that overweight and obesity are associated with an increased risk of new-onset asthma in nonallergic children (Gilliland et al., 2003). In German girls, the incidence of asthma (as diagnosed by a medical doctor) rose with increasing obesity, which did not apply to boys at the age of 6 to 7 years. Hay fever and eczema were unrelated to weight in both genders (Von Kries et al., 2001). Some authors, however, suggest that trends in overweight and obesity do not explain the increase in asthma and that the evidence indicates the association between asthma and obesity is only of recent origin. Obesity may be a marker of recent lifestyle differences associated with both overweight and asthma (Chinn and Rona, 2001a).

11.7 Hormonal Alterations; Puberty and Its Complications

Parents commonly consult a general practitioner or pediatrician when they believe that the sexual development of a child may be abnormal. This is a more common occurrence in obese boys. The genitals are often so immersed in superfluous fat that in spite of their growth being adequate, they appear to be retarded. Therefore, it is recommended that children and parents with such concerns consult a medical practitioner. As a result of visiting a practitioner, there is an increased chance that the child's obesity problem may be treated.

Obese adolescent girls (aged 17.1 ± 1.4 years) often have menstrual disorders, including oligomenorrhea, amenorrhea (or irregular menses), and hirsutism. Polycystic ovary syndrome (PCOS) may begin at the perimenarcheal age; therefore, the relationship between hyperandrogenemia and obesity in girls has been the focus of some studies. In a study by Malecka-Tendera et al. (1998) — having excluded subjects with any ovarial pathology — LH, FSH, testosterone (T), SDHEA and insulin were measured in the follicular phase or after 6 months of amenorrhea. BMI ranged from 18.3 to 34.5kg/m^2 and waist-to-hip ratio from 0.66 to 0.94. No correlation was found between the above-mentioned hormones. Adiposity and waist-to-hip ratio correlated significantly with the T level, but not with insulin. A significant positive correlation between BMI and T level was also found. These results suggest that in girls with menstrual irregularities, overweight is associated with hyperinsulinemia (as shown in other studies) and also with enhanced androgen production, which may be a risk factor for PCOS.

With respect to hormonal problems, the relationships may be double-edged. That is, some hormonal abnormalities can result in obesity, and in turn, obesity can significantly deteriorate hormonal activities in the developing organism. However, clinical cases of obesity caused by hormonal dysfunction in children are quite rare and the majority of cases have other pathologies, most commonly resulting from an energy imbalance.

11.8 Orthopedic Problems, Body Posture, and Movement

The structural consequences of obesity can include the orthopedic conditions of Blount's disease, Legge-Calve-Perthes disease, genu valgum, flat-footedness, and subtalar pronation. In addition, obesity has frequently been associated with the infantile form of Blount's disease (*tibia vara*). The increased stress on young bones resulting from excess weight may act on an underlying varus deformity and result in changes that are characteristic of Blount's disease. Dietz, Gross, and Kirkpatrick (1982) reported a similar incidence of the disease in obese children, for example, a slipped capital femoral epiphysis.

Numerous aspects of growth, development, and maintenance of body tissues are mechanically related. Inappropriate loading of the skeletal framework, particularly in areas of epiphyseal growth activity, can alter the pattern of growth in these critical regions (Micheli, 1983). An increase in compression on one side of an epiphyseal plate may alter growth on that side, while normal proliferation occurs on the opposite side (Le Veau and Bernhardt, 1984). The end result of such unequal loading is a distortion in the normal angle of the epiphyseal plate. This may lead to unequal loading being experienced elsewhere and the direction of normal growth being altered (Frost, 1972, 1979).

Genu varus often produces additional lower extremity exacerbations that include compensatory pronation, talar adduction, and a degree of in-toeing. Additional to the abnormal loading forces mentioned, there is the potential for a predisposition to the early onset of osteoarthritis (Le Veau and Bernhardt, 1984).

A study in Spanish children showed that along with an increased BMI, the intermalleolar distance was higher in overweight children than in normal-weight children. Fifty percent of the overweight children showed an intermalleolar distance of more than 10 cm, a value considered abnormal. These findings indicate that the incidence of genu valgum is much higher in overweight children and may contribute to reduced physical activity (Bonet-Serra et al., 2003).

Both cross-sectional and longitudinal studies (Felson et al., 1988) corroborate obesity, or as yet unknown factors associated with obesity, as causes of knee osteoarthritis. The biological explanation for the link is unclear, but obesity may initiate cartilage breakdown or promote joint destruction after the incipient lesion. It is evident that osteoarthritis does not remit but possibly either remains stable or progresses with time (Hills et al., 2002).

Foot structure and plantar pressure can also be influenced by increased weight (Hills et al., 2001). Rear-foot dynamic forces generated by subjects in a study (Dowling, Steele, and Baur, 2001) were significantly higher in obese versus nonobese subjects, as were mean peak dynamic forefoot pressures. Foot discomfort–associated structural changes and increased forefoot plantar pressures in the obese foot may also hinder the involvement of obese children in exercise and physical activity. Another study from the same laboratory found that excess body weight had a significant effect on foot structure evaluated using a pedograph (Footprint angle, Chippaux-Smirak Index scores). Obese children displayed structural foot characteristics that if excessive weight was to persist, may develop into problematic symptoms (Riddiford-Harland, Steele, and Storlien, 2000). These findings have important implications for preventive measures early in life to avoid articular problems such as osteoarthritis. The role of weight loss in the alleviation of symptoms has not been assessed in a systematic fashion. An untested hypothesis in relation to osteoarthritis and the knee (Felson et al., 1988) found that osteoarthritis in the knee is caused by the increased force per unit area in the knees of obese individuals.

The consequences of the tendency for the foot to pronate may also result in a flattened foot and hypermobile forefoot (Wearing et al., 2004). The minimization of foot stability in these conditions requires greater muscle activity for normal weight acceptance and transfer. Alterations in leg musculature, specifically the triceps surae and tibialis anterior muscles, tend to exaggerate the existing pronation (Hills et al., 2001).

Body posture in obese children is also a common problem. However, some deviations of the vertebral column and the position of the scapulae may be less noticeable as they are covered by a larger thickness of subcutaneous fat. Very often, the muscles of the abdominal wall are also flabby; therefore, the prominent belly of the obese child is not only the result of fat storage but also of muscle weakness. Inadequate body posture can cause a hyperlordosis. The level of the shoulders is often uneven, and the head and neck are in a poor position, which predisposes the individual to a poke neck. Obese children are also subject to the same range of postural deviations as normal-weight children. As the development of musculature in obese children is mainly sound, the deterioration of body posture can be rectified by appropriate instruction and exercises. Generally, obese children and adolescents are less fit and active than nonobese individuals of the same age, and this has major implications for the musculoskeletal system, particularly overloaded joints during activities of daily living that require weight bearing (Bar-Or, 1998).

Obesity has a negative effect on the static postural control of teenagers. Stabilometric data on surface, length, and spontaneous sway in the lateral (X) and anteroposteror (Y) axis with open and closed eyes in two conditions on firm floor and foam floor conditions have been assessed. A decrease in static and dynamic balance capacity of obese subjects has been observed; however, the effect of fat distribution in individuals has not been considered (Bernard et al., 2003). Similar disparities were found in a recent study to compare static and dynamic balance tasks in obese versus nonobese prepubertal children (Deforche et al., 2004).

In a study of obese children, Goulding et al. (2000) have reported a spinal overload with a lower vertebral bone mineral content for bone area, body height and weight, and stage of pubertal maturation. Spinal area was low in overweight and obese girls compared with girls of healthy weight, but overweight and obese boys had enlarged their vertebral area appropriately for their increased body size. This indicates that during growth overweight and obese children may not increase their spinal BMC to fully compensate for their excessive weight (Goulding et al., 2002), a mismatch between body weight and bone development during growth.

Bone mineralization and strength were also evaluated in obese children aged 6 to 17 years by qualitative ultrasound (QUS) of bone speed and sound (SOS). Tibial and radial SOS was correlated with pubertal stage and chronological age. No significant correlation was found between endurance time as an indicator of fitness and bone SOS. Bone strength measured by QUS was reduced in obese children, but was affected by the degree of obesity (Eliakim, Nemet, and Wolach, 2001). In obese preschool children 3 to 5 years of age, total body bone area (TBBA), total body bone mineral content (TBBMC), and tibial cortical bone measures along with anthropometric characteristics of fatness, diet, physical activity, and strength were measured. Higher TBBA and TBBMC in children with greater body fatness indicate a reduced mineralization of bone and that obesity in preschool children may have a negative effect on total body bone mass accretion. A smaller tibial periosteal circumference and thus cross-sectional area with higher percent of body fat (without increased body weight) can also lead to biomechanical disadvantages and lower activity (Specker et al., 2001). However, bone mineral density was not influenced by obesity in Turkish children, but higher values were observed in obese children in puberty, which may be due to hormonal changes (Hasanoglu et al., 2000).

There is an increasing interest in the physical challenges for the obese associated with the execution of activities of daily living. However, there is a dearth of information related to the structural and functional limitations of obese state. Therefore, the implications of the persistence of the obesity on the musculoskeletal system, particularly during weight-bearing tasks such as walking, are poorly understood (Hills et al., 2002). Work to date has addressed the locomotor characteristics of obese children (Hills and Parker, 1991, 1992, 1993; Hills, 1994) and adults, plantar pressures under the feet of obese individuals (Hills et al., 2001), the influence of obesity on foot structure and functional performance of children (Dowling, Steele, and Baur, 2001; Riddiford-Harland, Steele, and Storlien, 2000; Riddiford, Steele, and Storlien, 1998), and potential relationships between obesity and osteoarthritis. Due to the enormity of the obesity epidemic, and the relative paucity of information available, there is an urgent need to focus more attention on the physical consequences of repetitive loading of major structures, particularly in the lower extremity.

Low levels of muscular strength and/or power of the lower limbs may have implications for impairment of motor function. Such deficiencies may limit involvement in activities of daily living, including walking and running, and be associated with heightened fatigue and risk of injury (Hills, 1994; Hills et al., 2001). Riddiford, Steele, and Storlien (2000) investigated the effects of obesity on the strength and power of 43 obese (BMI: 24.1 ± 2.3 kg m^{-2}) and 43 nonobese (BMI: 16.9 ± 0.4 kg m^{-2}) healthy, prepubescent children (8.4 ± 0.5 y). Children were limited in activities that required them to move their body weight (including vertical and standing long jump) but were not disadvantaged in upper-limb strength and power activities (such as basketball throw for distance and arm push/pull ability). Similar findings were reported by Hills and Parker (1993). More work is required to profile children of different weight categories undertaking a range of physical activities. Results would be invaluable in the design of appropriate intervention strategies (Hills et al., 2001).

11.9 Dental Caries

The relationship between dental caries and eating habits (24-hour recall and food frequency recall) has been studied in Brazilian children aged 1 to 12 years. Forty-two percent of children were born with an adequate birth weight, and most of them had a mixed diet prior to 6 months of age. The main food provided after weaning was cow's milk in 40% of cases. The frequency of food intake was 5 times per day in 45% of the children. Thirteen percent of children studied were obese and most of those ate white sugar and candies at least once a day. The prevalence of caries was 75%. These results indicate that children ingested more energy than needed, but the data were insufficient to relate obesity to dental caries. However, the high intake of sugar provides an indication that this might be a factor in the increased prevalence of dental caries. Other factors such as regular dental hygiene and composition of saliva may also be involved.

11.10 Immune Function

Obesity during growth can also alter the immune function (Boeck, Chen, and Cunningham-Rundles, 1993) including impairments in host-defense mechanisms. Total salivary IgA, serum C3 complement (C3c), and immunoglobulin A (IgA) were assessed in obese children aged 6 to 13 years. Comparisons with laboratory reference values for normal healthy children revealed that the data distribution showed higher frequencies near the zone of the highest reference values for serum IgA and C3c. When results of IgA in the saliva were expressed as a percentage of the normal value, 49.5% of the study population presented data lower than 76%. These results show a compromised secretory immune system without the incidence of clinical symptoms and infection, whereas humeral immunity might not be affected (Pallaro et al., 1998). Further assessments of salivary IgA and serum C3c IgA in obese schoolchildren revealed also a compromised secretory immune system without incidence of clinical symptoms and infections, whereas humoral immunity might not be seriously affected (Pallaro et al., 2002).

11.11 Sleep Disturbances

A link between sleep quality and obesity was followed in a tri-ethnic cross-sectional sample of adolescents 11 to 16 years of age (Heartfelt study) following total sleep time and sleep disturbance time obtained by 24-hour wrist actigraphy. Obese adolescents experienced less sleep than nonobese adolescents. Sleep disturbances were not directly related to obesity in this sample but influenced physical activity level, which diminished by 3% for every hour increase in sleep disturbance (Gupta et al., 2002).

Obstructive sleep apnea (OSA), which often appears in obese children (Erler and Paditz, 2004), is also associated with metabolic characteristics: its severity is correlated with fasting insulin levels, independent of body mass index. Insulin levels may be further elevated as a consequence of OSA in obese children (De la Eva et al., 2002). In contrast with adults, test position is important when evaluating obstructive sleep apnea, and obese children breathe best when in a supine position (Fernandes-do-Prado et al., 2002). Polysomnography has showed obstructive sleep apnea syndrome (OSAS) in some Singaporean obese children (Chay et al., 2000). During the early stages of narcolepsy there appears to be a tendency for increased weight gain in children (Kotagal, Krahn, and Slocumb, 2004). Sleep-related breathing disorder was associated with elevated blood pressure and obesity in preadolescent children; its control may be important for the reduction of lifelong hypertension risk (Enright et al., 2003). An association between sleep-related breath disorders and increased blood pressure was found in white and Hispanic children in Tucson (Enright et al., 2003). There is a putative link between childhood narcolepsy and obesity (Kotagal and Krahn, 2004).

11.12   Experimental Model Studies

Studies on the effect of increased fatness on health parameters using laboratory animals have been undertaken mainly in adult genetically obese animals. Rarely has the development of obesity been followed in normal animals from the early periods of life, except for those made obese through increased dietary intake using the cafeteria diet and hypokinesia.

An experiment by Plagemann et al. (1992) confirmed the pathological effects of excess fatness developed as a consequence of early postnatal overfeeding in Wistar male rats from small (3 to 4 pups, overnutrition) as compared to normal-sized (12 pups, normonutrition) and large (20 to 24 pups, undernutrition) litters. Serum insulin levels were significantly increased in overnourished pups from the smallest litters as compared to the other groups at the age of 15 days. These hyperinsulinemic rats had greater food intake and weight gains during the suckling period until adult age. The degree of overweight and obesity correlated significantly with basal hyperinsulinemia and increased blood pressure in small-litter adults. In addition, the early-overnourished animals developed an increased type 1-like diabetes susceptibility to a sub-diabetogenic dose of streptomycin in adulthood. These results indicate the essential importance of food intake very early in life and predisposition to obesity, increased diabetes susceptibility, and also for increased cardiovascular risk in later life. Animals (Wistar male rats) from small, normal-sized, and large nests had different weight and fatness in adulthood and developed different sensitivity to isoprenaline application, resulting in experimental cardiac necrosis and death. Animals from large nests with least adiposity survived best with least cardiac damage, and vice versa for fatter animals from small nests (Pařízková, 1977).

These conclusions are in agreement with the results of experiments following a reverse situation. Rats kept marginally malnourished from lactation until puberty and later realimented showed a range of different characteristics. Animals grew more slowly, showed a higher level of spontaneous physical activity (running in rotation cages), and were subsequently leaner in adulthood. However, they had the same sized vital organs (heart, adrenals, and so on) and were more resistant to experimental cardiac necrosis induced by isoprenaline in adulthood (lower spontaneous mortality, smaller damage of the heart muscle). In other experiments, the percentage of fat correlated with cardiac damage induced by isoprenaline as related to the level of physical activity (exercise and/or restriction of activity) (Pařízková, 1996a; Pařízková and Faltová, 1970; Pařízková et al., 1982).

11.13 Developmental and Nutritional Characteristics of Long-Living Populations

A long-living population in Abkhazia (living at a mean altitude of 600 m above sea level) was studied by Russian and U.S. scientists in the 1960s and 1970s. Children were never forced to eat more than they chose to spontaneously. Children grew more slowly and had smaller skinfolds, and overeating was considered unacceptable at any age. All subjects were highly active from childhood to old age and had lower body weight and less fat in adulthood, along with favorable serum lipid profiles and a more positive health status. The population achieved a higher age (higher ratio of nonagenarians) as compared with a genetically identical population living in bigger cities nearby and following quite a different lifestyle and nutrition. This involved eating more than was needed, with a food intake of undesirable composition, and with restricted physical activity (Kozlov, 1987; see also Pařízková, 2000; Pařízková and Chin, 2003).

11.14 Summary

Health risks have been considered more serious when an increased storage of fat occurred during the growth period. This applies especially for the abdominal, visceral adipose tissue, which is a predictor of cardiovascular diseases, diabetes, and other diseases. The TC, LDL-C, TG, TC/HDL-C ratio and fasting insulin levels are increased and correlate with BMI and adiposity.

There is a marked increase of BMI between the postpubertal period and 25 years of age among those who subsequently died earlier, those who developed cardiovascular diseases, and particularly those who developed diabetes. In contrast, those who reported cancer had a lower BMI throughout. The deviations of lipid profile have been studied jointly with hematological (for example P-selectin, D-dimer), body composition, and hormonal characteristics as related to cardiovascular risks. Other studies showed that in obese subjects, insulin, PAI-1, and fragment 1+2 of prothrombin were positively correlated with BMI. Fibrinogen and factor VII levels were associated with fatness. Apo-E polymorphism seems to influence some lipid profile abnormalities associated with increased fatness; however, clustering of risk factors and insulin resistance (IR) seem not to be dependent on Apo-E polymorphism. C-reactive protein concentration was also correlated with cardiovascular risks, but only HDL-C, heart rate, and blood pressure remained statistically significant after adjustment for weight and ponderal index.

Especially in children of hypertensive parents, obesity was related to an increased blood pressure in the growing obese. The risk of hypertension increased across the range of BMI values, and there was no threshold in connection with other metabolic and hormonal abnormalities. Increased blood pressure (BP) was manifested during rest and physical activity. Increased systolic BP was associated with hyperinsulinemia, hyperleptinemia, and visceral fat accumulation. Waist circumference was independently associated with cardiovascular risk factors, especially diastolic BP and IR, and independently of age and degree of sexual maturation. Variability of BP during daytime and sleep was greater in the obese. Arterial stiffness may be an indicator of early vascular changes. Aortic strain, pressure-elastic modulus was significantly different in obese hypertensive subjects along with increased BMI and TC. Endothelial dysfunction was also correlated with fatness.

Hyperinsulinemia often results in type 2 diabetes, which has been increasing in particular populations, including obese Pima Indian children. Such individuals may have an increased parasympathetic drive to the pancreas, which could result in hypersecretion of insulin and increased prevalence of obesity. Dependence was shown on early AR and weight gain between birth and 1 year. These results indicate the effect of growth rates *in utero*, weight gain in infancy, and age of AR. Experiments in laboratory animals have shown the effect of increased early nutrition on hyperinsulinemia, diabetes susceptibility, blood pressure, greater weight and fatness, and susceptibility of the cardiac muscle to experimental cardiac necrosis later in life.

Insulin resistance (IR) correlated inversely with intramyocellular triglyceride stores (IMCL). A threshold value for visceral adipose tissue (VAT), VAT/SAT (subcutaneous AT), and sagittal abdominal diameter as a risk for metabolic derangement (insulin, TG, alanin aminotransferase) was defined in the adult obese. These values were lower with regard to biochemical complications in boys.

Obese children also show a greater risk for multimetabolic syndrome (MMS), which correlates with other anthropometric and metabolic risk factors. Hepatic problems were also revealed increasingly in obese children as nonalcoholic hepatosteatosis. In addition, respiratory diseases and asthma appear more frequently in obese children, as do hormonal problems and earlier menarche.

Orthopedic and bone problems are stressed by obesity: Legge-Calve-Perthes disease, genu valgum, flat-footedness, subtalar pronation, and Blount's disease (*tibia vara*). Intermalleolar distance increases with increasing BMI. Foot structure and plantar pressure can be increased and result in foot discomfort and potential structural changes. Body posture deviations are less apparent because of the thicker fat layer, and static postural control is also affected. Measurements of bone mineral content have shown that during growth obese children do not increase their bone mineral density to fully compensate for their excess weight. Dental caries was related to diet and sugar consumption, but may also be associated with other factors such as hygiene and saliva composition.

Increased adiposity is also associated with impairments of host-defense mechanisms. Measurements of salivary IgA and serum C3c IgA showed a compromised secretory immune system without the apparent consequences in regard to clinical symptoms and infections. Sleep disturbance is also linked to obesity; obstructive sleep apnea often appears in obese children and is associated with other metabolic deviations. Experimental studies have further elucidated the relationships between adiposity and metabolic disturbances.

Observations in long-living populations have revealed the relationship among slower growth, leanness, better health, higher physical fitness, and longer life expectancy. This was in significant contrast to comparable ethnic groups, particularly those living in cities at lower altitude, with reduced levels of physical activity, a different inadequate diet, and poor lifestyle habits.

Part 2

Treatment and Management Principles

12

Treatment and Management

Due to the multidimensional nature of obesity, the condition is often described as complex and particularly resistant to treatment. This may be due to the failure, in most situations, to provide the necessary multidisciplinary support. Similarly, the longer an individual is obese, the more difficult it may be to change his or her diet and exercise behaviors, and it may be therefore less likely that the condition will resolve spontaneously.

Effective long-term treatment options for overweight youngsters are critical for a successful reduction in the prevalence of adult obesity and its associated co-morbidities. The involvement of a team of health professionals using a range of behavior management techniques increases the chance of a successful outcome, that is, the maintenance of a desirable body weight and composition.

It has been recommended that in a multidisciplinary approach to weight management, diet, exercise, and psychological support should be the three key components. These components should be provided together as they are interrelated and interdependent, and have mutually supportive features. In most cases, weight-control programs for obese children during continuing growth in height should focus on weight-maintenance strategies as opposed to weight loss (Hills and Byrne, 2001). The particular features of these individual approaches, as well as any combined approach, depend on the degree and duration of obesity and the age of commencement of the condition. The past and present health and fitness level of the child and family background are also important. Further, the possibility of considering the whole environment of the child during the treatment period plays an essential role. Wherever possible, the overweight child should maintain a similar weight while growing at the expected rate, provided that the degree of obesity is not so severe that more intensive treatment is required. A severely restricted or crash diet has the potential to jeopardize the normal growth and development of both muscle tissue and bone.

In addition to the potential physical concerns as a function of inappropriate weight loss, the effects of a failure to lose weight should not be underestimated. Parallels have been identified between unsuccessful weight loss attempts and psychological problems, including a predisposition to eating disorders (Golan et al., 1998; Nuutinen and Knipp, 1992a,b). A common problem in self-managed weight-loss attempts in young people who are poorly informed is the use of unhealthy eating practices and inappropriate exercise. Therefore, the need exists for specific assistance from relevant health professionals. For dietary issues, a nutritionist or dietitian should be involved, and an exercise physiologist should be responsible for the prescription of physical activity and exercise. Ideally, the management of obesity during growth and development requires the mobilization of a team of health professionals from medical, pedagogic, psychological, nutrition, and exercise backgrounds (Zwiauer, 2000).

A study comparing obese adolescents and their parents (followed during behavioral treatment over 6, 60, and 120 months) showed weight maintenance in adolescents but a failure to maintain weight loss in parents (Epstein et al., 1995a). Logistic regression analyses showed that children were more likely than their parents at each point in time to have percent of overweight decreases greater than 20%, with over 20% of the children and less than 1% of the parents showing changes this large. Child-only programs of obesity behavioral treatment are usually less effective compared with programs that target the parents, who, it is noted, could benefit in a similar way with regard to increase in adiposity reduction (Golan, Weizman, and Fainaru, 1999).

The effect of a weight-loss intervention can be very different in individuals due to the degree of obesity and its duration. In addition, hormonal, biochemical, and functional parameters, along with family history and genetic predisposition, play a role. During recent years, these issues have been the focus of attention of groups such as the European Childhood Obesity Group (ECOG, Burniat, 1997; Frelut, 1997, Burniat Cole, Lissau, and Poskitt 2000). The specifics of the treatment and prevention of obesity in childhood has also been discussed in many meetings (Wabitsch, 1997b). The individual approach to the treatment of obese individuals of any age, gender, and environmental background has been stressed in adults (Rollnick, 1996), but particular effort must be made during the growing years to reduce excess weight and fatness. Some reservation in the area stems from the frequency of weight gain after weight loss in reduction treatments that occurs especially in severely obese adolescents (Rolland-Cachera et al., 2004).

Attitudes toward obesity and its treatment may be biased and thus cause problems with respect to the management of obese individuals during growth and development. "Dispelling the myths" about children's obesity (Bandini and Dietz, 1992) may represent a critical step in both the prevention and the treatment of obese children. Believing that all obese individuals overeat, eat too much junk food, and do not move enough suggests that the obese are social deviants, helping to justify the intense discrimination against them. Another myth is the inability to treat obesity. This notion has the potential to remove health-care professionals from the responsibility of understanding and caring adequately for obese children.

An understanding of the problems associated with childhood obesity is still lacking and needs to be improved and expanded. It is still poorly understood why in a family, one child is obese and the other not, in spite of the same environment and similar genetic background. More recently, there has been further examinations of these problems, with special genes being investigated and their role defined in greater detail (Clement and Ferre, 2003; Farooqui et al., 2003; Tremblay et al., 2003). The principles of obesity prevention achieved particularly by increased physical activity and monitored diet have also been examined (Baranowski et al., 2000).

The starting point in the rectification of the problem is to use all the available knowledge on the complex mechanisms of obesity development and to implement this knowledge as early as possible in life. The process must respect individual peculiarities. Therefore, any intervention must be the result of a careful and detailed profile of each child, including the history, genetic background, degree and duration of obesity, health and fitness status, and psychological status. Evidence-based clinical guidelines are crucial tools for health and other practitioners to effectively treat and manage childhood obesity. An increasing range of material has been developed at a national level in various countries (Barlow and Dietz, 1998; INSERM, 2000; Australian NHMRC, 2003) and also a recent comprehensive review in the area by the International Obesity Task Force for the World Health Organization (Lobstein, Baur, and Uauy, 2004).

Prevention seems to be the best solution for obesity management (Dietz and Gortmaker, 2001), commenced in the family, school, and other institutions that take care of children. The Kiel Obesity Prevention Study (KOPS), which was started in 1996, enrolled a representative sample of 5- to 7-year-old children; 20.7% were evaluated as obese, and 31% of normal-weight children were considered to be at risk of becoming obese. An inverse social gradient for children's obesity was revealed, similar to other studies; health-related behaviors and parental fatness also had a strong influence on obesity development. Positive changes were observed with regard to health-related behaviors after one year of combined school- and family-based interventions, which had the significant effects of age-dependent increases in median triceps skinfolds and percentage of fat in overweight children (Muller et al., 2001). The results of KOPS seem to be promising; better school education and social support are considered efficient strategies for obesity prevention. Early introduction of obesity management, especially in children from at-risk families with high BMI or with high birth weight, has also been stressed in 6- to 7-year-old children in Hong Kong, which concerned, inter alia, also sleep duration and parental smoking (Hui et al., 2003).

More studies have addressed the effect of reduction treatment. However, in nearly all cases, the design, duration, mode of operation and groups followed from the point of view of age range, gender, stage of sexual maturation, obesity duration, result achieved and its maintenance, and other factors are far from being homogeneous. Drawing general conclusions is difficult, although some key insights can be gained from many individual studies.

12.1 Assessment of the Obese Child

The following list of assessment items is often referenced in the provision of an authoritative understanding of the status of each child or adolescent. An overview of the behavioral and psychotherapeutic approaches in the management of childhood obesity has been presented by Flodmark and Lissau (2002). The author uses this approach in a clinical setting. The influence of the family should never be underestimated, from both an historical and a treatment perspective. Therefore, family members have the potential to be key players during the assessment and subsequent treatment and management phases. Due to the wide variability in individual differences, each program, while following the same central themes in assessment, must be individualized (Pařízková, Maffeis, and Poskitt, 2002). Variability must also extend to the respective families of obese children. The ability of practitioners to gain family involvement and support during the treatment and management phases may be one of the most influential factors in the likelihood of a successful outcome in the longer term (see Chapters 4–11):

Physical growth history: An historical overview of size and shape during the growing years starting with birth weight, comparisons with siblings, and patterns of growth of parents.

Anthropometric and body composition profile: Height, weight, BMI, circumferences, limb lengths, skinfold measurements. (Note: Skinfold measurements are unreliable in more obese individuals.)

Nutritional profile: Assessment of energy intake, eating practices and regime during the day, food preferences and aversions. An understanding of family eating practices is particularly useful at this stage.

Psychological characteristics: Status of the child, his/her reaction to behavioral intervention.

Functional and fitness assessment: Indication of response to exercise through an assessment of health-related components of physical fitness.

Family interview: Group meeting and discussion with all family members. This should be followed by the administration of psychological questionnaires including body image and body satisfaction instruments.

Health status: Hormonal and biochemical characteristics.

12.1.1 Treatment Strategies and Markers of Success

Methodological approaches of aspects mentioned earlier were given in previous chapters. As indicated previously, it is often extremely difficult to compare the results of studies in this area.

In the management of most individuals, the essential initial element is a modification of the diet. This management component is addressed later in this chapter in more detail. Individual studies often fail to report the true nature of energy intake in the obese, as the consumption of food and drink is commonly underreported in this population. The opposite is true for physical activity. It is customary for the obese to overestimate energy expenditure when self-reporting physical activity participation. Further, it is unusual for health professionals to know the full details of the historical nature of the health, nutrition, and physical activity status of the obese patient or subject.

The natural trend is for the young individual to increase and not reduce total body weight. The cornerstones of obesity management during growth are significant modifications of eating and activity behaviors, the combination of which results in a more active and healthy lifestyle. Any proposed change in lifestyle during the growing years must be cognizant of the peculiarities of the individual, such as his or her period of growth, gender, and environmental, social, economic and psychological factors. In obese infants and school-age children, the support of parents in the weight-management process is indispensable. With adolescents who may be more motivated and have greater potential for self-management of their condition, parental support and encouragement is also of great importance but self-control should be fostered in the individual (Zwiauer, 1998).

Less severe obesity can be managed by monitoring a reduction of energy intake and appropriate adjustments in the composition of the diet. However, in more severe cases, a very low energy diet may be implemented. Irrespective of the level of obesity, an increased energy output is essential for long-term success. The promotion of physical activity followed by an individualized prescription of exercise must be incorporated wherever possible. With very large young people, the same degree of caution should be exercised in relation to activity and ideally provided by an exercise physiologist with the joint supervision of a medical practitioner to avoid accidents and overloading children.

The response of children to a standardized treatment approach is variable (Dietz and Robinson, 1993). Nuutinen and Knip (1992a) considered the characteristics of children who had various degrees of success after reduction treatment. Weight, body composition, and insulin levels were the main outcome variables. Those who were successful at 1 year of treatment had greater weight loss, lower loss of lean body mass, and lower fasting serum insulin levels. Predictors of better success in weight loss at 2 years were the decrease in BMI of the mother and documented energy intake over the first year.

A retrospective review and comparison of subgroups defined by age and frequency of visits to an obesity treatment center was conducted to determine if the timing and frequency of interventions influenced the outcome of treatment in obese children aged 1 to 10 years (Davis and Christoffel, 1994). Children were seen within one year and with one or more subsequent visits in the next year in a nutrition evaluation clinic and an outpatient clinic at a metropolitan hospital. At the time of the initial visit, a comprehensive history and physical examination by a physician, registered dietitian, and social worker were undertaken. A sound diet and exercise plan was suggested. A subsequent visit occurred after one month, with later intervals tailored according to individual need. A comparison of the outcomes of treatment in four groups subdivided according to age and frequency of visits showed that the most successful treatment of preadolescent obesity may be possible in the preschool years with frequent visits to the clinic or center. Therefore, to treat early and often may be the best method (Pařízková and Chin, 2003).

A multidisciplinary intervention program (Blecker et al., 1998) was most successful in long-term weight maintenance for children who were only mildly obese at the beginning of the treatment program. More than 70% of boys and 40% of girls grew out of their obesity if they could self-monitor their lifestyle with a simple checklist on a permanent basis. This was also revealed in a study of Japanese children involved in a multidisciplinary program. This approach has the potential to be used in a number of settings, including with various medical practitioners and without the need for special facilities (Asayama et al., 1998b).

Analyses of changes in obesity prevalence as well as experiences with different treatment modalities have revealed that it is possible to provide recommendations for both treatment and the prevention of obesity during growth. A study by Flanery and Kirschenbaum (1986) examined the effect of four classes of variables associated with weight-reduction programs. These included self-control techniques, degree of social support, attribution style, and self-reinforcement style in obese children. The results of this study conducted in two localities suggested that obese children who terminated ineffective problem-solving efforts quickly and who had more adaptive weight-reduction attribution might be more likely to succeed in long-term weight reduction. Differential results in the two samples suggest that variables investigated in this study may play a greater role in weight maintenance rather than in initial behavioral change.

For an intervention to be effective, it is important to know the reliable predictors of treatment and the likely reaction of the obese individual. In a study of prepubertal American and Caucasian boys aged 9 to 11 years, total energy expenditure (TEE) by doubly labeled water (DLW), resting metabolic rate (RMR), the thermic effect of food (TEF), and substrate oxidation after the meal were assessed (DeLany, Harsha, and Bray, 1998). The primary endpoint was a two-year change in the percentage of body fat measured by DXA. The best predictor of weight gain after two years was a high protein oxidation, followed by low energy expenditure and high RQ during the TEF. It was possible to conclude that energy expenditure, resting metabolic rate, and components of substrate oxidation are predictors of an increase in body weight and fat mass during late childhood. With this information, it may be possible to select individuals with an increased risk of remaining overweight.

The level of hyperinsulinemia is also considered a marker of success in the treatment of obesity (Zanelli et al., 1993). Groups of obese children aged 5 to 16 years were assessed longitudinally and screened for insulinemia and glycemia after an oral glucose tolerance test, plasma levels of total cholesterol, HDL-C, and TG. The sample was divided into subgroups on the basis of insulinemia and was similar according to all variables tested, except for weight loss and plasma triglyceride levels. The hyperinsulinemic group had a lower percentage reduction in excess weight, and the results in this group were not dependent on the duration of treatment. This did not apply to the normo-insulinemic group of obese children.

As mentioned previously, various approaches are used in an attempt to encourage weight loss in children and adolescents, so results have not always been comparable or similarly successful. Reported results are as variable as the studies are different. Comparisons of study outcomes must include consideration of the changes in body weight, BMI, and body composition, as well as other outcome measures. For example, an educational strategy to improve diet may have positive results in childhood obesity, as was the case in a Milan (Italy) population with young people (aged 3 to 18 years) in which mean prevalence of obesity was 13.4% (Ceratti et al., 1990).

The current knowledge and understanding of various approaches in the treatment of pediatric obesity has been reviewed by a number of authors (Glenny et al., 1997; Epstein et al., 1998; Caroli and Burniat, 2002; Summerbell et al., 2003; Yanovski and Yanovski, 2003) and most recently by Lobstein, Baur, and Uauy (2004). Generally, the most effective combined therapy, using the principles of the improvement of energy balance by diet and exercise and behavioral modification, is recommended for children and youth (Pařízková, 1977, 1996b; Pařízková, 1998a,b). This approach is also the most effective for adults. However, weight-management treatment in obese growing subjects requires special approaches tailored to individuals in this age period (Pařízková, Maffeis, and Poskitt, 2002).

Recommendations for the improvement of childhood obesity treatment programs reported in the literature include the application of behavioral choice theory, improving knowledge of response extinction, and recovery with regard to behavioral relapse. These are some of the greatest problems of obesity treatment in children and adults. The individualization of the treatment and integration of basic scientific information with clinical research outcomes are additional recommended components of therapeutic procedures for obese children (Epstein et al., 1998).

The maintenance of a successful outcome in reduction treatment is a significant challenge in adults and the same applies to children, even when weight loss may often be achieved more easily (Dietz, 1986, 1990, 1993, 1998a,b,c; Epstein, 1993; Epstein et al., 1986, 1989, 1990, 1998; Pařízková, 1963c, 1977, 1993a,b, 1998a,b). A study of obese children aged 6 to 16 years indicated that a weight loss of at least 10% of the initial value after two years of treatment was the criterion of a "successful loser." Approximately half of the children succeeded in meeting this criterion. In children who were successful, body weight decreased by 24.7%, along with a significant decrease in TC, TG, and insulin; an increase of serum level HDL-C; and an increased ratio of HDL-C/TC. These positive results were maintained after 5 years of the study period. In normal-weight children, serum lipids and insulin remained stable during this period (Nuutinen and Knip, 1992a). Similarly, an effective weight-reduction program using a family-oriented approach and/or group approach had the best results (Foreyt et al., 1991). In addition, the provision of resources such as a manual on dietary change and overall lifestyle improvement including exercise was better than the group that only received written information. This program was included in "Cuidando El Corazon," a weight-reduction intervention for Mexican American subjects.

Findings of another study (Fripp et al., 1985) suggest that if aerobic conditioning is used to modify the health risks of atherosclerosis, it is likely to be accompanied by a reduction of body weight. Importantly, without a reduction of excess fat, health cannot be effectively promoted. A counterargument in the consideration of best approaches to obesity management in children incorporates the numerous negative examples regarding the fear of obesity and an exaggerated reaction to it by an excessively reduced diet and high levels of exercise. These phenomena may be a more common occurrence in adolescent girls, with the potential for the development of symptoms similar to anorexia nervosa. A case of a girl aged 7 years showed an excessive reduction of food intake and elimination of carbohydrates and an excessive involvement in exercise (Tsukuda and Shiraki, 1994). Height velocity for this individual reduced from 6.0 to 4.1 cm.year^{-1}, compared to the values in control girls of the same age of 5.5 ± 0.74 cm.year^{-1}. The individual's eating behavior was finally normalized without specific psychotherapy. Such situations must be prevented because of possible longer-lasting health, functional, and psychological consequences. These problems may be considered comparable or even more serious than problems resulting from obesity. Concerns regarding the treatment of childhood obesity were raised for these and related reasons in the earlier work of Woolley and Woolley (1983).

Young people are also exposed to a wide range of inappropriate health messages through the various forms of mass media. For example, one of the more common trends in recent years has been the societal tendency to glamorize thinness. When the characteristic feature of the human race is diversity in body size and shape, this "message" is potentially problematic. A strategy to assist young people in coping with a wide range of potentially misleading messages is to provide them with the skills to critically appraise advertising. There is a wonderful opportunity for society to profit in a positive fashion through advertising to promote healthy eating and physical activity behaviors, and to make them economically and financially rewarding to counteract the widespread prevalence of poor or inappropriate lifestyle practices.

12.1.2 The Role of Family Support

The family of an obese child must play a lead role in the treatment process if the individual is to maximize the opportunity of a successful outcome (Golan and Crow, 2004; Golan and Weizman, 2001; Lobstein, Baur, and Uauy, 2004). In families where obesity is more pronounced, Kalker, Hovels, and Kolbe-Saborowski (1991) found that children were able to reduce their weight more than average during treatment but regained the weight during the subsequent 3 to 5 years. The highest levels of overweight were recorded after that time. The level of obesity of the other members of the family, whether the individual was an only child, or the gender of the obese children did not influence the initial decision to stop or continue with the treatment. Boys were more successful in weight reduction than girls based on mean scores both after 3 to 6 months and also after 5 years. However, this difference was not significant. Children without a family history of obesity were significantly less overweight at the beginning compared with those with a familial obesity, and similarly, they showed the best short- and medium-term results. Thus, in spite of good short-term results, obese children of obese parents should be regarded as those at greatest risk of weight regain and therefore should be checked and treated on a regular basis over a long period during the growing years. This issue was discussed in detail in Chapter 3.

Many claim that it is too difficult or even impossible to achieve permanent change using standard procedures of obesity treatment. Therefore, the potential effect of the family must not be underestimated, especially for younger obese children. The prevention of obesity in such children can be most successful if initiated with the simultaneous prevention and treatment of obesity of a parent and/or older siblings. An early start is the best guarantee of an adequate result in the longer term. Epstein et al. (1986b) have suggested that in relation to weight loss in weight-management programs, outcomes are related to the weight of parents and the present status of the obese child.

Epstein (1997) has also suggested that a family-based intervention program should be introduced to rectify energy imbalance in slightly older obese prepubertal children (approximately 8 to 12 years of age). The involvement of at least one parent as an active participant in the weight-reduction process can improve both short- and long-term effects of weight regulation. There is a dual benefit when family and friends support a child in behavior change, as those providing a supporting role also benefit.

Other positive changes have been reported in parent-directed weight-reduction programs with young children. For example, the degree of compliance in children was significantly correlated with the change in percentage overweight in Taipei children (Chen, Ku, and Wu, 1993). A number of longitudinal studies over 1, 5, and up to 10 years (Epstein et al., 1986a, 1994) have also illustrated the importance of parents. The results after 1 year showed that the amount of relative weight change was related to the initial treatment success, the number of children in the family, and the gender of the child. Children who were initially more successful had fewer siblings and were female. These results suggest that family size may interact with the treatment to determine weight change (Epstein et al., 1986a). When nonobese siblings are present in the family, the adherence of only one family member is very difficult to achieve.

Multivariate regression analyses of changes in relative weight and fitness after 5 years of treatment in obese children showed two factors independently related to fitness change; maintenance of weight loss from the end of 6 months of treatment to the 5-year follow-up, and the initial level of physical fitness. Children with the lowest levels of fitness at the beginning of the treatment and who were able to maintain weight loss up to 5 years showed the largest improvement (Epstein et al., 1988). Another family-based behavioral treatment study (Epstein et al., 1990) conducted across a 5-year period with obese children aged 6 to 12 years provided the following results. Treatments with conjoint targeting and reinforcement of child and parent behavior, plus reciprocal targeting and reinforcement of children and parents, were associated with the best outcomes for the child. Predictors of child success included self-monitoring, changing eating behavior, praise, and change in percent of overweight of parents. Predictors for successful parental outcomes were self-monitoring of weight, baseline parent percent of overweight, and participation in fewer subsequent weight-control programs. Similar conclusions were gained in a 10-year longitudinal study. Long-term change in children depends on the mode of treatment and evidence converges on the importance of the family and other sources of support for a change to adequate eating and physical activity (Epstein et al., 1990; Epstein et al., 1994; Nuutinen and Knip, 1992a).

Wadden et al. (1990) considered the effect of a 16-week program on obese adolescent girls who were treated with different levels of parental participation. The greater number of sessions attended by a girl's mother, the greater the weight loss of that girl. Weight loss was associated with significant improvements in body composition, serum TC, and psychological status. Other studies by Epstein (1993, 1994) have demonstrated the essential role of an active approach of mothers and fathers in helping their obese children.

Parents should be active participants in all aspects of the treatment and management of their obese child to maximize the impact of both diet and exercise (Flodmark and Lissau, 2002). Epstein (1993) has suggested that the motivational structure within the family that supports or discourages behavior change may be just as important as the specific behaviors that the weight-management process is attempting to modify. As might be expected, when parents and children are treated together, better results are gained than when children are targeted alone.

A study by Golan and Weizman (1999) assessed the role of parents in the treatment of obese children aged 6 to 11 years. With the experimental group of children, parents were agents of change whereas in a comparable group, a conventional approach was used. Anthropometric and biochemical measurements and questionnaires to assess sociodemographic characteristics, diet, and physical activity in the family were completed at the beginning and end of the study. Mean percentile weight reduction was significantly higher in children in the experimental group (14.6%) than in the control group (8.1%). This study provides further substantiation of the essential role of parents in the rectification of obesity during growth.

In obese children treated on an outpatient basis, best results in a reduction program were obtained in subjects aged 4 to 14 years with two or more siblings plus an adequate adherence to the prescribed diet and good family support. In this study, the gender, level of obesity of other family members, initial age, and previous food and exercise behaviors did not have a significant effect (Flodmark et al., 1993).

12.1.3   Individual vs. Group Approaches to Obesity Treatment

The results of treatment can vary according to whether treatment is provided on an individual or a group basis. In a one-year treatment program, Nuutinen and Knip (1992b) found that both groups had a similar weight reduction, linear growth. and lean body mass development. Similarly, the serum level of HDL-C and HDL-C/TC increased and TG decreased significantly in both groups. However, fasting insulin levels decreased significantly only in the group treated as individuals.

In Singapore, where a high prevalence of obesity has been reported (Ray, Lim, and Ling, 1994), three subgroups of obese preschoolers (with mild, moderate, and severe overweight) were studied. The latter group was referred to dietitians for management while nursing staff using preplanned counseling sessions managed the other two groups. There were differences among groups with respect to family history of obesity and hypertension. After one year of the intervention program, 40.4% of the children improved in their obesity status and 20.2% reached normal-weight status. All groups significantly improved their health status.

Suttapreyasri et al. (1990) studied the response of obese children in Bangkok using several training methods. After 3 months of training, the knowledge on obesity increased significantly using each model, and weight reduction was significant in the group that was provided with lectures and rewards to decrease body fatness. After 6 months, each group showed similar increases in height and weight, but the group given lectures and rewards had the lowest increase in weight.

In very severe cases of obesity in adolescents, a closely monitored program such as an inpatient approach must be considered as for similar cases in adults. The results of a follow-up lasting 33.3 months, with a mean duration of inpatient treatment of 6.8 months, showed that long-term inpatient treatment had a positive effect on weight change. Successful outcomes were induced using a permanent change in lifestyle brought about by a combination of nutritional therapy, psychotherapy, and exercise (Siegfried et al., 1998). However, inpatient treatment of subjects who are obese but without co-morbidities is particularly difficult, especially due to the facilities required and the expense of such treatment.

Self-training was shown to be as an efficient approach to treat obesity in obese 12- to 16-year-olds who stayed in the medical center for at least 4 months. Eighteen boys were trained with a self-training method, adapted progressively to each boy and controlled. The training took place within a 10-week period with five 30- to 40-minute sessions a fortnight. Morphological, functional (aerobic capacity and muscle strength), and psychomotor qualities were followed. After 3 months' training and after comparison with the control group, a significant improvement in psychomotor capacities, a major tendency for the improvement of the aerobic capacity, and very positive effects on the psyche were found (Dupuis et al., 2000).

Some programs did not prove to be efficient enough; intervention in teacher training, modification of school meals, the development of school action plans targeting the curriculum, physical education, tuck shops, and playground activities had little effect on children's behavior other than a modest increase in consumption of vegetables. Sedentary behavior and global self-worth was higher in the obese children of the intervened group; there was no difference in BMI, other psychological measures, or dieting behavior between the intervened and nonintervened group (Sahota et al., 2001).

12.2 The Effect of Diet

Considerable attention has been paid to the factors that determine food habits during the early years of life. Further consideration has been given to the possibility of influencing food preferences and eating patterns in a desirable way through health promotion. The prevention or delay of adult-onset diseases may be facilitated by interventions in early childhood. Numerous common chronic diseases that fit into this category include ischemic heart disease, cerebrovascular accidents, hypertension, malignancies, and also obesity (Kemm, 1987).

The importance of the diet during early life is of central significance as this period is assumed to be the most critical and sensitive. Establishment of proper dietary habits during childhood can have long-term positive consequences with regard to weight control and prevention of obesity (Westenhoefer, 2002). Food intake and its composition during this period of growth can influence metabolic development and predetermine some of the future metabolic processes (Pařízková, 1998a,b). However, while the importance or significance of the potential benefits for young children may be undisputed, there are still some shortcomings in research in the area, including negative consequences of dietary controls (Caroli and Burniat, 2002).

12.2.1 Dietary Allowances for Obese Children

The definition of food intake, including energy and macro- and micro-components of recommended daily allowances (RDAs) for obese children and adolescents, is a unique problem. Along with the reduction of stored fat, fat-free mass and functional capacity should increase to attain an optimal health status (Schoeller et al., 1988). A 2-decade study spanning the period from birth to 21 years (Rolland-Cachera et al., 1990a,b) revealed that 41% of children who were fat at 1 year of age were still fat in adulthood. It was also revealed that one can be obese without being hyperphagic (at least at the period when children were followed up). Therefore, the definition of a reduction diet must be qualified and an individualized approach used whenever possible, taking into account individual energy expenditure, such as for growth, BMR, and physical activity (WHO, 1985). Although the evaluation of BMI is suitable, periodic checkups of body composition status aimed at the provision of information, changes in fat-free mass, or a marked slowdown in height are recommended.

A monitored reduction in food intake is acceptable in obese children as it is in adults. However, the appropriate definition of the actual allowance for an obese child is quite difficult to quantify. Total food consumption should be less than before but should still include all of the necessary items required for the adequate growth and development of lean body mass. Again, this varies in different periods of growth in both genders and depends on the initial degree of obesity and health status of the individual; this means that each category and/or individual has a different RDA of food. The preparation of meals on a daily basis can also be a difficult task for families who are not specialists in nutrition. In addition, in families in which not all members are obese, it can be a problem to prepare meals separately for individuals, especially children. The effect of inadequate diets may not manifest immediately but may be delayed when the rectification of the child's status could be more difficult.

Numerous dietary regimes have been developed but generally only the basic characteristics of the approach are reported. A reduction diet for a child is not simply a scaled-down version of food usually consumed by youth and adults. The diet must consist of reductions in the amount of high-risk items, such as saturated fats, sweets, and highly processed food that is often high in fat and sugar. At the same time, adequate amounts of essential vitamins, minerals, fiber, and polyunsaturated fatty acids should be included to meet the RDAs for the age and gender of the individual.

Caution should be exercised where any form of dietary modification is used and height velocity should be monitored during periods of weight management, as changes in velocity are more likely in growing individuals who lose, maintain, or increase weight more slowly than average. The same rule should apply to the health status, functional capacity, physical performance, and psychological status. Greater attention needs to be given to the identification of the optimal diet to support linear growth during weight loss. Dietz (1983) has suggested that a safe approach to employ in dietary restriction is to limit the amount of high-fat food in the diet. This may result in a reduction in total caloric intake by approximately one-third. Attention should also be given to a reduction in the consumption of snack foods such as ice cream, potato chips, and soft drinks (Dietz and Hartung, 1985).

A study of Japanese fourth and fifth graders (Saito and Tatsumi, 1994) showed a significant decline in obesity levels after 3 months of therapy using a low-carbohydrate, high-protein diet and exercise. After the educational program, dietary intake decreased, especially due to a decreased carbohydrate intake. Nutrient intakes were in the appropriate range for boys, but energy and iron intakes were lower than the RDAs for girls while protein intake increased. This diet and exercise treatment program was very effective as evidenced by the decrease in obesity level from 30% and above to 10.4% for boys and to 7.5% in girls. Recommendations for dieting practices and their improvement were considered in another follow-up (Ikeda and Mitchell, 2001); reductions of energy especially at the expense of, for example, fat, cholesterol, and simple sugars were suggested.

Children's eating patterns should be addressed with other components of a total weight-management program; these components include parental involvement, reduction in energy intake, and increased physical activity and exercise (Dietz, 1993; Epstein, 1996; Epstein et al., 1986a,b, 1990, 1998). Family eating and exercise patterns play a significant role in the etiology, treatment, and management of childhood and adolescent obesity. Eating is often considered an important indicator of the emotional state of family members and of interactions between parent(s) and child(ren). Optimal nutrition depends on the development of a positive relationship between parent(s) and the child(ren). The eating practices of children are enhanced when parents recognize and respond appropriately to the needs of the child (Satter, 1996).

For some parents, concerns about overfeeding and causing obesity in their children are pervasive. While an appropriate awareness of food consumption in both type and quantity is necessary, being so concerned that food is withheld and hunger not satisfied in children can be problematic. This practice may be more prevalent if parents are anxious or concerned about their own eating practices. There is a real need for sensitivity on the part of parents to a child's likes and dislikes and feeding cues. The promotion of a positive feeding environment in the home that discourages rigidity and inflexibility regarding eating practices and behavior should be a central focus.

12.2.2 The Effect of Low-Energy Diets

The aim of weight reduction in obese children is to achieve a loss of excess fat and preserve an adequate growth in height and lean body mass. However, when the degree of obesity is already severe or morbid, a greater restriction of energy is necessary. A special protein-sparing, low-energy diet was used at the Hospital for Sick Children in Toronto for severely obese adolescents (Bell, Chan, and Pencharz, 1985). The regime provides 2.0 to 2.5 g of protein per kg of ideal body weight, plus adequate fluid and nutrient supplements. The amount of meat, poultry, and fish that supplies this allowance of protein was determined using a protein-equivalence system developed for the diet. The system allows both dietitians and patients to plan meals that minimize energy intake while maintaining protein adequacy and diet variety. When this diet is prolonged beyond the recommended 3 to 6 months, limited carbohydrate may be added in the form of selected vegetables. This type of diet must be properly supervised, but its safety and efficacy have been demonstrated in adolescent individuals.

In obese youth, the protein-sparing modified fast diet produced significantly greater changes in percent of overweight at 10 weeks (−30% vs. −14%) and at 6 months (−32% vs. −18%). At 10 weeks, a significant loss of adipose tissue with preservation of lean body mass occurred in the protein-sparing modified fast group. A transient slowing of growth velocity was seen at 6 months in both dietary groups compared with the values at 14.5 months. Growth velocity approached normal levels at 14.5 months compared with standards for North American children. When dietary groups were combined, the blood pressure decreased significantly at all points of the study. The initial average values of serum TC also significantly decreased, and no biochemical or clinical complications were observed. The results indicate that it is possible to use hypocaloric diets without negative consequences for growth, but such diets should not be used without careful medical supervision (Figueroa-Colon et al., 1993). Another longitudinal study (Epstein, Valoski, and McCurley, 1993) also confirmed that moderate dietary restriction in overweight children with adequate dietary guidance does not have a negative long-term effect on children's growth.

A study by Stallings et al. (1988) considered the treatment of obese adolescents with the protein-sparing modified diet (PSMF) (880 kcal.kg^{-1}.day^{-1} and 2.5 g protein.kg ideal body weight^{-1}.day^{-1}) for 3 months. Approximately three-quarters of the subjects were followed up after 1 year and 48% had sustained weight loss, with the percentage of ideal body weight for height decreasing from 154 to 125 over this period. Total body potassium (K) decreased 13% and total body nitrogen (N) decreased 14.3% over the year of study. The protein-sparing diet did not prevent some loss of K and N during this treatment; however, the decrease did not exceed their normal predicted values.

The protein-sparing modified fast diet and a hypocaloric balanced diet with different dietary strategies was administered to a group of obese children aged 4 to 14 years. During the first 10 weeks, a group of children was placed on a protein-sparing modified fast diet (2520 to 3360 kJ), and another group of children and adolescents was placed on a hypocaloric balanced diet (3360 to 4200 kJ). Subsequently, all participants had a hypocaloric diet and the energy level was increased from 4200 to 5040 kJ in a 3-month period and maintained for 1 year. Both diets produced significant weight loss during the first 6 months.

Figueroa-Colon et al. (1996) used a clinic-based hypocaloric diet intervention in children aged 8.8 to 13.4 years in New Orleans. During the first weeks, super-obese children were placed on a 2520 to 3360 kJ (600 to 800 kcal) protein-sparing modified fast diet. Subsequently, the diets of all children were increased in a 4-month period by 420 kJ (100 kcal) every 2 weeks until a 5040 kJ (1200 kcal) per-day balanced diet was attained. At 6 months, the super-obese dieters on the protein-sparing modified fast diet had a significant weight loss from baseline (-5.6 ± 7.1 kg) with a positive growth velocity Z-score. Blood pressure and serum lipids decreased, and no complications were observed. The diet was effective in the super-obese children in the medically managed clinic program implemented in a school setting. The efforts of committed clinic staff, school officials, peers, and family involvement were crucial to the success of this intervention program over a period of 6 months.

Obese children have also been successfully treated using a classical hypocaloric diet (Burniat and Van Aelst, 1993). At the beginning of the follow-up, the energy intake of obese children was $98 \pm 24\%$ of RDAs, with $38.4 \pm 4.2\%$ of lipids, $47.8 \pm 4.5\%$ of carbohydrates, and $13.8 \pm 2.5\%$ of protein. The food consumed by the obese children contained a small amount of fiber and total water. The reduction diet included 1200 to 1800 kcal.day^{-1}, or about 65% of RDAs, with 20% protein, 30% lipids, and a total water volume > 1.5 ml.kcal^{-1}. After at least 6 months, the children exhibited a decrease in their excess P50 BMI from $155 \pm 22\%$ to $133 \pm 16\%$. An evaluation of the dietary intake after treatment showed a significant improvement. Total energy intake was lowered to 75% of RDAs, the percentage of lipids to $33.5 \pm 5.3\%$, and total water was 1.28 ± 0.37 ml.kcal^{-1}. The percentage of proteins was increased while the percentage of carbohydrates remained changed. This study revealed that the classical hypocaloric balanced diet had a significant effect on obese children, although the improvement of their nutrition did not accurately follow dietary recommendations for the particular age groups (Burniat and Van Aelst, 1993).

The effect of a balanced low-caloric diet and very low-caloric diet of different duration in subjects of different ages was summarized and the results evaluated by Caroli and Burniat (2002), but in many cases the weight loss was not specified. Standard protein-sparing diets and modified fasts have been suggested; intended energy and protein intake was 10.6 kcal/kg ideal body weight/day, 66% protein, 24% fat, and 10% carbohydrate of total energy, P/S (ratio of polyunsaturated to saturated fat) 0.6, at least 1.5 L of water/day and 15 to 20 g fiber/day. Weight loss and other metabolic modifications showed both positive and negative effects of diet reduction treatment.

Spieth et al. (2000) assessed a low-glycemic index (GI) diet compared with a low-fat diet in obese children over 4 months. There was a greater decrease in BMI in the low-GI group, which suggests that such a diet may be a

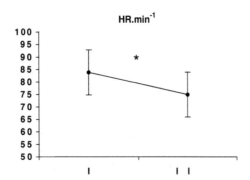

FIGURE 12.1
Changes in heart rate (HR) after a low-calorie diet (I, LCD = 525 kcal.day^{-1}) and after weight loss (II, –5.7 ± 1.6 kg). * indicates (p < 0.05). (Based on data from Zwiauer et al., 1989.)

promising alternative to the standard diet treatment for obese children. The GI diet was used in another study that emphasized selection of foods with a low to moderate GI with 45–50% energy from carbohydrates and 30–35% from fat. At 12 months, BMI and percent of body fat decreased more in the experimental group compared to the conventional group. Glycemic index was a significant predictor of treatment response among both groups, whereas dietary fat was not (Ebbelink et al., 2003). Avoiding drinks with high-energy content may also help to prevent increased adiposity (Bellisle and Rolland-Cachera, 2001; James et al., 2004). The sweet taste of carbonated beverages is very attractive to many young people, but overconsumption can increase energy intake undesirably.

Very low calorie diets (VLCDs) can be risky in the treatment of obesity in children, even when they contain a high-quality protein. This was shown in a study with a group of obese children monitored for the appearance of cardiac arrythmias by frequent 24-hr Holter recordings. After weight loss, cardiac arrythmias appeared in some patients. This can be potentially dangerous for the health of obese children (Schmidinger et al., 1987).

General concerns have been expressed for the marked reduction of food intake in obesity treatment. However, Zwiauer et al. (1989) conducted a study to consider cardiac function in a group of obese children with a daily intake of 500 kcal across a 3-week period. Twenty-four-hour electrocardiograph recordings (Holter ECGs) were made and analyzed in the group. Weight loss during this period was 5.7 ± 1.6 kg. Average and minimal heart rate decreased constantly throughout the study period (Figure 12.1). During the second week, maximal heart rate increased significantly but returned to baseline values in the third week. No dysrrhythmias were monitored either before, during, or after the period of therapy. These results indicate that a low-calorie diet (500 to 700 kcal.day^{-1}), with an appropriate macro and micronutrient composition, is a safe therapeutic approach for obese children and adolescents.

The composition of diets, such as those with a low-fat content, may be problematic in pediatric nutrition as already mentioned. The effect of obesity on the availability of essential and long-chain polyunsaturated fatty acids (LC-PUFAs) was followed up in a group of children. The results of the study suggested that obese children do not require LC-PUFA supplementation to low-fat diets during reduction treatment (Decz, Molnar, and Koletzko, 1998).

However, an improvement in the diet of children can be achieved by reducing a proportion of fat intake. For example, skim milk can be used instead of higher-fat alternatives. This is an economical, single-food strategy that makes it possible to achieve contemporary RDAs of macro- and micro-nutrients, and maintain nutritional adequacy. It is more of a challenge, for example, when replacing meat higher in fat with a lean alternative. In such cases, some slight deficiencies, such as vitamin E deficiency, have been reported (Peterson and Sigman-Grant, 1997). A concerted effort is needed to replace the common but unsuitable components of a high-fat diet with healthier alternatives (Sigman-Grant, Zimmermann, and Kris-Etherton, 1993).

An adequate dietary intake in terms of quantity and composition, modified according to the needs of the individual and program, is the most indispensable tool and most often used approach to improve body weight and composition. Where inpatient support is not available, dietary counseling at schools or other institutions is highly advisable. However, some problems can occur when attempting to restrict food intake, including undesirable changes in relation to height velocity (Dietz and Hartung, 1985; Pařízková and Rolland-Cachera, 1997).

There is some variability in results in studies that have considered a slowing of growth after treatment of obesity using a restricted diet. For example, a study by Epstein et al. (1990) showed that after 5 years of treatment (from 6 to 12 years of age) obese children still remained taller than the norm (65th percentile). A study of Russian children showed that dietetic management produced a different effect in obese children, which attests to the heterogeneity of the disease. Therefore, conducting more detailed analyses of the causes of obesity and suggesting that a more exact diagnosis should be done prior to involvement in such programs (Kniazev et al., 1985).

This approach was used in a group of obese children during a 2-year period in a school health-care setting (group II), as compared with a group of severely obese children with intensive treatment (group I). The age range of children was 6 to 16 years. They were treated over 1 year and observed for another year. Food intake data was collected using a 4-day record method. At baseline, there were no differences in food consumption or nutrient intake between obese and normal-weight children. The group with intensive therapy (I) significantly decreased fat intake during treatment, which was permanently maintained throughout the observation period. Weight loss was 16.2% of the initial value, in contrast with group II, in which no change was revealed. Body fat and relative weight was significantly correlated with the decrease in energy intake. Both the dietary counseling group in the school

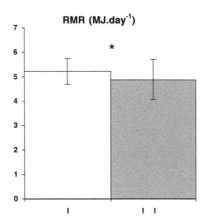

FIGURE 12.2
Changes in resting metabolic rate (RMR) before (I) and after (II) weight loss (-5.4 ± 1.2 kg) during 6 months of a mixed hypocaloric diet. * indicates ($p < 0.05$). (Based on data from Maffeis, Schutz, and Pinelli, 1992a.)

health-care setting and the control group displayed no change in daily fat intake. The conventional approach for obesity treatment appeared to be far less effective as shown in group II (Nuutinen, 1991). In another study, dietary instruction lasting 13 weeks partly rectified the degree of obesity (as evaluated by Rohrer's Index) and some serum biochemical characteristics in children of the third to sixth grade in Taiwan (Chang, Hu, and Wang, 1998).

Body composition and resting energy expenditure (REE) in obese adolescents changed significantly following weight loss due to a low-energy, high-protein diet (800 kcal to 3349 kJ.day^{-1}) in obese adolescents. Total body potassium (TBK) as well as extracellular, intracellular, and total body water (ECW, ICW, TBW) did not change significantly after weight loss, indicating a preserved body composition. The REE decreased with weight loss; however, when expressed as kcal.kg^{-1} body weight and/or fat-free mass^{-1}, no significant changes were revealed (Stallings and Pencharz, 1992). The hypocaloric diet decreased RMR in obese adolescents after 6 months of mixed hypocaloric diet resulting from a weight loss of 5.4 ± 1.2 kg (Figure 12.2) (Maffeis, Schutz, and Pinelli, 1992a).

Nitrogen (N) balance was studied in a group of obese children after a liquid formula VLCD containing 1339 kj (44 g protein, 33 g carbohydrate, 0.9 g fat) was consumed, resulting in a weight loss of $15.3 \pm 4.6\%$. There were no complaints of hunger or discomfort, and no serious side effects were observed. Half of the patients achieved N balance during the second week and all but one in the third week. Great inter-individual variance was found in the rate of N loss during the course of the study. No significant correlation was revealed between cumulative N balance and weight loss and initial body weight. Blood parameters remained unaffected except for blood glucose and urea, which slightly decreased. Uric acid concentrations increased slightly; in some patients it increased more than 8 mg.day^{-1} and was therefore treated

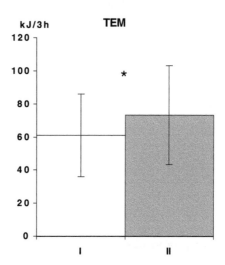

FIGURE 12.3
Changes in the thermic effect of mixed liquid meal (TEM) before (I) and after (II) weight loss by a hypocaloric balanced diet. * indicates ($p < 0.05$). (Based on data from Maffeis, Schutz, and Pinelli, 1992b.)

by allopurinol. Total serum protein decreased and serum albumin values did not change. This type of VLCD proved to be efficient from the point of view of rapid weight loss. A marked improvement of N-balance in 3 weeks could be achieved with the VLCD containing 1 g.protein.kg ideal weight^{-1}.day^{-1}. This amount of protein seems to be indispensable for achieving a sparing effect in growing subjects during weight reduction by VLCD (Widhalm and Zwiauer, 1987).

The effect of a low-calorie balanced diet (LCBD) was assessed in Japanese children aged 3 to 15 years using bioelectrical impedance analysis (BIA) (Kohno, Tanaka, and Honda, 1994). Forty-one percent of obese males and 13% of obese females increased their obesity index after temporary improvement of obesity status after 1 year. Fat and lean body mass did not significantly change, irrespective of the increment of obesity index. This was due to the increase of lean body mass during growth. These observations indicate the importance of a range of body composition measurements.

Maffeis, Schutz, and Pinelli (1992b) indicated that the thermic response to a meal (TEM), which is lower in obese children than in controls, significantly increased after a slimming diet up to the values of controls, that is, to 73 ± 30 kJ. These results support the hypothesis of a moderate thermogenic defect in some obese children, representing a consequence rather than an etiological factor of obesity during growth (Figure 12.3).

Total antioxidant capacity (TAC) and plasma levels of lipid soluble antioxidant vitamins (a-tocopherol and b-carotene) are decreased in obese children. The effect of reduction treatment lasting 20 weeks on TAC was followed up in obese children aged 16.7 ± 1.2 years. After a weight loss of 10.4 ± 4.6 kg, the plasma level of TAC normalized in contrast with those subjects who maintained or even increased their body weight during the same period (Molnar et al., 1998).

12.2.3 Administration of Supplementation in Reducing Diets

The use of supplements in conjunction with a weight-reduction diet can help to reduce the energy content, promote satiety during meals, and curb hunger between meals (Kimm, 1995). With respect to the prevention of obesity, it is recommended that fiber intake during growth be increased gradually up to the RDAs and assist children to adapt to eating sufficient fresh fruit and vegetables. A safe range of dietary intake of fiber for children over age 5 years is up to 10 g per day. This range is considered safe even for children and adolescents with marginal intakes of some vitamins and minerals, and provides enough fiber for normal laxation. This is a difficult task for many people, especially considering the relative ease of availability of various types of junk food, which rarely include sufficient fiber and other healthy items. However, a diet too high in fiber is contraindicated during growth, although such a risk is limited given the nature of common diets available in industrially developing countries. The possible prevention of some chronic diseases, including obesity, can also be considered due to an increased fiber intake (Williams, 1995).

The effect of a diet with unprocessed wheat bran was studied in obese children. Blood glucose and immunoreactive insulin (IRI) concentrations were measured during an oral glucose tolerance test, oral glucose alone, or combined with 15 g of unprocessed wheat bran. The latter combination significantly reduced body weight, blood glucose, and plasma IRI concentrations at 30 min of the tolerance test. These results support the inclusion of bran in the diet of obese children during reduction treatment (Molnar, Dober, and Soltesz, 1985). Other results indicate the importance of an increased ratio of carbohydrates in children's diet, and a reduction in energy intake at the time of the main meals in the prevention of obesity (Maillard et al., 1998).

Vido et al. (1993) assessed the inclusion of glucomannan (1 g twice a day) in the diet of a group of children with an average age of 11.2 years and a placebo in the diet of the control group. During the 2-month study period, all children followed a normo-caloric diet. At the beginning of the study, the drug and placebo groups were comparable. At the end of the study, the mean overweight of the drug group decreased from 49.5 to 41% and that of the placebo group from 43.9 to 41.7%. Decreases in both groups were significant. The only significant between-group differences were a reduction of serum lipids (a-lipoprotein and an increase of b-lipoprotein and triglycerides). Children on the placebo diet only displayed a decrease of triglycerides and Apo-b-lipoprotein.

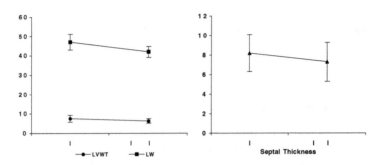

FIGURE 12.4

Changes of intraventricular septal thickness (ST, mm) before (I) and after (II) weight loss (–13.9 ± 4.3 kg) in obese adolescents after a 14-week diet. (LVWT, left ventricular wall thickness; LVV, left ventricular volume). (Based on data from Archibald et al., 1989.)

12.2.4   Risks of Hypocaloric Diets

An uncontrolled restriction of food intake can cause deficiencies in obese children. This phenomenon was followed in a group of obese children and adolescents before and after a 13-week treatment with a hypocaloric balanced diet (HCBD) or a 10-week treatment with a protein-sparing modified fast diet (PSMF). The energy intake provided by HCBD and PSMF was calculated to be 60 and 25%, respectively, of the recommended dietary allowances (RDAs) for age and gender. No further supplementation was provided. The composition of the diet was assessed using a visual memory system for dietary intake recall before starting the weight-loss system. Both diets produced significant weight loss with a considerable reduction in the arm muscle area of the PSMF group. After treatment, no significant changes were observed in serum Fe, ferritin, and transferrin in either group, whereas erythrocyte zinc content increased significantly in the HCBD and the PSMF groups, along with an improvement in the erythrocyte index. A significant increase in plasma zinc was also observed in the PSMF group (Di Toro et al., 1997).

12.2.5   The Effect of Hypocaloric Diets on Cardiocirculatory Parameters

Echocardiography was used to assess changes in cardiac characteristics in a group of obese adolescents after weight loss (Archibald et al., 1989). The group lost a mean of 13.9 ± 4.3 kg representing a decrease of 15.5 ± 5.0% of initial body weight. Serial measurements of intraventricular septal thickness (ST), left ventricular wall thickness (LVWT), and left ventricular volume assessed by standard m-mode echo-cardiographic methods over 14 weeks showed only slight nonsignificant changes (Figure 12.4).

In another study (Pidlich et al., 1997), surface electrocardiographic (ECG) parameters were followed in obese children aged 12.2 years, before and after a conventional low-calorie diet containing an average of 525 ± 109 kcal. The

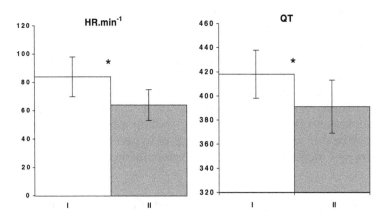

FIGURE 12.5
Effect of weight reduction (–5.7 ± 1.6 kg) on heart rate (HR) and surface electrocardiogram (QT interval, msec) of obese boys and girls (average age 12.2 ± 1.7 years), before (I) and after (II) reduction. * indicates ($p < 0.05$). (Based on data from Pidlich et al., 1997.)

mean loss of body weight was 5.7 ± 1.6 kg. All electrocardiograms were within normal limits; however, a change in the ECG pattern was noted after weight loss. Heart rate and the QT interval decreased (Figure 12.5), and there was a tendency toward a rightward shift of the front-plane QRS axis and a leftward shift of the horizontal-plane QRS axis. Therefore, weight reduction in obese children and adolescents is associated with significant changes in ECG pattern.

The effect of weight reduction on blood pressure using a hypocaloric diet has also been confirmed in obese children. A significant reduction in both systolic and diastolic blood pressure was noted. A long-term dietary intervention study in a group of obese adolescents showed a marked increase in erythrocyte sodium levels and maximal frusemide-sensitive sodium and potassium fluxes, but no changes in cell potassium or water and no effect on lithium–sodium counter-transport. These parameters are sensitive biochemical markers of human essential hypertension. A correlation between the decrease in percentage of body fat and the increase in cell sodium content suggests a link between the metabolic effects of reduced food intake and control of erythrocyte cation handling. Changes in body weight, especially weight loss, are important in studies of erythrocyte transport in spite of the fact that the mechanisms linking dietary energy restriction and changes in erythrocyte cation metabolism are unknown (Weder et al., 1984).

The effect of sodium intake on the regulation of blood pressure in obese adolescents was followed after a 2-week period on a high-salt diet (greater than 250 mmol. Na.day^{-1}) and a low-salt diet (less than 30 mmol.Na.day^{-1}) (Rocchini et al., 1989). When the obese adolescents changed from the high-salt to the low-salt diet, the obese group had a significantly greater mean change in arterial pressure (–12 ± 1 mmHg) than did the nonobese group (+1 ± 2 mmHg), ($p < 0.001$). The variables that best predicted the degree of

sodium sensitivity were the fasting plasma insulin level, the plasma aldos-
terone level (while on the low-salt diet), the plasma norepinephrine level
(while on the high-salt diet), and the percentage of body fat.

In a study by Rocchini et al. (1989), after 20 weeks of treatment, the subjects
who lost more than one kg of body weight had a reduced sensitivity of blood
pressure to sodium difference from value during a high-salt diet to a low-
salt diet. These results support the hypothesis that the blood pressure of
obese adolescents is sensitive to dietary sodium intake and that this sensitivity may be due to the combined effects of hyperinsulinemia, hyperaldosteronism, and increased activity of the sympathetic nervous system.

12.2.6   Changes in Respiratory Parameters after Weight Reduction

As mentioned in Chapter 6, a number of respiratory parameters are changed
in obese children and adolescents. A group of children and adolescents with
medium to severe essential obesity were followed before and after a reduction diet lasting 6 months. More than one-third of the subjects showed
pathological values of peak expiratory flow (PEF) and/or forced expiratory
volume before dieting. All female subjects normalized their respiratory
parameters after 6 months of the reduction (that is, forced vital capacity —
FVC, and also PEF and FFV), while 5 of the 7 males still had pathologic
respiratory indices in spite of comparable weight loss (Brambilla et al., 1992).
These results indicate that obesity can cause a significant number of pathological changes in respiratory parameters in growing individuals. Improvements are not guaranteed when excess weight is reduced using a diet-only
approach.

Morbidly obese children commonly suffer from sleep-associated breathing
disorders that appear to be reversible after a reduction of weight (Lecendreux
et al., 1997). Hypopnea, obstructive sleep apnea, and the respiratory disturbance index significantly improved after a reduction of weight, but central
sleep apnea did not (Lecendreux et al., 1997).

12.2.7   Changes in Biochemical and Hormonal Parameters
           after a Restricted Diet

The positive effect of weight reduction on serum lipids has been repeatedly
confirmed in numerous studies using various programs of obesity treatment.
For example, family-based behavioral obesity treatment lasting 6 months
showed greater weight-reduction changes in obese children compared to a
control group (Epstein et al., 1989b). Simultaneously, a reduction of fasting
serum triglycerides and TC levels along with an increase of HDL-C were
found. After 5 years of followup in a small sample of children comprising
the experimental group, an improvement in relative weight and fitness from
6 months to 5 years was also associated with an improvement in lipoprotein
profiles.

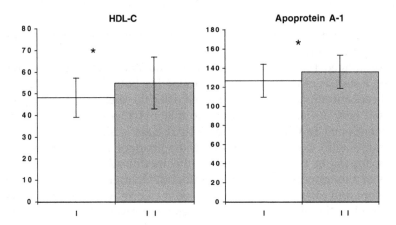

FIGURE 12.6
Changes in serum lipids (HDL-C, Apoprotein A-1) in obese boys aged 5.3 to 9.9 years, before (I) and after (II) reduction dietary treatment. * indicates (p < 0.05). (Based on data from Ferrer-Gonzales et al., 1998.)

A study of obese children aged 5.3 to 9.9 years of age in Spain showed increased serum lipid levels (total and lipoprotein cholesterol, triglycerides, apoprotein A1 and B) (Ferrer-Gonzales et al., 1998). After diet treatment lasting 6 months, the values of total body weight, BMI, and skinfolds (triceps and subscapular) decreased significantly. In subjects who responded well to this treatment, increased serum levels of HDL-C and Apoprotein A1 were found (Figure 12.6). The results indicate that prepubertal obese patients show alterations in lipid profiles. This is not correlated with anthropometric parameters, but a reduction in BMI and skinfold thickness also improved lipid profiles. Initial pathological serum lipid levels in subjects who responded well to the treatment were normalized, but in those who did not reduce weight, no positive changes in serum lipids were revealed.

A longitudinal study of obese children with initially increased serum lipid levels and plasma insulin concentrations but a lower HDL-C/TC ratio showed a decrease in relative weight by 15.8% over the first year of reduction treatment with a parallel decrease of TG and plasma insulin. the HDL-C and HDL-C/TC ratio increased simultaneously. These changes remained stable over the second year of observations. At 5 years, the obese subjects still had a reduced weight (12.8% lower than initially) and a higher serum level of HDL-C (Knip and Nuutinen, 1993).

Similar results were gained in a study of the effect of a weight-reduction regimen by diet in grossly obese children aged 15 years (Zwiauer, Kerbl, and Widhalm, 1989). Mean weight loss was 9.6 ± 2.1% of the initial body weight. Highly significant decreases in TC, LDL-C, HDL-C, TG, HDL3, and Apolipoprotein B concentrations were also observed, while HDL2 concentrations remained almost constant. These observations showed that the decrease of HDL-C that occurs after weight loss due to treatment of obese adolescents with a hypocaloric diet does not result in a decrease in the anti-atherogenic HDL2 subfraction.

A special study of the effect of a reducing diet, either with or without enrichment by polyunsaturated fatty acids, was conducted across 8 weeks in children aged 12.5 ± 1.2 years (Zwiauer and Widhalm, 1987). The results showed a similar reduction in weight following both diets. TC, LDL-C, and Apo-B concentrations were also reduced after the diet enriched by polyunsaturated fatty acids, but there were no major changes in HDL-C levels.

As mentioned in Chapter 9, the GH-IGF axis is significantly altered in individuals with exogenous obesity. Most changes in the peripheral IGF system appear to be independent of the modifications of GH secretion. Results of a longitudinal study in prepubertal children with exogenous obesity before and after weight reduction on a calorie restricted diet revealed that not all of the observed abnormalities were reversed with a significant reduction in the BMI SD score (Argente et al., 1997b).

Wabitsch et al. (1996) has repeatedly studied changes in IGF and BP after weight reduction. It was shown, for example, that obese girls aged 15.0 ± 1.1 years, with BMI 31.1 ± 3.8 $kg.m^{-2}$ had increased levels of IGF-1, IGFBP-1, IGFBP-2, and IGFBP-3 and normal values of IGF-2. After weight reduction by 8.1 ± 2.0 kg, IGF-2 and IGFBP-2 increased, and IGF-1, IGFBP-1, IGFBP-3, and the ratio of IGF-I/IGFBP-3 decreased significantly. Fasting insulin levels were positively correlated with IGF-1 but inversely with IGFBP-1 and IGFBP-2. IGFBP-2 was associated with several metabolic parameters, namely, an inverse correlation with uric acid and triglyceride levels. The ratio IGFBP-2 to IGFBP-1 was inversely correlated with total cholesterol and LDL-C. In addition, IGFBP-2 was inversely correlated with the waist-to-hip ratio. The results indicate that the decrease in IGF-1/IGFBP-3 after weight loss could be partly responsible for the impaired growth velocity revealed in obese growing subjects during treatment with restricted diets. Low values of IGFBP-2 and high IGFBP-1 levels are associated with an unfavorable atherogenic risk profile (Wabitsch et al., 1996).

A lower body weight after reduction therapy is usually accompanied by a decline in serum insulin concentrations. In a study by Chalew et al. (1992), BMI decreased significantly from 39.1 to 34.7 $kg.m^{-2}$ after a low-calorie diet lasting 5 to 8 weeks. Insulin also decreased significantly, but these changes had little effect on the integrated concentrations of growth hormone (IC-GH). Factors other than circulating insulin levels are likely to play a major role in mediating the reduced levels of GH usually found in obese children.

Overweight children aged 12.5 ± 1.9 years placed on a short-term weight reduction in a camp setting showed decreased plasma leptin levels from 16.5 ± 9.8 $ng.ml^{-1}$ to 10.0 ± 8.6 $ng.ml^{-1}$ after a significant fall in BMI. Plasma apoA-1 and HDL-C were independent predictors of leptin concentrations during weight loss. HDL-C transports a variable portion of leptin in circulation (Holub et al., 1999).

The results of a hypocaloric diet were addressed in obese children in two visits to an outpatient department at intervals of 1.5 and 4 years. The group of children with a successful response to the hypocaloric diet treatment (a significant loss of weight) showed a decrease in the plasma levels of Apoprotein A1 and B, triglycerides, nonesterified fatty acids (NEFA), and insulin together with an increase in the level of HDL-C. These changes were not significant in the group of obese children who did not lose weight. For obese children who had high levels of TC despite reduction treatment, the pathologic plasma profile did not show any change while the group with a high level of insulin showed a significant increase of apoprotein A1 and B, and TC and HDL-C. The group in which insulin levels became normal after treatment showed a good development of the biochemistry parameters studied (Bueno-Lozano, Balsamo, and Cacciari, 1991). Weight loss due to a reduction diet decreased insulin resistance and increased insulin sensitivity in children aged 10.1 years (Hoffman et al., 1995).

A significant reduction in serum triiodothyronine (T3) concentration, along with a REE decrease, was found after 6 weeks of a weight-reduction program in obese children. The T3 concentration reduction, which was parallelled by FFM loss, could be responsible for RMR reduction (Kiortsis, Darach, and Tarpin, 1999).

The effectiveness of a family-based, multidisciplinary, behavior-modification program was also adapted for obese adolescents with insulin-dependent diabetes mellitus (IDDM). The measurement of skinfolds and glycated hemoglobin revealed the positive results of reduction therapy, including an improvement of body image and self-esteem in these adolescents (Thomas-Dobersen, Butler-Simon, and Fleshner, 1993).

As indicated by the above-mentioned results, there appears to be a certain bias when a restricted diet is used. There is a risk of a slowdown of growth in height and lean body mass and also changes in other parameters that are not always desirable. Therefore, another approach is preferred. That is, energy intake should not be drastically reduced but rather an increase in total energy expenditure is preferred. A prescribed diet should certainly be introduced, but the intake needs to be checked and the composition of food monitored. Along with diet, a system of exercises plus an overall increase in physical activity level and modified lifestyle should be used.

12.2.8 Changes in Immunological Parameters after a Hypocaloric Diet

Some of the changes in immunological parameters due to obesity were mentioned in Chapter 11. Kravets and Kniazev (1989) studied immunological parameters and serum lipids in obese children aged 3 to 14 years who were treated using a hypocaloric diet enriched by polyunsaturated fatty acids (PUSFA from nonpurified oil, 0.5 to 1.0 g of weight as an additive to vegetable and meat salads, twice a week). A statistically significant increase in the relative content of T-lymphocytes and theophylline-resistant lymphocytes with simultaneous reduction of null cell number was revealed. This might be associated with their stimulating effect on the differentiation of young precursors-lymphocytes, or with the release of T-lymphocyte receptors due to normalization of lipid metabolism, as found in other studies. This study showed the positive effect of a diet with PUSFA that acted as an immuno-stimulant on the general condition of children.

12.3 Exercise Management

The effect of exercise alone on obesity has less of an impact than low-calorie diets (Bar-Or et al., 1998). However, such diets are not always considered suitable to treat obesity during the growing years (Dietz, 1991, 1993; Pařízková, 1972, 1977, 1996a, 1998a,b,c). The importance of physical activity to health, and specifically to weight management, is undisputed. The increasing prevalence of overweight and obesity is always attributed to a number of factors, the most important of which is the decline in physical activity participation by children and adolescents with a concomitant increase in inactive behaviors (Lobstein, Baur, and Uauy, 2004). As mentioned in Chapters 1 and 2, sedentary leisure pursuits such as television and video viewing and playing computer games, the effect of which was shown, for example, in the longitudinal Framingham Children's Study (Proctor et al., 2003), are commonly coupled with the consumption of energy-dense snack foods high in fat and sugar. These practices, along with the use of cars or public transportation instead of walking, as well as an extensive array of labor-saving devices in the home and workplace, have resulted in reduced energy expenditure in daily tasks. These changes have had a significant impact on individuals of all ages.

After 2 years of a comprehensive family-based behavioral weight-control program (dietary and behavior change) 8- to 12-year-old obese children substituted nontargeted sedentary behaviors for some of their targeted sedentary behaviors. The decrease in sedentary activity was accompanied by a decrease of percent of overweight and body fat and improved aerobic fitness; self-reported sedentary activity decreased and physical activity increased. The results support reducing sedentary behaviors as an adjunct in the treatment of pediatric obesity (Epstein et al., 1982, 2000; Epstein and Roemmich, 2001; Robinson, 2001).

The effect of TV viewing on physical activity in obese children was followed during 12 weeks; TV viewing was contingent on pedaling a stationary ergometer for experimental subjects, but not for control subjects. The intervention group had a significantly increased pedaling time but decreased TV-viewing time, and experienced a significantly greater reduction in total body fat and percent of leg fat. Total pedaling time during intervention correlated with greater reduction in percent of body fat. Contingencies in the home environment can therefore be arranged to modify physical activity and TV viewing (Faith et al., 2001).

The incorporation of exercise in weight-control programs increases the chance of success (as determined by weight loss or weight maintenance (Epstein and Goldfield, 1999) along with numerous additional benefits. Individuals can increase their energy expenditure, protect against the loss of fat-free mass, and improve cardiorespiratory fitness, muscular strength, endurance, and self-esteem through appropriate and regular physical activity. Other positive benefits of regular physical activity may include appetite control, an increased likelihood of maintenance of weight loss, desirable changes in body composition, and potential changes in fat cell development (Walberg and Ward, 1985). Physical activity also has the capacity to improve lipoprotein profiles and normalize carbohydrate metabolism (Bar-Or and Baranowski, 1994). An increase in energy expenditure through physical activity is critical in view of the sedentary lifestyles pursued by many individuals and the documented reduction in metabolic rate coincident with diets low in energy. A similar positive effect of exercise was also shown in subsequent studies (Maziekas et al., 2003).

Exercise in isolation, or combined with a reduction in energy intake, is recommended in the treatment of obesity, particularly in cases where an individual may benefit from improvements in energy efficiency (Blanchard, 1982). Increased energy efficiency is characterized by a normal energy intake; therefore, it may be dangerous to attempt to modify the diet further and thereby potentially compromise an individual's health status.

A more marked reduction in energy intake alone can cause the loss of lean tissue as well as fat (Dietz, 1991, 1993; Pařízková, 1963a, 1977). There is also the potential for basal metabolic rate (BMR) to reduce, as tissues are broken down to provide energy. The loss in protein may be derived from muscle tissue and/or skeletal tissue. There is some evidence to suggest that hypocaloric diets that contain a large proportion of carbohydrate might minimize the protein deficit. However, both the sensitivity of different tissues to carbohydrate intake and the degree of protein loss from all tissues are uncertain (Davie et al., 1982).

Exercise can contribute to the maintenance and potential increase in lean body mass while maintaining a decrement in fat mass. When diet alone is the focus of weight reduction, up to 25% of lean tissue may be lost (Stern, 1983). This loss may be reduced to approximately 5% by adding exercise (Brownell and Stunkard, 1980).

Longitudinal studies have showed that an adaptation to a higher level of activity during childhood can result in reduced deposition of fat (Moore et al., 2003), and also predispose the subject to more intense and a better regime of physical activity later in life due to an improved fitness level. A significant proportion of obese children may be at an increased risk of greater adiposity because of lower energy expenditure (Trost et al., 2003). Longitudinal observations by the Bogalusa Heart Study revealed that children who spent most time with television viewing had the greatest increase of fat over time (Proctor et al., 2003).

Interestingly, there have been relatively few intervention studies that have considered the benefits of strength training in obese children, which being predominantly static in nature, may be easier for subjects with excess fat. The best results for changes in BMI, body composition, physical fitness, behavioral improvement, and psychological status were gained in summer camps where both diet and physical activity are monitored (Pařízková, 1972, 1975, 1977, 1995, 1996a,b, 1998a,b,c). Treuth et al. (1998) assessed fitness and energy expenditure following a school-based, low-volume strength -training program. Obese prepubertal girls in this study demonstrated gains in strength but no significant increase in energy expenditure. The authors recognized that energy expenditure might be further enhanced with a more intensive strength-training program and/or in combination with aerobic training. In this study, more attention was given to the influence of the activity on energy expenditure, as measured by 24-hr calorimetry and doubly labeled water, although aerobic capacity was also assessed (Treuth et al., 1998).

Bar-Or (1995) has suggested that resistance training in children is safe as long as the necessary safety precautions are adhered to. It is important that an experienced adult supervise such training. Weight-bearing exercise, which is commonly difficult for subjects with excess weight and fat, has also been considered alongside resistance training. The benefits of weight-bearing activities during the formative years have been well established, but less attention has been paid to the effects of such activity for those who are overweight or obese. There are numerous ways in which innovative activities that combine resistance with loading can be used with great effect. Examples of the types of tasks that can be employed with children are outlined in Chapter 13.

Resistance training loads in lower extremities enhanced the muscle strength of flexors and extensors in normal-weight children, but may be insufficient to do so in overweight children (Falk et al., 2002). Other types of strength training along with diet had positive effects on TC, the LDL/ HDL ratio, and LBM, but no significant effect on BMI (Sung et al., 2002).

A range of studies have shown that exercise alone can reduce body weight, both in experimental animals and humans. Gradual reductions in weight are possible with modest modifications to activity patterns. It may be postulated that an early exercise intervention with growing individuals may produce a greater opportunity for the enhancement of weight reduction and, most important, an exposure to the necessary skills and practices required to enjoy and sustain a long-term commitment to physical activity (Hills, 1995). Motivation to move plays an essential role in the introduction of the increased physical activity and exercise regime for an obese child unaccustomed to greater workloads (Sothern et al., 1999b). Also, structured exercise using resistance training of various sorts can be applied in a multidisciplinary outpatient treatment program for obese children and youth (Sothern et al., 1999a).

Wilmore (1983) reviewed studies of exercise and obesity with physical activity as the sole focus and reported that loss of body weight was minimal

(Epstein, Koeske, and Wing, 1983). There is general agreement that while weight loss is low, there are usually increases in lean body mass along with reductions in body fat during growth. Although exercise may have a negligible impact on total energy expenditure when basal requirements account for a major proportion of energy utilization (Stock and Rothwell, 1982), there is a contribution to prolonged post-exercise metabolic rate that may influence weight loss.

A multiple regression model was used by Barbeau et al. (1999) to analyze the results of the effect of 4 months of exercise training (4 days per week, 40 min per session, heart rate 157 ± 7 beats per min, energy expenditure 946 ± 201 kJ per session). Body fat decreased, bone mineral density increased, and most important, the frequency of exercise and decrease in energy intake resulted in an increase in vigorous activity.

Increased physical activity can be augmented through an increase of common everyday activities such as walking and stair climbing. In adults (Blair et al., 1992), 30 to 40 min of activity such as walking, working in the yard, or doing housework can significantly reduce cardiovascular disease risks. Such modifications may be more effective than programmed exercise for long-term weight prognosis. Exercise programs should promote increased energy expenditure, the loss of body fat, and the maintenance of lean body mass, and also lead to permanent increases in habitual physical activity. Greater benefits in both weight loss and adherence have been reported in studies that have used behavioral approaches to weight management. The program Hip Hop to Health is an obesity prevention strategy for minority-group preschool children (Stolley et al., 2003).

As mentioned earlier, weight-control programs for children have traditionally been employed in a variety of settings with the involvement of a range of health professionals and other adults. Sole practitioners and various group approaches have included school personnel, such as physical and health educators, medical practitioners, exercise physiologists, nutritionists, dietitians, and parents. A team approach to weight management is generally superior to an ad hoc approach and is likely to help maximize the potential long-term success for the patient.

Physical activity and exercise is therefore considered to be an important component of a weight-reduction program, mainly in combination with a diet. However, in adulthood, the efficiency of physical activity alone as a means of significant weight reduction is doubted, as it is hardly realizable on a desirable level due to age and possible co-morbidities. This is of special concern especially considering the long-term effects of obesity (Westerterp, 1999). This also applies to excessively obese youth, who resemble older individuals rather than others of corresponding chronological age. Experience shows that even in the individuals who are very disciplined, resistance to fat loss generally occurs before their body composition is comparable to that of normal-weight individuals (Tremblay, Doucet, and Imbeault, 1999). However, even a small weight loss can reduce health risks resulting from obesity.

The evidence of the effect of exercise alone on obesity and its role in the prevention of excess fatness is still inconclusive. As mentioned previously (Chapters 4 to 6), some authors have not found a significant relationship between physical activity, energy expenditure, and overweight and obesity. In most cases, such studies of physical activity and energy expenditure were limited to a brief, short-term analysis rather than the more desirable longitudinal approach.

Other studies have provided evidence of the positive outcomes of increased physical activity and exercise, especially in the treatment of the obese (Epstein, 1995). This has been best illustrated by longitudinal studies lasting several years in the same growing individuals over longer periods of development (Kemper et al., 1990, 1999; Pařízková, 1972, 1977, 1998a,b,c).

As mentioned in Chapter 1, there are numerous methodological problems and constraints concerning the measurement of physical activity levels during growth and development (Saris, 1986). These problems may be magnified, for example, when methods more appropriate to older individuals are used for children and thus provide unreliable data. Therefore, the evaluation of the effect of physical activity and exercise has the potential to be biased. It was mentioned in Chapter 5 and 6 that the effects of physical activity and exercise, and significant adaptation to them, are related to the frequency, intensity, duration, and type of activity, which are all dependent on the individual characteristics of the subject. All these prerogatives are mostly described insufficiently, and exercise is understood as one simple issue, without proper specification. For example, psychological and emotional involvement and supervision by pedagogues also play a significant role. This may be able to explain inconsistency in results. In many cases, due to further confounding factors such as genetics or diet, the range of physical activity level in subjects with different adiposity is not sufficiently large to show a significant relationship.

The growing organism is in a unique situation with respect to physiological control. A restricted energy intake is not recommended due to the potential negative effects on the growth and maturation processes. In contrast, an increase in the level of activity is easier to achieve in most children compared with obese adults. This is particularly the case when there is no excess deposition of fat. In the case of severe or morbid obesity, the situation is more similar to that in older individuals. For such individuals, special restricted diets must be introduced along with a modified exercise program.

When defining an adequate physical activity and exercise regime for children, it is necessary to consider that spontaneous physical activity and the type of games preferred change during growth (Hills and Wahlqvist, 1994a,b; Hills, 1995). There are differences in children's play as a function of age, growth, and developmental stage. It is important to recognize the potential contribution of games and play to the maintenance of energy balance and a desirable body composition in young children. Three kinds of play physical activity with consecutive age peaks can be distinguished. The first, rhythmic stereotypes, peaks in infancy and is hypothesized to improve control of specific motor patterns. This is followed by exercise play, which peaks in the preschool years and is related primarily to strength and endurance. The evidence for possible benefits for fat reduction and thermoregulation is less clear. Finally, rough-and-tumble play is characteristic of the childhood years and peaks in middle childhood. This type of play has a distinctive social component and primarily serves dominance functions (Pellegrini and Smith, 1998). The latter two forms of play are more prevalent in males. The role of these types of children's activities in the maintenance of a desirable body composition warrants further analysis.

12.3.1 Relationships between Body Composition and Fitness during Growth

A parallel study of the development of aerobic fitness, blood pressure, and BMI (Shea et al., 1994) revealed significant interrelationships, indicating the possible implications for the development of interventions directed to the primary prevention of hypertension. A study was undertaken of free-living children aged 5 years at baseline who were followed over a mean of 19.7 months. Aerobic fitness was assessed during a treadmill test. Mean systolic blood pressure was 95.3 mmHg (SD $\pm$ 8.38) and increased by 4.46 mmHg per year. Mean diastolic pressure was 53.9 mmHg (SD $\pm$ 5.81) at baseline and did not change significantly. Children in the highest quintile of increase in aerobic fitness had a significantly smaller increase in systolic blood pressure when compared to children in the lowest quintile (2.92 vs. 5.10 mmHg.year^{-1}; p < 0.03). Children in the lowest quintile of increase in BMI did not significantly differ in the rate of increase in systolic blood pressure compared to children in the highest quintile (3.92 vs. 4.96 mmHg.year^{-1}). In a multiple regression model including baseline systolic blood pressure, aerobic fitness, height, BMI, and other co-variates, a greater increase in fitness (p < 0.01) and a lesser increase in BMI were associated with lower rates of increases in systolic blood pressure. In a similar multivariate analysis, an increase in fitness was also associated with a lower rate of increase in diastolic blood pressure (p < 0.02). These data indicate that the development of an increased level of aerobic fitness, along with reduced adiposity (which is usually the result of an increased level of physical activity and exercise), can contribute to a reduced deposition of fat, lower BMI, reduced risk of hypertension, and reduced metabolic health risks (Sudi, Gallistl, and Trobinger, 2001).

Trends in relation to the development of spontaneous physical activity and fatness, for example, during the preschool years, show a clear relationship in normal-weight children. The natural trend for changes in subcutaneous fat in children is as follows. When the level of spontaneous physical activity is high, there is the maintenance of the same amount of subcutaneous fat in girls and a slight decrease in boys (Pařízková et al., 1983, 1996), which precedes the adiposity rebound (Rolland-Cachera, 1995; Rolland-Cachera et al., 1984, 1988, 1990a,b). Longitudinal observations (8 years) of the development of body composition and aerobic power runs parallel in growing boys indicating the peak of natural physical fitness and lowest deposition of fat during puberty (Pařízková, 1963a,b, 1977).

12.3.2   The Effect of Regular Exercise during Growth

The significant effect of physical activity from an early age was shown in the Framingham Children's Study in which children aged 3 to 5 years were followed longitudinally together with their parents (Moore et al., 1995). Physical activity was monitored using an electronic motion sensor. On average, girls who had a higher than median activity level increased their triceps and subscapular skinfolds by 1.0 mm, while inactive girls gained 1.75 mm. Active boys lost an average of 0.75 mm in the triceps skinfold while inactive boys gained 0.25 mm. When age, television viewing, energy intake, baseline triceps, and parent BMI were adjusted for, inactive preschoolers were 3.8 times as likely as active preschoolers to have an increasing triceps slope during follow-up. As predicted, a lower level of physical activity already had a considerable effect on fatness.

A number of studies (Pařízková et al., 1985b; Pařízková, 1996a,b, 1998a,b,c) have demonstrated the significant effect of increased physical activity in preschool children. Children who were more spontaneously active had a lower BMI, smaller deposition of fat, higher cardiorespiratory fitness, and significantly increased serum level of HDL-C (Figure 12.7).

In a study of French children aged 10 years, Deheeger, Rolland-Cachera, and Fontvieille (1997) considered physical activity, body composition, and food intake. Validated activity questionnaires covering the previous year, nutritional intake (dietary history method), and anthropometric measurements (including triceps and subscapular skinfolds) were assessed. BMI, arm muscle, and arm fat areas were calculated from these measurements. Anthropometric measurements and dietary intake were recorded in the same children at the age of 10 months and every 2 years from the age of 2 years. At the age of 10 years, more active children had a significantly higher energy intake due mostly to a higher energy intake at breakfast and in the afternoon. Greater energy intake was mainly due to a higher ingestion of carbohydrates. The intake of fat was similar in both active and less active children, as was protein. In spite of the higher energy intake in the active group, BMI values were the same in both active and less active children, but body composition values were different (Figure 12.8). Active children had less fat and a higher ratio of lean, fat-free mass. Adiposity rebound (AR) occurred later in active children. Body fatness was positively related to the time spent watching television and playing video games. The higher level of physical activity resulted in an improved growth pattern and a more desirable body composition with less fat, in spite of a higher intake of energy.

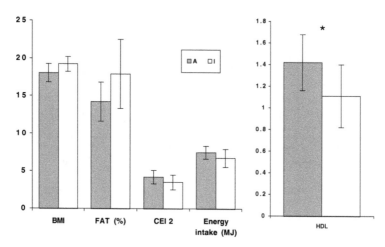

FIGURE 12.7
Body mass index (BMI), percentage of stored fat (% fat), cardiorespiratory efficiency (CEI 2), energy intake and serum HLD-C level (mmol/l) in active (A) and inactive (I) preschool children (CEI 2 = kpm/HRw – 10 × HRr; kpm = body weight × height of step × 150; HRwr = heart rate during 5 min mounting the 30-cm high step, and during 3-min recovery; HRr = heart rate at rest, 150 = 3 mounts/min × 5). * indicates ($p < 0.05$). (Based on data from Pařízková, 1996b.)

Previous longitudinal studies have followed the effect of increased exercise on the development of body composition in healthy adolescent boys aged 10.8 to 17.7 years with normal nutritional status. Subjects varied significantly with respect to the physical activity regime that was controlled and supervised. The most active group of boys was enrolled in regular sports training (track and field, basketball) for at least 6 hours per week. Training was supervised, and boys achieved a high level of exercise intensity across the whole school year. In contrast, the least active group participated in physical education at school (as did more active boys) and less than 2 hours of unorganized physical activity per week. Under such circumstances, both groups of boys developed an almost identical BMI, but in the active group, the absolute and relative amounts of lean body mass were significantly larger than in the least active boys. Consistent with this result, the relative and absolute amount of stored fat was also lower in the active boys (Figure 12.9). These differences were significant from the second and third year of the study. The most active boys also reported eating more than the least active boys (Pařízková, 1968a,b; 1970; 1977; 1982a,b).

In summary, the active group was significantly leaner and the least active group was considerably fatter. These results were confirmed over a longer period of development with sustained differences in the physical activity pursuits of the different groups. It must be stressed that the differences in the level and intensity of exercise undertaken were marked. Aerobic power was also highest in the boys who performed the greatest amount of exercise. This value did not decrease after puberty as in the least active boys. These

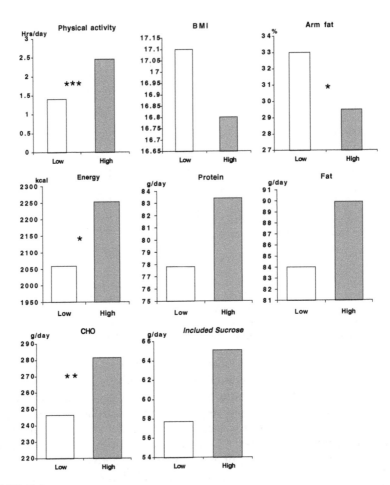

FIGURE 12.8
Differences in physical activity, anthropometric characteristics (BMI, arm fat), and intake of energy and macronutrients in 10-year-old boys with low and high physical activity level (hours per day). * indicates ($p < 0.05$); ** ($p < 0.01$), *** ($p < 0.001$). (Based on data from Deheeger et al., 1997.)

results are evidence that the level of physical fitness of the less active children has already peaked and begun to decline in adolescence (Pařízková, 1963a; 1970; 1977; 1982a,b; 1985; Pařízková and Carter, 1976). No comparable data are available for similar long-lasting (8 years) studies involving the same adolescents with such different physical activity interventions during which body composition (using hydrodensitometry), VO$_2$ during a maximal workload on a treadmill and physical performance were tracked etc. (Pařízková, 1977, 1998b; Šprynarová, 1984).

Numerous other studies have demonstrated the significant effect of organized, supervised, and sufficiently intensive exercise under the guidance of physical educators or trainers on body composition in normal-weight adolescents. Such changes are commonly paralleled by adjustments in aerobic

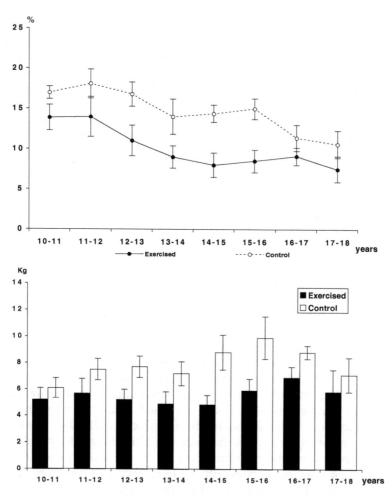

FIGURE 12.9
A longitudinal study of the development of stored fat: top (percentage); bottom (densitometry) in regularly exercised and control inactive boys. The differences between groups are significant from the 2nd until the 8th years. (Based on data from Pařízková 1961a, 1963a, 1968b, 1970, 1976, 1997.)

power and functional capacity (Owens, 1998). In motivated self-monitoring children and adolescents, sufficient activity may be achieved without any external support. However, during growth, this type of self-imposed discipline is rare and some assistance is preferable. For most children and adolescents, continued participation would be sustained only under proper professional supervision of physical educators and/or exercise physiologists. More research is needed to optimize the exercise prescription in children specific to the enhancement of improvements in body composition and functional capacity. Guidelines for exercise prescription along with suitable activities are provided in the following chapter.

12.3.3 The Effect of Sports Participation

Studies of young athletes show that energy balance is maintained under conditions of higher energy output, for example in gymnasts, hockey players, skiers, sprinters, divers, and runners (Pařízková and Heller, 1991). Energy intake was consistently higher than the RDAs for normal youth of the same age with the exception of female gymnasts and sprinters. Protein intake in athletes was usually markedly higher. However, BMI was average (that is, around the 50th percentile), and there was a significant reduction of stored fat in the young athletes when compared to untrained individuals. Lean body mass in relative and absolute values was greater than in inactive peers of the same age. With respect to fatness and aerobic power, the best results were found in young athletes adapted to weight-bearing activities in dynamic (track and field, and running) and endurance sport disciplines. These youngsters were members of sport schools, but not junior champion athletes.

A study of energy balance using heart-rate monitors to register heart rate during the training day was conducted on male gymnasts who had a higher level of general fitness, including aerobic power. The experimental period lasted 1 week during a sport training camp in the mountains where the exercise intensity was even higher than during a normal school year and was supplemented by other activities such as hiking. Energy expenditure (EE) was derived using regression equations established for each individual on the basis of the relationship between heart rate and oxygen uptake during treadmill testing. Simultaneously, energy intake (EI) was measured using food diaries supplemented by interviews, and a computer program was developed to provide detailed analyses of local foodstuffs. BMI was comparable to normal-weight boys of the same age. The energy balance during 1 week showed correspondingly increased values for both EI and EE. When EE is low, such a balance is more difficult to achieve, and commonly EI does not correspond to EE (Pařízková and Heller, 1991).

This study illustrates that energy balance can be achieved without negative changes in body composition and BMI, even with a higher energy intake compared to RDA. Despite an ability to balance energy values and an abundance of dietary intake, deficiencies in micronutrients and imbalances in macronutrients were found.

Energy balance studies using the DLW technique have shown that the RDAs for young athletes may be too high for normally active children and adolescents living in affluent societies (Thompson, 1998). Commonly, the process of adaptation to an increased workload includes an increase in metabolic efficiency. Some measurements in adults have shown that energy intake does not always increase correspondingly to energy output without any negative consequences with respect to BMI, body composition, and level of performance. It is unusual for athletes in intensive training to have an inadequately high intake of energy. A higher intake of energy in an active, well-adapted athlete can be problematic if the intensity of training fluctuates.

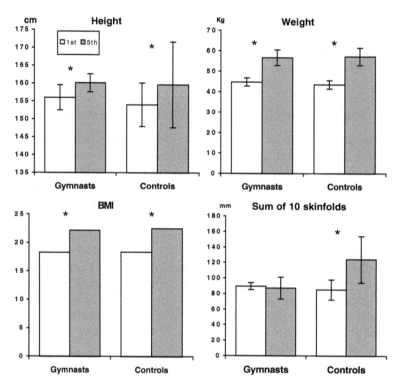

FIGURE 12.10

Differences in developmental height, weight, BMI, and sum of 10 skinfolds at the beginning and after 5 years of a longitudinal study in gymnasts with regular training and in control girls without training. Only sum of 10 skinfolds after 5 years is significantly higher in control girls without training compared to gymnasts. * indicates ($p < 0.05$). (Based on data from Pařízková, 1977.)

A 5-year longitudinal study has shown the same increase in height, weight, and BMI in female gymnasts and a control group of untrained girls. The latter group showed a significant increase in the sum of 10 skinfolds. In the trained girls (Figure 12.10), the weight increment consisted of additional lean, fat-free body mass (Pařízková, 1963b, 1968, 1977, 1986).

Other observations in young female athletes aged 11 to 15 years (Lopez-Benedicto et al., 1988) have revealed a decreased body fat, lower levels of serum free fatty acids (FFA), and higher levels of HDL-C and Apo A1. Female gymnasts are characterized by an especially low percentage of body fat. The most significant correlations were found between body composition and Apo A1, and Apo A1/Apo B in swimmers and control girls in whom the range of body fatness was much larger than in gymnasts. These examples show a beneficial effect of exercise, provided it is regular and sufficiently intensive. As yet, there has been no clear indication of whether exercise training increases fat utilization in obese adult subjects at rest, during exercise, or across a 24-hr period. With regard to this problem under conditions of developed obesity, further studies are needed (Hoppeler, 1999). Aerobic training induced an increase in the response of plasma and subcutaneous adipose tissue concentrations of glycerol to β-adrenergic stimulation in adult obese subjects, in spite of the lack of changes in body weight and aerobic power (Štich et al., 1999).

12.3.4 Studies of the Effect of Exercise on Experimental Animal Models

The classic study of Mayer et al. (1954) showed that rats that exercised daily for up to 1 hr decreased food intake and body weight when compared to sedentary control rats. When the exercise duration increased beyond 1 hr, food intake was increased but only to the extent that body weight was maintained. At exhaustive levels of exercise (6 hr), both food intake and body weight decreased. Longitudinal physical conditioning studies in humans also show no change in caloric intake with mild to moderate intensity exercise training (Chin et al., 1992). Evidence from a study of rats running voluntarily in rotation wheels showed an increase to 130% of energy intake as compared to sedentary rats. In contrast, when considered on a short-term basis, exercise suppressed food intake to prevent a potentially dangerous disruption of energy substrate homeostasis. Both exercise and food intake increased FFA and glucose in the blood of the laboratory animals. These changes, combined with the exercise-induced alteration in glucagon, corticotropin-releasing hormone (CRH), and body temperature, may contribute to the short-term anorexic effect of exercise (Scheuring et al., 1999).

As shown in another experimental model, the effect of the adaptation to exercise (that is, increased energy output) was a decreased ratio of % depot fat and a different metabolic activity of the adipose tissue. The release of FFA *in vitro*, both spontaneously or after various doses of adrenaline added to the medium, was significantly higher from the adipose tissue of the animals adapted to daily exercise since weaning (daily running on a treadmill) (Figure 12.11). This was compared to control and/or hypokinetic animals (restricted to small cages). The intake of food was always highest in the exercised animals. The effect of exercise is relatively smaller, but reduced activity is relatively greater in growing animals. The reverse situation is apparent in adult or older animals, that is, a relatively greater effect of exercise and smaller or no effect of hypokinesia (Pařízková, 1968a, 1977). The restriction of activity has a more significant effect on metabolic activity of the adipose tissue in a developing organism during growth resulting in an increased deposition (Pařízková, 1977). This results from the natural trends in physical activity during ontogeny. During growth, spontaneous activity is generally high and decreases with aging. Therefore, hypokinesia has a more marked effect during growth (Pařízková, 1968b).

The activity of lipoprotein lipase (LPL) was significantly higher in the heart and skeletal muscle of exercised animals. The inflow rate of applied FFA labeled with ^{14}C was spontaneously greater to the heart and skeletal muscle of the exercised animals but lower to their adipose tissue (Figure 12.12). In

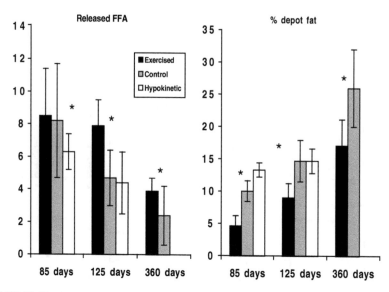

FIGURE 12.11

The comparison of released free fatty acids *in vitro* (incubation 60 min; FFA meq/1 ml medium/ 1/g adipose tissue) from the epididymal adipose tissue of exercised (daily run on a treadmill 2 h), control, and hypokinetic male rats (kept in small spaces 12 × 8 × 20 cm since weaning) aged 85, 125, and 360 days. * indicates ($p < 0.05$). (Based on data from Pařízková, 1977.)

the animals adapted to hypokinesia the situation was the reverse; that is, the highest inflow rate of labeled FFA was to the adipose tissue. Under the same conditions, the expired $^{14}CO_2$ by the animals adapted to regular dynamic exercise was significantly greater (even under conditions of anesthesia and complete physical rest) compared to control, inactive rats, or to hypokinetic animals adapted to the restriction of activity. These data indicate a greater ability to utilize lipid metabolites, which results in a lower deposition of fat. The adaptation to regular exercise changes not only body composition and the ratio of stored fat, but has more profound consequences with respect to the metabolic activity of tissues, especially the adipose and muscle tissues of experimental animals (Pařízková, 1968a,b; 1977; 1978b). The results of some studies executed in trained and untrained adults are in agreement with the conclusions from this experimental model.

12.3.5 The Effect of an Interruption to Regular Exercise on Body Adiposity

The effect of exercise and sports training on the fluctuation of fat percentage with a change in the intensity of physical activity and training has been studied. A more detailed 5-year longitudinal follow-up of the female gymnasts mentioned earlier (Figure 12.13) revealed the following results. Girls were measured several times during the year (at the beginning of the school

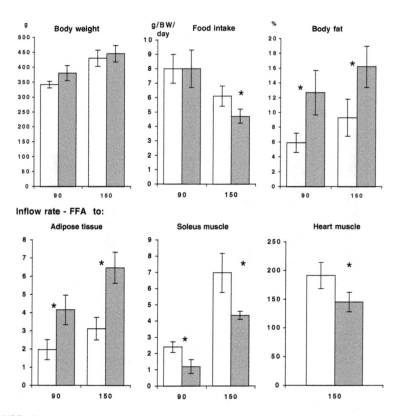

FIGURE 12.12
Comparison of body weight, food intake, percentage of body fat (%), and inflow rate of applied
labeled fatty acids (14C; mmol.g^{-1}.min^{-1}) to adipose tissue, the soleus muscle, and the heart in
exercised (clear) and control, inactive (shaded) male rats aged 90 and 150 days. * indicates (p
< 0.05). (Based on data from Pařízková, 1977.)

year when the usual level of intensity of gymnastics was maintained, then
before a summer camp in which training intensity was increased). The
changes in body fat in response to a change in intensity of activity were
rapid (Figure 12.13). Energy intake was also significantly higher during the
period of intensive training when fat decreased, then declined significantly
during the period of inactivity when fat increased (Pařízková, 1977; Pařízková
and Poupa, 1963). The reduction in training intensity and energy expenditure
was sufficient for an increased deposition of fat, in spite of a reduced energy
intake. Girls in this study were not elite athletes but pupils of a sport school.
Similar changes are even more apparent in some former athletes of any age
who stop their exercise training (Pařízková, 1982a,b, 1985, 1986).

Corresponding changes are also seen following injury. A failure to maintain the usual level of sports training may result in an enhanced deposition
of fat. When such a situation lasts for an extended period of time, the
development of obesity is a risk. For example, a longitudinal follow-up of
an adolescent football player who interrupted training because of a shoulder

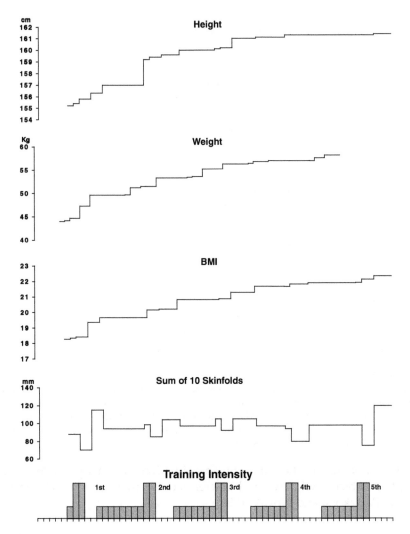

FIGURE 12.13
Development of height, weight, BMI, and sum of 10 skinfolds in female gymnasts assessed longitudinally over 5 years fluctuating training intensity. (Based on data from Pařízková, 1977.)

injury showed the development of obesity, a deterioration of aerobic fitness, and dyslipoproteinemia (Kaplan, 1992).

An excess deposition of fat may occur in individuals who have adapted to an increased aerobic workload, had a permanently high-energy output, and then decreased their activity level suddenly (Figure 12.14). An increase in body weight, BMI, and adipose tissue may result even when food intake decreases simultaneously. The data of Jeszka, Regula, and Kostrzewa-Tarnowska (1999) has shown that young ballet dancers have lower proportions of fat and a high negative energy balance. Food intake based on 24-hr recall data was lower than energy output (24-hr monitoring of heart rate) compared to

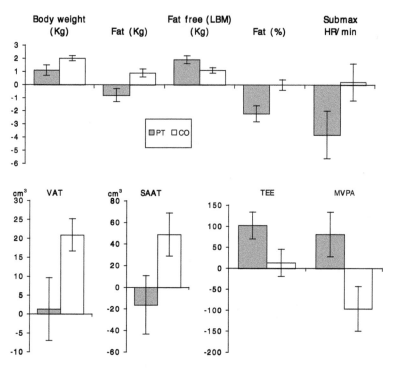

FIGURE 12.14

Effect of 4 months of physical training (PT) in obese children compared to control subjects (CO); changes in body weight, body composition, heart rate during submaximal work load (submax HR.min⁻¹), visceral adipose tissue (VAT), subcutaneous abdominal adipose tissue (SAAT), total energy expenditure (TEE), and moderate to vigorous physical activity (MVPA) over 4 months. (Based on data from Gutin et al., 1995, 1997, 1998.)

control schoolgirls of the same age. This situation was only possible in well-adapted subjects who were characterized by increased metabolic efficiency (Pařízková and Novák, 1991).

12.3.6   The Effect of Exercise in Obese Children and Youth

The classical observations of Mayer (1974) showed that when lean and obese children claimed the same physical activity and exercise (as reported by questionnaire data) over the same time period, filming them showed much less real motor activity and movement in the obese. Even when exact measurements of the energy expenditure were conducted using the DLW technique, only information on the total amount of energy output per day, but not about the fluctuating intensity of workload and its peaks during various periods of the day, could be determined.

A certain level of intensity that achieves well-defined threshold intensity for a sufficient duration and frequency during micro- and macrocycles can produce changes in body composition and aerobic power, or improvement of some motor skills and physical performance level, and thus improve so-called metabolic fitness. These principles also apply to obese children. Stimuli that do not meet or exceed the necessary threshold values cannot cause significant physiological change. There appears to be contradictory conclusions on the effect of physical activity and exercise with respect to fatness and fitness, with some studies confirming a positive effect while others do not; a possible reason for such was given earlier in the section titled "Exercise Management."

Many obese individuals of all ages may be active but generally for very short periods of time and at an intensity that is too low. This level of effort does not increase the pulse rate above certain critical levels (which vary for different age groups). Importantly, such lower level activity does not significantly increase the intensity of workload and energy output of the organism over a certain period of time, which is a necessary stimulus for the development of the systems involved in the improvement of functional capacity and physical fitness. When the fitness level of an individual is not improved, exercise remains a difficult and unpleasant task for the obese child, and the level of spontaneous physical activity and willingness to exercise remains low. As a consequence, any loss of fat mass may be minimal or nonexistent.

The challenge in weight-management programs is to encourage an increase in energy output in individuals whose previous experience of physical activity may not have been pleasant. Therefore, it is critical that particular care be taken to plan and implement an appropriate physical activity and exercise regime (Hills and Wahlqvist, 1994). The prescription issue is considered in some detail in the following chapter. It is important to remember that much of the increased energy output in overweight subjects is due to the higher energy costs of weight-bearing activities, as a function of the higher load caused by excess body fat. This might modify the balance between EE and EI and prevent excess deposition of fat, provided that this increased strain does not reduce spontaneous PA. The level of motor activity of an obese child during an average day is usually much lower than in normal-weight peers with a failure to achieve the necessary level of exercise in spite of an increased daily energy expenditure (Pařízková, 1982a,b).

Specificity in terms of the nature and intensity of exercise and training is essential for weight management. A 5-month longitudinal study on the effect of a strength-training program on obese prepubertal girls showed a significant increase in muscular strength and VO_2 peak values ml.min^{-1} (based on a treadmill test). However, this was not true when VO_2 was a covariate for total and/or fat-free body mass. The same applied to resting metabolic rate (REE) measured by room respiration calorimetry. There were no changes in total energy expenditure (TEE), activity-related energy expenditure (AEE), and physical activity level (PAL), either unadjusted or adjusted for total and/or fat-free body mass. This long-term, school-based strength-training program favorably influenced muscle strength but did not increase the daily energy expenditure in obese girls (Treuth et al., 1998). These observations provide further justification for well-designed exercise programs aimed at improving body composition through a reduction in excess fat.

The effect of physical education on fourth- and fifth-grade elementary school students has been studied by Sallis et al. (1993). Project SPARK compared the results of three different offerings of physical education: (1) usual physical education classes, (2) classes using classroom teachers, and/or (3) with physical education specialists. There were no significant group differences in triceps and calf skinfolds and/or in the sum of these skinfolds. However, there was a trend for higher skinfolds in group 1. After intervention at 2 years, there was a tendency for lower levels of fat in groups 2 and 3, but the differences were not significant (Sallis et al., 1993). The intensity of exercise may not have been sufficiently different among groups.

A study of energy expenditure in preadolescent children over 4 years showed that the main determinants of change in fat mass adjusted for fat-free mass were gender (greater gain for girls), initial fatness, and parental fatness. None of the components of energy expenditure (total and physical activity related energy expenditure measured by DLW) were inversely related to changes in fat mass. That is, reduced energy expenditure was not the cause of the increased stored fat (Goran et al., 1998).

There is widespread consensus that interventions to manage obesity should be implemented as early as possible. This approach has been employed in a number of studies in preschool children in various countries. As mentioned previously, the effect of a higher level of spontaneous physical activity is apparent in preschool-age children. HDL-C serum level was significantly higher in active preschoolers compared to their inactive peers, along with a trend for a lower BMI, a lower percentage of fat, and greater cardiorespiratory efficiency as assessed by a modified step-test. Percent of body fat correlated significantly with TC and TG levels. Active preschoolers also showed a trend for a higher energy intake (Pařízková, 1996a; Pařízková et al., 1986).

In Thailand, the effect of a school-based exercise program was tested in children in the kindergarten system (daycare centers). Exercise consisted of a 15-min walk prior to morning classes and a 20-min aerobic dance session following the afternoon nap, 3 times per week, over 26 weeks. The prevalence of obesity at the end of the study decreased in both groups who exercised (from 12.2 at baseline to 8.8% of cutoff values for triceps based on National Center for Health Statistics guidelines) and control groups (from 11.7 to 9.7%). Differences between groups were not significant. Girls in the exercise group had a reduced likelihood of an increasing BMI slope than the control girls. The study concluded that exercise can prevent BMI increases in girls and prevent obesity in preschoolers (Mo-suwan et al., 1998).

From a physiological perspective, the greater strain of participation in physical activity by the obese results in an increase in heart rate. A lower ventilatory threshold in the obese causes higher energy demands for the same activity compared to lean children. Further, this feature also contributes to obese individuals displaying more fatigue, greater stress, and heart rate increases during the same running workload. Each of these factors may contribute to a reduction in spontaneous physical activity and a preference for quieter and more sedentary activities for the majority of time (Maffeis et al., 1997, 1998). This creates a vicious cycle and the chance of further decreases in activity levels that are already low.

Despite some pessimism with respect to the effect of exercise in the treatment of obese children, the role of physical activity and exercise has been stressed in many contexts as a suitable component in the management and treatment of the condition during childhood (Abrosimova et al., 1984; Rippe and Hess, 1998). Data on dietary intake and activity regimes in children and adolescents (Bordi et al., 1995; Dietz and Gortmaker, 1993; Dietz et al., 1991, 1993, 1998a,c) have shown that the main lifestyle change in industrially developed countries has been a lower level of activity in all age categories commencing with young children. There is widespread acceptance of the link between activity and health as purported in the statement "America needs to exercise for health" (Booth and Tseng, 1995).

In obese Chinese children, the exercise prescription deemed suitable to reduce weight and fatness has been defined according to the level of aerobic power development in local children. This equates with 50% of VO_2 max, 1 hr per day for 12 weeks with a frequency of 5 days per week. The exercise should be rhythmical and aerobic such as running and various endurance game-type activities, for example, football (Ding, 1992).

Gutin (1998) has also demonstrated the effect of exercise as a function of alternating periods of training and detraining. After the initial 4 months of training, percent of body fat decreased but increased after another 4 months of interruption to training. In the reverse situation, the group with no training during the initial 4 months maintained and/or slightly increased percent of fat, but decreased after another 4 months of training. The Amsterdam Growth and Health Longitudinal Study (AGAHLS) showed a significant inverse relationship between the development of fat mass and the level of physical activity corrected for dietary intake. Therefore, the level of fat mass provided was predictive of activity status. As is the case in childhood, the promotion of physical activity in adolescence appears to play a significant and effective role in the early prevention of obesity (Kemper et al., 1999). Some dependence of child eating and obesity on genetic factors and the environment was shown in Project Grow-2-Gether (Faith et al., 2002).

The effect of reinforcement on the behavior of obese children should not be underestimated. Following an individual choice between sedentary activities or movement-based physical activities, obese subjects were either positively reinforced for decreases in high-preference sedentary activity or were punished for high-preference sedentary activity, had access to high-preference sedentary activity restricted, or had no contingencies on activity (control group). Preference for sedentary activity decreased in the reinforced group, but increased in the restriction and/or control group.

12.3.6.1   Changes in Body Composition and Fitness after Exercise Intervention

Other studies have supported the significant effect of exercise on body composition in physically active children (Hills, 1991; Hills and Byrne, 1998a; Gutin et al., 1995). Black obese girls aged 7 to 11 years were subdivided according to physical activity and exercise regimes. Body composition, measured by DXA, skinfold thickness, and circumference measurements, and the level of physical performance (evaluated during submaximal treadmill testing) showed a significant improvement. An increase in aerobic fitness and a 1.4% decrease of stored fat was reported after a period of an organized aerobic training lasting 10 weeks with 5 sessions per week. The results were compared with a group that was engaged in weekly lifestyle discussion without formal physical training. The status of the latter group with respect to most fitness and body composition parameters measured remained unchanged (Gutin et al., 1995). This study demonstrated that it is possible to manage fat deposition and physical fitness through an organized and controlled physical training in terms of intensity and frequency, even without a diet intervention. It was also shown that the increase in visceral adipose tissue (VAT) was significantly less in the physical training group as compared to the control group (Owens et al., 1999).

Another study showed that exercise results in a considerable weight loss with a normocaloric diet. Weight-management treatment was provided to a group of Cuban children who used a diet with the energy content corresponding to the expected body weight for height. Growth and puberty occurred normally under these conditions of obesity management, and lean body weight and muscle area of the mid-upper arm increased. A substantial loss of fat, as indicated by a reduction of fat weight, relative fatness, and fat areas of the mid-upper arm, was also achieved. Body weight for height shifted to lower percentile channels. These results underline the favorable effect of this approach of obesity treatment that does not alter the normal course of development in obese children during the most rapid period of growth (Amador, Flores, and Pena, 1990). The potential bonus at this time is to profit from the reverse of the commonly observed decrease in fatness during this period of development (e.g., Pařízková, 1963a, 1977). This preadolescent period is one of the most preferable growth periods for obesity treatment because the interest in spontaneous physical activity is still high and a decrease in lean body mass that often occurs when reduction therapy is applied later is absent (Pařízková, 1977, 1998b).

Body composition also changed significantly in a group of obese children provided with physical training over a 4-month period compared with a control group with no training (Figure 12.15). A marked decrease in total and visceral adipose tissue was apparent after physical training (Owens et al., 1998). The results of this and other studies using organized and sufficiently intensive exercise reveal the positive effect of an increased energy output in obese and also normal-weight children. The decrease in heart rate was most pronounced in subjects with the greatest weight loss. Maximal

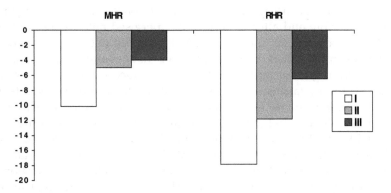

FIGURE 12.15
Effect of weight loss in obese children on the decrease of maximal (MHR) and recovery heart
rate (RHR); (I) the change in children with greatest, (II) medium, and (III) least weight loss.
(Based on data from Gutin et al., 1997.)

and recovery heart rate also decreased following weight loss in obese children (Owens et al., 1998).

Four months training has been found to increase bone density more than
during the subsequent 4 months without training. There were no differences
in dietary intake during these periods (Gutin et al., 1999a). The same period of
training (i.e., 4 months) did not result in significant changes in hemostatic
factors (fibrinogen, plasminogen activator inhibitor 1, and D-Dimer). Children
with greater adiposity and concentration of hemostatic factors before the period
of physical training showed greater reduction in hemostatic variables after
physical training than did children with lesser values (Ferguson et al., 1999b).

The physical activity regime provided for obese children needs to be well
planned and implemented in order to achieve maximum benefits regarding
loss of fat mass and potential readjustment of BMI and functional capacity.
The effect of an increase in exercise and a decrease in sedentary behaviors
was followed in children aged 8 to 12 years (Epstein et al., 1995b). After 4
months, significant differences in the reduction of the percentage of overweight were observed between the sedentary and the exercise groups. After
1 year the sedentary group had a greater decrease in percentage of overweight
than the combined and the exercise groups and a greater decrease in percent
of body fat. All groups increased their fitness level. Children in the sedentary
group increased their tolerance of high-intensity activity and reported lower
food intake than did children in the exercise group. These results confirm that
the reduction of time spent in sedentary activities without greater energy output can considerably increase weight loss during growth.

12.3.6.2   *Hormonal, Circulatory and Metabolic Changes after Exercise-Induced Weight and Fat Reduction*

Participation in a light training program can improve the situation of obese
children with respect to glucose homeostasis, insulin dynamics, and risk

factors for coronary artery disease. A study of obese adolescents aged 13.3 ± 1.4 years before and after 15 weeks of supervised mild intensity exercise found that body weight, fatness, and VO_2 peak did not change when compared to the initial values. However, relative changes after training appeared in mean serum glucose and peptides, fasting glucose (–15%), total glucose response (–15%), peak insulin response (–51%), total insulin response (–46%), peak C-peptide response (–55%), and total C-peptide response (+53%). Systolic and diastolic blood pressure was also reduced as well as the serum level of LDL-C. Increases in hepatic insulin clearance (decreased insulin levels along with C-peptide levels) might also be the result of the adaptation to an increased training load. While the intensity was low, the duration was sufficient to provide an improvement. These results confirm that in obese children, health risks may be reduced by exercise even without more marked weight and fat loss (Kahle et al., 1996).

The failure to achieve weight loss might not be a sign of weakness in the management program but the result of changes in body composition. There was a simultaneous increase in lean body mass at the expense of fat. This result highlights the importance of testing other parameters, at least for the encouragement of the obese individuals. This finding also supports the rationale for weight stabilization in many children. If this is achieved with exercise and increased EE, improvements are enhanced, with the probable outcome being a significant improvement as the individual grows into his or her final height. Also, leptin concentration was found to have decreased during 4 months of physical training and increased again after 4 months without training. Fat mass was highly correlated with baseline leptin and greater reductions in leptin during the 4 months of training were seen in children with higher pretraining leptin levels, and in those whose total mass increased least (Gutin et al., 1999a).

As a safe, feasible, and efficient form of exercise, a resistance and strength training program (which included also diet and behavior intervention) for 7- to 12-year-old obese children was tested. Weight, percent of ideal body weight, and BMI were reduced significantly after 10 weeks, and did not increase at the 1-year follow-up; this was similar to the other group treated with diet, walking, and behavioral intervention. Fat-free mass did not reduce in the resistance training group, which suggests that the addition of specific exercises may improve the results of treatment, especially in severely obese subjects (Sothern et al., 2000b).

A 2-week training program for obese children in a specialized institute and 6 weeks at home resulted in weight reduction and improved exercise lipid use, indicating an increase in their ability to oxidize lipids during exercise. This increase was no longer found in those who were treated by diet alone (Brandou et al., 2003). This has been previously shown in experimental animals (Pařízková, 1977) and was also indicated in obese subjects.

12.3.6.3   The Effect of Exercise on Cardiocirculatory Parameters

Participation in an exercise-training program across a period of 1 year resulted in a significant decrease in body weight, degree of obesity, and resting heart rate in obese children. Left ventricular wall thickness did not change. The total voltage in SV1 + RV5 decreased after 3 months of training but returned to pretraining voltage after 1 year of training. There was no change after 2 years of training. In summary, these results indicate that after 1 year of exercise training, resting heart rate decreased while left ventricular end-diastolic dimension and left ventricular mass increased (Hayashi et al., 1987).

The effect of a 4-month physical training on left ventricular (LV) structure and function along with body composition and hemodynamic changes was followed in obese children. Echocardiography and DXA was utilized; at baseline, elevated LV mass was associated with excess general and visceral adiposity, and elevated cardiac output. Although physical activity significantly reduced total and visceral fat, no significant changes in LV or hemodynamics were found (Humphries et al., 2002).

The beat-to-beat variability in electrocardiogram intervals (heart-period variability) is a marker of cardiac autonomic activity that can predict arrythmias and mortality rate in animals and adults. This parameter was followed in obese children before and after a period of sports training over a 4-month period (5 days per week, 40 min per day) during which weight reduction occurred (Gutin et al., 1997). Cardiovascular fitness was assessed using submaximal heart rate during supine cycling. Resting heart-period variability was measured in the same position, and body composition was evaluated by DXA. A pretraining to post-training change score was computed for each variable. A lower submaximal heart rate and percent of body fat were found in the group who reduced weight and fat due to training compared to the group of obese children without training during the same period. All changes in the trained group indicate that physical training alters cardiac autonomic function favorably by reducing the ratio of sympathetic to parasympathetic activities.

In another study group of children treated by exercise, in addition to reductions in body weight and fat, multiple risks of coronary heart disease were lowered. This was not apparent in obese children treated only by diet and behavioral therapy (Becque et al., 1988).

The effect of a regimented training program was followed in obese boys aged 10 to 11 years over 4 weeks with 5 one-hour sessions of 45 min cycling per week at 50 to 60% of a predetermined maximal oxygen capacity (VO_2 max) (Blaak et al., 1992). The aim of the study was to determine whether there would be an increase in the level of spontaneous physical activity of the obese subjects. No significant change in body weight, percentage of fat, sleeping metabolic rate, spontaneous activity (assessed by heart rate recording), and activity questionnaires was observed after 4 weeks. There was a

12% increase in average daily metabolic rate as measured by DLW, half of which can be explained by the energy cost of training and the rest by an increase in energy expenditure outside the training hour. These results indicate that training leads to a considerable augmentation in the overall energy expenditure in obese children without a change in their level of spontaneous physical activity.

As indicated in an earlier section, many studies of obese children using hypocaloric diets have reported decreases in serum lipids along with weight and fat loss. A minimal decrease of fat-free, lean body mass is also often reported. Following the restriction of food intake, HDL-C commonly does not change or decrease, as is the case for TC, LDL-C, and TG. These results were not found after a long-term supervised aerobic exercise program with obese children aged 11 years. The activity program was undertaken over 1 year during daily school life. The intensity of training consisted of running 20 min, 7 times per week, at a pace that corresponded to the blood lactate threshold. No dietary intervention was used in this study. After 1 year, the obesity index had decreased significantly. Weight loss was due only to stored fat reduction as confirmed by the simultaneous increase of lean, fat-free body mass. One of the most important results was a significant increase of HDL-C serum level in both boys and girls after the first year, an increase of 16% and 19%, respectively, with a slightly lower value in the second year. After 2 years, a significant decrease of TG was still found in obese girls. Serum TC was unchanged in both genders after 2 years. This study provides a clear indication of the benefits of a long-term supervised aerobic exercise program in obese children with respect to weight loss, positive body composition changes, and concomitant improvement of lipoprotein metabolism (Sasaki et al., 1987).

Secular changes were shown in blood pressure during childhood from 1948 to 1998; however, these positive changes, i.e., its reduction in 5- to 34-year-olds of both sexes and from a range of ethnic groups in high-income countries, may be plateauing with regard to an increased prevalence of, for example, childhood obesity (McCarron, Smith, and Okasha, 2002). Central adiposity and vascular dysfunction was favorably influenced by circuit training along with fitness level and muscular strength in a recent study (Watts et al., 2004).

12.4   The Results of Combined Treatment by Diet and Exercise

During recent years a multicomponent program using diet, exercise, and behavioral intervention has been proved as mostly efficient and long-lasting. The combined approach of a comprehensive behavioral lifestyle program including increased exercise, a protein-sparing modified fast, and a balanced hypocaloric diet has been suggested by numerous authors over many years

(Bar-Or, Dietz, Epstein, Pařízková, etc.). This multidisciplinary approach is normally most effective in weight reduction of youth (Sothern et al., 1993). The physician and the physical education specialist are essential in the treatment of obesity (Ward and Bar-Or, 1986). In order to achieve a long-standing control of overweight, a combination of the changes in eating and activity patterns using behavior modification techniques is recommended (Bar-Or et al., 1998). A combined focus is also best for preventing obesity in the earlier age groups. Another structured multidisciplinary program of exercise and diet was shown to decrease body weight and BMI and improve physical fitness (Eliakim et al., 2002).

The combination of an increased energy output and reduced energy intake has been repeatedly recommended as the best means of obesity management during growth and development (e.g., Dietz, 1993; Epstein, 1983, 1995, 1996; Korsten-Reck et al., 1990, 1998; Peja and Velkey, 1988; Ulanova et al., 1985; Ylitalo, 1982; Hills and Byrne, 2000; Hills and Parker, 1988). In adults, the same approach may be difficult to implement, particularly in the presence of co-morbidities. The implementation of a well-planned exercise and physical activity program can provide a significant benefit in relation to weight loss, and improvement in fitness, motor skill, and posture. This approach has been used to great effect in many countries (Pǎrízková 1972, 1982a, 1989; Pařízková et al., 1995, 2003).

In a study of Japanese children, more than 70% of boys and 40% of girls grew out of obesity if they could self-monitor their lifestyle with a simple checklist on a permanent basis. Instructions included that meals should be eaten 3 times per day on a regular basis with 1 snack per day. Children were advised to avoid extra dishes, juices, oily and greasy food additives, sugar, and candies. and they were told to consume in excess of 200 ml of milk per day. The energy density of the diet was not prescribed. Children were also instructed to play no more than 1 hour of video games alone at home per day. Each child (or family) was instructed to keep a checklist to evaluate (yes or no) if they could observe the 7 items (3 meals and 1 snack a day, no night eating, video games, and housework duty) on a daily basis. The subjects visited the outpatient clinic at 3-month intervals for anthropometric measurements and reported on their checklist scores. Advice and instruction was provided for the family at each visit. The mean duration of the treatment was 526 days, with children being an average age of 8.95 years. This serves as a model for a combined mode of treatment and management commonly used within a pediatric department without special facilities (Asayama et al., 1998b). Personal involvement plays an essential role in the outcomes of this process.

With regard to physiological acceptability during the period of growth and development, this combined method of treatment needs to be promoted. The decrease of weight, BMI, excess fat, and serum lipids, and the increase of aerobic power, physical fitness, and most often, HDL-C, were revealed after this treatment in obese children and adolescents. In another study of obese German children, physical training improved long-term weight control. In conjunction with such a program, it is important to assess the psychosocial background as a clue to lack of motivation in some children (L'Allemand, Mundt, and Gruters, 1998).

A nonrestrictive approach to diet is tolerated by many as it may establish more favorable conditions for the changes in lifestyle necessary for permanent improvement of the morphological and functional status of the child. Such an approach can also be more easily applied under the conditions of the outpatient treatment (Amador et al., 1990). Some therapeutic procedures using a restricted diet alone have resulted in slightly reduced growth, especially with respect to body height. The advantages of treatment with a diet adequate for preservation of growth and maturation rates of children during early stages of obesity have also been demonstrated.

Comparisons have been made between procedures comprised of diet, exercise and training, education, and psychological support. The only difference between these two approaches was the energy content of the diet. The first diet was restricted to 0.17 MJ.kg^{-1} of expected body weight for stature, while in the experimental group the diet was fitted to the physiological requirements for age, gender, and physical activity (0.25 MJ.kg^{-1}). The results showed that the consumption of restricted diets for 6 months impaired the velocity of growth, maturation, and lean body mass accretion. The incidence of dropout was slightly higher in the restricted group with no relapses registered in the other groups. In the combined approach it was sufficient to reduce "risky" foodstuffs (fat, sugar, and delicacies) without a marked restriction of food intake. This group used exercise of a sufficient intensity over an extended period of time.

Findings on the results of obesity treatment indicate that fitness changes are greater for subjects provided exercise alone, or exercise combined with diet, in comparison with subjects provided no exercise, or diet alone (Hills and Byrne, 1998, 2000). This approach seems to be mostly encouraging for prevention and treatment of obesity during growth (Epstein and Goldfield, 1999). Decreasing TV, videotape, and video game use may be a promising approach to reduce childhood obesity; BMI, skinfolds, and waist circumference were decreased after an intervention that reduced TV viewing and meals eaten in front of the TV set (Robinson, 1999). The effectiveness of combined treatment programs could be predicted by leptin assays, i.e., in subjects with relative hyper- or hypoleptinemia compared to obese children with normal baseline leptin levels, the effect can be decreased (Miraglia-del-Giudice et al., 2002a).

Obese children treated by inpatient multicomponent 10-week treatment without stringent energy restriction showed reduced weight and BMI, developed higher self-esteem, and were more capable to cope with external eating stimuli. It was noted that the subjects did not develop anorexia or bulimia nervosa. Such a multicomponent program is a valuable option for treatment of obese children (Braet et al., 2003), provided that enough financial resources and willingness for long inpatient programs are assured.

12.4.1 Changes in Body Composition and Fitness Following Weight Reduction

The relative success of a combined diet and exercise therapy should be judged using stringent measurements of body composition. Some studies have shown that during weight loss, particularly in more severely obese children and during the later stages of puberty, lean, fat-free body mass may be lost in greater quantities (e.g., Pařízková, 1963b; 1968b; 1977; 1998b). These results may also be due to a simultaneous loss of body water that can indicate a loss of not only fat but also fat-free tissue. A residential treatment 10-week program using moderate dietary restriction, physical activity, and psychological support decreased overweight, reduced fat, and improved maximal performance level by increasing performance time and peak power without an improvement in absolute VO_2 (Deforche, De Bourdeaudhuij, and Hills, 2003). An individualized training program reduced body weight, but decreased FFM and LBM compared to a program with dietary advice alone. Bioimpedance analysis showed smaller changes in LBM in exercised children; the changes in body weight after 1 year were inversely correlated with changes in FFM after 12 weeks of intervention. This has important implications as a loss of FFW during weight reduction may be a risk factor for regain of weight (Eliakim et al., 2002; Schwingshandl et al., 1999).

Rolland-Cachera et al. (2004) considered the results of a 5-month weight-reduction program on obese children. The program consisted of exercise and a low-calorie diet but with either a high or a moderate protein content. The protein content of the diet did not affect weight loss and change of BMI, which was reduced in both groups.

Body composition measurements using DXA before and after a combined diet and exercise program in 12.8 ± 2.6 year-old children revealed that total weight and fat mass decreased, but fat-free body mass was maintained. The results were not dependent on age, race, gender, or stage of development (Figueroa-Colon et al., 1998).

A comparison of the results of a study consisting of diet only, and/or diet combined with aerobic exercise (approximately 250 kcal per session) showed a greater decrease of overweight in the combined group after 4 months. This decrease was $-25 \pm 13.5\%$ compared to $-15.8 \pm 10.8\%$ in children treated by diet only. Treatment compliance was also better in the group using both exercise and diet (Reybrouck et al., 1990).

Aerobic power ($VO_2.min^{-1}.kg$ body weight^{-1}) increased significantly along with a decrease of BMI and percentage of body fat in adolescent boys after 7 weeks of treatment in a summer camp (Figure 12.16) (Pařízková, 1972, 1977, 1998c). The program included a monitored diet (1700 kcal.day^{-1}) with sufficient liquids (unsweetened) and an all-day exercise program with sports activities suited to children with varying degrees of obesity (Pařízková, 1977, 1998a,b).

As a function of the intervention, improvements in functional capacity were found with respect to the economy of work during standard workload

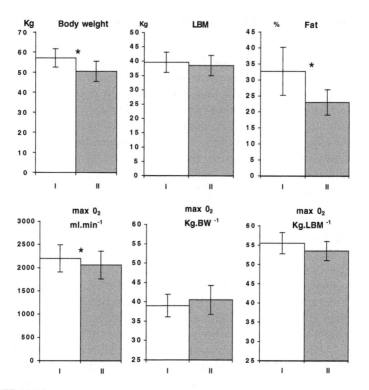

FIGURE 12.16

Changes in morphological characteristics (body weight, lean body mass (LBM), percentage of stored fat (%) and oxygen uptake in absolute and relative (O_2 ml.min.kg^{-1} body weight, and/ or kg lean (LBM), fat-free body mass during maximal workload on a treadmill in obese pre-pubertal boys and girls before (I) and after (II) reduction treatment by monitored diet and exercise in a summer camp. * indicates ($p < 0.05$). (Based on data from Pařízková 1968a; 1972; 1975; 1977.)

testing on a cycle ergometer. The economy of work and energy efficiency is lower in obese children compared to normal-weight children (Pařízková, 1963, 1972, 1977). Following a reduction of weight and fat through exercise and diet in a summer camp, the energy cost of the same activity and work-load was significantly decreased. The heart rate during the same workload was lower (Figure 12.17), oxygen uptake decreased, and a higher economy of work and mechanical efficiency was recorded. Vital capacity also increased significantly after a combined treatment program (Figure 12.18) (Pařízková, 1977, 1993b). Similar results were gained during further follow-ups. The heart rate responses during a standard workload on a bicycle ergometer test before and after weight reduction are displayed in Figure 12.19. These results confirm that both peak performance and standard workloads (characteristic of tasks in everyday life) can be executed more favorably after the reduction of excess fat (Hills and Parker, 1988; Deforche et al., 2003).

Significant changes in functional parameters and body composition have been shown in relation to changes in the intensity of exercise in summer

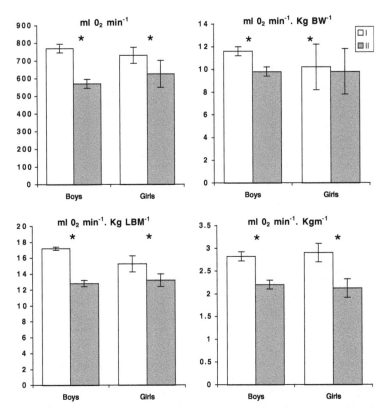

FIGURE 12.17

Changes in oxygen uptake in absolute and relative values (O_2 ml.min1.kg^{-1} body weight, and/ or lean body mass, LBM, and ml O_2.min^{-1}.kgm^{-1} of performance) over a standard workload in obese pre-pubertal boys and girls before (I) and after (II) reduction treatment by monitored diet and exercise in a summer camp. * indicates ($p < 0.05$). (Based on data from Pařízková 1968a; 1997; 1993b.)

camps. The camps feature a combined diet and exercise program run each school year over 4 consecutive years. The combined effect of exercise of an adequate intensity on adiposity and fitness is shown in Figure 12.20. During the earlier period of obesity treatment (11 to 12 years of age), there was a reduction in percentage of stored fat but FFM did not decrease. However, there was some reduction of lean body mass later. In spite of LBM being greater in obese than normal-weight boys in a longitudinal study during the same growth period, it is preferable not to lose LBM. Therefore, it is more beneficial to start at a younger age during the initial phases of obesity. The change in ventilation, oxygen uptake, and energy cost of the same standard workload were similar to results in other studies of obese children.

Both the amount and distribution of fat changed after the treatment in summer camps. The centrality index (subscapular/triceps ratio) was evaluated in obese girls and boys during a 3-year longitudinal study. The results of this index indicate that the reduction of fat was always relatively greater

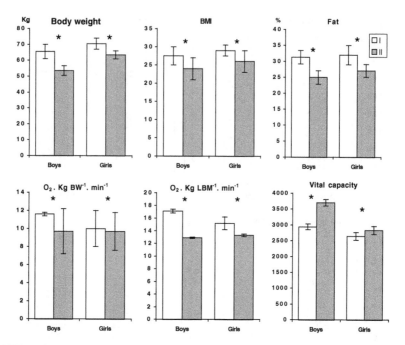

FIGURE 12.18

Changes in body weight, BMI, percent body fat, and oxygen uptake as related to total body weight and/or lean, fat-free body mass, and vital capacity over a standard workload in obese pre-pubertal boys and girls before (I) and after (II) reduction treatment by monitored diet and exercise in a summer camp. * indicates (p < 0.05). (Based on data from Pařízková 1968a; 1977; 1993b.)

on the trunk than on the extremities of the obese girls (Figure 12.21) (Pařízková, 1993b). Similar changes in the centrality index were observed in obese boys of the same age.

A 12-month reduction program that consisted of individual nutritional counseling, guidance on physical activity, and supportive therapy found weight loss in the majority of children. VO_2 max.kg lean body mass^{-1} (LBM) increased from 44.2 to 47.1 ml.min^{-1}.kg LBM^{-1} (p < 0.025). There was no change in time allocated to physical activity during the weight-reduction period, but the children's participation in training teams of sports clubs increased. These data also indicate that obese children are less fit than children of normal weight, which is especially apparent with aerobic power. A loss of body fat improved the level of physical fitness significantly (Huttunen, Knip, and Paavilainen, 1986).

The effect of diet-plus-behavior (DB) treatment and DB-plus-exercise treatment (EDB) were compared with respect to changes in basal metabolic rate (open-circuit spirometry) and body composition (hydrostatic weighing). Dietary management and restriction was based on the dietary exchange program and behavior management, including record keeping, stimulus control, and reinforcement techniques. Aerobics 50 min per day, 3 times per

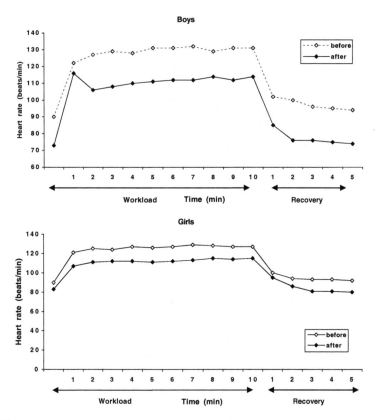

FIGURE 12.19

Changes in heart rate of obese boys and girls during standard, submaximal workload on a bicycle ergometer before and after weight reduction treatment by exercise and diet in a summer camp. (Based on data from Pařízková 1972; 1993b; 1997.)

week, comprised the exercise component. Results revealed small but statistically significant improvements in body composition for both groups. However, no significant differences were found between groups. All control subjects gained a significant amount of body weight (Katch et al., 1988a). Following weight reduction, RMR and FFM decreased, although no differences were found in RQ when comparing obese and control children (Maffeis, Schutz, and Pinelli, 1992a).

A weight-loss program including exercise (Rocchini et al., 1988) resulted in desirable improvements, including a decrease in resting systolic blood pressure and exercise diastolic and mean blood pressure. In addition, obese adolescents showed structural changes in the forearm resistance vessels. These structural changes were reversed to a large extent in the weight-loss program.

Blood pressure distribution in a group of obese adolescents was shown to be skewed 1SD to the right of normal children ($p < 0.01$); after weight reduction resulting from a program of energy restriction and behavioral

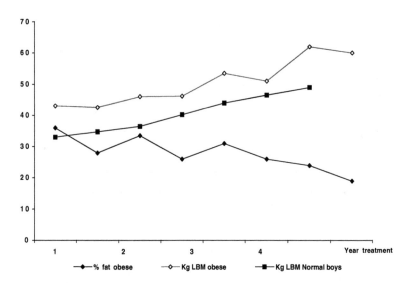

FIGURE 12.20

A 4-year longitudinal study of body composition changes (lean, fat-free body mass and % stored fat, measured by hydrodensitometry with simultaneous measurements of air in lungs and respiratory passages) after weight decreases in obese boys following four consecutive treatments through monitored diet and exercise programs in summer camps, and after weight increases during the school year (lean body mass kg in obese boys, lean body mass kg in normal-weight boys during the same growth period (longitudinal data), and percentage of stored fat in obese boys. (Based on data from Pařízková 1997; 1998b.)

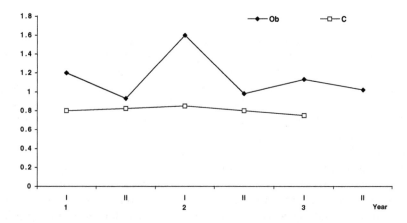

FIGURE 12.21

A longitudinal study (11 to 14 years) of centrality index changes (subscapular/triceps ratio) in obese girls over 3 years, before (I) and after (II) the reduction therapy by diet and exercise in a summer camp compared to values for normal-weight girls (C). (Based on data from Pařízková, 1998b.)

change alone and/or combined with exercise, this distribution was no longer different from that in normal-weight adolescents (Rocchini et al., 1988). Hemostatic risk factors for cardiovascular diseases were also influenced by short-term energy restriction combined with exercise in obese youth (Gallistl et al., 2001c).

Other studies have shown that behavioral and public health models, including dietary and exercise interventions, can have long-term effects in obese juveniles. A modest effect on body weight, fatness, and blood lipids was found, and the impact of the interventions endured the 5-year follow-up period (Johnson et al., 1997).

A multicomponent and multidisciplinary after-school intervention program in adolescent post-menarcheal girls showed successful results. This was especially the case with respect to reducing the rate of weight gain, reducing body weight by 11.5%, maintaining the pretreatment amount of lean, fat-free mass and improved eating and exercise behaviors. Changes in food habits included reducing energy dense foods, reducing frequency and amount of food ingested, and eating more slowly. Encouragement and praise from the group leaders played an essential role in weight control. The greatest obstacles to success were boredom, hunger, lack of family and peer support, and having food in sight (Hoerr, Nelson, and Essex-Sorlie, 1988).

Similarly, positive experiences with a combined treatment and management approach were found in other populations, for example, in Brazilian obese adolescent females. Greater weight loss and a more favorable change in serum lipids and body composition were found in groups using a combined physical exercise and dietary education (Cezar et al., 1998).

The combined effect of diet and exercise was also studied in two groups of obese girls (Epstein et al., 1985). Treatment in the first group consisted of diet only; in the second group treatment consisted of regular supervised exercise (walking or running 3 miles, 3 times per week). Both groups of girls significantly reduced percent of overweight after 2 months of this treatment. However, after a further 4 months, girls who exercised still had a reduced percent of overweight and improved their level of physical fitness. The percent of overweight in girls in the diet-only group decreased during the first period from 0 to 2 months but not from 2 to 6 months.

The effect of a weight-reduction program on body composition in obese children and adolescents across the pubertal barrier was conducted (8.5 to 14.8 years). Lean body mass (LBM) was estimated from the resistance index (RI) and was obtained by bioelectrical impedance analysis (BIA) before and after the 3-week program of weight reduction. All individuals lost body fat during the treatment, whereas the change of lean body mass was heterogeneous. The individual change in body fat was inversely correlated with change in lean body mass. A number of subjects were reevaluated after 4 months. The regain in body weight during this period was inversely correlated with the change of LBM during the weight-reduction period. These results indicate that changes in LBM during a weight-reduction program can predict the short-term results in those children who manage to maintain or even increase LBM and lose weight only through a decline in stored fat. Changes in LBM during weight reduction seem to predict the long-term outcome, that is, loss of LBM is associated with greater regain of total body weight in the longer term (Schwingshandl and Borkenstein, 1995).

The effects of lifestyle modification and exercise in a 1-month YMCA program on body composition and serum lipids were studied in a group of obese sedentary children. The measurements at entry, after the intervention and subsequently, 1 and 4 months after completion showed a nonsignificant decrease in body weight and sum of two skinfolds and a significant increase in the number of sit-ups and distance covered in a 9-min run. There was no change in flexibility and a nonsignificant decrease in TC (Cohen, McMilla, and Samuelson, 1991). A longer program would be necessary to consider the continuity of positive changes in morphological, motor, and serum lipid parameters.

Another combination of therapeutic approaches for obesity treatment was used in Cuban children. Children were divided into four groups (diet, exercise only, diet and exercise, and control group). In both genders there was a significant positive effect of exercise on body weight and efficacy index, and a significant interaction between fiber intake and exercise in girls, but not in boys. These results suggest a possible effect of fiber in the diet that may be accentuated by exercise (Pena et al., 1989).

12.4.2   Serum Lipid Changes

A combined treatment was used in long-term observations of German children aged 9 to 12 years. Children who maintained the nutritional habits introduced during the program and who remained active in sports were able to maintain a desirable body weight (Korsten-Reck, Bauer, and Keul, 1994; Berg et al., 1994). Whether short-term benefits gained in childhood will continue into adulthood and help to reduce the cardiovascular risks later in life needs to be assessed by further research. A combined reduction therapy using diet and exercise has a significant effect on serum lipids.

A group of obese boys was followed before and after 4 weeks of weight management. A hypoenergetic diet (0.18 MJ.kg^{-1} expected body weight for age) and exercise reduced the values of relative fat body weight (calculated by regression equations for 5 skinfolds) and TC, TC/HDL-C ratio. TG decreased but did not reach significance; however, it had a better correlation with the reduction of adiposity (delta% body fat) than the two previously mentioned variables. The increase in lipolysis during the 4-week study is expressed in the significant increase of free fatty acids (FFA) and its correlation with delta% body fat ($r = -0.714$). There was a trend for an increase of HDL-C and a significant inverse correlation with delta% body fat ($r = -0.804$). This study also confirms the efficacy of treatment by diet and exercise simultaneously to improve not only body weight and composition but also serum lipid profile and therefore reduce health risks. Treatment efficacy and delta FFA were lower in subjects with lesser adiposity as related to muscle mass at the middle third of the upper arm (measured through the energy/

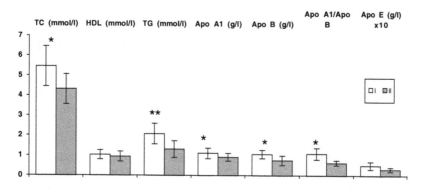

FIGURE 12.22

Effect of energy restriction over 4 weeks on total (TC) and HDL cholesterol (HDL-C), triglycerides (TG), apolipoprotein-A 1, B and E, before (I) and after (II) reduction treatment. * indicates (p < 0.05); ** (p < 0.01). (Based on data from Endo et al., 1992.)

protein index) (Hermelo et al., 1987a). These conclusions concur with other results from experimental models mentioned previously (Pařízková, 1977).

Children treated by diet and moderate exercise during 15 days of hospitalization were assessed with the diet of one group supplemented with fiber. Weight loss was observed in both groups along with the reduction of TC and LDL-C. Triacylglycerols, VLDL-C, and HDL-C did not change in this short time frame (Sterpa et al., 1985).

The effect of a hypoenergetic diet (0.18 MJ.kg⁻¹ expected body weight for age) combined with physical exercise and psychological support was reported in another study of obese children aged 10 to 14 years. Significant changes in total body weight and composition (using skinfold measurements) occurred along with changes in serum lipids and physical fitness evaluated by the efficiency index (EI). Significant correlations were found between the EI values and changes in TC and TC/HDL-C ratio. Although the increase in HDL-C was not significant, the values were highly correlated with EI during the first and second assessments. Differences were found in the magnitude of increase in free, nonesterified fatty acids (delta FFA), which suggests that lipolytic mechanisms were not uniformly impaired. Treatment efficiency and delta FFA were lower in subjects with less adiposity as related to muscle mass at the middle third of the upper arm (measured via the energy/protein index) (Hermelo et al., 1987b).

After 4 weeks of combined therapy (energy-restricted diet and exercise), the weight loss achieved in a group of obese children was 8.4% of the initial body weight (Endo et al., 1992). The values for serum lipids were higher than in normal-weight control children before the reduction treatment and were significantly changed after the treatment. HDL-C was low before and unchanged after treatment. Serum apolipoprotein A-I level was normal before treatment and significantly reduced after weight reduction (Figure 12.22). Serum apolipoprotein B level was significantly higher before treatment as compared to controls and decreased to the normal range after treatment. The ratio of apolipoprotein B to apolipoprotein A was significantly high at admission and decreased significantly after treatment. Serum apolipoprotein E level was normal but also decreased after treatment. The benefits of an improved serum lipid and apolipoprotein concentration are also important in reducing the risk of the future development of atherosclerosis. Exercise treatment, which also reduced serum lipids and lipoprotein, insulin, and glucose concentrations, is effective only when continued; the benefits of such treatment are lost when children interrupt their increased physical activity and exercise (Ferguson et al., 1999a). Lipid profiles improved after weight loss due to combined treatment; this differed according to gender. The TC, LDL, TG serum level decreased. Girls tended to be more susceptible to a decrease in LDL level, which might result in an increased cardiovascular protective effect (Sothern et al., 2000a).

There is considerable support for the continued use of exercise in combination with diet for treatment and management of obesity in children and adolescents. However, the limited number of well-controlled studies indicates the need for more research in this area. The potential impact of exercise programs in the prevention and treatment of obesity during growth has been extensively reviewed (Epstein, Coleman, and Myers, 1996; Goran, Reynolds, and Lindquist, 1999; Van Mil, Goris, and Westerterp, 1999). Similarly, the role of the family has been highlighted in the combined treatment by diet and exercise. Future work must address the specifics of exercise prescription, including the effect of the intensity, type, duration, and frequency of various exercises. As mentioned before, the insufficient information on these factors makes it difficult or even impossible to compare and analyze the results of available studies.

12.4.3 Hormonal, Metabolic, and Hemostatic Changes as a Result of Diet and Exercise

Significant weight loss and decreases in serum leptin and fasting insulin concentrations occurred as a result of combined obesity treatment (Falorni et al., 1997a). There was also a correlation between the reduction of relative body weight and of serum leptin but not of fasting insulin. A significant reduction of IGFBP-3 and an increase of the IGF-1/IGFBP-3 molar ratio were also found after weight loss in obese children and adolescents.

Obese Czech children aged 9 to 16 years were admitted to a facility for the treatment of obesity using both monitored diet and exercise suited to more severe cases of obesity (Lísková, Hosek, and Stoicky, 1998). Serum leptin decreased significantly after the reduction of weight and BMI along with a reduction in lipoproteins and apolipoproteins and systolic and diastolic blood pressure (Figure 12.23). Risk factors for cardiovascular disease and diabetes were therefore also reduced.

In a study involving systematic physical activity together with energy restriction in obese 14-year-old boys, Rychlewski et al. (1996) determined

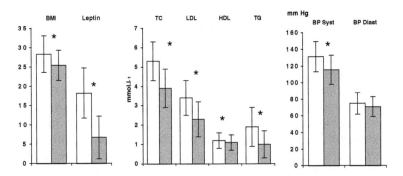

FIGURE 12.23

Changes of body mass index (BMI), serum leptin level, total (TC) and LDL-cholesterol (LDL), triglycerides (TG; mmol/l), systolic and diastolic blood pressure before (I) and after (II) 1 month of treatment in a spa, with a diet consisting of 5.217 MJ/day (protein 23%, fat 30%, carbohydrates 47% of energy). Energy expenditure (EE) elevated by 10 MJ/week by exercising 25 min/day at 70% of maximal heart rate. * indicates (p < 0.05). (Based on data from Lísková, Hosek, and Stozicky, 1998.)

immunoreactive insulin (IRI), C-peptide, fructosamin, and binding of 1251-insulin. Management of exercise and diet resulted in a decrease in body weight, a reduction in stored fat, and an increase in physical efficiency. Insulinemia and insulin-resistance as measured by the amount of 1251-Insulin binding was also reduced by 20%. Over the 3-week period, the obese boys had a daily physical workload on a bicycle ergometer with a load of 1 Watt.kg body weight^{-1} lasting 30 min. The diet during this period equated with 1300 kcal.day^{-1}. Testing involved a bicycle ergometer protocol at an intensity of 75% VO_2 max. As shown in a further study, after a 10-week multidisciplinary program, weight and fat loss IRI decreased significantly, whereas C-peptide reactivity (CPR) in obese children did not change. CPR/IRI molar ratio, considered an indirect estimation of hepatic insulin clearance (HIC), rose significantly after weight loss. Results of this study suggest that hyperinsulinemia in obese children and adolescents is caused by decreased HIC (Escobar et al., 1999).

The relationships of the changes of subcutaneous fat (using the Lipometer) and its distribution on the trunk and extremities, along with fat mass, waist and hip circumference, and their ratio, and changes of metabolic factors (TG, TCh, insulin, glucose) in 3-weeks treatment by diet and exercise were followed in children 11.9 to 12.0 years of age. Reduction treatment reduced body adiposity, as well as most of the metabolic parameters. The results suggested that the changes in the atherogenic and metabolic risk factors are largely independent of the concomitant loss of subcutaneous fat. The reduction of body mass explained only a small part of the variability in changes of insulin (Sudi et al., 2001c).

Glucose-induced thermogenesis was tested in obese children aged 14.3 ± 0.3 years before and after 6 weeks of treatment by diet (5441 to 6279 kJ.day^{-1})

and aerobic exercise training (walk, jog, calisthenics, swim) and compared to controls (Nichols, Bigelow, and Canine, 1989). The thermic effect of 100 g glucose tolerance test (calculated as the area under the response curve for 3 hours in excess of resting metabolic rate) was similar in obese adolescents before treatment and controls. After treatment this value was lower in obese subjects. The area under the response curve for glucose was elevated in obese subjects before treatment compared to controls. Before treatment, the insulin response was similar in obese and controls, but it decreased in the obese after treatment. The improvement in peripheral insulin sensitivity after 6 weeks of obesity treatment by exercise and diet and after weight loss was not accompanied by favorable changes in carbohydrate-induced thermogenesis in obese adolescents.

Plasma leptin, TC, and apolipoprotein (apo) A-I and B were measured in obese children aged 12.5 ± 1.9 years before and after 3 weeks of weight reduction in a special camp (Holub et al., 1998). Binding of endogenous and exogenous radio-labeled leptin to lipoproteins was studied by stepwise and continuous density gradient ultracentrifugation. As in other groups, plasma leptin level was significantly higher in obese than in nonobese subjects and decreased from 16.5 ± 9.8 ng.ml^{-1} to 10.0 ± 8.6 ng.ml^{-1} after weight reduction ($p < 0.001$). In a multivariate regression, relative BMI and apo A-I was significant predictors of baseline leptin and accounted for 38% ($p < 0.003$) and 15% ($p < 0.006$) of the variance of baseline leptin concentrations in obese children. The change in plasma leptin associated with weight loss was independently predicted by a difference in plasma HDL-C explaining 29% of the variance of leptin changes ($p < 0.0032$). A substantial portion of both endogenous and exogenous labeled leptin was recovered with the HDL-C fraction. Therefore, plasma apo A-I and HDL-C are independent predictors of leptin concentration during weight loss, respectively. HDL-C also transports a variable portion of leptin in the circulation (Holub et al., 1999).

Important changes in the levels of insulin, cortisol, growth hormone, thyroxin, triiodothyronine, along with nonesterified fatty acids (NEFA), glucose, lactate, b-hydroxybutyrate (b-OHB), and triacylglycerols (TG) in the blood were followed up in a group of boys aged 13.7 years during a period of weight reduction. Boys were examined at the beginning (I), then after a 10-day stay in an inpatient department (II). The reduction treatment then continued in a spa. The initial assessment was executed with an 11 MJ diet (approximately 110 g of protein, 100 g of carbohydrate, and 80 g of fat). The energy was then decreased to 5.2 MJ (110 g of protein, 100 g of carbohydrate, 45 g of fat). In addition to the diet, supervised low to moderate aerobic activity was performed 4 hours per day. A blood sample was obtained after 10 days (II), with the final sample after 52 days or at the end of the treatment in the spa (III). The changes in the above-mentioned indicators are provided in Table 12.1. All parameters decreased after the first 10 days of treatment when the daily weight loss was 300 g except for the serum level of NEFA and b-OHB. After the following period, insulin did not change, but a significant decrease throughout the period of treatment was observed for the concentration of

TABLE 12.1

Changes of Body Weight, Hormonal, and Biochemical Parameters in Adolescent
Obese Children Aged 13.7 ± 1.3 Years during Three Periods of Reduction Treatment

	I		II		III	
	X	SD	X	SD	X	SD
Body weight (kg)	77.4	12.0	74.4	10.9	68.2	11.2
Insulin (mU/l)	15.4	5.6	12.7	5.0	13.0	7.4
Cortisol (mmol/l)	746.0	456.0	648.0	648.0	539.0	357.0
Growth hormone (ng/l)	8.2	12.2	2.1	1.2	15.7	21.2
Thyroxin-T4 (nmol/l)	108.0	33.0	107.0	36.0	94.0	29.0
Triodothyronin-T3 (nmol/l)	2.89	0.64	2.15	1.0	1.9	0.49
Glucose (nmol/l)	5.46	0.061	4.09	0.45	5.32	0.87
Lactate (nmol/l)	1.13	0.35	0.82	0.24	1.25	0.51
NEFA (nmol/l)	0.27	0.06	0.36	0.08	0.24	0.10
β-OHB (nmol/l)	0.65	0.28	4.48	2.06	0.49	0.25
Triacylglycerols (nmol/l)	1.35	0.81	0.78	0.24	0.81	0.81
Protein (g/l)	79.0	3.6	79.4	3.4	77.7	3.4

Source: Based on data from Šonka et al., 1993.

cortisol, thyroxin, and triiodothyronin. The substrates showed a different
pattern of change after the treatment following an important modification
of their levels during the first 10 days. An opposite trend followed so that
the initial level was similar to that obtained on day 52. This was the case for
glucose with lactate presenting similar shifts but was not significant. The
level of NEFA and β-OHB displayed a mirror-like picture. The changes in
growth hormone level were not significant (Šonka et al., 1995).

A 6-week diet and exercise program in overweight and obese adolescents
showed decreased body weight, BMI, and fat percentage significantly along
with the reduction of waist and hip circumferences, waist-to-hip ratio, and
blood pressure (Figure 12.24). IGF-1, IGFHP, leptin, and insulin concentrations decreased also during the program (Kratzch et al., 1997).

Obese children were evaluated before and within 48 hours after the completion of a 5-month exercise training program (ETP, 3 aerobic sessions per
week, each increasing the energy expenditure by approximately 300 kcal)
and a moderate diet restriction. Weight gain after ETP was minimal, and
improved insulin tolerance and an unexpected increase in the response of
gastric inhibitory polypeptide (GIP) was revealed. Even after ETP, obese
children continued to secrete more insulin than normal-weight children.
Glucose tolerance, similar to pre-ETP for obese subjects and controls, did
not change following ETP. An improvement in glucose utilization in obese
children following ETP was associated with an increase in GIP secretion.
This finding contrasted with reports that energy restriction would improve
glucose utilization with decreased insulin and GIP secretion. This study
demonstrated an uncoupling of GIP and insulin secretion and suggests shifts
in peripheral tissue sensitivity to insulin-induced glucose uptake. These
shifts may, in part, be influenced by GIP (Kahle et al., 1986).

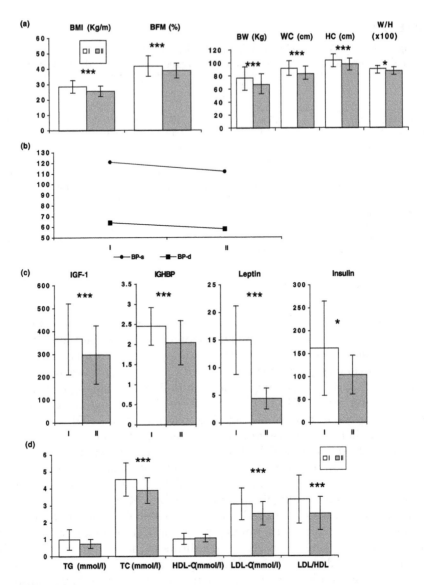

FIGURE 12.24

Changes of (a) anthropometric (body mass index (BMI), percentage stored fat (%), body weight (BW), waist (WC) and hip (HC) circumference and their ratio (WHR); (b) blood pressure; (c) IGF-1, IGFHP, leptin, insulin; and (d) serum TG, TC, HDL-C, LDL-C, and LDL-C/HDL-C ratio in overweight and obese adolescents before (I) and after (II) weight reduction by 6 weeks of exercise and diet. * indicates ($p < 0.05$); *** ($p < 0.001$). (Based on data from Kratzsch et al., 1997.)

Body weight correlates significantly with insulin levels and blood pressure in obese and nonobese adolescents. Following weight loss, a decrease in insulin levels and blood pressure was observed. The reduction of blood pressure during the weight loss correlated significantly with the change in both insulin and body weight (Rocchini et al., 1987).

The influence of physical training (PT) on components of insulin resistance syndrome (IRS) was examined in obese children aged 7 to 11 years. This was under two conditions of reduction therapy: (a) 4 months of PT followed by four months without PT, or (b) 4 months without PT followed by 4 months of PT. The results were analysed using ANOVA. A significant interaction indicated that the changes over time were different for the two groups. During the 4 months of PT compared to the period without PT, there were significant decreases in the TC/HDL-C ratio, TG, insulin, and percent of body fat. Following periods without PT there were increases in insulin and percent of body fat. Thus, PT improved some components of IRS in obese children, with some benefits being lost following its interruption (Gutin et al., 1998).

A further study confirmed higher fasting plasma concentrations of IRI and C-peptide, and also a lower C-peptide to IRI molar ratio in obese children aged 11. 4 ± 2.5 years compared to normal children of the same age (Knip, Lautala, and Puukka, 1988). Obese children also had reduced erythrocyte insulin binding over the physiological range of circulating insulin concentration. A negative correlation between insulin tracer binding and the relative weight was revealed. This weight-reduction program resulted in a decrease in mean relative weight score, and after treatment, obese children decreased fasting blood glucose levels. The same applied to IRI concentrations at 90 min following an oral glucose load when compared to the onset of therapy. No significant differences between the insulin-binding characteristics at the beginning and at the end of the reducing therapy were found.

In another study, French obese children were tested after the completion of a 3-month inpatient weight-reduction program. The initial GH-U concentration in the urine (pmol/mmol creatinine) was 0.0256 on admission, and 0.0352 on discharge ($p < 0.0001$; normal values 0.031 ± 0.019). Using a two-level hierarchical model with adjustment for age, gender, and initial BMI, the increase in GH-U was facilitated by enhanced physical activity depending on the time spent by a child participating for more than 1 hour above the average (Lehingue et al., 1998). After GH excretion, the restoration of its values was correlated with various anthropometric parameters so as to define which one could be a predictor for GH increase after weight reduction. GH restoration was significantly related to hip, not waist, circumference decreases. This suggests that in this respect, subcutaneous fat is more important than visceral fat (Locard et al., 1998).

Urine secretion of GH (GH-U) increased after an inpatient slimming program in obese children. A mean decrease of 0.90 SD for BMI was accompanied by a 34% increase in GH-U. Time spent in physical activity was the only component of the program found to be related to the magnitude of GH-U increase (Lehingue et al.,, 2000).

The effect of an 8-week reduction treatment (1000 kcal.day^{-1}) on thyroid-stimulating hormone (TSH) and prolactin (PRL) responses to thyrotropin-releasing hormone (TRH) was followed in obese subjects aged 8.5 to 17.4 years, before and after reduction of weight. In females at baseline, fT4 serum levels were significantly higher than in control girls with normal weight and fell significantly following weight reduction with rT3 increasing following weight loss in the whole group. Other changes also appeared in the TSH and PRL peaks after TRH following weight loss in girls, as well as in other parameters in the whole group. However, the results of this study suggest that thyroid function is normal in obese adolescent subjects and not influenced by the restriction of energy intake. This occurred even though a reduced hypothalamus dopaminergic tone on pituitary thyreotrophs and lactotrophs could cause subtle alterations on TSH and PRL release, partially influenced by gender and the level of sexual development (Guzzaloni et al., 1995). A reduction of overweight achieved with a normal energy diet showed a significant decrease in thyroxin, triodothyronin (T_3, T_4), and leptin serum concentrations, which were higher in obese children, but there was no significant change in TSH (Reinehr and Andler, 2002). There is thus no necessity to treat the increased serum TSH.

Weight loss due to reduction treatment also had an effect on adrenal androgens in obese boys who were followed up before puberty (group I) and at the first stage of sexual maturation. Pregnenolon and dehydroepiandrosteron plasma levels were significantly higher in both groups (I and II) of obese boys when compared to normal-weight controls. These values decreased to normal values following weight reduction, apart from pregnenolon in the prepubertal group I. Progesterone was significantly increased in both groups, and was normal following weight reduction. Also, 17-OH-progesterone plasma levels showed no significant difference between obese and control groups. Androstenedione was higher in the prepubertal obese group I before the treatment, and then showed normal values after weight reduction. No significant difference was found in the other groups. Testosterone and estradiol showed normal values in the two groups both before and after weight reduction. Cortisol showed a similar pattern. It can be concluded that cortico-adrenal activity is increased in obese boys while the same was found in obese girls. The increased secretion of adrenal androgens might be due to an increased secretion of cortico-adrenal stimulating hormone, or to an enhanced adrenal sensitivity to the hypothetical hormone. These results could also explain the precocious menarche that often occurs in obese adolescents (Pintor et al., 1984).

The level of serum interleukin-6 (IL-6) was followed along with indices of obesity, leptin, estradiol, systolic and diastolic blood pressure, and heart rate at baseline and after 3 weeks in obese children with 3.5–8 MJ daily energy intake with exercise. All parameters decreased significantly. Percentage of fat, BMI, and leptin were not related to IL-6 in the program, but IL-6 correlated significantly with indices of obesity, BMI, and leptin after weight loss (Gallistl et al., 2001a).

Homocystein (tHc) is associated with indexes of obesity and insulin resistance in obese children. After a weight-reduction program including physical activity, BMI, fat mass, percentage of fat mass, insulin, and C-peptide decreased significantly, whereas homocystein and vitamin B_{12} showed significant increase. Folate and LBM did not change. Changes in tHcy during weight reduction were significantly associated with baseline LBM, and were inversely related to changes in LBM during weight loss. Children who increased LBM showed lowest increases in tHcy compared to children who lost LBM. In multiple-regression analysis, only baseline LBM contributed independently and significantly to changes in tHcy (Gallistl et al., 2001b).

Protein utilization was also influenced by an increased physical activity program that was used in children either alone (walking program 5 days per week, 2 to 3 miles per day), or in combination with diet. ^{15}N glycine was used to assess protein synthesis and breakdown as well as the net turnover (NET) and N flux. When only diet was used, NET decreased, protein synthesis decreased, and protein breakdown did not return to baseline levels (Ebbelink and Rodriguez, 1999). Abnormalities of protein metabolism concerning whole-body protein turnover (WBPT), which occur early in childhood obesity, were found to be modifiable by lifestyle changes (e.g., exercise and diet) (Balagopal et al., 2003).

Energy restriction and increased physical activity also improved the hemostatic risk profile in obese children and adolescents. Fibrinogen, factor VII coagulant activity, von Willebrandt factor antigen, and soluble P-selection decreased significantly after combined treatment by diet and exercise in white boys and girls 11.9 to 12.0 years old, along with positive changes of weight and adiposity (Gallistl et al., 2001c). The changes in fibrinolytic prameters (including tPA-Ag and plasminogen activator inhibitor type 1 – PAI-1) associated with weight loss can occur independently of simultaneous decrease of adiposity; improvement in metabolic state and additional changes of parameters that were not ascertained and related to physical activity and energy restriction could have influenced the improvement of fibrinolytic parameters (Sudi et al., 2001b). Also, other authors found positive changes of PAI-1 after weight loss due to similar treatment, especially in children who had higher initial levels of PAI-1, and who reduced most their BMI (Estelles et al., 2001). Levels of PAI-1 correlated with TG and insulin, but not with TC and glucose levels.

12.4.4 Changes in Cardiocirculatory Characteristics and Motor Performance

Weight and fat loss after 7 weeks of treatment by diet and exercise in a summer camp improved the level of cardiorespiratory fitness through an increased aerobic power. Similar results were found in repeated follow-ups before and after similar treatment in both boys and girls (Pařízková, 1977, 1993a, 1998b).

In another study, preadolescent obese subjects were assessed before and after a 6-month behavioral weight-control program. Significant improvements were found for both weight and fitness level, which was also reflected by changes in heart rate during exercise and a recovery period. The most successful children decreased their maximal and recovery heart rates, and the reverse was found for the least successful subjects. The severely obese subjects improved their fitness only when weight loss was substantial (Epstein et al., 1983).

An intervention study by Cohen, McMillan, and Samuelson (1991) showed a nonsignificant decrease in body weight and sum of two skinfolds, significant increases in the number of sit-ups (23 to 35), and distance covered in 9 min (1201 to 1419 yards). There was no change in flexibility and a nonsignificant decrease in TC (178 to 155 mg.dl^{-1}).

The effect of diet and exercise was assessed in an experimental group of obese children simultaneously with a control group without intervention. At the beginning, obese children were significantly inferior to normal-weight children in fitness items such as standing long jump, pull-ups, sit-ups, step-test, and total fitness scores. No differences in lying trunk extension and standing trunk flexion for body flexibility were observed. Obese children were superior in static strength, that is, hand-grip strength and back strength. The deterioration of physical fitness was due to the enhanced deposition of fat rather than to increased body weight alone, which was more pronounced in boys than in girls. The results in the experimental group showed significant improvement in fitness of most items, especially in abdominal muscle endurance and aerobic capacity. This treatment did not limit growth velocity or reduce the development of lean body mass (Suzuki and Tatsumi, 1993). Similar findings were reported following a 16-week diet and exercise intervention in obese prepubertal children (Hills and Parker, 1988; Hills, 1990).

12.4.5 Changes in Bone Mineral Density

Growth is usually accelerated in obese children. Bone mineral content (BMC, measured by DXA) was studied in obese children before and after a weight-reduction program, including moderate energy restriction and exercise lasting 9.3 ± 3 months. Before weight loss, 25 OH vitamin D was below safety levels in some children. PTH, osteocalcine, and 1.25 OH vitamin D were normal in all subjects. However, bone density of the lumbar spine was lower. During weight loss, BMC increased and became similar in the subgroups supplemented and nonsupplemented with the above-mentioned vitamins. BMC was correlated with height increase, but not with plasma content or the increase of any biological parameters measured (Frelut et al., 1998). Additionally, Gutin et al. (1999a) observed increased bone density after physical training.

12.5 Hormonal Therapy

Obesity during childhood is associated with several abnormalities of the growth hormone (GH) axis, including decreased spontaneous secretion, decreased response to exogenous secretagogues, and changed pulsatile pattern of GH secretion. A study was conducted in which prepubertal severely obese boys aged 10 to 12 years were treated during 6 months with GH, and followed for an additional 6 months. Diet or exercise interventions were not used. Body fat percentage decreased significantly after GH treatment. Iv glucose tolerance tests showed an increased responsivity of the acute insulin secretion. In isolated adipocytes, the maximum isoprenaline and tributaline-induced lipolysis were increased approximately 2.5-fold. No effect was observed on basal and insulin-stimulated lipogenesis. These results indicate that GH treatment lasting 4 months reduced body fat in prepubertal boys; decreased the percentage of fat, possibly via stimulation of catecholamine-induced lipolysis; and occurred without negative effects on glucose homeostasis. GH has also been used for reduction treatment in other studies (Kamel et al., 2000).

Others refer to GH treatment in obese children as decreasing adiposity, reducing TG accumulation by inhibiting lipoproteine lipase, and enhancing lipolysis both via increased hormone-sensitive lipase activity and via induction of beta-adrenoreceptors (Su-Youn-Nam and Marcus, 2000). Fasting serum leptin was reduced after 3 weeks of GH treatment. Body fat percentage, but not BMI, also decreased; this suggests that GH treatment can have a direct effect on serum leptin independent of the effects on body composition (Elimam, Norgren, and Marcus, 2001).

Leptin ineffectiveness with regard to human obesity treatment may be caused by a lack of leptin availability at target sites in the hypothalamus; testing this hypothesis in an experiment, viral vectors to introduce the leptin gene into the brain for a sustained supply of leptin to the hypothalamus in rats were used. A single injection of recombinant adeno-associated virus encoding the leptin gene into the third cerebroventricle prevented the aging-associated gradual increase in body weight and adiposity in adult rats. When applied to prepubertal rats, significantly lower body weight gain and adiposity were maintained for up to 10 months. The same effect was achieved in high-fat-fed and obesity-prone rats, and reduced blood insulin, TG, and FFA. Central leptin gene therapy may herald the development of newer therapeutic strategies (Kalra and Kalra, 2002). However, beneficial effects of daily subcutaneous injections of leptin were recently reported in several children (O'Rahilly et al., 2003).

12.6 Pharmacological Treatment

Drug therapy in obese children has been considered; however, no pharmacological agents are currently approved or recommended for the treatment of pediatric obesity (Daniels, 2002; Yanovski and Yanovski, 2003). A recent review has been written by Molnar and Malecka-Tendera (2002). Generally, the oral administration of appetite suppressors has been recommended as inappropriate. The occasional poor results of other therapeutic approaches, especially under the conditions of outpatient or school-based treatment, drug treatment for resistant, very severely obese cases, have been observed. In São Paolo, Brazil, the results of diet and exercise therapy were compared to the results of the same therapy supplemented by 30 or 60 mg (according to age) of the racemic form of fenfluramine (D.L-fenfluramine) in two groups of obese youth. The groups did not differ in baseline mean age, BMI, or percentage of ideal weight, and were followed up over 1 year. Part of the exercise and diet (placebo) group was unwilling to continue in their therapeutic program. The subjects of the drug group lost significantly more weight, as expressed by the reduction of BMI values (29.2 ± 4.5 to 23.1 ± 3.9 kg.m^{-2}) as compared to the placebo-treated group (BMI 29.9 ± 4.3 to 28.6 ± 4.1 kg.m^{-2}). Dry mouth and drowsiness were the most common complaints, occurring in about 18% of the subjects during the first 2 weeks of therapy, and disappearing with a reduction of D.L-fenfluramine dosage (Madeiros-Neto, 1993). However, few studies have been conducted using drugs for the treatment of childhood obesity. The use of fenfluramine showed undesirable side effects, for example, heart valve problems, and is no longer recommended and on the market, even for adults. It applies even more to children, and in spite of problems not being reported in the study by Madeiros-Neto (1993), the use of similar drugs is not recommended.

A pilot study in obese adolescents has shown caffeine/ephedrine (Letigen) as a safe and effective component of the treatment of obese adolescents, who lost significant amounts of weight and fat. This decrease was significantly greater than in the subjects treated by a placebo. Adverse effects were negligible and did not differ in the Letigen and placebo groups (Molnar et al., 1999).

Leptin injections have resulted in the reduction of body weight in primates, although human clinical trials have not been reported until recently. No similar effect has been shown in the obese of all ages (Schonfeld-Warden and Warden, 1997). As mentioned previously, GH has also been used for reduction treatment (Kamel et al., 2000).

Therapeutic trials are currently under way to evaluate some agents, for example, Orlistat and Sibutramine. Controlled clinical trials are necessary for the evaluation of the effect of drugs for weight management during growth. It should not be assumed that the risks and benefits associated with these drugs are the same for children as for adults (Daniels, 2002). A pilot study with Orlistat treatment showed that obese prepubertal children were able to reduce their fat intake to avoid gastrointestinal side effects. The results of this study suggest that Orlistat may be a suitable component in a behavior-modification treatment program for weight reduction in obese children (Norgren et al., 2003).

12.7 Surgical Interventions

Gastric surgery has also been used in adolescents aged 11 to 19 years. Subjects were interviewed an average of 6 years postoperatively. The mean preoperative

BMI was 47 whilet at follow-up, BMI averaged 32. Two-thirds of the patients weighed within 9 kg of their lowest postsurgical weight at the time of followup, and three patients had sought additional obesity surgery. Excellent psychosocial adjustment, improved self-esteem and social relationships, and a more satisfying appearance were reported by these patients, but compliance with exercise and dietary instructions was poor. Long-term patient monitoring and commitment are recommended, as for example, prescribed multivitamin and calcium supplements were taken only by a limited number of subjects (Rand and MacGregor, 1994). However, when gastric banding was used in another clinical study of seven obese adolescent boys, a long-term weight loss without daily vomiting was achieved only in one boy. Therefore, gastric banding was not recommended during adolescence (Hölcke, Norgeren, and Danielsson, 2004). However, laparoscopically performed gastric banding had a good result in a 13-year-old subject with morbid obesity and end-stage renal insufficiency, which caused lifesaving weight loss and hemodialysis (Knerr et al., 2003).

Plastic surgery was suggested for the improvement of the consequences of important weight loss (that is, more than 30 kg) in morbidly obese adolescents. Abdominal and mammary ptosis and adipose gynecomastia on the trunk, and wing-like arm deformities and lipomeria of the medial aspect of the thigh on the limbs, were observed. At the facial and neck level, usually no changes were found. Irritations with maceration and skin surinfection (Malandry et al., 1998) that can result in a sepsis were also revealed. Psychological complications due to such a situation are commonplace, so the intervention with the help of plastic surgery has to be considered, especially in more serious cases. The procedures are almost the same as in adults, with this complementary treatment being determined by close cooperation between pediatrician and plastic surgeon (Malandry et al., 1998).

12.8 Intragastric Balloon Therapy

This form of intervention was reported in five morbidly obese adolescents aged 11 to 17.7 years with a BMI between 30.3 to 52.7 kg/m^{-2} who previously failed to lose weight with a conventional weight-loss program. Balloons filled with 4 to 600 ml saline solution were given during general anesthesia. Vomiting and abdominal distension lasted only 1 day. Weight loss after 3 months was between 3.5 to 14.5 kg; however, after another 6 months, all subjects had regained the initial weight lost, or gained more weight than before the treatment. The feeling of abdominal distension and early satiety lasted only 1 to 2 weeks. In two subjects, spontaneous deflation of the balloon occurred with a spontaneous loss per annum in one of them after 6 months. No further complications were observed after the removal of the balloons at 6 to 7 months, but the results showed that gastric balloons had only a transitory effect on weight loss in morbidly obese adolescents and that other approaches should be used (Bollen et al., 1998).

12.9 Alternative Approaches

In addition to the combination of diet and exercise, auricular acupuncture was used in weight-reduction treatment in obese subjects aged 16 to 70 years in Taiwan. The rate of effectiveness was 86.7% and weight rebound was only 6.7%. The effectiveness of weight reduction was significantly correlated with the compliance of participants with each therapeutic method and not with age. No side effects were reported (Huang, Yang, and Hu, 1996).

The efficacy of acupuncture as a method for weight reduction was assessed in obese children. Electro-acupuncture had a beneficial effect on various pathogenic components in obese children. This was manifested by a cessation of subjective complaints, increased weight and fat loss, increased performance level and increased efficiency of the cardiovascular system, and a decrease in serum lipids to normal values. Therefore, the authors recommended this method in comprehensive treatment of children with constitutional exogenic obesity (Gadzhiev et al., 1993).

12.10 Psychological and Behavioral Treatment

A cognitive-behavioral training program, which includes in a more marked way well-established behavioral methods, was also used together with diet and exercise (EG) for weight reduction at the age of 9 to 19 years, as compared to group of obese children treated only by diet and exercise (CG). The effect of 6 weeks' inpatient rehabilitation was followed with regard to somatic and psychological changes in both EG and CG. Significant improvements in self-reported eating behaviors and self-reported quality of life were achieved, and the prevalence of obesity tended to decrease more in EG than in CG (Warsburger et al., 2001).

Treatment oriented not only to somatic but also psychosocial approaches comprised nine outpatient sessions during 3 months, and resulted in a decrease of BMI and body fat mass (measured by BIA). Psychosocial variables were raised on the basis of the scale "self-portrait" on Seitz and Rausche's personality questionnaire for children. After treatment, anxiety and inferiority improved significantly, and also higher values in the scale "over-estimation of the self" were obtained (Lehrke and Laessle, 2002).

12.11 Summary

For obesity treatment, various approaches are used, most often diet, exercise, and psychological intervention. In addition, hormonal, pharmacological, and surgical methods are used. The results of studies are again not homogenous depending on the characteristics of subjects (e.g., initial age, degree of sexual maturation, gender, duration of obesity), and combination and duration of treatment. Therefore, to start with, a proper characteristic of subjects as individuals (anthropometric, nutritional, functional, psychological as described before) is indispensable. Treatment can have, however, both desirable positive as well as negative consequences, so the choice of adequate means should be cautious. Family support during treatment is an essential factor for the success of permanent weight loss. Individual treatment gives mostly better results than a group approach, depending on the character of subjects, and the same holds true for inpatient or outpatient (that is ambulatory, school-based, etc.) treatment.

A diet that is based on the individual characteristics and medical history of the child, which results from the WHO recommendations (considering also physical activity and energy expenditure) is most often used. In the case of moderate obesity, "growing up" to an adequate value of weight can be accepted, but mostly special recommendations are used. Reduction of energy intake, mostly of fat and sugar, is used, and the increase of healthy foodstuffs (e.g., vegetable, fruit, skimmed milk products) is recommended. Very low calorie diets (VLCD) are acceptable for morbid obesity but must be used under medical supervision. Positive changes as followed in subjects of preschool, school, and adolescent age — reduction of body weight, BMI and of total, subcutaneous, visceral fat accompanied by the change of serum lipids (decrease of TC, LDL-C, TG, Apo B, and increase of HDL, Apo A 1), decrease of insulin, and IGF 1, BP 1, BP 3, IGF 1/IGF 3 level and other factors — were found after dietary treatment. Negative consequences of reduction treatment include slowdown of growth in height and of lean, fat-free body mass along with further changes. Supplemented diets (PUFA, fiber, etc.) were used in some studies with positive results. Leptin level decreased along with insulin level and insulin resistance, and insulin sensitivity increased. Also, T3, REE, RMR, along with FFM, decreased.

Exercise used alone often does not change BMI and body weight in a marked way, which can be due to a simultaneous increase of lean, FFM, and reduction of fat. Dynamic, aerobic exercise increasing energy expenditure (EE) is preferable, but could be difficult for more obese subjects, so, for example, resistance training is also used, which improves somatic parameters and metabolic fitness. Longitudinal studies showed many positive effects of regular and sufficiently intensive exercise, even with increased energy intake (EI), for example, increase of lean, FFM without changes in

BMI, improved aerobic capacity, and of other parameters of physical and motor performance. Optimal balance between EI and EE can be more easily achieved with increased than with lowered values. Other longitudinal studies showed that interruption of exercise was followed by increased deposition of fat, often with decreased energy intake. Animal experiments contributed to the understanding of adaptive mechanisms for exercise (for example, a higher lipolytic activity and higher use of lipids as energy source, even at rest, and during workload was found).

The effect of exercise was apparent in obese subjects, who were losing weight and excess fat, experienced improved aerobic and motor fitness, better economy of work, improved serum lipid profiles, hemostatic variables, bone density, decrease of leptin and insulin, and peak C-peptide response, to name a few examples. Cardiorespiratory parameters also improved. The best solution was the combination of diet and exercise therapy with psychological intervention (which alone can have significant positive effects) as all mentioned consequences of dietary or exercise therapy were mostly more efficient and longer lasting. Along with improved serum lipid profiles and hormonal changes (e.g., decrease of T3, T4, GH U, adrenocortical activity, insulin, leptin, interleukin), increase in homocysteine, improvement of hemostatic risk profiles, increase of bone mineral content, along with reduction of BMI, FM, waist and hip circumference and their ratio, were observed. Physical and motor performance specially tested also improved along with better economy of work and reduced heart rate during workload.

Also hormonal therapy, for example, using growth hormone (GH) had positive results, indicating stimulated catecholamine lipolysis, and direct effect on leptin decrease. Leptin therapy has been largely ineffective in humans; however, some improvements after subcutaneous injections of leptin have been reported recently. Pharmacological intervention, in spite of some success in weight reduction, was not yet generally recommended in pediatric treatment. Surgical therapy as gastric banding showed some negative results before finishing growth, similarly as gastric balloon therapy; plastic surgery, however, can correct some negative effects of morbid obesity (abdominal and mammary ptosis). Alternative therapy as acupuncture was reported to give good results. In some cases psychological and behavioral therapy alone was used also with desirable results, especially when other approaches could not be applied.

13

Practical Programs for Weight Management during the Growing Years

Interventions in early childhood may have a substantial effect on the lifestyle behaviors of an individual, particularly with respect to dietary intake and physical activity or exercise (Dietz, 2004). There are numerous opportunities for young people to learn good eating habits — for example, using the medium of computer games at school and profiting from the topical nature of this technology. The effect of such proactive approaches can be substantial and capitalize on a high-interest factor for most children. The introduction of healthy food habits from a young age is particularly important for children who have had an impaired food intake (Turnin et al., 1998). The importance of the childhood diet in the prevention of adult obesity is essential and must start early (Scaglioni et al., 1999), as is the case for a proper involvement in physical activity (Molnar, 1999; Pařízková, Maffeis, and Poskitt, 2002; Suskind et al., 2000).

13.1 Arrangement of Weight-Management Programs for Obese Children

As mentioned in the previous chapter, the combined approach of diet, exercise, and behavior modification in weight management programs gives the best and often permanent results. It has also been demonstrated that for both diet and exercise regimes, it is essential to adhere to the monitored change on an ongoing basis. This may be difficult in a situation where only one individual in a family is attempting a lifestyle modification. The preference is for all family members to assist the child by following and benefiting from the same lifestyle changes.

As previously mentioned, an alternative approach is to employ an inpatient treatment program. This type of approach is rare given the cost and lack of suitable space; institutions may be unwilling or unable to commit the necessary resources. However, this approach is the most suitable for the treatment of morbidly obese children (Deforche et al., 2003). Summer camps or health clubs offer similar possibilities for obese children, particularly where the necessary supervision for both diet and exercise can be guaranteed (Gately, Cooke, and Mackreth, 1998; Gately et al., 2000). The better possibility for most obese children is a supervised activity program as a distinct component of a school or university clinic setting. The school-based approach may be an after-school or holiday period opportunity. In the university-based clinic of one of the authors, targeted KidFit activity programs provide an on-site opportunity for young people to be active in a fun, group setting. There are other examples of similar approaches. For example, pilot school obesity prevention programs with long-lasting multifaceted and sustainable activities involving children only have been suggested and resulted in positive behavioral changes (Warren et al., 2003). Other special programs such as the Chicago project, which uses an ecological approach to obesity prevention, have been cited (Longjohn, 2004). Some effort has also been directed to special populations such as the multicomponent program for obesity prevention (involving diet, exercise, family involvement, and school curriculum) in elementary schools serving American Indian communities (Caballero et al., 2003). Interventions aimed at reducing overweight and obesity should be culturally specific and target young children —for example, the New York City WIC population program (Nelson, Chiasson, and Ford, 2004).

Residential or inpatient programs in special centers that enable more consistent intervention, with regard to moderately restricted diet, physical activity programs, and psychological support, result in the decrease of fat and improving physical performance (Braet et al., 2003; Deforche, De Bourdeaudhuij, and Hills, 2003). A 2-month rehabilitation program in a specialized institute and following 6 weeks of continued diet and exercise at home decreased weight and increased the ability to oxidize lipids during exercise in obese adolescents (Brandou et al., 2003).

13.1.1   Ambulatory and Outpatient Programs

The combination of diet and sport has been used successfully as an ambulatory program for obese children. For example, an outpatient program attended by obese children aged 9 to 13 years over 1 year consisted of a diet of 1200 kcal.day,$^{-1}$ exercise 3 times per week, and psychological support. The results of this therapy were an increased level of physical performance, improved coordination and endurance, and greater self-confidence. A reduction of approximately 20% of the initial weight was achieved but only in the age range of 12 to 13 years. The younger children achieved only a smaller reduction. During the initial period of this study, HDL-C decreased but increased within 4 to 5 months to exceed pretreatment levels. No vitamin deficiencies were reported (Korsten-Reck et al., 1990).

Primary (elementary) school-based programs have been well defined as effective means of preventing obesity during childhood. For example, Sahota et al. (1998) included dietary interventions with nutritional education incorporated in the curriculum. Policy changes included snacks consumed during breaks, "Fit Is Fun" programs with improved playground facilities, the development of after-school physical activities, and such activities as cooking, health weeks, and competitions. The program was extremely popular with the participants, and it was recommended that similar programs could be of great assistance in the prevention of obesity.

The effects of various levels of physical activity have also been reported in Italian children aged 9 to 14 years (Di.S.Co. project: experimental community project for preventing chronic-degenerative diseases). The program included nutritional habits and status, anthropometric parameters, and motor abilities. This study underlined the widespread trend of poor nutritional habits (including of those enrolled in regular sports activities) and a poor attitude toward voluntary physical activity. The school has a privileged opportunity to help in the promotion of healthy lifestyles and the correction of poor habits starting from the early period of growth (Caldarone et al., 1995), and there have been a range of programs to increase physical activity and exercise since (Fox, 2004).

Group programs that do not rely on the use of special diets and standardized training programs but that instead concentrate on changing food and physical activity habits can also be very effective. For example, Vitolo et al. (1998) used programmed monthly meetings of obese Brazilian children aged 13 to 15 years with pediatricians, nutritionists, physical educators, and psychologists. The result was a decline of BMI from 36.0 to 30.3 $kg.m^{-2}$ after approximately 9 months. The key to success in this approach was the management of children in a group setting and a sharing of experiences.

Outpatient programs should aim to maintain a permanent increase in energy expenditure through participation in a mixture of organized (structured) and unstructured exercise. This should be over and above the non-negotiable habitual or everyday physical activity. Children should be stimulated and encouraged to undertake as much as possible of usual physical activities such as walking, climbing steps, household tasks, work in the yard, and so on. If this is achieved, it is possible to increase the level of functional capacity and physical fitness, which then makes it possible to adhere to exercise and sport programs more readily and comfortably. In addition, the enhancement of body awareness plays an important role in adherence to regular physical activity (Fox, 2004). Examples of body awareness activities for young children are provided later in the chapter.

Long-lasting changes in eating habits that result in weight and fat reduction may have a greater chance of success through individual consultations and regular checkups of parameters such as BMI, skinfolds, serum lipids, and other biochemical parameters. Tracking of functional testing during standard and maximal workloads on a bicycle ergometer or treadmill is also particularly valuable and enables a fine-tuning of exercise prescription.

Consultations with staff of the ambulatory center should wherever possible include the parents to assure the maximum involvement and cooperation of the family. Eating habits and food choice should be controlled with the help of interviews and the completion of diaries over a 3- to 10-day period. This approach is difficult in young children and so should involve parents. Meaningful records from children may be possible only in late childhood and adolescence due to an inability of younger children to accurately record detailed responses because of lack of experience and developmental age. Discussion of results should occur with the child and at least one, but preferably both, parents. Greater success is possible in modifying the nutritional habits of children if parents have an adequate and well-balanced approach to their own eating.

Outpatient treatment programs have been utilized more often recently and should focus on specific living conditions and eating behaviors of the family, as well as the age and self-control of both the child and other members of the family, especially the father (Weyhreter et al., 2003).

Family pediatricians should take responsibility for the management of obese children in their offices. A 12-month study showed that when a positive, long-lasting active contact with obese children and their families was maintained, individual children's ability to lose weight was enhanced (Nova, Russo, and Sala, 2001). Children who completed the family-based behavioral weight-control program with regular visits and treatment interventions were successful in moderating weight gain, and there appeared to be positive effects on the children's mood and eating-disorder symptoms (Levine et al., 2001). The importance of the involvement of parents in the treatment and management of obese children is clearly demonstrated in the findings of Wake et al. (2002), which indicated that parents often underestimate the degree of obesity and resulting health risks, and do not show concern.

13.1.2 Treatment in Summer Camps

A combined approach to weight management using both diet and exercise can be implemented and controlled in healthy obese individuals with inpatient treatment. However, a better and more natural option for children (other than school-based programs) is to participate in summer camps. Such camps have been run successfully in several countries in the past. For example, in the former Czechoslovakia starting in the 1950s (Pařízková, 1963a,b, 1972, 1977; Kalvachová et al., 1986; Lísková, Hošek, and Stožický, 1998) camps were used to great effect and saw improvements in body composition and functional capacity of many of their participants (Pařízková, Maffeis, and Poskitt, 2002).

In the United Kingdom, a 3-year follow-up of an 8-week diet and exercise program for children attending a weight-loss camp was completed by Gately, Cooke, and Mackreth (1998). A group of children entered the program in 1994, and then returned in 1995, 1996, and 1997. Body weight and height were assessed during each program, in which energy intake was restricted to 1600 kcal per day and the daily exercise prescription was five 1.5-hour sessions. This program was structured using fun and skill-based activities, which provided children with the necessary motor abilities to participate in physical activity with peers when they returned to their home environment. Educational information on nutrition, exercise, and lifestyle was also included. BMI decreased from 30.2 (pre-1994) to 25.5 kg/m^2 (1997). Seventy-seven percent of subjects had reduced their BMI after the 3-year program. These results indicate that a program that concentrates on increasing the skills and improving the motor habits necessary for participation in sport activities helps produce successful lifestyle alterations. This program, initiated by the Leeds Metropolitan University, continues and was reimplemented in the summer of 1999 for children aged 11 to 17 years using the same principles, with additional data provided by Gately et al. (2000).

The effectiveness of the complex treatment of obese children in a sanitarium-type camp has also been ascertained in Russian children (Lebedkova et al., 1984). The results of similar summer camps for obese children have also been reported from other countries (Southam et al., 1984) and have involved 4-day stays, with 4 hours daily spent learning and practicing eating and exercise skills conducive to weight loss. In conjunction, the parents of obese children involved met weekly to discuss the program content and to explore their role in the management of their children's weight. A significant reduction in body weight, percent of overweight, and skinfold thickness was achieved. Improvements were also shown in self-reported personal habits and participants' knowledge of weight-management concepts. The results of this form of obesity management reveals that an intensive program of eating and exercise behavior instruction, practice, and monitoring can be particularly effective under conditions similar to a home setting, which may have special importance for children of this age range (Southam et al., 1984).

A study by Jirapinyo et al. (1995) reported on the impact of a 4-week camp on Thai children with moderate or severe obesity aged 8 to 13 years. Dietary restriction during the time at the camp and dietary self-control at home were incorporated. Various types of exercise, including swimming and group therapy, were included in the program. Weekly sightseeing trips outside the camp added to the interest and motivation of children; in fact, this feature was attractive for all participants. After the program, children lost on average approximately 5% of their initial weight; most of the weight loss was due to the reduction of stored fat and not of lean body mass. The conduct of the camp-based program did not cause any complications. These results provide further justification of the suitability of this approach for the treatment of childhood obesity, especially during the initial periods.

Treatment in a summer camp using a group approach to management also resulted in a more marked and longer lasting weight loss in a group of obese Belgian children (Braet, Van Winckel, and Van Leuwen, 1997). This work continues to provide evidence of the success of such interventions in Belgium (Deforche, De Bourdeaudhuij, and Hills, 2003). A further example is a study of Polish obese adolescents treated in a 3-week long summer camp using energy restriction (5.51 MJ.day⁻¹) and exercise, which resulted in a significant weight loss and positive changes in body composition. However, in this study the results were gender dependent, with better results for boys than girls (Jeszka, Regula, and Kostrzewa-Tarnowska, 1999).

A number of pediatric weight-loss programs have also been reported in Taiwan. In a "pediatric-obesity club," four fundamental components — diet, exercise, behavior modification, and the involvement of parents — were included in a treatment program. In this family-based, parent-directed program, 11% of the participants showed a decrease in the degree of obesity after a 1-year follow-up, compared to 3% of a control group. In another individualized outpatient counseling clinic, the success rate was 59% after 1 year. Although the continued long-term effectiveness of this approach cannot be determined, it seems that a realistic and culturally sensitive weight-reduction program should be developed for each country. There is an urgent need for Asian countries such as Taiwan to develop such programs as early as possible because the prevalence of obesity is on the increase (Chen, 1997; Pařízková and Chin, 2003).

13.1.3   School-Based Programs

Schools have the opportunity, mechanisms, and personnel to deliver nutrition education, to promote physical fitness, and in many cases, to provide a school food service capable of preparing an adequate diet suitable for the prevention of excess deposition of fat. A 2-year longitudinal study on the effect of an enhanced physical activity program and modified school lunch program was conducted of elementary school children in Nebraska (Donelly et al., 1995). At year 2, lunches had significantly less energy (9%), fat (25%), and sodium (21%), and more fiber (17%). Physical activity in the classroom was 6% greater in the intervention groups, but physical activity outside school was approximately 16% less for the pupils comprising the intervention group compared to control pupils without intervention. No significant differences were found for body weight, stored fat, cholesterol, insulin, and glucose. However, HDL-C was significantly greater and TC/HDL-C was significantly less for the intervened pupils compared to the controls. This finding indicates that the total volume, and especially the intensity and mode of exercise during selected periods, might significantly influence at least some parameters in spite of the lack of differences in the total amount of activity. A regular intervention in the management of physical activity programs is necessary in order to make these programs more efficient on a broader scale. A school-based randomized controlled trial was prepared for prevention of obesity in American Indian schoolchildren (Caballero et al., 2003).

Bar-Or et al. (1998) has rightly suggested that schools are in a strong position to encourage and provide physical activity opportunities for all children but particularly for the overweight and obese. Logically, staff with the necessary expertise, whether this be physical and health educators, school nurses, or sports coaches, are well placed to provide innovative and targeted assistance. Further, most schools have a range of physical facilities and equipment on-site without the need to consider a move to other venues. Most schools are also underutilized, certainly outside of school hours.

There are also great opportunities to use break times for physical activity during the school day as well as before and after school and in specified time slots on weekends. The school academic year is also very short, with long holiday periods dotted throughout. Such times provide prime opportunities during which activity programs could be offered.

One contributing factor to the increase in overweight and obesity in the pediatric years has been the demise of physical education at school. School physical education, if used effectively, is a major avenue for the promotion of physical activity among children. During the childhood years (approximately 5 to 7 years of age), the young start to make comparisons between their physical performance and that of their peers. Children are conscious of the potential rewards associated with success in physical activity, such as feelings of competency and mastery, improvements in self-esteem, and the accolades of others. It is important that children's perceptions and considerations of the value of participating in physical activity be recognized (Hills, 1995). These include fun and enjoyment, health and fitness, the desire to learn new skills, the chance to achieve, and friendship and cooperation.

13.2 Principles of Weight Reduction Diets for Obese Children

In the treatment and prevention of childhood obesity, an adequate and monitored food intake is essential. Taking into account the physiological situation of a child during growth, dietary treatment should be aimed mainly toward an improvement in the composition of the diet. This includes the recommended ratio of the main macronutrients, an adherence to recommended daily allowances (RDAs), and monitoring of the energy content of ingested meals. As mentioned in Chapter 7, in more severe cases of childhood obesity, hypocaloric diets or special protein-sparing diets restricted in energy have a place in obesity management.

Every child has a unique personality, and this relates to and includes nutritional and motor components. The term "nutritional individuality," coined by Widdowson (1962), reflects the individual variability that exists in approaches to nutrition. The more that is known about a child and his or her eating habits, the greater the chance of having an impact in the rectification of the child's health problems, including obesity. A sound knowledge and understanding also minimizes the chance of making fundamental errors of judgment that may be critical to the success of the treatment process. The relationships between present diet and, for example, the risk for cardiovascular diseases in children from predisposed families are not always clear.

However, families need guidance to change dietary patterns to prevent further future diseases and health complications (Kelley et al., 2004).

General guidelines for treatment should reflect the combined needs of a compatible reduction of excess fat and preservation or an increase of lean body mass, with a continued increase in height. These features, along with an improvement in functional capacity and other necessary qualities of the organism, should be the major goals. Another important treatment principle is to respect food and physical activity preferences. For example, no child should be forced to eat meals and foods they dislike because an adult deems this to be appropriate. It is far more preferable, although potentially difficult, to structure a diet according to the child's preferences. It may be necessary to patiently experiment in order to find what is believed to be the most acceptable to the child. If this is achieved, there is greater hope of the child adhering to the modified diet, and the result might be a long-lasting or permanent change in eating behavior.

13.2.1   Definition of a Reduction Diet

RDAs for normal healthy children and adolescents have been defined with respect to the individual age categories and gender from birth to the late teens. This means that it is not possible during growth to give one detailed general RDA and recipe aimed at weight, BMI, and fat reduction, with respect to energy, macronutrients, and vitamin and mineral composition for all obese youth. This is often expected but is not possible if the goal is a positive, lasting result of individual reduction treatment. One suggested procedure for defining an adequate diet is described next.

One of the most important principles is the use of an individual approach according to the child's health status, physical fitness, and psychological traits. Consequently, a medical examination by a pediatrician as well as consultations with a nutritionist and other specialists are necessary. Physical activity habits and exercise recommendations should also be considered. In addition, co-morbidities need to be identified and, where necessary, treated simultaneously.

A comprehensive analysis of the history of food intake, including the dietary habits of the individual, should be undertaken prior to prescribing a recommended diet. A range of options is available. The most suitable and feasible option is the inventory method, which uses daily diaries over 1 week and preferably during at least 3 weekdays and 1 weekend day. The food frequency method can also be used. Similarly, these assessments should be representative of the usual dietary regime of the child. When necessary, more sophisticated and demanding approaches may need to be implemented.

On the basis of such analyses, an individualized dietary intake should be defined for each child. The composition of the diet should correspond to the RDAs of WHO, EU, and the U.S. Academy of Science, which all recommend 12–13% of total energy intake from protein, up to 30% of fat and 50–60% of carbohydrates. Proteins should comprise 50% from animal origin and 50%

from plant origin. Also, the composition of fat should include one-third from saturated, one-third from monounsaturated, and the rest as polyunsaturated fats. Carbohydrates should be mostly complex polysaccharides (dark bread, cereals, and so on), and 10% of the energy intake should be sugar (WHO, 1985).

Depending on previous practices, some food items may need to be reduced, especially if they were ingested in excessive quantities before. According to numerous authors, this mainly concerns fats (especially saturated fats) and simple sugars. The combination of these items in sweets is a significant risk for the deposition of excess fat. However, the level of physical activity should also be taken into account (see Table 5.1 and Table 5.2), even though it is usually low in obese youth. Thus the energy content and composition of the diet for each individual can be assured. Such foods should be replaced by other items, such as fruits and vegetables. An individual approach considering the age, gender, degree and duration of obesity, and energy output is also necessary. Table 5.3 provides an example for an obese child. Diet and nutritional management, especially concerning energy and the main macronutrient intake of the child, should follow the results of treatment and be modified according to the results achieved. This means that food intake becomes less restricted and monitored when some positive change of BMI and fatness have been achieved, and when the subjects are able to exercise more, for example.

Vitamin and mineral content in the diet should always correspond to the RDAs for the particular age and gender of the child. In the case of a more markedly reduced food intake, which provides a certain risk of some deficiencies, these items may need to be supplemented.

The frequency, timing, and regularity of meals and the consumption of the necessary major nutrients during the day are very important. For example, skipping breakfast and ingesting the majority of energy during the second half of the day, particularly having a large meal for dinner, may provide a higher risk for obesity in some individuals. A regular intake of meals, which may be at least five smaller meals, starting with an adequate breakfast in the morning and including a good lunch and a light evening meal, should be the goal. Better control over the time of eating may be just as important for many children as any individual component of the prescribed diet. For example, discouraging eating prior to going to bed, when there is little further potential to increase energy expenditure until the following day, is an important goal. Similarly, limiting the size of bites and also the speed of eating are important eating behaviors to change if needed (Brownell, 1984; Brownell and Kaye, 1982; Epstein et al., 1982, 1990, 2001; 1984; Mahan, 1987).

The consumption of regular snacks, particularly those high in energy such as chips, corn, and sweets, must be progressively reduced. This is also the case for all delicacies and foods high in saturated fats. These foods must be limited and/or eventually eliminated as their intake correlates with an increase in weight (Nicklas et al., 2003). The same applies to the consumption of food and drinks that commonly contain a high amount of sucrose. These habits should include the replacement of high levels of soft drinks by eating more fruit that is not too sweet (apples, grapefruit, oranges, strawberries, kiwi fruit) and vegetables (tomatoes, raw cucumbers, cabbage). These changes may be difficult as children are not accustomed to eating these food items because they are "addicted" to various widely advertised energy-dense snacks. However, when some weight and fat reduction is achieved (i.e., BMI is closer to normal values), due to the concurrent growth process and energy and substrate needs for the recommended increased exercise, the individual may modify the intake of the above-mentioned items, in particular sweets, because children usually feel the elimination of sweets is very undesirable.

Drinking an adequate amount of fresh water (when available) or gaseous water with lemon juice or a small amount of nonsweetened fruit juice is also a priority. Obese children need to be properly hydrated, but at the same time it is necessary to prevent an increased intake of energy from inadequate beverages. The same principle applies for normal-weight children, especially in parts of the world where water losses from the body are increased due to the climate. An adequate intake of liquids is critical.

A general principle for the use of reduction diets for obese children is to only make the necessary reduction in energy intake on the basis of energy needs of each particular child. When the degree of obesity, overall health, and functional status is well defined, energy intake should be lower than for a child with normal weight. In special cases of severe or morbid obesity, a protein-sparing, very low energy diet or classical hypocaloric diet is warranted. On the basis of a number of studies, the use of such an approach over a short period of time does not have negative consequences. The implementation of such restricted diets is mainly recommended if another health problem exists concurrently with obesity. Restricted diets must be used only under strict medical supervision, preferably in a controlled environment, such as an inpatient department in a hospital or children's clinic. Under normal family or school conditions, severe dietary restrictions should be avoided.

The purpose of this volume is not to provide a list of special recipes for individual meals for obese children of different ages and degrees and duration of obesity, but rather to define and specify the main guidelines. Fundamentally, it is necessary to appreciate that a detailed and unified approach common for all children who need to reduce excess fat cannot be prepared. To ensure the successful impact of a diet, the nutritional and physical individuality of each child or adolescent must be respected. This includes the conditions and dynamics of the obese individual's family and the broader environment. For example, it is counterproductive to insist that a child eat a food that he or she has hated since early childhood. The choice of meals, especially at the beginning of treatment and management, should be adjusted for each obese individual.

Similarly, a diet aimed at reducing body fat in a younger child with a moderate degree of obesity would be quite different and much easier to define than a diet for an older individual with more developed, longer-lasting obesity. The avoidance of difficult cases of prolonged obesity in children and adolescents is another argument for the effective prevention of obesity during growth.

The role of the family and an appreciation, knowledge, and understanding of the whole environment is essential (Golan and Crow, 2004). As mentioned on numerous occasions throughout this volume, there may be a much greater challenge to treatment and management when only one child in the family is obese and other members are of normal weight. The role of the mother or responsible adult who is preparing the meals is a pivotal and often difficult one. From the commencement of management, at least as a start, meals should be the same or similar for the whole family so as not to make the child feel segregated and mistreated. When all members of the family, especially siblings who are not obese, have some solidarity and accept the fact that they should eat the same or similar meals as their obese brother or sister, the process of management may have more chance of success. The diet should serve as a good model for all members of the family; after all, food habits may have been suboptimal for others. They, too, may be at risk of obesity in the longer term if poor dietary practices were to continue. There is always the possibility of supplementing the energy intake of other family members as necessary when the obese child is not present. After a period of time, the obese child may more readily accept his or her special position and be happy to eat a different meal than others if this is necessary. This degree of acceptance and attitude is more likely when the child is supported and treated appropriately from a psychological perspective and, most important, self-identifies with the necessary regime of changing nutrition and physical activity (Pařízková, Maffeis, and Poskitt, 2002).

13.2.2 The Effectiveness of Reduction Diets

Weight regain can occur, as shown by some studies. The influence of weight-reducing diets (studied using the same amount of energy but different proportions of protein and carbohydrate) on body weight and composition was followed after the end of treatment and then after 2 years (Rolland-Cachera et al., 2004). A weight loss of 30.3 kg was compensated by a weight increase of 21.3 kg, and BMI z-scores returned to baseline levels after 2 years. For all measurements, no dietary group differences existed at baseline or at any time during intervention or follow-up. Energy intake, physical activity, and snacking did not change positively. Substantial weight loss was obtained with a moderate energy-restricted diet with normal fat content. After weight loss, mean weight increased in spite of moderate energy intake, together with the drift toward obesity-associated behavioral patterns. The causes of the inability to permanently change nutritional behavior should be studied further. The obesogenic environment, such as food advertising, should also be considered (Ashton, 2004).

The yo-yo effect is less frequent in children and youth during continuing growth, but may appear from natural causes, such as the acceleration of growth during certain periods. However, mainly in adolescent girls the fluctuating effort to lose weight can result in the yo-yo phenomenon, which may lead to anorexia, bulimia, and similar problems. In this respect, the effect of mass media may also be undesirable.

A proper adjustment of the family diet to prevent obesity or to assist in the treatment of a mild degree of obesity in a young child by appropriate and smaller dietary modifications is needed. In summary, the examination of energy balance and turnover is critical. A modest reduction in the energy intake and a substantial increase in energy output through physical activity and exercise are desired. This lifestyle approach provides the best guarantee against obesity development. Dieting, especially alone, is not "natural" for a growing child, so the increase of energy expenditure along with a monitored diet seems to be the best way to achieve lasting results.

13.3 The Behavioral Aspect of Dietary Therapy

Psychological intervention has been identified as an important part of the equation of treatment and management and includes participation by the family of an obese child. This also involves dietary behavior and addresses not only the amount of food according to the RDAs on energy and individual items but also recommendations for the selection and preference of special foods, as well as regime of dietary intake during the day, as related to other activities (see Chapter 7).

The utilization of behavior management may well have an important place in the process, but does require the necessary understanding of the techniques involved and must be seen as a component rather than the stand-alone option or answer. Successful behavior management requires a combined approach, cognizant of the complexity of the condition and its multifactor etiology. A comprehensive approach is necessary as the human mind cannot simply be subdivided into various parts in which different types of treatment and management are used. Behavioral therapy has an important place in management but may be more effective when considered in the broader context (Flodmark, 1999; Flodmark and Lissau, 2002). The attitude of the child and of his or her family with regard to the nutritional regime aimed at a decrease in body weight and fat is a significant aspect that can either enhance or reduce the effect of the treatment.

13.4 Defining General Principles of Physical Activity and Exercise for the Obese Child

An increased energy output through physical activity and exercise is an essential component of the weight-management process (Fox, 2004; Maziekas et al., 2003). The choice of activities must reflect the physical capabilities of each individual but be dominated by dynamic, weight-bearing aerobic exercise. This may be challenging or in some cases extremely difficult in children with excessive fat deposition. This type of activity increases the aerobic power and enhances the increased mobilization and utilization of lipid metabolites. Including ordinary activities such as commuting to school are also considered very important (Tudor-Locke et al., 2002b; Hills and Cambourne, 2002). In some populations, such as in China, children's walking and biking are much more common, with a more limited time spent TV viewing. More assessments should be conducted to monitor the effect of this situation, including the increased mechanization in many countries where habitual physical activity has been more common than in North America (Tudor-Locke, Ainsworth, and Adair 2003).

A dynamic, weight-bearing workload is possible in growing individuals with a mild degree of obesity. In cases where obesity is more advanced, the starting activities may be limited to exercises in the swimming pool, which allow the individual to benefit from the Archimedes principle. After some initial success in weight reduction and an improvement in the level of fitness in the aquatic activities, the larger individual would benefit from a progressive introduction of specific exercises in a lying or sitting posture. Depending on the age and interest of the individual, this may include work on a bicycle or rowing ergometer, or resistance-training exercises supplemented by some weight-bearing activities.

As soon as appropriate for the individual, but usually following further improvement in body composition and functional capacity, it is possible to include a proportion of the mainstream exercises and sport activities as would be prescribed for normal-weight children. This approach also serves to assist in the maintenance of the results achieved during the earlier phases of the weight-management program (Pařízková, Maffeis, and Poskitt, 2002). The level of overall free-living physical activity should be checked as exactly as possible to enable the evaluation of both distance covered (pedometers and accelerometers) and if possible the intensity of the activity (heart-rate monitoring) (Tudor-Locke et al., 2002).

Given the differences in the initial level of health, functional capacity, and physical performance, plus the different level of adaptation to a workload, the prescription for individual children is quite variable. Some obese children have good levels of motor and physical performance but many have an insufficient, low level of fitness. Because of the individual variability in health and fitness, it may be appropriate for children considered as candidates for weight management to be examined by a team of health professionals (pediatrician, physical educator, exercise physiologist, and psychologist). With the help of the child or adolescent, an appropriate exercise prescription can be defined. Inadequate and unrealistic workload demands on an obese child at the commencement of treatment and management can completely discourage the individual and jeopardize the potential for a positive outcome of the weight-management process.

Weight reduction during growth and development is not a natural trend for a young person. It is necessary to be conscious of this and guard against any compromise to the normal development of height, lean, fat-free body mass including all individual systems. This also has implications for physical fitness and performance, which usually improves following weight loss. The aim in the weight-management process should be to optimize these functions, which is possible when using the right factors. The most important goal should not be forgotten. The aim of a weight-management program should not, in the first instance, be only to decrease body weight and fat, but rather to improve functional, motor, psychological, behavioral, and all other aspects.

13.4.1 Aims of Physical Activity and Exercise Interventions

The primary aims of intervention for children and adolescents should be to promote confidence and enjoyment in physical activity and enhance the physical well-being of an individual with the attainment of a desirable body composition. During growth, such an approach is of primary importance as it is necessary to influence the child to self-identify with all aspects of the weight-management process (Pařízková, Maffeis, and Poskitt, 2002). Physical activity interventions can be more difficult when compared to dietary interventions because the latter can be considered a regular part of everyday living and is incorporated into the family, school, and other life domains; this is mostly not the case for exercise under present conditions, especially in greater urban agglomerations. Therefore, physical activity interventions require more inventiveness, organization, and perseverance.

The objectives for improved opportunities in physical activity may be encompassed in the characteristic needs of children:

- The need for vigorous activity to promote optimal growth and development
- The need to maintain a desirable body weight and composition
- The need for regular physical activity along with a nutritious and well-balanced diet
- The need for physical and motor skill development to enable enjoyable participation in physical activity

- The need for involvement in group activities with peers of a similar size and shape to provide support and the opportunity for social interaction

The overweight or obese youngster should be mainstreamed into school and community activities at the earliest possible opportunity.

13.4.2 Attitudes of the Child

The expected outcomes for overweight and obese children who participate in a quality activity program can be summarized on the basis of relevant attitudes, knowledge, and skills, and which also apply to their attitudes with regard to diet. A positive emotional attitude of the child toward increased exercise might be critical to success in fat reduction.

A psychological focus should be incorporated in any interventions so the child achieves the following:

- An appreciation of one's own body as unique and desirable
- An understanding of the health benefits of a nutritious diet combined with regular physical activity
- An improvement in self-esteem and body image
- A tolerance and understanding of the capabilities and interests of others

13.4.3 Knowledge

The child should be provided with the necessary knowledge and understanding of the weight-management process, and the same information should be provided to all family members. Information may be provided from a physical educator, another teacher, teacher, parent, family member, or a friend. Knowledge and understanding should encompass the following:

- An understanding of a range of physical activities that suit the individual's interests and capabilities
- An understanding of one's body, its growth, development, and physical limitations as related to the diet
- A comprehension of the importance of regular physical activity

13.4.4 Skills

The achievement of an adequate level of motor and related skills is indispensable for the maintenance of a consistent and meaningful involvement in physical activity. An allied goal is to develop and maintain a reasonable level of health-related fitness with the following components in particular: cardiorespiratory endurance, flexibility, a desirable body composition, and muscular strength and endurance. Other goals include the following:

- Acquire motor skills: balance, agility, coordination, and speed
- Develop social skills: ability to accept oneself, and to tolerate and cooperate with others
- Develop a range of related sport and physical activity skills

In order to maximize the opportunity for individual and group success in the activity setting, the following guidelines are essential:

- Work hard to construct and maintain an appropriate psychological climate.
- Ensure that the appropriate design and delivery of activity sessions is of central importance.
- Ensure that group participants are sensitive to individual needs.
- Recognize good performance and measurement of personal improvement on an individual rather than a collective or comparative basis.
- Evaluate sessions and take special note of activities that were more or less popular.
- Keep in mind that a key to the receptiveness of participants is their perceived readiness to be involved and attempt particular types of activities.
- Work to ensure that opportunities for success in the physical activity setting are related to an emphasis on short-term goals and attempt to maximize motor skill development and learning.
- Evaluate individuals based on improvement and effort rather than solely on performance and ability.

Of overriding importance for the child is enjoyment and fun related to a perception of competence and accomplishment. The attractiveness of the activities and the nature of the activity setting have a major influence on the children's enjoyment. The interest taken by the teacher or responsible adult and their empathy for each individual are further influencing factors.

A major aim is to have children make a commitment to physical activity and value the physical activity choices they make. If innovative opportunities are provided to enhance activity and sessions are social experiences, in the longer term, there might be less of a reliance on clinic initiatives. The more home-based activities that are attempted and maintained, the more likely that self-responsibility will be maximized.

Responsible adults need to capitalize on the basic interest of children in movement, and this focus on movement should be started from a very young age. The center of this interest should be on the enhancement of fundamental motor skills. In time, when these skills are well developed, they can be extended progressively to sports-specific skills. A lack of skills interferes with the interest in exercise of an obese child, who is usually less proficient in many motor skills as compared to normal-weight peers.

To a large extent, particular aspects of the physical activity program should be well understood by the individual child. For example:

- The expectation of increased energy expenditure and the degree of tiredness and fatigue one might experience
- The purpose of the activity program
- The importance of being provided with feedback
- There is a graded increase in health and fitness expected but children should be aware that they should not experience excessive discomfort.

Aerobic exercise should be a specific focus of group activity programs and individual home-based programs with as much variety incorporated as possible. Examples of core activities include swimming, cycling, riding stationary bicycles, walking and jogging, treadmill walking and running, stair-climbing, and a wide range of active games. Water-based activities, particularly for those who are comfortable with the aquatic environment, can be particularly valuable. The benefits provided by enhanced buoyancy mean that even nonswimmers can be provided with a meaningful activity session. Aerobic work should be combined with a cross section of games, skill work, gymnastics, dance, and movement activities that are enjoyable.

Benefits cannot be maximized without careful planning and design and implementation of a quality program. High priority should be given to developing appropriate attitudes about physical activity and the associated health benefits. Understanding and emotional involvement is helpful for all children, which is always assisted by gradually improving skills.

The overweight child is at a distinct disadvantage when participating in most physical activities, especially when relocating the total body weight. Difficulties in participation tend to be a common reason for obese individuals to withdraw from vigorous activity. If this happens, it helps to perpetuate low levels of physical fitness and reduced motor skill development. Therefore, activities in a program should focus on increased levels of participation in conjunction with opportunities to enhance motor skills.

13.4.5 Factors to Enhance Program Design and Implementation

A number of additional factors may enhance program design and implementation:

- There should be a gradual progression from activities that promote a low level of energy expenditure to activities at a higher level. This should involve the provision and encouragement for maximal participation by every child.

- Caution must be taken to prevent injury in the activity setting. This consideration is important throughout the program but more critical in the early stages.

- Exercise must be vigorous enough to affect a training load on the cardiorespiratory system. Therefore, the intensity of exercise must be closely monitored in aerobic activity.

- Every attempt should be made to make activities enjoyable and, as a consequence, self-motivating.

- Overweight and obese individuals often recount poor experiences of physical activity, particularly where nonobese children have been present. While a major goal should always be to provide the necessary skills to facilitate the mainstreaming of the obese child in physical activity settings, initial success is enhanced when groups of overweight individuals work together.

- Water intake should never be restricted since this could result in dehydration.

13.4.6 Exercise Prescription

The current guidelines for exercise prescription for weight management in children and adolescents are general in nature; therefore, much work remains to be done to identify more specifically the amount, type, and intensity of exercise necessary to produce weight loss while maximizing desirable metabolic adaptations (Hills and Byrne, 1998; Lobstein, Baur, and Uauy, 2004).

Exercise prescription or exercise dose generally involves four integral components. The *mode* or type of exercise is reflected as cardiorespiratory (aerobic) training, resistance weight training, walking, swimming, or cycling. The *frequency* of exercise, or how often one exercises, is usually represented as the number of days per week or number of sessions per day an individual participates in. The *duration* of exercise, or period of time, is represented as total energy expended (kJ) or total energy (kJ.kg body weight^{-1}). *Intensity*, or how hard one works, is quantified as %VO$_2$ peak or maximum, % maximum heart rate (MHR), % heart rate reserve (HRR), rating of perceived exertion (RPE), lactate threshold, and metabolic equivalent (MET) (Hills and Byrne, 1998c; Hills, Byrne, and Ramage, 1998).

The goal for all overweight and obese children should be to increase their energy expenditure in an adequate way, that is, with an achievement of the necessary threshold intensity tolerable by the child. For those who have been largely inactive, a short dose of activity may be all that they are able to tolerate in the short term. The aim is to progressively increase the volume of exercise that can be managed and ideally to have this sustained over an increasingly longer period of time. Depending on the physical condition of the individual, a start may be made with as little as one or two brief sessions of 10 to 15 min per week.

13.4.6.1 *Medical Examination and Preparticipation Screening*

Prior to undertaking an exercise program, all prospective participants should obtain a medical certificate or referral from their medical practitioner, specifying nutritional and health characteristics of the child. One of the most important factors is to gain the interest of the child and ensure his or her motivation and self-monitoring in the recommended exercise program. Therefore, the recommended exercise must be tolerable and acceptable for the child with regard to character, duration, and frequency, as related to personal characteristics (e.g., health status, level of functional capacity, and adaptation to physical workload).

As is the case for dietary intake of an individual, it is not possible to provide a unique and homogeneous recipe for the exercises that will result in an improvement in body composition. It is possible to provide a general overview and instructions for use by a trained adult or parent to introduce an appropriate mode of exercise. Generally, guidelines and recommendations are superficial — for example, aerobic exercise at a certain ratio of aerobic power with no further details provided. This is one area of great need for future research.

13.4.6.2 *Mode of Exercise*

Exercise should have a significant cardiorespiratory element. Potential dynamic activities include walking, jogging, treadmill walking and running, swimming, stair-climbing, bench stepping, and skipping. Children should be encouraged to start with brief sessions and gradually increase the length of sessions over time. A longer-term goal is the encouragement of increased habitual physical activity, with additional activities as often as possible, ideally on a daily basis. The choice of activities should be based on the likes and dislikes of individuals, along with enjoyment an appropriate challenge. Activities that foster a combined improvement in motor skill are favored.

There is no selective effect of training mode on body composition changes if total work output is equivalent. However, the individual variability in the overweight and obese means that there are differences in the suitability of exercises.

Walking is one of the most effective modalities for children, adolescents, and adults, particularly in the early stages of a program. There were given numerous advantages of this modality, including a lower risk of musculoskeletal injury than running, convenience, the ability to produce a training effect if used appropriately, and the fact that no particular skill is required. While skill level may appear to be unimportant, the efficiency with which one walks is very much associated with ability and management of the extra load to be carried. Particularly with the immature child, extra care and attention may need to be provided in order to maximize the value from a relatively simple loco-motor task (Hills, 1994; 1995; Bar-Or et al., 1998).

Exercise performed in water has the advantage of the buoyancy effect and a reduced loading on joints. This enables a more rapid progression in terms of total volume of exercise and less risk of injury (Hills and Byrne, 1998). Other water-based activities (in addition to swimming) include kickboard exercises, aqua-aerobics, and deep-water running.

Resistance training is recognized as an essential element of weight-man-agement programs for people of all ages. The growth and maintenance of metabolically active tissue is critical and integrally linked to regular involve-ment in physical activity.

13.4.6.3   Frequency of Exercise

An ideal initial frequency of exercise would be three to four times per week, but additional benefits may be gained by exercising more frequently, even daily where possible. As mentioned earlier, it is important not to be over-zealous in attempting to commence regular physical activity. Individuals too often begin a program full of enthusiasm and with the best of intentions but stop soon due to soreness, injury, or tiredness.

13.4.6.4   Duration of Exercise

Any increase in activity beyond the level of commitment prior to commencing a program is a good start. For many children, particularly those who have not been completely inactive, approximately 20 to 30 min of sustained activity per day is a good starting point if the aim is to improve cardiovascular fitness. This time frame assumes that one is active for the full period of time and that the heart rate is elevated to an appropriate training level. If the child has been extremely inactive, a shorter time frame may initially be needed.

Exercise sessions may be structured in a variety of ways but ideally should include the following components:

- Preparatory warm-up exercises and endurance tasks
- A range of games and motor skill, dance, and gymnastic activities
- Games and sports skills incorporating a cool-down period

13.4.6.5   Intensity of Exercise

A substantial training effect can be accomplished by exercising in an appro-priate heart rate range. As fitness improves, the heart rate response lowers for a given workload or activity. As for other components of the exercise prescription, there needs to be a progressive increment in work output to provide an overload of the cardiorespiratory system to gain an improvement.

Intensity of exercise is by far the most difficult to quantify and is a particular challenge for young people. The better approaches for the determination of intensity of exercise are heart-rate monitoring and rating of perceived exertion. Ideally, one might suggest that an allied goal of activity participation is to understand the physiological response of one's body. Young people, particularly those in late childhood and adolescence, can be trained to measure heart rate with a reasonable degree of accuracy, but this ability is a particular challenge for some. Although the use of heart-rate monitors is a logical alternative, this technology may be available only in a clinic setting. The Borg RPE scale has also been used to determine exercise intensity in obese children (Ward and Bar-Or, 1986), but it is not in widespread use.

Working with children to increase their knowledge and understanding of the physical responses to exercise is challenging. Knowing one's own body provides enormous benefits when prescribing exercise. Too often we rely on others for advice, and this is certainly the case for young people. We need to balance the adult prescription mentality with objective indications of intensity from children. This includes the opportunity for children to make decisions about how hard they work. In this way, adult imposition that may include greater expectations of work output than are desirable could be minimized (Hills, 1995).

In a simplistic sense, exercise intensity for weight loss may involve exercising at an intensity as high as possible for the available time period. This may suit some young people but may be fraught with problems for others, including potential cardiovascular and musculoskeletal risk and adherence to activity.

Exercise prescription for weight management may be described as a conundrum. The total volume of energy expended will determine the amount of weight loss, not the composition of the exercise (Hills and Byrne, 1998). For all obese individuals, but particularly children and adolescents, the real challenge is to individualize the exercise program wherever possible in the knowledge that this will influence the individual's tolerance, interest, and adherence to physical activity in the longer term.

13.5 Exercise Program

The exercise program consists of the following considerations:

- A physical fitness or conditioning component
- Participation in appropriate physical activities, sports skills, and recreational pursuits
- Guidance in lifestyle habits that encompass exercise and diet

13.5.1 Conditioning Program

The capacity for exercise varies widely between individuals. This is even the case with individuals of a similar age and physical status. For this reason, it is important to structure activities based on each individual's response to exercise. Activity sessions may include the following sequence of activities:

- Warm-up activities
- A set of stretching exercises
- A cardiorespiratory conditioning period
- Muscular strength and endurance activities
- Dance, gymnastics, or other motor skill activities
- Games and sports skills incorporating a cool-down

13.5.2 Warm-Up Period

The focus during this period should be on low-intensity activities involving large muscle groups. This period serves to elevate the heart rate in preparation for more vigorous activity to follow.

13.5.3 Stretching Activities

An extension of the warm-up activities should include simple stretching exercises. Other tasks are chosen to complement the specific focus of the main section of the activity session to follow.

13.5.4 Cardiorespiratory Endurance and Strength Activities

These activities form the bulk of the exercise program and are designed to improve the efficiency of the heart, lungs, and associated blood vessels. A range of strength tasks is incorporated using a combination of partner resistance and gym equipment.

13.5.5 Dance, Gymnastics, and Other Motor Skill Activities

Obese individuals should gain an exposure to a wide cross section of experiences in these areas on a rotating basis. Dance is often a good choice because it is very attractive for children and adolescents. The various forms of dancing to popular music can be quite energy demanding, and so it is particularly suitable for an increased energy expenditure. An exposure to simple gymnastic activities and more structured classical gymnastic exercise can be especially helpful for the training of the individual muscle groups and also improve body posture. Activities in these areas can be planned to suit obese individuals of various ages.

13.5.6   Sports and Recreational Skills

Activity opportunities should include a diversity of skills designed to improve a child's or adolescent's involvement in individual and team physical activity tasks. Obese children should be encouraged to swim, since the excess body fat of the individual enhances buoyancy and facilitates this sort of activity, and swimming can involve all major body parts. This form of exercise can be undertaken year round if one has access to an indoor swimming pool, and is particularly suitable for a growing child. A wide variety of exercises can be conducted in the water and with or without equipment (Hills and Byrne, 1998).

Bicycle ergometer work can supplement the exercise program at the beginning of the program prior to the use of resistance training exercises. Road cycling is a good alternative, but only if safety is not compromised. Cycling as an exercise may be problematic for some individuals if the position of the chest is cramped and does not permit adequate breathing and the development of the chest muscles. In all activity tasks, the development of optimal breathing is one of the main aims of the exercise program for the obese.

Genu valgum, a common condition in obese children, may be exacerbated, particularly during activities such as skating. This type of activity is not recommended under such circumstances or until weight loss and the adoption of the necessary skills. The careful introduction of cross-country skiing may also be a goal as the young person gains some success in the program. All weight-bearing activities such as running, jumping, and other track-and-field events can be gradually implemented. Various games are also an excellent choice depending on the individual's enjoyment of this form of exercise. Enjoyment of particular activities helps to maximize adherence to such a program, provided that there is suitable peer company.

13.6   Lifestyle Habits

The conscious modification of a number of key habits can help to reduce the tendency toward inactivity. Suggestions for adjustment include using stairs instead of escalators and elevators, and walking children to school or to stores instead of driving. Parents may rotate responsibility for supervising a group of neighborhood children walking to and from school if safety is an issue (Hills and Cambourne, 2002). Another suggestion is to take a brisk walk whenever convenient during the day. Encourage and support the young person in anything that incorporates an increase in physical activity, and attempt to practice and reinforce activity skills that have been introduced in this book.

Some of the suggested activities may be unrealistic and therefore compromised due to safety concerns, especially in larger urban areas. This need not be a drawback but rather a challenge. Activity that is organized and supervised by appropriate adults is often a more suitable choice.

13.7   General Guidelines for Exercise Participation

13.7.1   Clothing

Clothing is important for a range of reasons, not only from the point of view of the suitability for exercise activities. Particular clothing can also play a role in adding to the attractiveness of an activity. This may be a strong factor in the pleasure gained by a young person in a range of settings, either in the gym, sports facility, or in the playground. This may be more of an issue to the participant than other instructions and advice they receive.

Clothing should be attractive to the child but of paramount importance is that items are comfortable and loose fitting. A concern for many overweight and obese individuals is self-consciousness. Empathy for this concern and doing everything possible to allay fears related to clothing, or lack of it, such as at the swimming pool, should be a high priority. Choose clothing with pleasant colors and with a style that is fashionable if this can help to improve the likelihood of continued participation and enjoyment.

Children and adolescents should be discouraged from wearing any plastic or rubberized clothing while exercising. This practice is potentially dangerous as the normal heat regulation of the body can be impaired. Resultant problems could include sharp increases in body temperature, dehydration, and possible heat exhaustion (Bar-Or et al., 1998).

13.7.2   Exercise Surface

Although the chosen activity will be the major determining factor with respect to exercise surface, every attempt should be made to avoid repetitive exercises on hard surfaces. Excessive loading and jarring on such surfaces, particularly if combined with poor footwear, can predispose one to injury, which should be avoided at all costs (Flynn, Lou, and Ganley, 2002). Where possible, preventive strategies could include working on a grassy area to avoid the risk of jarring injuries.

13.7.3   Appropriate Time to Exercise

This is a very individual issue. Participation is the most important issue, not when exercise is to occur. Time of day for exercising is often determined by the adult rather than the child's preference and the time that the chosen activity session or program is offered, for example, during or after school, in the evenings, and during holiday breaks. Avoid exercising in extreme weather conditions, particularly periods of high temperature and or humidity. However, it is recommended that individuals exercise as often as possible under any suitable conditions.

13.7.4 Possible Complications Resulting from Exercise

There is always a possibility, especially in a more obese, clumsy child with too much enthusiasm at the beginning of a new regime, for illness or injury to occur. Physical activity should be modified, reduced, or eliminated according to ability and/or the severity of injury or sickness. Always consult a medical practitioner when in doubt. When the child has suffered an injury, look for opportunities to maintain fitness by completing alternative modes of activity. For example, if an individual is unable to bear weight and walk or run because of an injury to the lower limb, swimming or cycling may be good alternatives.

13.8 Motivation

Too often, exercise programs are started with the very best of intentions only to fail due to a lack of interest on the part of the individual. Many things can be done to help maintain one's motivation for activity. The fundamental starting point is to determine the likes and dislikes of the child. Capitalize on the activities that they like and use opportunities to attempt such tasks as the stepping-stone to new experiences. Commitment to activity is likely to be much greater along with the chance to downplay the common excuses for inactivity, such as it's "too hard, too boring or too embarrassing" (Bar-Or et al., 1998):

- Choose realistic and achievable short-term goals that are not performance based. This may relate to the total activity time and the type(s) of activity.
- Exercise at a regular time of the day and make this part of the child's daily routine.
- Exercise with a partner, in a small group, with the family, or with similar peers.
- Monitor the changes in one's body, for instance, have participants write down how they feel and record any obvious physical changes they can notice.
- Consider a system of reward for improvements in behavior. For example, improvements may include reductions in inactive behaviors such as television viewing, attaining a goal of being active on a predetermined number of occasions across successive weeks, or

completing a given distance in their aerobic activities (Hills and Byrne, 1999).

- Avoid a preoccupation with weight. Do not equate the loss of a certain amount of weight with success, or thinking of losing weight quickly as the only desirable outcome. For many children, weight loss may not be a sensible goal. Depending on the age and stage of physical maturation, most children and many adolescents may have considerable potential for further growth. Any minimization in potential for growth in height, a potential risk on a restrictive diet, should be avoided at all costs. If weight loss is a viable and necessary option, a logical approach is to remember that if weight has been accumulated over a period of time one should consider any reduction in excess over a similar period of time.

- The approach of accepting a deposit or bond at the beginning of an exercise program that will be repaid on the successful attainment of a goal, or similar forms of contract, can be detrimental if too much of a focus is placed on the reward at the expense of any meaningful change in behavior. Nevertheless, young children and older individuals alike do love to have their achievements acknowledged. Simple rewards in recognition of the individual's efforts and achievements such as T-shirts and movie tickets, or an educational item like a book, can be powerful motivators.

- Behavior modification techniques need to be prominent in all work with children. Counseling should include techniques that will assist in behavior changes that are desirable in relation to dietary and physical activity changes.

13.9 Self-Monitoring

A point system to reward time spent in physical activity may be one way to encourage modifications in behavior as a step toward self-monitoring. Role models also have an important place in the growth and development of children and adolescents. Useful modeling of behavior may be provided by peers, siblings, parents, and significant others, such as teachers and coaches (Bar-Or et al., 1998).

Children should be given examples to encourage both participation in activity and improvements in eating behavior. For example, if uncontrolled eating is a problem, identify and then eliminate the troublesome cue or cues. Assistance from family members to help young people learn to avoid temptations is paramount. Avoiding stores on the way home from school, discouraging excessive television viewing, avoiding the consumption of foods low in nutritional value, encouraging good eating habits and practices, and avoiding fast food are all possible strategies.

Considerable attention has been given to the settings in which the greatest opportunity exists to help large numbers of children who are overweight or obese. University- or hospital-based clinics have a rather limited impact, even if these clinics also provide the opportunity for group activity programs to complement the individualized approach. Generally, such centers attract the more difficult individuals or the more obese children and adolescents. The limited number of centers providing a comprehensive and integrated program, along with the potential cost, may also be a limitation to larger numbers of individuals accessing such facilities.

13.10 Home-Based Exercise Programs

Home-based programs provide numerous challenges. A desirable outcome is for the child or adolescent to take an increased responsibility for his or her well-being. Very young people may have a limited capacity to take on such a role, but nevertheless such responsibility should be fostered at an early age. The ability of individuals to self-manage their condition, preferably with the support of a program planned for them, is associated with their level of motivation and the support and encouragement they are given. Opportunities for support include parents, siblings, and/or health professionals who may take on the role of a personal trainer. As for clinic-based programs, the latter option, while the most desirable, is not feasible except for a relatively small proportion of the population due mainly to the cost involved.

Home-based programs may work for some individuals, but the number may be limited to those who have committed family members to assist as role models. Even with supportive family members, they need support by way of knowledge and understanding and appropriate educational materials. The author has had some experience in this area and has found that home-based activities can be a strategic component of a weight-management program, particularly when running in tandem with a clinic or school program. When parents have an integral role to play in such programs, their usefulness in the home setting can be maximized (Golan and Crow, 2004; Hills, 1995). With a written home program, parents can assist by providing supervision and assistance if instructed by other staff — for example, a physical educator or a clinic staff member — and can verify work completed by children by signing off sheets as part of a contractual arrangement.

A good model for an integrated approach to school or clinical setting complemented by home activities may be as follows:

- Initial screening, assessment, and support provided through an activity program in a university clinic or school setting.
- Personalized sessions with relevant health professionals depending on need, such as a medical practitioner, dietitian, exercise physiologist, and/or clinical psychologist. An individualized exercise prescription and dietary plan is required.
- Group activity program.
- Home-based program to complement the above.
- Educational material to support both settings. This should be resource material of particular benefit to all family members, potentially in the form of a consolidated booklet or book with material specific to the individual provided. This option may include completion exercises related to the program activities, material that complements the theory and practice of nutrition and physical activity, diaries, questionnaires, growth charts, and a "passport to health" that is the property of the individual child.
- Educational seminar sessions on topical issues related to growth and development, body image, self-concept, self-esteem, nutrition, physical activity, and other relevant topics.

13.11 Recommendations for Leisure-Time Activities

Video games and television programs have attracted considerable attention during recent years and have been considered one of the main reasons for the progressive reduction in physical activity and exercise from the more common levels in young individuals some decades ago (Vandewater, Shim, and Caplowitz, 2004). This also includes TV advertisements for foods (Halford et al., 2004a,b). As shown by some authors, a reduced level of sedentary activity of young people can result in an improvement in BMI, a loss of excess fat, and an improvement in the general health and functional status of obese children (Eisenmann, 2004) starting at an early age (Abbott and Davies, 2004).

Especially in the early stages of treatment, it is recommended that the obese child become involved in some type of organized, regular physical activity. During such a monitored program, the time for activity is better utilized provided that adequate supervision and guidance from qualified staff is available. Unfortunately, there is a shortage of specialized staff available to provide the special approach that obese children require. Pedagogic experiences with normal-weight children are of course the basis of physical education for all children, but physical education is not readily available to all young children as it should be. Without the guarantee of a quality physical education program and the specific requirements for a special population such as the obese, an increased demand is placed on the organization (school, clinic, hospital, health, and fitness center). Special programs are also more expensive but do provide a better guarantee of a safer and sustainable benefit.

Individual exercise and special sport activities implemented later must be chosen cautiously for obese children. Such children can be easily discouraged when they are unable to participate or are not achieving any noticeable results. Exercises must be selected according to the degree of obesity and its duration, and according to the age and gender of the child. As mentioned earlier, health status and initial functional capacity levels provide the necessary details to determine a starting point for the preparation of the well-planned exercise program.

Parents have a preference for supervised activities because many are afraid to let their children run freely without supervision in parks or playgrounds due to safety reasons. The possibility of long-term health benefits from a comprehensive weight-management program with exercise as a central feature should be a persuasive factor in the encouragement of the family to participate actively in management of their child's weight.

In more severe cases of childhood obesity, it is necessary to decide whether the individual should participate in the usual physical education classes at school. Very obese children often have some additional health problems. Further, many obese individuals will try anything to avoid physical education with their normal-weight peers, who can treat their obese classmates in a cruel and discouraging way. This is a major factor in the reduced interest in exercise.

The authors' experiences have shown that when children participated in physical education programs in summer camps where only obese children were present, their inhibitions disappeared. The children are able to achieve some level of physical performance and are competitive among themselves in the sporting activities. Correspondence to parents is evidence of the acceptability of such camps to obese children; one child wrote that "I feel very happy here and would like to stay here even longer." Camps lasting approximately 7 weeks resulted in the loss on average of 10% of the children's initial weight and fat, an improvement in performance, and an increased self-esteem (Pařízková, 1977, 1998b,c). It is regrettable that this sort of weight-management program is usually too expensive for the majority of families. Therefore, outpatient programs and participation in physical education classes for obese children during the school year are the most appropriate choices. However, even these opportunities are not very common in the majority of countries and especially in the bigger urban areas where they are most needed. Long ago, on the occasion of the XIIth International Congress of Pediatrics (Mexico City, 1968), Doxiadis (1968) suggested a specially arranged city agglomeration. His suggested plan consisted of more individual centers — city cells — from which there is always adequate space

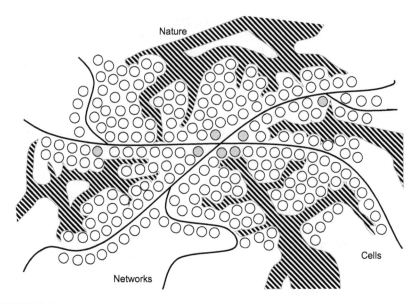

FIGURE 13.1
An "ideal" construction of a city to maximize access to open areas for physical activity. (Adapted from Doxiadis (1968), a diagram as part of a presentation titled "The city and the development of the child, a basic concept for our cities." XII International Congress of Pediatrics, Mexico City.)

as they are sufficiently close to the natural environment (Figure 13.1). While this may be an idealistic suggestion, such an arrangement may be realized in the future in an increasing number of settings and contribute to the healthy development of children.

13.12   The Role of the Teacher and Physical Educator

The personalities of those who organize, supervise, and guide physical education and exercise for obese children are pivotal and must be similar to the role of the family. The individual should be patient, knowledgeable on all developmental aspects and problems of the obese child, kind and joyous, and sensitive to reinforcing children even when they make mistakes. It is also very important to stress all successes, although they may be minimal in the eyes of others.

Adults who have had experiences with elite athletes of all ages are typically not suitable for the monitoring of exercise and physical education for obese individuals. Work and experiences with a select group of high achievers in the physical activity domain often means that such teachers and coaches do not have empathy for the plight of the obese individual. Many often believe that "obesity is always the result of laziness and gluttony," and that it is necessary to be tough with those who are obese. Such an approach may work in some cases, but for the majority of obese children, who are frequently shy and may have an inferiority complex, this type of approach completely discourages exercise. Nevertheless, it is possible to provide some teachers with the necessary skills to adapt their attitudes in order to work effectively with obese children.

13.13 Suggestions for a Balance between Physical Activity and Exercise

A sample program may include the following:

- Morning exercise for 10 to 15 min (may include stretching and muscular strength and endurance activities).
- Afternoon and/or evening (preferably both) of preparatory warm-up exercise lasting 15 to 30 min.
- A minimum of two hr of games, exercise, sport activities, walking and running in the open air (each weekday).
- Twice a week, participation in normal physical education classes whenever possible, modified to suit the obese.
- During weekends, at least 5 to 6 hr of physical activity of any sort, including games, exercise, and sport. Whenever possible this should occur in the open air and away from pollutants, for example, in large urban areas. Parents, siblings, friends, and peers, or anybody suitable who is willing to cooperate, should participate.
- Exercise should involve all large muscle groups (including abdominal wall, chest, and back muscles mainly because of their contribution to improved body posture).

At the beginning of a program it is necessary to execute all movements slowly and in a controlled fashion. Movement that is correct and progressively becomes more economical and purposeful is the goal. Exercising in a setting where there are mirrors enables progressive improvement through the self-control of one's own performance. However, this might discourage some individuals, especially in the beginning of the intervention. Use of correct feedback, both visually and verbally, can also facilitate the progressive control of movement necessary to manage body posture and achieve a symmetric and stable gait. This work should not be exclusive to the obese but is also necessary for children of normal body weight. Any improvement in appearance is a bonus for an individual who may still have a long way to go in order to increase his or her interest in exercise.

13.14 Selected Exercises for Individual Parts of the Body

13.14.1 Body Posture

An appreciation of correct body position for sound posture is essential:

- Head is drawn up, with the chin and the neck at a right angle.
- Shoulders are spread and drawn back and down.
- Arms are hanging along the sides with elbows rotated out so that the thumbs are directed forward.
- Abdominal muscles are drawn in and buttock muscles are contracted.
- The pelvis is thus reinforced and is mildly drawn backward, flattening any exaggerated lordotic curve caused by a protruding abdomen.
- When standing, the feet should be oriented in such a way that body weight is evenly spread.
- The pronounced neck lordosis often found in obese individuals can be minimized by the contraction of muscles between scapulae and the vertebral column, especially between the 6th and 9th vertebrae.
- Simultaneously, the rib cage is lifted and the shoulders are drawn back and down. Therefore, the position of the chest is improved, which enables better breathing.

13.14.2 Breathing Exercises

Breathing exercises are suitable only when children have acquired an adequate body posture. During all exercises it is necessary to be aware of the flow of the air in and out of the lungs. Most children (not only those who are obese) breathe superficially, automatically, and typically without any conscious control of their breathing.

Conscious breathing is best taught in a lying position. Attention must be concentrated on expiration, and various rhythms are used. During these exercises the abdomen should be drawn in, the pelvis tilted back, and the small of the back pushed toward the ground. Expiration should always last longer than the inspiration as it has been shown that after a proper expiration, the lungs automatically inspire in a better manner. It is also recommended that the muscles of the ribs be exercised. The adoption of adequate breathing simultaneously improves body posture.

13.14.3 Other Exercises

For very obese children with a low level of fitness, it is best to prescribe exercise in an aquatic environment. Following some improvement in performance, it is recommended that exercise occur in a lying position, on the back or on the abdomen. This can progress into sitting and kneeling positions. This progression reduces the load of one's own body weight that interferes with weight-bearing activities such as walking and running as well as when exercising in a standing position. Again, it is important to start with a slow rhythm and to properly explain how to perform all exercises. Instruction should also include how the individual will benefit from such an exercise, and what should be avoided to execute all movements properly.

The coordination of exercise and breathing rhythm is essential. Relaxation after exercise when the muscles are mostly contracted is indispensable. Exercise is performed four to six times at the beginning, later eight to ten times. A kind and empathetic approach helps obese children at the beginning to gain confidence. The creation of a nice and enjoyable ambience enables a better response from all involved.

All exercise can be executed in a right or wrong way. The latter not only results in limited benefits but could also cause some harm. Therefore, an experienced teacher or exercise physiologist should be responsible for exercise prescription for obese children, or there may be some risk of injury if inappropriate procedures are introduced.

13.14.3.1 Exercises for the Vertebral Column

Better functioning of the vertebral column involves the strengthening of the muscles of the abdominal wall, and the relaxation and lengthening of the contracted muscles of the shoulders and back. One then needs to relax the hip joints and simultaneously to strengthen the muscles around the joints. It is good to start in a lying position. At the beginning it is recommended that the supervisor assist the exercising child, for example, to help him or her to get up from the lying position to the sitting position by pulling the child's hands. During all exercise, it is necessary to watch for free breathing, to ensure that the children consciously control their breathing, do not hold their breath, and concentrate on expiration. The elaboration of the so called muscular corset, which helps to position the vertebral column in a desirable posture, is a suitable task (Åstrand and Rodahl, 1977).

A number of exercises for the improvement of the posture of the vertebral column in a lying position on the back and/or on the sides are available, involving various movements of the legs and the arms. Other sets of exercises can be executed in sitting, kneeling, or standing positions. Each exercise must be followed by appropriate relaxation.

13.14.3.2 Exercises for Upper and Lower Extremities

When exercising the lower extremities, strengthening of the thighs needs to be stressed. In spite of their large circumferences, thigh muscles are often too weak and flaccid in obese children. It is helpful to stand on the spot and lift alternate knees in a controlled fashion or to exercise with a rope. From standing, the next progression would be to jogging on the spot and completing similar movements. Exercises should be limited in number at the beginning, gradually increasing over time. Skipping can also be useful if it is low and elastic. These exercises can be supplemented by leg flexion and extension movements on appropriate machines, squats, and stepping up and down on a bench while maintaining an adequate body posture and breathing frequency.

Movements of the upper extremity should be executed with the remainder of the body stable in the standing, sitting, kneeling, and lying positions. The progressive isolation and control of major muscle groups from the shoulders should be the goal.

13.14.3.3   *Exercises for the Pelvis*

Conscious control of the position of the pelvis is critical for body posture and the position of the internal organs. Good postural control can be achieved by utilizing a set of exercises in the standing, sitting, lying, and kneeling positions.

13.15   Encouraging Obese Children to Adhere to Regular Exercise

The following should be considered to encourage obese children to adhere to regular exercise.

- Irrespective of the modest beginning and initial results, it is important to demonstrate some positive improvement after a short period of time. There may not be any absolute change in body weight or BMI, but this may be caused by the simultaneous decrease of fat mass and increase of lean, fat-free body mass. Therefore, an evaluation of body composition measures including circumferences can be used to great effect. Reductions in centimeters at particular sites can be motivational and enable increased comfort for example in the clothes one wears. The lack of change in body weight may also be due to a simultaneous growth in height. All changes should be shared with the child and used as a major educational opportunity. Positive comments are of paramount importance to the child.
- It is necessary to persuade the obese child that only a permanent adherence to increased physical activity and an exercise program will provide a lasting reduction of overweight and excess fatness along with an increase in the level of physical performance and fitness. The opportunity for personal involvement of the obese child or adolescent in the weight-management process through an appropriate psychological approach is the best way to ensure successful treatment. It may

also be useful to identify a group of charismatic individuals well known as local identities to provide some "star" quality.

- An enjoyable atmosphere in a nice environment needs to be fostered with a kind and friendly physical educator. With quality staff, best results can be achieved. However, a degree of discipline is also necessary and must be adhered to. The recognition of issues and concerns can help to increase the interest in physical education classes and also enhance and make the involvement in spontaneous exercise during leisure time more favorable.

- Positive evaluation and encouragement should be provided for each child on an individual basis. The presence of the other participants, or family and friends, is very important to most young people. This helps to encourage the child to continue to exercise and to maintain any increase in physical activity levels.

In summary, when no effect is obvious, one needs to determine whether to speak about the issue or not, or alternatively, to find something positive in the experience. Examples include the better performance of an activity or physical task, or the improvement of the silhouette or body posture. Some appreciation, praise, and encouragement are always very much appreciated.

13.16 Supportive Role of the Family

Parents and family members are usually the closest people to the child. Their emotional and psychological support is essential in all aspects of the weight-management process and the education of the child.

Do not expect something different of the overweight or obese child. In other words, anything expected of the overweight child should be expected of other family members. This applies to the consumption of food and all other activities. As mentioned in our discussion of nutrition, the best solution is for family members to actively participate, at least at the beginning of the new program. When all family members adopt and adhere to an active lifestyle, the more acceptable it is for the obese child. Exercising together with children is a good custom in families, as is spending leisure time walking and including all members of the family and vacationing together. Often, simple options are the most enjoyable to encourage an increase in activity. For example, a more modest program in a park or recreational area close to the family home can be sufficient as it is ideal to participate in at least some of these activities together. It is difficult or almost impossible to persuade a child to increase his or her physical activity output when looking at overweight parents who move only when they must.

Walking and suitable games can be shared on regular occasions but as frequently as possible. Even small competitions can be fun and enable the involvement of all participants on the basis of gender and age. When caring parents have more than one obese child, their role may be made easier. Greater problems may be related with diet and exercise when one child is obese and another is not. However, when siblings are supportive, results can improve depending mainly on the parents. A more active lifestyle can be useful for everybody, and it is always better to adapt the program to the necessities of the obese child and increase the level of physical activity and exercise than the opposite way.

The obese member of the family should never be ridiculed and criticized. This applies particularly to the siblings as well as peers at school. There is a risk that the obese child will be a target for joking and ridicule, some of which may be very unpleasant. This scenario rarely results in a defense reaction and an effort to improve status, with the aim to lose weight faster and achieve success in some other area. More commonly, it results in the spontaneous isolation and self pitying of the child with few positive outcomes with respect to the reduction of weight and fat.

Obese children commonly cannot avoid negative reactions at school. They should at least be able to feel secure, at ease, and well appreciated at home. This applies particularly to the development of the effort to adhere to the prescribed diet and exercise program. The encouragement, kind assistance, and help of family members can significantly support a greater commitment to exercise.

13.17 Sample Activities That Provide the Basis of an Activity Program for Young Children

13.17.1 Games and Game Skills for Children

An introduction to games and game skills should be considered in an orderly sequence of stages. Progression through these stages is directly related to stages of motor development of the individual child.

13.17.1.1 Stage 1 Skills

Opportunity should be provided for free play with large, soft, light balls. Other useful ideas include running games, singing games, and anything that fosters children's imagination.

13.17.1.2 Stage 2 Skills

Running and dodging

Hitting skills
- Hitting a ball off the top of a cone marker or off the ground.
- Continuous hitting of a balloon, trying to keep it in the air using either hand.

Catching
- Rolling a ball between partners who are stationary.
- Fielding a rolling ball.
- Catching a large ball (encouraging a basket catch on the chest.)
- Catching a bean bag with two hands and the next time with only with one hand.

Throwing
- Underarm roll, trying to control direction and distance.
- One-handed roll, concentrating on gripping the ball with fingers. Combine with stopping and catching skills.

Bouncing
- Various tasks bouncing and catching a large ball.

13.17.1.3 Stage 3 Skills

Running and dodging
Hitting skills
- Bouncing a ball and hitting or striking with hand or bat.
- Hitting a ball against a fence or wall.
- Hitting a ball from a stationary position, for example a T-ball stand.

Catching
- Catching a bean bag with one hand, alternating sides.
- Making two- and one-handed catches with various types of ball, for example, small to large.
- Add a partner or small group to test above-mentioned skills.

Kicking
- Try to kick a large ball off the ground, alternating feet, progressively incorporating target and distance goals.
- Use alternate objects for balls, perhaps empty milk cartons and bean bags.

Bouncing

- Bouncing a large ball with both hands sitting, kneeling, or standing.
- Throwing and catching a ball overhead.
- Bouncing and catching a ball on the move; start with walking, then speed up.
- Pat bouncing while walking, then running.

13.17.1.4 Stage 4 Skills

Running and dodging

Hitting skills

- Involving progressive increases in difficulty: hitting a stationary ball, hitting a ball pitched underarm, hitting a ball to a particular area of the field, experience hitting tasks using different bats and rackets.

13.17.2 Body Image or Body Awareness, Spatial Awareness, and Eye–Hand and Eye–Foot Coordination

All children need to be provided with activities to develop body image (or body awareness), gross and fine muscle coordination, and rhythmic coordination. Some children will learn more slowly, and some obese children will have difficulty in performing simple skills. Many children, of all shapes and sizes and as a function of lack of opportunity or time spent in physical activity, may have difficulties in one or more of these areas.

Body image or body awareness: How the child views him- or herself and the child's awareness of the relation of one body part of the body to another.

Spatial awareness: The child's awareness of his or her body in space and in relation to directions such as up, down, forward, and backward.

Eye–hand and eye–foot coordination: The child's ability to integrate muscles in tasks requiring the use of eyes and hands or hands and feet.

13.17.2.1 Body Image

Touch: Child touches different parts of the body, while standing, sitting.

Body movement: Child moves various parts of the body as the teacher names each; child crawls, moving arm and leg of one side simultaneously.

13.17.2.2 Spatial Awareness

Once a child becomes thoroughly aware of his or her own body, he or she must begin to use body parts to explore space. The child must feel what it is like to move through, in, out, over, around, and under various pathways and obstacles.

13.18 Summary

Defining programs for dietary intake, physical activity and exercise, and behavioral changes is a difficult task. The process should be individualized for each obese child and take into account the age, gender, and degree and duration of obesity. General guidelines can be more responsibly suggested, with the recommendation of ambulatory and/or individual programs, inpatient and/or outpatient treatment, school-based programs and/or summer camp treatment, and intervention. Not only the individual characteristics of a child but also the availability of these approaches most often lead to the choice of the manner of treatment. Proper anthropometric, functional, and medical characteristics are the starting point for the recommendation of a particular diet from the point of view of amount of energy, main components, and their ratio of mineral and vitamin content; the latter is mostly the same as for normal-weight children. The regime of food intake and its distribution as related to daily activities has to be considered. Diet should be generally acceptable and likeable, and should not include items that the child does not accept, but should exclude risky items such as saturated fats and too much simple sugars. On the other hand, healthy items such as vegetables, fruit, whole-grain breads and cereals, skim milk and cheese, and lean meat should be promoted.

The interventions of physical activity and exercise programs could be more difficult as they are usually not included in daily life as often as eating behaviors. Such programs must be defined and specified similar to diet, which has not commonly occurred in most cases. In this respect, it is necessary to apply attractive invention, and to increase motivation by a suitable choice of exercise activities and modification of the whole lifestyle. It is important to gain the interest and personal involvement of obese children using suitable and fun exercises, likeable personality of the teacher, an attractive setting and dress for exercise, and persuasive encouragement even in cases where no great success has been achieved. The gradual increase in the intensity, duration, and frequency of suitable exercise including all muscle groups, supporting body posture and adequate breathing, is a recommended way of involving the obese child in a regular and continuing regime of optimal exercise. These factors will enhance the opportunity to achieve desirable results with regard to weight, BMI, and excess fat reduction.

Diet, exercise, and behavioral changes should be applied simultaneously, and it is the role of the environment, first of all the family, that is essential. The optimal form of example for a child with regard to food intake, regime of eating, physical activity, and exercise must come from the parents and siblings (Stanton and Hills, 2004). This also applies to the peers of an obese child, but undesirable experiences such as ridiculing could take place that are mostly related to the motor abilities of the obese. For that reason, taking part in exercise lessons with comparable peers with similar physical characteristics and the same aims is generally recommended. For this purpose, summer camps as well as year-round lessons, sessions, seminars, and group activities are welcome.

14

Summary

14.1 Main Characteristics of Childhood Obesity

Childhood obesity has become a global epidemic, and the condition is now evident much earlier in life. The numerous co-morbidities typically associated with adult obesity are also now being recognized in childhood and adolescence. This suggests that research, clinical support, and preventive measures must be developed to identify and work with at-risk young individuals while providing appropriate support for the wider community with a lifestyle approach to weight management.

One of the main reasons for the limited success in the treatment and prevention of childhood obesity to date, despite considerable research and clinical experience in the area, is that all of the causes have not been satisfactorily explained. Genetic make-up includes not only specific genes causing family clustering of obesity but also the predisposition to a certain food intake. This includes the amount of energy and the composition of the diet influenced by specific food preferences and aversions. The same may also apply to the level of spontaneous physical activity. Some evidence suggests that the genetic predisposition to obesity may be related to both the total volume as well as type of physical activity an individual undertakes. In addition, susceptibility to the effect of both diet and physical activity level is considered to be genetically conditioned. The role of "thrifty genes" has been considered, with special attention having been paid to nutrition and physical activity regimes of children in many countries, the effects of which may have changed over time and interrelate with genetic predisposition. In contrast to the inborn classical genetic abnormalities and/or hormonal disturbance syndromes associated with an increased fat ratio, with prevalence rates as low as fractions of promiles of the population, simple obesity accounts for tens of percent of the child population at present.

The prevalence of simple obesity has increased predominantly in industrially developed countries such as the United States and Canada as well as in Western Europe, especially the United Kingdom, France, and Spain. However, children from higher socioeconomic groups in Third World countries such as Tobago, Papua New Guinea, and Jamaica are also at risk. The prevalence of childhood obesity in Asian, African, Middle Eastern countries, and

Oceania was initially low but has recently increased. This is particularly the case in larger urban areas where prevalence rates may be similar to that in some developed countries. As economic and social situations improve in these countries, the prevalence of childhood obesity is also increasing in other social strata. The same concerns exist for those of lower socioeconomic status in the industrially developed countries.

Childhood populations from developing countries who emigrated and became acculturated to their new country, or populations undergoing marked social and cultural changes (e.g., including the increase in childhood obesity in the former East Germany and in Canadian Inuits) provide some important examples of the etiology of obesity. The speed with which obesity has worsened in such areas suggests that environmental causes are more likely to have been responsible for the change rather than genetics. However, in some countries, obesity prevalence seems to have reached a plateau; however, this situation has been changing significantly until present.

A special type of obesity that occurs, although exclusively in countries of the Third World, is an accompanying stunting of growth (a lower height for age), which follows early malnutrition, or more specifically, undernutrition. The mechanism of this type of obesity has not been fully elucidated, but it seems that the adaptation to the restricted food intake early in life with a subsequent abundance of food can cause an increased metabolic efficiency, perhaps due to "thrifty genes" accompanied by an increased deposition of fat.

Research on genetic factors and obesity has developed significantly with family studies and considerations of the role of particular gene polymorphisms and mutations disposing certain individuals to greater and/or lower sensitivity to environmental factors. In particular, these factors include nutrition and physical activity level — that is, energy balance and turnover. It is well known that under very similar circumstances a single subject (even from one family) appears to store excess fat more easily than another. A number of gene disorders concerning melanocortin, Trp64Arg, UCP2,3, and many others have been studied; however, the analysis of results is still inconclusive so it seems to be premature to genotype obese subjects at present. Ongoing studies are sure to provide more evidence about the effect of genetic predisposition on obesity. Obesity is thus considered to be determined by several oligogenic genes, the expression of which is modulated by polygenic background and environmental factors.

However, analyses of research data to date may have been compromised (much more than is the case in adults), because studies in children have been undertaken with subjects of various ages who are categorized into age groups at different stages of sexual maturity. The timing of sexual maturation is also somewhat variable in different countries. Further, there has been a failure to report, or at least consistently report, the duration and severity of obesity and potential co-morbid conditions. The same shortcomings may apply to studies that have considered various treatment modalities. In addition, all children, in spite of their many common features, are unique individuals with "nutritional individualities," differing not only in dietary intake but also in the absorption, digestion, metabolization, and utilization of nutrients. Comparisons are therefore potentially compromised if appropriate consideration has not been given to these issues. Nevertheless, a number of important pointers have been gained, each of which can be used to influence the more effective treatment and also contribute to the prevention of childhood obesity.

Obesity is defined as an excessive accumulation and ratio of stored fat when compared to other tissues. In contrast, overweight refers to an increase of body weight above an arbitrary standard usually defined in relation to height. Overweight may not be always entirely caused by increased body fatness. Therefore, for the evaluation of obesity, the most important approach is the measurement of the amount of body fat, in both absolute and relative terms. A number of methods have been used in the assessment of body composition. The most important laboratory techniques used to date have traditionally utilized hydrodensitometry (underwater weighing), dual-energy x-ray absorptiometry (DXA), dilution methods using D_2O or T_2O, total body conductivity measurements (TOBEC), ^{40}K measurements, magnetic resonance imaging (MRI), and creatinine excretion. The field (or bedside body composition assessment techniques) have traditionally involved anthropometry. Most commonly, skinfold measurements have been taken and summed or converted using regression equations based on the relationships of subcutaneous and total body fat to percent of body fat values. Circumference measures from the hip, waist, and arm have been widely used to calculate fat and muscle areas. Waist circumference is now one of the most valued measures and is used to estimate intraabdominal or visceral fat. This measurement is now widely recognized as being preferable to waist/hip ratio. Bioelectrical impedance analysis (BIA) has also gained widespread acceptance recently, particularly in population studies and mainly due to its ease of use. Other more sophisticated techniques such as computed tomography (CT) have also been used; however, the degree of irradiation has prevented the more widespread use of this method during growth. Future technological development could reduce this limitation and provide for the more extensive use of this method. Unfortunately, none of these methods has been directly validated by anatomical or biochemical methods.

The parameter of most widespread use in the assessment of overweight and obesity is the body mass index (BMI). BMI growth charts have been developed in many countries on measurements from the local growing population — for example, in France, the United States, Sweden, the United Kingdom, and the Czech Republic. Cutoff points for BMI have been established that enable the more accurate determination of overweight and obesity at different ages. However, results may not be relevant in different parts of the world as the cutoff points were established on the basis of measurements in only a relatively small number of countries. BMI has also been validated using other measurements of body composition such as BIA, MRI, DXA, and densitometry. Correlations have always been significant, but individual methods do not give identical results. The accuracy of the estimation of body fat using BMI alone is compromised, particularly in cases of more severe obesity. Where appropriately trained testers are available, the more direct measurement of body fatness by measuring skinfold thickness is recommended. However, the skinfold measurement may be a spurious technique in individuals who are very obese. As a relatively simple index, BMI provides the opportunity for trend data to be used to track individual and group predisposition for the development of obesity with increasing age. One of the most important components in this respect is the adiposity rebound (AR), where BMI starts to increase again after a temporary decline during childhood. Compared to their normal-weight peers, AR occurs earlier in obese children and is an important predictor of the development of obesity in later years. In addition, BMI percentile crossover during growth is also a direct means of predicting later fatness.

With respect to other morphological features, obese children commonly show an accelerated growth in height along with increased weight. However, higher stature may only be temporary as not all obese children remain tall as adults. An increase in stored fat is often accompanied by an increased development of lean, fat-free body mass, an increase in some bone dimensions (for example, bi-iliocristal breadth in boys), and bone density.

Fat deposited in the growing organism is not only indicative of increased relative (percentage of fat) and absolute amounts (kg of fat) but also of a different distribution pattern. These differences are reflected in various patterns of fat deposition on the trunk and extremities as evaluated by various indices calculated from skinfold thickness measurements — for example, the subscapular/triceps ratio. Similarly, the amount of intraabdominal fat relative to subcutaneous fat is important and presents an increased health risk during childhood. Intraabdominal fat can be assessed by ultrasound, by MRI, and also by simple anthropometric measurements such as the waist-to-hip ratio or the distance between the tip of the abdomen and L4 to L5 measured by pelvimeter (sometimes referred to a sagittal diameter or depth). The waist circumference measure is the preferred individual circumference measure.

The distribution of body fat varies significantly in normal-weight boys and girls but does not show any significant gender differences between obese boys and girls. Characteristic trends include an increased deposition of fat on the trunk as related to the extremities, or increased intraabdominal fat as related to subcutaneous fat. This type of fat pattern is significantly related to a number of adverse biochemical and hormonal characteristics. These morphological features can also provide an estimation of the possible variability in health risk in different types of obesity during growth. Childhood obesity is certainly associated with morphological change but also with changes in many other parameters, such as nutritional, functional, biochemical, hormonal, and psychological areas, which vary markedly when comparisons are made with normal-weight peers.

Both energy intake and energy expenditure have been studied extensively. In the former, food habits and the composition of ingested foods have been considered. With respect to energy output, total energy expenditure (TEE), resting metabolic rate (RMR), and energy spent in physical activity (AEE) have been the main areas of focus. These assessments have not necessarily been undertaken to elucidate their role in the development of obesity, or in the prevention, treatment, and management of the condition. The main cause(s) of obesity is undisputed and always present as an excess of energy relative to body needs. An energy imbalance is of particular concern in genetically predisposed individuals from families with an increased prevalence and susceptibility. It must be remembered that obesity never occurs in conjunction with a markedly restricted food intake as frequently occurs in poorer countries of the Third World and where malnutrition is rife. Similarly, obesity never occurs among young athletes involved in intensive, dynamic aerobic sports and training.

Some studies have shown neither an increased energy intake nor decreased resting or total energy output due to inactivity in assessments of children. Other studies that have compared obese and normal-weight youngsters have found significant differences, including an increased food intake and reduced activity. The discrepancies between the results of individual studies might stem from differences in experimental design, limited observation periods, and different approaches to methodology, including evaluation.

Resting metabolic rate (RMR, or resting energy expenditure, REE) is related mainly to body size and lean, fat-free body mass. Therefore, comparisons between direct measurements and indirect derivations of REE in obese and normal-weight children have identified certain differences. Because regression equations using body weight and/or height were derived on measurements of predominantly normal-weight children (WHO, 1985), direct measurements of RER are recommended for the evaluation of REE in obese children. Higher absolute values of REE have been found in obese children, but when values are adjusted to fat-free body mass, these values usually did not differ. The thermic effect of food (TEF, or meal TEM, and/or diet-induced thermogenesis, DIT) and REE were not related to different types of fat distribution. TEF (DIT) as a percentage of REE (RMR) was lower in obese children.

Total energy expenditure (TEE) can be measured using a number of methods — for example, direct and indirect calorimetry. More recently, doubly labeled water ($^2H_2$ ^{18}O) has been used for the measurement of TEE over a number of days under free-living conditions. However, the cost of this method is prohibitive and it is nonspecific in the sense that it cannot provide details of specific components of daily activity characterizing varying intensity and peak values, but only the total energy expenditure. Consequently, field measurements are largely used. The better options in this regard have included heart rate monitors, accelerometers, activity-rating scales, and questionnaires. Results gained in studies from this area are inconsistent. In relation to TEE, some studies have not shown any differences while others have found a higher TEE in the obese compared to normal-weight subjects, along with a higher volume of sedentary activities in obese subjects. This finding may be explained by the increased energy cost of all movements of an obese child. During the same physical workload, energy expenditure is higher in the obese because they carry excess fat load, causing additional strain and discomfort. The same or higher TEE can thus correspond(s) to lower physical activity in the obese compared to normal-weight subjects. When this was considered, it was concluded that the physical-activity level was lower and the ratio of sedentary activities higher in the obese. In some studies, a significant negative relationship between activity and fatness was shown. In subjects with a low activity level, the ratio of stored fat was higher, and the reverse situation appeared in active subjects who were leaner pro- vided the range of values of these particular characteristics was sufficiently large. These relationships were apparent from a very young age and became more pronounced as children aged. Overall, more studies have shown greater inactivity in obese individuals, and this applied more frequently when one or both parents were obese.

Similar conclusions were also gained by following, for example, Pima Indian children who are genetically more predisposed to obesity. For exam- ple, the time spent viewing television (considered as a marker of sedenta- rism) predicted weight gain 8 years later. Another study showed that in spite of a comparable TEE, the level of physical activity and energy expended was lower in obese children. In obese children, sport grades in school were lower as was the involvement in sport training. The effect of physical activity and exercise was most markedly demonstrated by longitudinal studies of the same subjects, where the differences in both activity and fatness were sig- nificant.

Physical fitness and performance are the functional characteristics that differentiate significantly obese and normal-weight individuals. Individual items of functional capacity are affected by excess fatness in different ways. Aerobic power measured on a treadmill test is the same in absolute values or higher in obese compared to normal-weight subjects. However, maximum O_2 per kg of body weight is lower in the obese and is a true reflection of cardiorespiratory fitness of the obese. Values for ventilatory threshold (VT, defined as the highest oxygen uptake at which the pulmonary ventilation stops to increase linearly) are lower in obese children. Similarly, results in dynamic performance of an aerobic nature and endurance are also worse in the obese, that is, wherever relocation of total body weight is required, such as running and jumping. However, muscle strength, which is dependent on total and particularly lean body mass, is often the same or even higher in the obese. Performance in static tasks is most often not compromised by excess fatness. The same may also apply to some motor skills involving smaller muscle groups (such as in plate tapping) or the use of individual limbs (such as in throwing, which also involves an element of strength).

Lung function measurements such as forced expiratory flow, maximal voluntary ventilation, minute ventilation, vital capacity, expiratory reserve volume, residual volume, diffusing capacity, and other characteristics have shown altered pulmonary function, indicating that bronchospasm of smaller airways occurs more frequently in obese children. Decreased distensibility of the chest wall has also been considered. Polysomnography showed a positive relationship between the apnea index with fatness and a negative correlation between the degree of sleepiness on multiple sleep latency tests. Many obese adolescents also snore.

Blood pressure significantly correlated with percent of ideal weight, skinfold thickness, adiposity, and BMI, particularly after an extended period with obesity. Obesity is associated with increased posterior wall thickness and left ventricular internal dimensions of the heart (assessed by echocardiographic parameters). These characteristics have been found as early as at age 6 years.

Plasma hemostatic measures such as D-dimer, fibrinogen, and plasminogen activator inhibitor-I were associated with body fatness. These relationships show that general adiposity and visceral adipose tissue might play a role in regulating plasma hemostatic factors in obese children. BMI and fatness indicators correlated with the number of white blood cells, lymphocytes, and neutrophils.

The measurement of food intake has shown that children were able to select an adequate diet without adult supervision when given a choice of nutrients. Some studies have revealed that satisfactory mechanisms to preserve an adequate energy balance exist from an early age. However, this applies when satiety mechanisms with respect to the energy balance of an organism are involved under conditions of normal food. Various factors affecting food intake and choice early in life can change this situation. Studies in infants have shown that a vigorous infant-feeding style was associated with greater adiposity. Infant food intake and nutritive sucking behavior at 3 months of age contributed to the measures of body size at 12 and 24 months. Mothers who preferred a chubby child more often had obese offspring.

The composition of food also has a significant effect. The ratio of protein at the age of 2 to 3 years had a significant positive relationship with the age of the adiposity rebound (AR), and then with BMI and body fatness at the age of 8 years and older. No other relationships with respect to food intake were revealed in a longitudinal study of French individuals. This reinforces that the earlier the onset of AR, increased BMI, and fatness, the more probable obesity is later in life.

There is some, especially more recent, evidence that obese children overeat. However, measurements of food intake have been conducted in a similar fashion to measurements of physical activity and EE, that is, mostly when obesity was fully developed and the observations concerned short periods of time, commonly not with simultaneous EE measurements. Many studies have shown the same food intake in obese and normal-weight children. In some studies, the food intake correlated with body weight and height only in obese children, not in normal-weight children or mixed groups. Other studies have shown that when energy intake was expressed in relation to fat-free mass, it was lower in the obese. Further studies have shown that the composition of the diet may be more important for the development of obesity than total intake of energy; this especially concerned the intake of fat at any age. A positive association of fat intake and adiposity development was found in a greater number of studies. Children of heavier parents preferred more fat and mothers have a greater influence on their children's food intake. Family situation and habits had significant effects. Eating in the absence of hunger, eating faster, and ingesting more snacks were also revealed in the obese.

The child's eating style is also important. The eating index (reflecting the child's precision in the ability to adjust food intake in response to changes in energy density of the diet) was correlated with body stores of fat. Children with greater adiposity were less able to regulate energy intake accurately. TEF (DIT) was lower in the obese children when compared to their normal-weight peers.

Food consumption patterns during the day are also important. Fewer meals per day, skipping breakfast, and ingesting relatively more food in the second half of the day, especially at dinner, is more common in obese children. Severely or morbidly obese children also eat more restaurant meals, pizzas, snacks, and soft drinks. Such children also eat faster and do not slow down their eating rate toward the end of the meal. Gastric electrical activity, measured by electrogastrography, was no different in obese children.

The utilization of macronutrients and the oxidation of fat are associated with body fatness. Exogenous fat oxidation expressed as a proportion of total fat oxidation correlated significantly with the degree of adiposity. This can be considered to be a protective mechanism to prevent a further increase in body fat mass in the organism. Exogenous carbohydrate utilization was found to be significantly greater and endogenous carbohydrate oxidation significantly lower in obese subjects when compared to their normal-weight peers. Obesity in preadolescent children is associated with an absolute increase in whole-body protein turnover, which is related to an increased lean, fat-free body mass. Both factors contribute to the explanation of the higher REE in the obese compared to normal-weight children.

Body fatness was significantly associated with a change of a number of biochemical parameters, as is the case in adults, particularly with serum lipid levels. A positive correlation between TC and TG, and the percentage of stored fat was already found in preschool children. HDL-C was significantly higher in active preschool children with a trend for lower adiposity. A more favorable serum lipid and lipoprotein level were associated with lower levels of fatness and a higher level of physical fitness in children aged 4 to 5 years and older. Obesity was associated with unfavorable lipid profiles in adolescents in many countries (Italy, Poland, Czech Republic, France, United States, and many others). In obese children in Rome, a higher level of ApoB, TG, TC, and LDL-C along with lower HDL-C levels were found. A higher TC/HDL-C ratio was also found in obese children in Austria and in another group of Italian children in the lower quartile of polyunsaturated fatty acid intake. TC and TG had a significant positive correlation with BMI in boys, and in girls, only TG correlated with BMI. Central fat patterning is an important marker of serum lipid deviations.

In vivo lipolysis reflecting the mobilization of lipid stores from subcutaneous adipose tissue of obese children showed a decreased sensitivity to epinephrine. A decreased mobilization of TG may contribute to excess fat accumulation during growth. Both intra- and extracellular triglyceride stores in the soleus muscle were higher in the obese. Differences were also found in the rate of lipolysis, for example among African- and Caucasian-American obese children.

Hyperuricemia has been observed in obese children; homocystein and C-reactive protein (CRP) were also associated with adiposity. Some parameters concerning mineral metabolism were also altered. These include alkaline-phosphatase, osteocalcin, parathyroid hormone, calcitonin, hydroxyproline, and cyclic AMP. All were significantly higher in obese children with lower urinary excretion of calcium and phosphate. During an oral glucose tolerance test (OGTT) the changes of calcium, phosphate, serum parathyroid hormone, and calcitonin were different in obese children. In some studies, bone mineral content (BMC) was also lower in the obese. Total antioxidant capacity and plasma levels of soluble antioxidant vitamins were reduced in obese subjects. Concentration of alanin-amino transferase (ALT) and cholinesterase (ChE) correlated positively with BMI, W/H ratio, insulin, and insulin/glucose index.

As primary classical hormonal disturbances causing greater fatness are far less common than simple adiposity, hormonal status and some deviations in obese children are mainly considered as secondary, resulting from a changed metabolic status. Most studies have characterized the levels of several hormones along with other metabolic, biochemical, and morphological parameters in the obese and mutual relationships established.

Insulin-like growth factor-1 (IGF-1) was significantly greater in obese children, and this correlated with body mass index. Values of IGF-1 increased significantly during puberty and were higher in the obese in the earlier stages of sexual maturation. Levels of insulin-like growth factor binding protein-3 (IGFBP-3) were not different in some studies. Similarly, the IGF-1/IGFBP-3 ratio was not different when comparing obese and normal-weight subjects. IGFBP-1 level is strongly associated with insulin sensitivity and fatness in early prepubertal children.

Insulin sensitivity, IGF-1, and obesity are important predictors of IGFBP-1 levels in pubertal children. IGFBP-1 is suppressed by insulin and may increase free IGF-1 levels and thus contribute to somatic growth, which is temporarily accelerated in obese children. The IGFBP-1 level may be a useful predictor for the early identification of the development of insulin resistance. The free form of IGF-1 in circulation in obese children is normal.

Significant positive relationships were found between BMI and somatomedin-C/insulin-like growth factor-1 (SM-C/IGF-1), and between immunoreactive insulin (IRI) and SM-C/IGF-1. Other studies revealed a significant correlation between BMI and immunoreactive insulin. These data seem to indicate that SM-IGF-1 in obese children is regulated by IRI, which is related to BMI. This regulating effect of insulin may be important in obese children since human growth hormone (HGH) production for stimulating factors is reduced.

In prepubertal children with exogenous obesity, the GH-IGF-1 axis is significantly altered, even when most changes in the peripheral IGF system appeared to be independent of modifications of GH secretion. Increased IGF-1 may also contribute, due to negative feedback, to the reduced growth hormone (GH) synthesis and secretion in obese children. Simple obesity is associated not only with a decrease in GH synthesis but also with increased GH clearance, along with increased insulin and IGF-1 levels. Growth hormone response to provocative stimuli is blunted and nocturnal GH concentrations are reduced. Obese children also have significantly lower urinary GH levels than age-matched normal-weight children.

Obese children have increased growth hormone binding protein (GHBP) activity. It may be speculated that this phenomenon can contribute to the compensation from the reduced GH secretion and accelerated GH clearance. GH also regulates the synthesis of IGF-1 in adipocytes, the increased amounts of which and of GHBP could be secreted from large amounts of adipose tissue in spite of GH hyposecretion. Affinity of GHBP is increased in the obese, and is associated significantly with percent of body fat, waist and hip circumferences, waist-to-hip ratio, body weight, serum leptin concentration, uric acid, insulin, TC, LDL-C, LDL-C/TC ratio, TG, and height standard deviation score (SDS). Multiple regression analysis including age, gender, anthropometric variables, percent of fat, and waist circumference as independent variables still revealed a significant association between GHBP and leptin, TG, TC and LDL-C, and LDL-C/HDL-C ratio. Body composition and visceral adiposity appear to be dominant negative determinants of GH production since the relationships between GH secretion and age and testosterone are attenuated or abolished by increased fatness.

Procollagen C-terminal peptide (PICP) increases during puberty with a more rapid decrease in girls and in normal-weight subjects. The PICP association to IGF-1 in normal-weight children and PICP to IGF-1/IGF-1BP molar ratio in the obese supports the concept that IGF-1 influences skeletal growth. IGF BP-1, which supports growth, is associated with insulin sensitivity and fatness in the obese during early puberty. BMI and immunoreactive insulin, which are interrelated, are also significantly associated with somatomedin-c/IGF-1.

Insulin resistance (IR) and hyperinsulinemia coexist in obese children. Both increased insulin secretion and decreased insulin clearance contribute to hyperinsulinemia in obese adolescents. Significant correlations between fasting insulin, body weight, fat mass (mostly visceral), and blood pressure was also found. Further studies have confirmed that the most important metabolic complication of obesity is impaired glucose tolerance, hyperinsulinemia, insulin resistance, decreased insulin sensitivity, and eventually noninsulin dependent diabetes mellitus type 2 (NIDDM). A defect in oxidative and nonoxidative glucose metabolism was revealed in obese preadolescents at the higher infusion rate using an euglycemic hyperinsulinemic clamp. The assessment of circadian rhythms has shown that insulin rhythm was disturbed but the secretion of insulin is as pulsatile as in adults. Higher levels of insulin were found in the saliva of obese children. The ability to inhibit lipolysis by insulin is impaired. Along with increased BMI, insulin sensitivity correlates significantly with blood pressure, TG, subcutaneous fat, percentage fat mass, and stage of sexual maturation, as found in African-American girls aged 5 to 10 years-old. Type 2 diabetes can occur already in early growth.

A higher secretion of steroids was reported in obese children when compared to normal-weight children, but the differences were greatly reduced when the excretion rate was related to total body weight. Body weight was correlated with certain steroid groups and compounds representing the androgens, androsteron, then ethiocholanolon and dehydroepiandrosteron. Differences in steroid secretion may indicate certain alterations in the adrenal function of obese children, but there was no reason to expect any significant disturbances in their steroid metabolism. Another study showed that obese children had an increased excretion of cortisol metabolites, along with an increased secretion of androgen metabolites and pregnenediol, a metabolite of pregnanolon. In some obese children. a hypersecretion of some components of the steroid spectrum was more frequent in boys. The integrated concentration of cortisol is also reduced in obese children. Hyperphagia and obesity are the common characteristics of hypercortisolism.

Menarche has been related to a certain level of fat deposition during puberty and usually occurs several months earlier in girls who are obese. The changes in circulating leptin can serve as a hormonal sign that influences gonadotrophin secretion. LH and FSH responses to GnRH were negatively correlated with BMI and circulating leptin in perimenarcheal girls and young adult women. In other words, decreased LH and FSH responses to GnRH were associated with increased adiposity. These findings were in agreement with a negative neuroendocrine effect of excess leptin in obese girls on the central reproductive system. Precocious puberty in obese children is assumed to be related to excess weight. Along with accelerated growth, bone age may also be advanced in obese children. Hyperandronemia was found along with hyperinsulinemia in girls with precocious menarche and central fat distribution.

Obese children have significantly higher average concentrations of beta-endorphin along with increased insulin. Beta-endorphin increases more with increasing fatness than insulin and is significantly associated with energy and macronutrient intake. Only in obese subjects was a correlation between these two hormones evident. The level of beta-endorphin may be used as an indicator of appetite in overweight and obese children. The reaction of somatostatin following a liquid meal is the same in obese and normal-weight subjects, in spite of a higher response of integrated insulin in the obese. It was revealed that it is unlikely that mutations in the coding region of the long isoform of the leptin receptor are a common cause of juvenile-onset obesity. Another study in extremely obese children did not show leptin deficiency mutation.

Ghrelin seems to be down-regulated in the obese, which may be a consequence of increased IR associated with visceral fat accumulation and increased PAI-1 concentration. Fasting values of ghrelin negatively correlate with BMI and waist circumference, not with percentage of overweight or percentage of fat, whereas leptin positively correlates with all parameters: BMI, waist circumference, percentage of overweight, and percentage of fat. Plasma ghrelin concentration has been found to negatively correlate with fasting immunoreactive insulin (IRI) and positively with PAI-1 concentrations. Ghrelin gene variation can contribute to obesity in children.

Abnormal secretion of gastric inhibitory polypeptide (GIP) and glucagon-like peptide-1 may be involved in the pathogenesis of hyperinsulinemia in obese children. Adiponectin, which longitudinally decreased with increasing body fat, negatively correlated with percentage of fat and fasting plasma insulin concentration in Pima Indian children aged 5 to 10 years old. Thyroid-stimulating hormone, T-3 and T-4, were increased in the obese 4.5 to 16 years old, and were associated with the degree of overweight; no correlation with leptin was found. Thyroid-stimulating hormone was not related to hemostatic markers. Thyroid dysfunction may be associated with an unfavorable hemostatic status present during growth.

A multivariate regression analysis of the interactions between tumor necrosis factor α (TNFα, a polypeptide cytokine) and insulin on circulating leptin levels among nonobese and obese children showed that plasma insulin levels were significantly positively associated with leptin levels even after adjustment for BMI in nonobese children. Plasma TNF-α levels were positively associated with leptin levels even after adjusting for BMI in girls only.

Increased adiposity contributes to an increased level of PAI-1-Ag, which is associated with leptin and insulin, but not after adjustment for fatness. BMI was the main determinant for variability of leptin, which does not seem to be independently linked with fibrinolytic parameters characterizing health risks.

Psychological assessments have indicated that the onset of obesity can depend on psychological problems such as stress in the family, at school, and among the peer group. On the other hand, obesity that develops in the early years of life can also contribute to psychological problems during childhood and beyond. Younger children generally do not perceive they have a problem provided they are not ridiculed. Physical growth changes are slower and more gradual during childhood than during adolescence, which is the period where self-awareness of appearance and body shape is more important. In addition to biological changes due to puberty, psychological adjustments also complicate this period of life.

There are a number of psychological accompaniments of childhood obesity. A well-planned psychological approach can significantly contribute to the evaluation of the causes of obesity, as well as play a key role in the management of obesity in a particular child. Common features include a fear of participating with normal-weight peers in social activities, games, and recreational activities. Children often feel shy and self-conscious, and avoid situations in which they may feel vulnerable or threatened — for example, in the gym or wearing swimwear. Their avoidance of physical activities and exercise further worsens their health and social status. Studies that have considered preferences for various forms of disability have consistently rated obesity poorly. Young children rate the obese lowest when compared with other forms of disability. Bullying of obese children is much more frequent than of nonobese children, and can complicate the psychological development of the obese child.

Obesity can contribute to an altered body image and related concerns. Body image, the picture that a person has of his or her appearance, may be disturbed with fluctuating intensity, even over short periods of time. Under positive conditions, the child may not be troubled by the disability although concern may never be far from one's consciousness. When one has esteem-lowering experiences and is depressed, more emphasis may be focused on his or her obesity, and the body becomes the explanation and symbol of unhappiness. Body perception disturbance is a form of disturbed perception of body image and is characterized by denial that the individual is the size that he or she is. The obese most commonly overestimate their body width compared with normal-weight individuals. Obese individuals are often evaluated as gluttonous and lack self-control, undermining their body image and isolating them psychologically and socially. On the other hand, food may become the individual's hatred and result in anorexia.

Excess weight and fatness may result in various physiological handicaps and altered psychological characteristics. For example, studies using a hyperactivity subscale (Connor's Parents Questionnaire) on the effects of obesity on various behavioral characteristics showed that children can have abnormal scores. Results showed higher "sex problem" scores in obese girls. Further evaluations indicated subtle behavioral differences in obese children. and the proportion of obese children placed in special education and remedial class settings was twice that for children with normal body weight.

Increased BMI is associated with unfavorable changes in physical activity attitudes, activity preferences, perceived physical activity competence, self-concept, and body image. There also appears to be a concern with body weight and shape. In severely obese children in China, lower performance on IQ scores plus a higher Eysenck Personality Questionnaire (EPQ) score was found. Obese Chinese children also showed lower total IQ, speech IQ, operation IQ, and thyroid function along with increased baseline secretion of insulin and C-polypeptide. Gonad development and maturity occurred earlier in the obese. However, decreased thyroid function may indicate some hormonal abnormalities in these obese children. Observations of this kind have not been reported in other populations of obese children.

Patients with early onset obesity demonstrated a greater frequency and higher levels of emotional distress and psychiatric symptomatology than individuals with a later onset of obesity. Psychiatric problems in adulthood may be associated with early onset of obesity, serving as a predictor variable for possible psychological disturbances in obese populations later in life. On the other hand, it is false to assume that all obese individuals are psychologically and emotionally disturbed. Many obese individuals do not perceive any problems and appear to cope more efficiently by pursuing other spheres of activity. This may include greater diligence at school and prevalence of sedentary occupations (such as stamp collecting, playing a musical instrument, etc.). These types of activities do not require a level of activity and physical fitness that would be required for participation in sports.

Juvenile obesity is usually accompanied by a number of health problems, related to biochemical, hormonal, and other changes. Childhood obesity contributes to approximately 30% of adult obesity. Parents do not often report concern about obesity as a poor health problem of their children, which may contribute to a late intervention or possibly none at all. This results in negative delayed health consequences. An obese child who becomes an obese adult will have more severe adult obesity than one whose obesity begins during the adult years. In such cases, the morbidity and mortality from all causes is increased, and risk of cardiovascular diseases, cancer (mainly of the colon), diabetes, and arthritis is higher. Participants who died during a 40-year longitudinal study in Sweden and those who reported cardiovascular diseases were significantly heavier at puberty and in adulthood than those who remained healthier.

One of the studies revealed that in a group of obese children, 28% had hyperlipidemia, 25% had elevated blood pressure, and 30% had asthma. Of these children, 63% had an obese mother, 31% had an obese father, and 50% had one or more obese siblings. Unfit children appear to be at an increased risk of high levels of serum lipids. This is primarily due to an increase in body fatness. In another study, it was shown that each 10 mm increase in the sum of 10 skinfolds was associated with a decrease of 1.4 $mg.dL^{-1}$ of HDL-C. Circulating leptin levels were significantly correlated not only with body weight, body fat, systolic blood pressure, and fasting blood sugar but also with TC, LDL-C, and TG. Increased blood pressure was apparent under resting conditions, and abnormal blood pressure reactions appeared during workload. Heart rate during workload was also increased more in obese children compared to normal-weight peers, indicating a lower level of cardiorespiratory efficiency and fitness. Associated health risks are greater the longer the individual has been obese and particularly when children approach adolescence. Increased visceral fat showed greater health risk than total and subcutaneous fat.

As mentioned earlier, the overweight and obese have an increased insulinemia, insulin resistance (IR), and impaired glucose tolerance, and a greater risk of type 1 diabetes mellitus in early life. One study showed also that the prevalence of NIDDM was on average twofold greater from the age of 2 years onward when compared to normal-weight children of both genders. Insulin resistance with respect to glucose metabolism was evident in obese children, and hyperinsulinemia was related to the development of hypertension. Insulin resistance correlated inversely with intramyocellular triglyceride stores (IMCL). A threshold value for visceral adipose tissue (VAT), VAT/SAT (subcutaneous AT), and sagittal abdominal diameter as a risk for metabolic derangement (insulin, TG, alanin aminotransferase) was defined in obese subjects.

The prevalence of multimetabolic syndrome (MMS) is also seen in obese children and includes hypertension, hyperinsulinemia, hypercholesterolemia, hypertriglyceridemia, low HDL-C, and impaired glucose tolerance. These features were associated with resting tachycardia, low physical fitness and reduced α-tocopherol plasma concentrations. In obese children and adolescents, the development of a fatty liver (hepatosteatosis) has been observed, is related to hyperinsulinemia, and can be accompanied by further metabolic alterations.

The deviations of lipid profile as given above are predisposition for cardiovascular diseases, and have been also studied jointly with hematological (P-selectin, D-dimer, etc.) body composition and hormonal characteristics as related to health risks. It was shown that that in the obese subjects, insulin, PAI-1, and fragment 1+2 of prothrombin were positively correlated with BMI. Fibrinogen and factor VII levels were also associated with fatness. Apo-E polymorphism seems to influence some lipid profile abnormalities associated with increased fatness; however, clustering of risk factors and IR seem not to be dependent on Apo-E polymorphism. C-reactive protein concentration was also correlated with cardiovascular risks, but only HDL-C, heart rate, and blood pressure remained statistically significant after adjustment for ponderal index.

Especially in children of hypertensive parents, obesity was related to an increased blood pressure in the growing obese. The risk of hypertension increases across the whole range of BMI values, and there is no threshold in connection with other metabolic and hormonal abnormalities. Increased blood pressure (BP) is manifested during rest and physical activity. Increased systolic BP was associated with hyperinsulinemia, hyperleptinemia, and visceral fat accumulation. Waist circumference was independently associated with cardiovascular risk factors, especially diastolic BP and IR, and independently of age and degree of sexual maturation. Variability of BP during daytime and sleep was greater in the obese. Arterial stiffness may be an indicator of early vascular changes. Aortic strain and pressure elastic modulus were significantly different in the obese hypertensive subjects along with increased BMI and total cholesterol. Endothelial dysfunction was also correlated with fatness.

There is an increased chance of obese children and adolescents developing some respiratory symptoms, correlating with body weight and triceps skinfold. This is also related to some alterations in respiratory function mentioned previously.

Hormonal alterations include menstrual disorders (oligomenorrhea, amenorrhea, or irregular menses) and polycystic ovarian syndrome (PCOS), which may be manifested at a perimenarcheal age. A significant positive relationship was found between waist-to-hip ratio and testosterone (T) levels, but not with insulin. A significant association was also found between BMI and T. These results seem to indicate that in girls with menstrual irregularities, overweight is associated with hyperinsulinemia along with an increase in androgen production, which may be a risk factor for PCOS. It is also common for parents to visit a medical doctor with their obese sons because they think their sexual development is retarded. Most commonly, the problem is related to an increased amount of fat deposited on the lower abdomen that makes the evaluation of the degree of sexual maturation more difficult.

Obesity during the growing years is also accompanied by orthopedic problems. These include increased intermalleolar distance, flat and hyper-mobile feet that minimize foot stability. Knee osteoarthritis also develops prematurely in severely obese individuals. Blount's disease (tibia vara) is also the result of increased stress on young bone from excess weight. Genu varus and foot discomfort–associated structural changes often produces additional lower extremity exacerbations that include compensatory prona-tion, talar adduction, and a degree of in-toeing. A decrease in balance capac-ity and a negative effect on static postural control were also revealed.

Body posture can also be altered due to excess weight and weakness in postural muscles. Hyperlordosis and a protruding abdomen are the result of excess fat deposition, an inadequate position of the vertebral column, and the tone of the abdominal muscles. Shoulders are often uneven and a "turtle neck" may also develop. Protruding scapulae and the eventual deviations of the vertebral column are less apparent than in normal children because of the extent of the subcutaneous fat layer. Muscle weakness accompanying a low level of physical fitness is the main cause. Measurements of bone mineral content showed that during growth obese children do not increase their bone mineral density to fully compensate for their excessive weight. Dental caries were more related to diet and sugar consumption, but other factors such as oral hygiene and saliva composition should also be considered.

Increased adiposity is associated also with impairments of host-defense mechanisms. Measurements of salivary IgA and serum C3c IgA showed compromised secretory immune system without marked manifestation in clinical symptoms and infections.

Sleep disturbance is also linked to obesity; obstructive sleep apnea appears often in obese children and is associated with other metabolic deviations. Experimental studies elucidated further the relationships between adiposity and metabolic disturbances.

Observations in long-living populations revealed the relationship between leanness, modest diet, better health, higher physical activity and fitness, and longer life expectancy as compared with ethnic groups living especially in cities at lower altitude, with less physical activity and different diet and life habits.

14.2 Treatment and Management Principles

Long-lasting positive effects of reduction treatment of the obese during growth are very difficult to achieve; therefore, treatment for obese children and adolescents must reflect the multidimensional nature of the condition. A clear explanation of the pathogenesis of obesity is a very difficult task, and therefore a multidisciplinary approach is warranted. There are three key components of treatment during the growing years: diet, exercise, and psychological support.

Best results can be achieved through the cooperation of a team of specialist health professionals, including pediatricians, nutritionists, psychologists, and physical educators/exercise physiologists. To many people, such a team seems to be superfluous as the principles of treatment seem to be self-evident. However, if the treatment process were so simple, there would be a much lower prevalence of obesity and also a greater success in treating permanently obesity at all ages.

When obesity has not advanced to a serious level, a logical recommendation is to monitor the individual's lifestyle, starting with nutrition so that the child does not increase in weight and fatness. He or she would "grow into" an optimal height and desirable value for BMI in relation to age and gender. However, this approach does not always provide desirable long-term results and is only temporary. Moreover, parallels exist between unsuccessful weight loss attempts and psychological problems that may include a predisposition to eating disorders. These problems are not only a personal difficulty for a child or adolescent, but can also seriously jeopardize the possibility of successful treatment.

As mentioned previously, each child has a unique personality, in spite of the many common traits of obesity. The first step in the treatment process is for the child to be properly examined for general health, morphological, nutritional, functional, biochemical, hormonal, and psychological status. This is critical in children who have a greater risk of familial obesity. This individual approach is usually more efficient than a group one.

Behavior modification involves the consideration of the amount and composition of the diet along with changes in physical activity that should be addressed using an individualized approach and support. This is always easier when started at a younger age and as close as possible to the commencement of obesity. For this reason, more detailed examinations of children who may be at risk should be undertaken as to treat early and often may be the best approach. An individualized treatment strategy with an integration of basic scientific information with a clinical research outcome are the components of a therapeutic approach recommended for obese children. According to the individual child, there may be significant differences in the reaction to various regimes of treatment. The same treatment will not have the equivalent effect on every obese individual. On the other hand, very similar results may be achieved with quite different approaches. Some studies have followed up on markers of possible success in treatment. Results showed that the best predictors of weight gain after 2 years were high protein oxidation, low activity EE, and high RQ during the TEF. This has led to the conclusion that EE, RMR, and components of substrate oxidation are predictors of an increase of body weight and fat in late childhood.

The supporting role of family during the treatment phase is essential. Children with obese parents are generally fatter than children with normal-weight parents, and generally lose weight with greater difficulties. This indicates the important role of genetic factors as well as the family environment from the very beginning of life. Children of obese parents might lose more weight than the average, but they also regain weight more easily. Short-term results might be good, but such individuals are at a greater risk of not maintaining the positive results of the weight reduction treatment.

The treatment process, both as a group or as individual therapy, must attempt to profit from the cooperation of the family. A parent-directed weight-reduction program can facilitate positive changes in children with respect to weight and fat loss. The degree of compliance may also be expected to be much higher. It has been shown that the greater the number of sessions of group therapy attended by mothers, the greater the weight loss of the obese daughters being treated. Parents should therefore be direct participants in any intervention program. Children who were more successful initially in treatment had fewer siblings and were females. The situation can be different with older children as family size can interact with the treatment to determine the weight changes in other ways.

Other predictors of success include self-monitoring and personal involvement of the child being treated. In this respect, appropriate parental assistance and psychological treatment to rectify poor lifestyle behaviors are essential. The major focus should be on a combined approach to reduce inactive behaviors while providing assistance to improve physical skills and supporting sound nutritional practices. The support of a group of similar obese individuals can help to improve adherence and thus improve treatment results. However, an individual approach may be more suitable for others. Decisions need to based on the personal characteristics of children.

Arguably, the most important feature of weight management for the obese child is the dietary intake. The establishment of recommended dietary allowances for obese children is a difficult task. Such determinations need to be made according to the individual characteristics of the child (such as age, gender, degree of sexual maturation, duration and degree of obesity, physical activity level, and energy output). This is one of the reasons for a comprehensive health appraisal of each child. Dietary history must be assessed, at least to establish eating patterns across a typical week. This can be best achieved with the direct assessment technique of weighing food with the help of a dietitian, nurse, or comparably trained health professional. This is a very demanding and time-consuming approach and may be biased as individuals under direct control do not eat as they usually do, and/or are inaccurate in their record keeping. A combination of food diaries and/or food frequency records completed with the help of the parents and teachers, and supplemented by interviews, can accurately assess daily food intake and composition. Computer programs may also be used to assist with analyses as long as the program is representative of locally available foodstuffs.

The results of such individual analyses provide an indication of poor dietary habits and can therefore be of great assistance in the design of a special diet suitable for the obese child at his or her particular age. The recommended allowance of energy should encompass the desired components for growth but be sufficiently conservative to allow for the mobilization and utilization of stored fat with regular participation in physical activity. The aims of the weight-management process for the child are to mobilize stored fat while maintaining normal growth in height and fat-free body mass and to improve functional capacity.

In more serious cases of obesity, very low-energy diets may be used. This process should be reserved for a relatively small number of individuals and the energy intake defined as exactly as possible. RDAs for the amount and ratio of the individual macro- and micronutrients for a particular age and gender category must be adhered to. Special protein-sparing diets with an increased amount of protein (up to 2.5 $g.kg^{-1}$ ideal weight of the child) have been used with young people to promote significant weight loss and maintain fat-free body mass. However, some studies have shown that in spite of an increased intake of protein, total body potassium and nitrogen decreased, accompanied by a considerable weight loss. As lean body mass is generally greater in obese children, such a temporary loss may be tolerated if one considers other positive improvements in health status found at the same time. Nevertheless, the use of such diets, as is the case for the classical hypocaloric diet, should be conducted under medical supervision. The best scenario may be under inpatient conditions where physical activity can also be fostered. Very low-energy diets (VLED) have been also used in children but this approach is not recommended for growing individuals; they are justified in rare cases of morbidly obese with health complications, under conditions of inpatient treatment.

The composition of any diet used in weight management may need to be modified, particularly with respect to the content of saturated fat. Diets with a low fat and sugar content have resulted in a decreased energy intake and increased weight loss. Fat intake must not decrease under 30% total energy intake, especially during earlier periods of growth, to assure optimal somatic and nervous system development. Recommended allowances should consider not only age and gender, but also energy output; in very active subjects (however rare among obese), they might be not so strict. Some studies have shown that it is not necessary to supplement such a diet with polyunsaturated fatty acids (PUFA). Logical low-fat alternatives are skim milk and low-fat cuts of meat. However, the possibility for slight deficits in vitamin E needs to be considered.

Low-energy diets can result in significant changes in body composition and a decrease in BMI and REE. In some studies, no reduction of potassium and nitrogen was observed but such changes obviously depend on the degree of food reduction and changes in food composition. Nitrogen balance can fluctuate, but after a certain period it will stabilize. Nitrogen losses show great variability in individual subjects, even under comparable conditions.

This is further evidence of the individual nature of all components of life-style, including nutrition. In some studies, blood glucose, serum protein, and urea is reduced after such diets but serum albumin does not change.

The thermic effect of food (TEF or DIT) has been reported as being lower in obese children but can significantly increase after a reduction diet. This indicates a slight thermogenic defect in some obese children, representing a consequential rather than an etiological factor in such children. Total anti-oxidant capacity (TAC) and plasma levels of lipid soluble antioxidant vita-mins, which are also lower in obese individuals, have increased after reduction treatment using a hypocaloric diet. Some reducing diets have been supplemented by special ingredients, mostly fiber, wheat bran, or glucoman-nan. Weight loss with such supplementation has not differed from an unsup-plemented diet but some serum lipid features do change.

Therefore, hypocaloric diets can be a risk, especially for the potential deficiency in some essential items. However, some studies did not show any change after such diets in serum content of, for example, Fe, ferritin, and transferrin. A hypocaloric diet followed for 14 weeks did not have any significant effect on heart parameters, intraventricular septal thickness, left ventricular wall thickness, and left ventricular volume. After weight reduc-tion, reduced heart rate and QT interval was found in obese children. Systolic and diastolic blood pressure also decreased. The effect of sodium intake in the regulation of blood pressure was followed; the results supported the hypothesis that blood pressure of obese adolescents is sensitive to sodium intake. This sensitivity may be due to the combined effects of hyperinsuline-mia, hyperaldosteronism, and increased activity of the sympathetic nervous system, all characteristic of obesity.

A reduction in weight following a restricted diet also results in changes to some respiratory parameters such as peak expiratory flow and forced expiratory volume. With a diet-only approach, no changes may occur; how-ever, hypopnea, obstructive sleep apnea, and respiratory disturbance index may improve significantly. As is the case in adults, serum lipid profiles improve significantly after weight loss due to caloric restriction. TC, LDL-C, TG, and apo-lipoprotein B decreased, and apo-lipoprotein A, HDL-C, and HDL-C/TC increased. After weight reduction, IGF II and BP2 increased, and IGF-1, BP1, BP3, and IGF-1/IGF-3 decreased. The ratio of BP1/BP2 was ameliorated. The decrease in IGF-1/BP3 ratio after weight loss indicated a decrease in biologically active IGF-1, which may contribute to the explana-tion of impaired growth velocity in obese children after a restricted diet.

Similar changes were observed in another study; the ratio of IGFBP-2 to IGFBP-1 was inversely related to TC and LDL-C. IGFBP-2 was inversely correlated with waist-to-hip ratio. In other studies, a simultaneous reduction of TG, insulin, FFA, and apo-lipoprotein A1 and B was found. A significant decline in serum triiodothyronine (T3) concentration along with a decrease of RMR after weight loss due to a 6-week low-calorie diet was also observed. T3 concentration reduction combined with FFM loss could be responsible for a RMR decline.

Serum insulin usually decreases after weight loss along with the reduction of insulin resistance and increased insulin sensitivity. Leptin also decreases; for example, a significant reduction from 16.5 to 10.0 ng.ml^{-1} after a reduction of BMI was observed. Plasma apo-lipoprotein A and HDL-C were independent predictors of leptin concentrations during weight reduction. Similar favorable changes following weight reduction were also observed in children with NIDDM.

The use of physical activity and exercise without dietary change usually has slower effects on childhood obesity. Exercise contributes to the maintenance and further development of fat-free body mass. Therefore, it is highly recommended for the treatment of obesity during childhood, when a heavily restricted dietary intake can result in a slowing of growth in height and a reduction of muscle mass. The aim should be to increase habitual physical activity and then progressively add more intense exercise. This is possible in a range of settings such as in physical education classes and activity summer camps like those in widespread use in Europe and North America.

There is strong evidence of the positive effect of exercise on body composition provided activity is dynamic, weight bearing, and aerobic. Longitudinal observations of 8- to 14-year-old boys involved in various physical activities and exercise have shown significantly reduced deposition of stored fat and increased development of lean, fat-free mass along with changes in BMI and increased aerobic power in subjects who participated in a satisfactory level of sport training, especially during summer holiday camps lasting weeks.

Observations in experimental situations with laboratory animals have enabled the *in vitro* and *in vivo* measurement of selected characteristics of lipid metabolism modified by the adaptation to increased and/or decreased physical activity (usually running on a treadmill). Trained animals have shown an increased ability to mobilize and utilize fat metabolites, characteristics that were also evident under resting conditions. Consequent changes included a decreased deposition of fat in spite of a higher food intake. Limited observations in adult humans, with biopsies of adipose and/or muscle tissue, have supported these findings. In children, such studies have not been executed for obvious ethical reasons yet.

The effect of exercise in growing youth is marked when the intensity fluctuates or when activity is temporarily interrupted. Body weight and BMI usually does not change markedly, but subcutaneous and total body fat increases significantly following a reduction in TEE. The reverse is found when TEE is increased by exercise.

The effect of well-organized physical activity and exercise has been demonstrated in numerous longitudinal observations in obese children. Various strategies have been employed. A meaningful comparison of results is difficult as the subjects and mode of exercise treatment are invariably quite different. However, in many studies a significant effect of exercise has been shown in relation to a decrease in body weight, BMI, and fatness (decrease in visceral fat), along with an increase in aerobic power and physical performance, provided that the intensity, character, duration, and frequency were sufficient. These changes fluctuated when the intensity of exercise therapy changed. There is a direct relationship between dose and response in terms of body composition and fitness parameters.

Boys exposed to four annual doses of activity during various stages of the treatment of obesity and under conditions of variable intensity of exercise showed decreases in serum lipids and an increase in HDL-C compared to boys treated only by a restricted diet. Even mild exercise, which may not result in weight loss, can improve glucose homeostasis, insulin dynamics, and risk factors for coronary heart disease. Exercise also favorably alters cardiac autonomic function by reducing the ratio of sympathetic to parasympathetic activity. Exercise is important for all obese individuals but particularly suitable for milder degrees of obesity and also for the prevention of the excess deposition of fat because exercise impairment in such individuals would commonly be minimal. A 4-year longitudinal study was conducted in which obese boys were measured before and after each year's summer camp. Better results were obtained at the age of 11 and 12 years than at the age of 13 and 14 years regarding the parameters of greater decrease of body fat, weight, and BMI; none or a smaller decrease of lean, fat-free mass and greater functional improvement were noted.

Many studies have not shown the same levels of improvement, and have therefore suggested or inferred that the role of exercise is superficial. It is important to qualify and question such findings. Some of the contradictions may be due to an insufficient intensity of exercise, or a treatment program that was too short. In many studies, dietary intake was not checked. Rather than the exercise being problematic, energy intake may have increased.

In summary, the best way to treat childhood obesity is to combine diet and exercise treatment and provide psychological support. This means a repetition of old truths, but under changing new life conditions, unfortunately, these are still not yet satisfactorily adhered to. The reduction of excess fat can be more pronounced with a monitored approach and improvements in body composition, serum lipids, hormone profile, and cardiovascular fitness. Functional parameters and physical fitness level will also be maximized using such an approach.

With regard to practical recommendations, suitably arranged school programs seem to be one of the best approaches for the optimal intervention using diet, exercise, and overall lifestyle modification. Outpatient and especially inpatient opportunities are quite rare and very costly. Summer camps are used to good effect in many countries and have a strong tradition with good results. However, the number of such camps is also very limited given the increasing numbers of obese children. Such camps may also be considered unsatisfactory as the positive results gained during the camps are often lost during the following school year; however, when absolved repeatedly during growth, they result in positive and more lasting results.

Dietary strategies are an indispensable component of weight management for obese children and adolescents, but need to be well organized and follow appropriate appraisals of current status. Energy should be derived individually, according to the recommendations of the WHO, EU, National Research Council (U.S.), and similar sources of RDAs prepared for specific populations, with all respects as given above. The composition of the diet should follow the desired ratio of protein as 12 to 13%, fats up to 30% (with one-third saturated, one-third monounsaturated, and the remainder polyunsaturated fatty acids), and 57 to 60% of carbohydrates. According to the WHO (1985), simple sugars should not exceed 10% of energy intake. However, this should be even lower in the case of obese children and the intake of sweets replaced by more appropriate food choices such as fruit. But as mentioned earlier, RDAs especially for fat and sugar should be considered with regard to physical activity level (PAL) as recommended by the WHO. This might vary due to different increases in exercise.

Vitamins and minerals must also correspond to the RDA for a particular age and gender group. When hypocaloric diets are prescribed, some vitamins and minerals may need to be supplemented. There must also be a sufficient intake of beverages, excluding sodas and sweetened soft drinks. Good quality drinking water is most desirable, although this can be a problem in some urban areas. Water and a small quantity of unsweetened fruit juice can be used as an alternative. Mineral water must be used cautiously, and snack foods, sweets, and other highly processed and energy dense products should be significantly reduced or excluded.

Along with adequacy of food and drink, the frequency of meals and their daily distribution is also important. The most desirable number of meals per day is questionable (but at least five per day), and is very much an individual issue. Nevertheless, an adequate breakfast and lunch should be the aim. Fresh fruit, low-fat yogurts, tomatoes, and other vegetables should be encouraged as snack items. Dinner should be served early, and wherever possible, this should be at least 2 to 3 hours before bedtime and should not represent the largest meal of the day. A unified approach or recipe for success is not possible for all children. These guidelines should serve as an appropriate starting point for all children.

Other approaches have also been used in the treatment of childhood obesity. Drug therapy in excessively obese children has been reported without adverse health complications; however, this approach is not recommended for children despite some positive results of short-term observations. Gastric and plastic surgery has also been used in children and adolescents. Intragastric balloon therapy did not give satisfactory results, and there is a lack of suitability of this procedure during growth. Alternative approaches such as acupuncture have also been used and positive results reported.

Practical approaches concerning physical activity must also be prepared according to the individual needs of the child. The medical checkup should consider the functional capabilities of the child and be part of the determination of whether the child can and should participate in the normal physical education program at school. Differences of opinion exist regarding the merits of obese children participating in physical education. Some would argue that an avoidance of physical education is recommended in the case of more severe or morbid obesity, particularly when the individual has more serious accompanying co-morbidities and orthopedic defects. Such children are likely to avoid physical education anyway if they perceive the setting to be threatening. A separate opportunity to move and experience physical activity with peers of a similar size and shape may be an excellent interim step to the longer-term aim of future mainstreaming of such children into normal activity settings, including at school.

Physical activity and exercise should be commenced in a controlled fashion. In the more serious cases of obesity, it is often best to start activity in an aquatic environment. The buoyancy provided by body fat helps to compensate for one's weight and enables a concentration on specific body movements. Progressively, it is recommended that various exercises be completed in a lying position on the back or on the abdomen and then move to sitting and kneeling positions. Individual exercises should be thoroughly explained and supervised, and technique should be checked and corrected where necessary. All activities should be completed slowly and safely in a nonthreatening environment. When some success is made in the activity setting or perhaps a combination of weight loss and motor improvement is noted, it is important to progress to the usual form of physical education and related activities as soon as possible. As mentioned earlier, the best procedure in the short term is for obese children to exercise together so they do not feel inferior to normal-weight peers who can behave quite cruelly with a lack of understanding and empathy for their bigger classmates.

Initially, exercise should aim to develop the cardiorespiratory system and increase the aerobic power of the child. A higher level of aerobic functioning facilitates the mobilization and utilization of fat metabolites, and therefore such activity is highly suitable for reduction treatment. After an initial period of preparatory exercises when the child has adapted to a higher work output and improves his or her skills, has increased habitual physical activity, and has lost some weight, it is recommended that children run. This may initially occur in an intermittent fashion and be interspersed within games. Swimming is most suitable at the beginning of treatment or for maintenance following weight loss, as it is a useful all-round exercise. However, it does not contribute greatly to weight loss. The continuous development of skills is a necessary precursor to an optimal involvement of the child in other exercises, games, and sport activities. Dance is also a very desirable supplement to an exercise regime as it can be made attractive for all children. The present styles of dancing guarantee a considerable increase in energy expenditure with the necessary intensity. Stretching activities should always be included in such a program.

In time, other disciplines such as track and field can be introduced and participation in various games such as football and basketball can be encouraged. Cycling is not highly recommended due to the increased risk of injury. However, using a bicycle ergometer for supplementary exercises at the beginning of the treatment process can be useful.

The enhancement and improvement of motor skills should be a goal for all children, as a predisposition of greater partiality for exercise and increased physical activity. In reality, obese children fare poorly in most activity tasks, but this is mainly attributed to the lack of opportunity or a reduced chance to try. A major challenge for all obese or overweight people is to manage their own weight in the available space during weight-bearing activities. Improvements in motor skill can be slow and in the obese may be achieved only following the loss of a considerable amount of weight. Muscle strength is usually greater in the obese children, but specific strength of certain muscle groups can contribute to an improvement in body posture and the reinforcement of the supporting musculature of the vertebral column to prevent back pain. However, this also concerns children and youth of normal weight.

Children should be knowledgeable about everything they do, including the purpose of exercise. They should be encouraged even when no great results are apparent and stimulated to personally become involved in their physical activity regime. Self-monitoring of physical activity and exercise along with a proper diet and food patterning is the best way not only to achieve the weight loss but also to permanently maintain the desirable body composition improvements. Common everyday physical activities such as walking, climbing steps, working in the yard, and so on can contribute to an increase in energy expenditure.

The prescribed exercise should include the involvement of all muscle groups. A conditioning program should include a warm-up period, exercises for the development of the cardiorespiratory system, stretching, and skill activities. The home environment, gym, or playground should be pleasant and attractive in order to provide an enjoyable atmosphere. The choice of an appropriate time to exercise during the day is also important, especially after a period of adaptation. However, this depends on the program of the child at school, in the family, and so on.

Breathing exercises and special exercises aimed toward improving the support of the vertebral column and posture should be included. The particular choice and mix of activities depends on the individual child, his or her personality, degree of obesity, health status, and level of physical fitness. The program should be modified according to all these characteristics in an attempt to achieve the best long-lasting results.

Finally, the role of the family must again be stressed. The best way is to adapt activity, similar to the focus with nutrition, to the needs of the child and to undertake at least part of the exercises and physical activities together. It is absolutely critical to avoid any ridiculing of the child for his or her effort. On the contrary, encouragement, praise, and appreciation are necessary ingredients for everyone. Obese children have enough negative experiences in the school and other environments; at least with the family they should feel at ease all of the time. It is highly desirable that the teacher who oversees the physical education of obese children should be an understanding and personable individual.

The main aim of all work in the treatment and management of obesity is to achieve not only a reduction in weight, BMI, and excess fat but to improve the overall health status and well-being of the child. The development of optimal somatic characteristics, metabolic fitness, increased functional capacity, improved physical performance, and health, and an increase in self-esteem, are further goals for obesity management during growth. They should be aimed toward the future physical, social, and psychological well-being of each child.

15

General Conclusions and Perspectives

To conclude with some final comments, it is necessary to remember that there are numerous unanswered questions and unsolved problems, mainly due to the multifactorial nature of obesity. First, the role of both endo- and exogenous environmental factors in the onset and development of obesity during growth has not yet been satisfactorily elucidated. This applies in spite of extensive research that has been conducted during recent years — for example, to consider genetic, hormonal, and social factors that may explain the origin and development of obesity. These issues have been investigated in cross-sectional and longitudinal studies. The latter set of studies have provided the most valuable information; however, definite conclusions cannot be defined yet. Further studies concerning other key factors such as diet and physical activity have also been conducted. It is certainly the case that the problem of childhood obesity cannot be solved by a single-factor analysis. In addition, mutual relationships between the influences of various factors over time may also play very important roles. Despite significant advances in our understanding, it is necessary to consider that there may be more that is left to be explained and solved than has been elucidated to date.

When childhood obesity is generally defined, it can be concluded that an excess deposition of fat in childhood is a phenomenon that is not consistent with the natural trends of growth. Under normal, physiological conditions, this period of development is characterized, as compared with adulthood and advanced age, by a lower ratio of stored fat and higher ratio of lean, fat-free body mass. This applies to those with normal weight and BMI in the individual age categories. Two periods, the period just prior to the adiposity rebound (AR) occurring at the preschool age and then during the prepubertal period, are characterized by quite a low deposition of fat. These periods are also defined as sensitive and critical periods of development. With increasing age, fat is deposited in greater quantities, even when BMI remains the same. Therefore, childhood obesity does not correspond with expected trends during growth. The phrase "fattening is aging" is justified and is already evident during childhood and adolescence.

Excessive adiposity is associated with some other functional, biochemical, and hormonal changes that are in line with the conclusions on the above-mentioned body composition changes. The young growing organism is also characterized by a higher level of aerobic power, expressed as the uptake of oxygen during a maximal workload, related to body weight (max $O_2.min^{-1}.kg^{-1}$). This parameter is considered one of the essential physiological characteristics of the cardiorespiratory, efficiency, fitness, and functional capacity of the organism, irrespective of activity status. Aerobic power deteriorates under normal conditions with increasing age and is considered a marker of "positive health." The increased value of aerobic power is now recognized as a marker of optimal health status, physical fitness, well-being, and reduced health risks of any individual.

The highest values for aerobic power are achieved during prepuberty and puberty, and gradually decrease throughout adulthood and old age. The level of aerobic power is lower in the obese compared to normal-weight children. When this functional parameter is related to lean, fat-free body mass, it is usually the same, but under conditions of more severe obesity, it may be lower. This differential is reflected in significantly lower performances in dynamic, weight-bearing activities in obese children, who run and jump with a lower level of ability than their lean peers. With respect to physical performance, only muscular strength and some skills involving smaller muscle groups of the extremities are not influenced by obesity in children and youth. More detailed research concerning functional capacity in individuals during different periods of growth and obesity development could provide a key to the prevention and treatment of the condition. A certain level of functional capacity and skill is a predisposition for a more active lifestyle and exercise.

A high level of spontaneous physical activity associated with higher aerobic power is one of the important characteristics of a growing, leaner organism. The frequency of involvement in spontaneous activity generally decreases later in life, with individuals showing more of a preference for sedentary activities. This is apparent in normal-weight youngsters of all species who clearly demonstrate spontaneity of movement and a more playful nature than older individuals. This difference is also associated with a relatively higher energy intake (as related to total and/or lean, fat-free body mass). A higher level of energy turnover in the growing organism therefore occurs. For that reason, it is more natural to increase the energy expenditure than to decrease energy intake in the treatment of obesity. However, in obese children, the level of physical activity is usually lower compared to normal-weight children, in spite of the same or even higher total energy expenditure. This is not caused by higher motor activity, but by a higher cost of any movement during usual daily activities. Also, energy intake has often been reported as being the same or even lower than in lean peers. More recent studies however have shown increased energy intake when following subjects over longer periods.

Excess fatness is also associated with increased levels of serum lipids, i.e., total cholesterol (TC), LDL-C, and triglycerides, and with lower HDL-C and ApoA 1. This is another characteristic of older organisms compared to those undergoing growth. Insulin levels are higher and insulin sensitivity is lower in obese individuals, with the level of growth hormone being lower and its clearance higher, which results in its reduced levels. Leptin levels are higher, and this correlates with total body fat. The obese also show higher IGF levels. The interaction of hormonal activities during the process of excess fat deposition, as well as during its reduction, will be another interesting problem to be elucidated further and in greater detail.

Hormonal and biochemical changes are significantly associated with more frequent and earlier health problems in obese children and youth. This mainly concerns the increased risk for cardiovascular diseases; the early onset of atherosclerosis (which has been defined as a pediatric problem), hypertension, and the like. Type 2 diabetes mellitus, which usually appears much later in life, is also more frequent in obese children than in their normal-weight peers. All these problems usually appear in the obese much earlier than in lean individuals. Childhood obesity is significantly related to adult obesity, and the morbidity and mortality of the above-mentioned diseases is more frequent at an earlier age in those who are already obese in adolescence and earlier. More long-term epidemiological and clinical data on this topic are desirable. Naturally, leanness does not always guarantee optimal health. Nevertheless, excessive adiposity is always an unwanted risk factor.

Psychological problems manifest more often in obese children and youth, with later psychiatric complications appearing more frequently in individuals with an early onset of obesity. With respect to the human psyche, excess fatness also precipitates certain types of deterioration that are usual in older individuals. The same applies to orthopedic problems, arthritis, and the deterioration of body posture and the vertebral column. The role of excess adiposity during childhood in the facilitation of the development of all of these health risks should be further explained, especially from the point of view of their prevention.

Changes caused by obesity during growth are, in certain aspects, very similar to those caused by aging. Excess adiposity speeds up the aging process, including deterioration in health status. As life expectancy is usually shorter in the obese, it is possible to consider the status of an obese individual during growth as of somebody who is, from certain points of view, older than his or her chronological age. In conjunction with the mentioned deterioration of the status of an obese child, the causes and mechanisms should be intensely studied with intervention occurring as early as possible. When intervention is not guaranteed, the situation usually worsens with increasing age. Spontaneous rectification of this problem occurs only too rarely.

The role of genetics in the development of obesity is undeniable and significant, and has already been studied from many points of view. The research in this area has been largely developing, and will surely give more answers and solutions to the obesity problem in the future than it has up to now. Genetic factors can condition not only the predisposition for certain morphological features concerning obesity but also food preferences and aversions, reaction to overfeeding, patterns of substrates oxidized, the level of spontaneous physical activity and reaction to workload, and the overall functional capacity, including the aerobic power and skeletal muscle oxidative potential. Greater sensitivity to such environmental factors as diet or physical activity is also considered to be due to genetic factors. Some of the above-mentioned aspects were recently studied in greater detail, but with respect to available research data, a complex study covering more of the mentioned aspects in their mutual relationships with obesity has not been conducted sufficiently over longer periods of growth. It was, for example, shown that an obese child has more adipocytes in his or her adipose tissue from a young age, with this difference progressively increasing until young adulthood. Such studies would be demanding but indispensable for the elucidation of the role of the individual factors and their interplay during obesity development.

However, as realized from a number of recent scientific studies on the rapidly increasing prevalence of obesity, the causes of this undesirable phenomenon cannot be the result of the changes of the genetic make-up, but result in greater sensibility to the effect of other factors. Environmental causes are mainly considered responsible for increasing obesity beginning during the growth period. Lifestyle has significantly changed over the last few decades and runs parallel with the increased prevalence of obesity.

Little data exists on overeating in obese children. Also, studies have most often revealed the same or even increased energy expenditure in the obese compared to normal-weight individuals. However, data exist on decreased levels of physical activity, a preference for sedentary activities, and reduced participation in sport activities and exercise in the obese compared to their normal-weight peers. This apparent contradiction can be explained by the fact that even the most common daily activities are executed in the obese at a higher energy cost due to the excess load of the increased ratio of stored fat. This makes motor activity more of a challenge and usually results in a spontaneous reduction of movement and interest in exercise and sports, highlighting the vicious cycle of increasing adiposity. Some studies provide inexact results, especially when using questionnaires to describe these activities; the same type and duration of physical activity reported by the obese and lean children are considerably different, especially with respect to the intensity of the exercise undertaken. This can play a most important role in the differences between these groups. This also needs to be studied in greater detail and considered not only during stabilized periods of obesity but during the onset and initial phases of its development.

As shown by some studies, the effect of physical activity on body fatness, aerobic power, serum lipids, health status, and the like can be guaranteed only when a certain level of intensity of exercise over a specified period of time is achieved. Also, particular types of exercise are more desirable. In particular, dynamic, weight-bearing activities of an aerobic nature of sufficient intensity can stimulate the cardiorespiratory system; increase the utilization of energy from food, especially that from fats; and facilitate the mobilization of lipids from fat deposits, and their increased utilization during muscular work. Most of the studies on energy expenditure describe the total energy expended during a certain period of time (most commonly average values per 24 hours), but do not provide meaningful information regarding whether the necessary intensity was achieved. This can be determined by measuring changes in heart rate; however, more commonly this technique has been used only as an indicator of gross energy expenditure. The use of more precise methods to determine heart rate and/or the energy expenditure peaks over shorter intervals during an extended measurement period may provide useful answers regarding questions on exercise intensity and its efficiency. Obese children do not always show a lack of motor activity, but it is most commonly performed slower and in a less intensive manner, due to the strain and higher energy cost compared to lean individuals. Such activity does not generally have a sufficient and significant effect on body composition and fitness. The development of more sophisticated methods will enable researchers to follow in greater detail the characteristics of daily workload and activity and help to better understand the differential effect of physical activity in individual cases followed during sufficiently long periods of time.

Similar problems appear in studies of dietary intake. Research data are largely representative of the period when obesity has stabilized rather than the period of its onset. Fewer studies have information regarding the composition of the ingested food, including macronutrient intake. Food patterning, frequency of intake, and distribution of meals with respect to energy content across the day have also received relatively little attention, despite the fact that such diet characteristics may play a very important role in the development of obesity during the growing years.

The onset of obesity can occur very early in life: however, the impact of some of the causal factors may not be manifested immediately, but rather later during development or adulthood. Paradoxically, it has been shown that both early overnutrition and undernutrition early in life can facilitate the development of obesity later in life. This also concerns the fetal period and the different dietary intake and nutritional status of the pregnant mother. Nutritional status can be partly reflected in the weight increments during pregnancy, which varies considerably in different countries ranging from relatively low to much higher average values. The problems of delayed effects of early stimuli on the growing organism, which most commonly include nutritional issues, have been increasingly discussed; for example, in two recent congresses on the fetal origins of adult diseases, which also concerned obesity (in Mumbai, 2001). A number of factors have been implicated, including the mother's level of education, nutritional and social status, and economic situation. The custom of "eating for two" does not take into account that the two in question are not comparable with respect to body size and therefore energy needs. One of the key findings in this area is that the number of adipocytes depends on early nutrition, during both the fetal and the early postnatal period.

There are also marked inter-individual differences in the composition of mother's milk. For example, the fat content and other characteristics of milk can vary according to the nutrition of the mother during and before pregnancy, which can also play an important role in food intake very early in life. There have been no longitudinal studies to consider the potential influence of the child's dietary intake and nutritional status in the predisposition to increased adiposity.

With regards to early nutrition, breast and/or bottle-feeding has an essential role. Many studies have shown that breast-fed children are less often obese at later ages than bottle-fed children. This has been explained, inter alia, by the differences in composition of mother's and cow's milk. Cow's milk contains, from the point of view of ratio of macronutrients, greater amounts of proteins and less of lipids and carbohydrates. It is also thought that a breast-fed baby stops accepting the mother's milk when satiated, meaning that the baby does not overeat. Under conditions of bottle-feeding, the mother often wants the bottle finished, which may result in the infant being fed more than he or she really needs.

Pediatricians and researchers have also found very different feeding behaviors following the first acceptance of mother's milk and/or bottled milk. These differences may be related to the early development of adiposity. While studies in this area continue, there is a question as to whether longitudinal follow-ups will be possible based on the availability of the subjects studied and their willingness to participate in such studies over many years. Excellent examples of longitudinal studies include the Bogalusa Heart Study, the Framingham Study, the Quebec Family Study, and the Amsterdam Growth and Nutrition Study, among others. Although longitudinal data from these studies have greatly contributed to our understanding in the area, the interpretation of this data is often challenging given the substantial number of intervening factors during development that affect individuals of various genetic backgrounds and were not followed and analyzed. A longitudinal study to consider the effect of various factors, including food intake from the time of pregnancy and the early periods of life until adulthood, could solve a number of important questions but may be unrealistic from an ethical and logistical perspective. Without such knowledge, however, many of the problems that may be manifested in the onset and development of obesity from an early age cannot be readily solved.

On considering the WHO's RDAs for energy intake, it was shown that during the first year of life it is recommended that children ingest approximately 10% more energy compared to their energy expenditure calculated by doubly labeled water. When children consumed a lower energy intake than published RDAs, they still grew normally. Under conditions of bottle-feeding, a greater surplus of energy intake can be expected. It would be interesting to follow children fed in this way over much longer periods to verify the effect of early overnutrition on the facilitation of obesity later in life.

From the point of view of food intake, recent trends in U.S. children and also those from most developed countries, including France, are undesirable. During the first years of life, the ratio of energy consumed from lipids most commonly increased while energy from carbohydrates decreased, with energy from protein remaining about the same. A desirable trend for this period of development would be an increase in the proportion of food intake from carbohydrates (except simple sugars) and a decrease in the proportion of total energy from lipids. There should also be a corresponding adherence or a lower proportion from protein in the diet of children (provided it meets RDAs). The role of an increased ratio of dietary proteins as a cause of premature onset of the adiposity rebound (AR), which can be the forerunner to greater adiposity later in life, has already been demonstrated in some longitudinal studies. Studies of this type are still very rare, and it is extremely difficult to compare results. Therefore, further longitudinal studies in different countries are warranted, ideally using the same longitudinal design, choice of parameters, and homogeneous and comparable samples of participants. The composition of the diet and specifically the relationship between macronutrients seems to play a more important role in the onset and development of obesity than simple overeating and an excess energy intake. It would be interesting to have longitudinal data on the energy expenditure and physical activity level in children with an earlier AR compared to those with AR occurring later. In this respect, not only the total amount *of* energy expended but also how it is spent — that is, considering the intensity and character of exercise — is essential and warrants detailed consideration.

There is some evidence regarding individual variability with respect to genetic contribution of mechanisms to accommodate the amount and composition of food ingested, and also with different patterns of physical activity (poor or better capacity in motor tasks). All subjects have a nutritional (e.g., differing diets, digestion, absorption, metabolization, and utilization) and motor (differing frequency, intensity, duration, and type of physical activity) individuality. This originates from both genetic factors and environmental influences at the beginning of life and is further developed beyond birth. For example, it is interesting to consider the reaction of young children to a previous meal's varied energy intake and that of the next meal. The interference of adults, especially of the mother, is again essential. Adults can help to facilitate the development of both adequate and/or inadequate food habits from early childhood. However, this does not apply in all cases as it seems that some children are born with a different appetite and with different preferences and aversions, which may be very difficult to modify. With regards to motor activity and its genetic predisposition, the effect of early encouragement and/or restriction of a child's initiative in this respect can markedly change motor and physical activity development later in life. This should also be studied in greater detail and for prolonged periods of time.

The role of the family environment, type and amount of food offered, the behavior of other family members, physical activity regime, leaving more freedom for the child to eat and move according to his or her likes and dislikes, could influence significantly both current and future food and motor habits. George Bernard Shaw once said that the two most important professions in the world do not require any systematic education, professional preparation, and qualification: politics and parenthood. Unfortunately, this is sometimes reflected in a very undesirable way.

The above-mentioned factors can also have a different influence during the various periods of growth. Critical periods (which include the period after birth, or preschool age) have been defined during which the effect of any factor, both positive and negative, has a more far-reaching effect in both the short and long term. The influence of such factors may not be immediately apparent, but after a period of latency may be manifested as a delayed effect.

Precocity of the AR is a good predictor of later obesity. The same applies to BMI that crosses percentiles during growth. This can start sooner or later depending on the child and preceding effects of further stimuli. The relationship to the actual level of spontaneous physical activity level (PAL) and energy output can also play an important role. The elucidation of these mechanisms — which can change, with respect to a different genetic basis, the present and future characteristics of the growing organism, including the predisposition for greater or lower adiposity — still remains to be answered. The solution in humans is particularly difficult due to the large interfering variability of all characteristics and situations in which children grow up.

The last of the sensitive, critical periods are prepuberty and puberty. During these periods, various stimuli can also change more profoundly and with more lasting effects on the various characteristics of the adolescent. In this respect, there are more experimental data on the delayed effect of diet and physical activity covering longer periods, as it is easier to follow individuals during more advanced periods of growth, at least until young adulthood. For example, the correlations between the values of various parameters such as BMI are always higher and more significant when measured over shorter periods of life, also due to the reduced possibility of the interference of other conditions of life.

Questions also relate to the prevalence, trends, and origins of obesity in individual countries. As mentioned in previous chapters, numerous data are available, but the lack of consistent criteria, procedures, and methods of measurement makes it difficult to make definite conclusions on the possible differences and/or similarities in obesity prevalence in various parts of the world. Some progress has been made, especially with regard to the use of BMI; however, there is still some reservation regarding the use of the same criteria of BMI in some populations whose data were not used for their definition. This concerns the majority of Asian populations, for example.

The increase of childhood obesity does not seem to be homogeneous. Existing evaluations show for example that the prevalence of obesity increased most in the United States (+60%), less in the United Kingdom and Japan, and least in France (+28%). As mentioned previously, in France but also in other countries, the prevalence of very severe obesity increased until recently relatively more (nearly four times) than the prevalence of moderate obesity (more than once). Obviously, some individuals are more sensitive to environmental factors than others, which might be due to the combination of hereditary factors and inadequate energy balance and turnover. For example, children of obese parents prefer more fatty foods and thus have a higher energy intake and as a result may become obese more easily than children of lean parents with adequate and balanced food intakes.

As mentioned previously, in certain countries the increasing prevalence in obesity occurs more often in the more severe degrees of obesity than in the milder forms. At least in some countries, the average values and the range of "normal" BMI have not changed, but the prevalence of severe and/or morbid obesity has increased more markedly. The average values of BMI in the childhood population in a particular country can be influenced by this phenomenon, but the differentiation has to be defined. This was considered as a special characteristic of the present situation, caused by a cluster of factors. They included familial and hereditary situations along with an impaired dietary intake (excess energy, particularly due to an increased fat intake, mainly saturated fat) and restricted physical activity. A low PAL and the consumption of energy-dense food is especially risky, particularly for those individuals disposed by some genetic mutations and predispositions. Changes in trends for different types and degrees of obesity during childhood deserve special attention. Despite the fact that morbidly obese children still represent such a minority in the growing population, they are at the greatest health risk both in the short term and in the future, and therefore deserve great attention. More detailed analysis of this phenomenon is also necessary.

In an attempt to solve these problems, it is necessary to examine both of the critical components of energy balance and turnover: diet and physical activity level. In the United Kingdom, the prevalence of childhood obesity increased between the years 1950 and 1990, and the energy and fat intake decreased after a peak in 1970. This may be explained in part by a decreased level of physical activity. However, very few studies have followed simultaneously using reliable methods and procedures and during a longer period, both dietary intake and energy expenditure, especially that due to physical activity and exercise.

As shown by some studies in younger U.K. children (1.5 to 2.5 years of age), nutritional intake has decreased by approximately 18%. However, the intake of protein has increased by approximately 13%, while fat has decreased by approximately 5%. The intake of carbohydrates has changed only very slightly. Other studies in Belgium, Denmark, Italy, France, and Spain have predominantly shown that the composition of diet could only poorly explain an increased deposition of fat. However, in the United States there is evidence that increased portion sizes and an increase in the overall amount of food purchased are associated with the trend for childhood obesity; this concerns mostly fast food and soft drinks with undesirably high-energy density along with attractive taste and packaging.

An important problem in conjunction with these comments is that, as mentioned previously, reported measurements in studies have mainly been conducted over short periods of time (approximately one week), and during the period of stabilized obesity. The information gained does not always correspond, and may not always provide objective and realistic results about, the initiating phase of obesity development. In this respect, it would be necessary to measure these two items of energy balance simultaneously and long enough during the previously mentioned sensitive, critical periods, when a temporary imbalance and decreased turnover of energy could cause more marked effects that could last until the later periods of development.

The answers to all questions may be particularly difficult in humans because of the need to measure over more prolonged periods of life and to implement methods that are reliable and acceptable for subjects. Ensuring the necessary cooperation of a homogeneous group of a high number of subjects willing to participate regularly in such a study is a very difficult task. The use of payments for participants may introduce bias as it would be preferably only those interested in and needing money who would participate.

The dropout of subjects from such studies is always large, especially in healthy subjects who do not need, for example, any medical or dietetic assistance. This can be partly compensated for by recruiting a sufficiently large sample, but then there is always a risk of not having a similarly homogeneous group at the beginning and the end of such a study, even when taking into account only those who both started and finished the study. Large cohort studies are organizationally and financially costly. Nevertheless, such studies are indispensable for the solution of both the prevention and the treatment of obesity, especially of that starting in early life. Under present conditions, it would be desirable to analyze all that has been revealed by individual studies conducted in various countries, in spite of the heterogeneity of practically all their aspects. Facts and analyses of those that used more advanced methodology are valid.

Individual scientists and clinicians in individual countries cannot realize the validation and further development of the research on childhood obesity. To start with, further surveys and analyses are necessary, as the number of studies has been recently increasing. This has indicated that the attention has recently focused on the problem of childhood obesity much more than previously, and ad hoc summarization does not give a true picture of the present knowledge. Until recently, scientific observations concerned only smaller groups of subjects, especially when more sophisticated methodical approaches were implemented.

Complex information on prevalence and distribution of childhood obesity in the individual continents, countries, social classes, and population groups on the one hand, and studies examining the causes and mechanisms resulting in obesity during growth using more sophisticated laboratory and clinical approaches in sufficiently large samples on the other hand, are indispensable for the necessary complex analysis. Thus, the more efficient prevention as well as treatment of excess fatness can be conducted.

Examples from certain parts of the world have identified some of the important aspects of optimal growth patterns that can predispose a child to better health, functional status, and longevity. The growth and development characteristics in populations with a high proportion of long-living subjects (over 90 years, and in good health) excluded excess deposition of fat during development, increased food intake, excess animal proteins and fat, and restriction of physical activity. On the other hand, longer periods of breast-feeding, slower growth rates, eating fresh food, increased physical and social activity, and greater workload from childhood until advanced age were the most important characteristics of those who could achieve higher age with participation in full activity. Health parameters, serum lipids, psychological and social parameters, and the like in such a population were on a more desirable level than in similar ethnic groups in Abkhazia with comparable genetic traits living under the conditions of city life. In spite of the undeniably more fixed positive genetic make-up, the way of life and overall characteristic development deserves special attention, as possible factors contribute to the reduction of obesity and the achievement of a positive health prognosis until advanced adulthood. However, since the end of the 1970s, when this follow-up was conducted by Russian and U.S. scientists, the lifestyle has changed markedly, and it would be impossible to repeat such measurements.

Present conditions facilitate the prevention and treatment of many diseases and pathological situations, but seem to cause other problems that used to be previously much less frequent when different life conditions were customary. The present diet and physical activity regimes do not correspond to the needs of the human organism according to the phylogenetic trends. This particularly applies with respect to the conditions of life in large urban settings and when considering children; recent trends in childhood obesity prevalence seem to attest to that. Moreover, the lifestyle in the industrially developed countries and their large cities has been introduced and exported, along with technological progress, to the countries of the Third World. As mentioned before, the situation, also with respect to obesity, has significantly worsened over the past one to two decades, and has started to have similar conditions as for the industrially developed countries. Obesity accompanying stunting is another example. This trend is highly undesirable and can be avoided.

Prevention is always better than cure. According to the recent knowledge on the effect of various factors influencing the growing organism in early periods of life, efficient interventions should be implemented from the very beginning of life. Lifestyle should be arranged in such a way that the development of obesity would be interfered with and prevented by efficient arrangements of dietary and physical activity regimes. There is evidence that this should start with the pregnant mother's way of life and continue from the beginning of postnatal life. In spite of this not always completely guaranteeing the prevention of increased adiposity, it could at least reduce the risk of obesity. This may appear to be simply a repetition of old truths but under new and changing circumstances; however, according to increasing obesity this is fully justified.

A concentrated effort is required to conduct a study involving a common program developed through consensus from not only representative scientific and medical but also governmental and community institutions in as many countries as possible. It is critical that data collection, storage, and analysis be organized on a higher level and a larger scale than ever before. Moreover, there is also interest in the countries where no systematic follow-ups have been conducted to date. Some initiatives in this respect have recently been developed. Research projects concerning early nutritional and other determinants of the development of obesity have been undertaken, with the aim of trying to identify the main causes of childhood obesity and its prevention. Recent research has stimulated even more new questions than giving answers, and only a broad international collaboration and cooperation can contribute to a better set of global solutions to the problem of childhood obesity.

References

Abbott, R.A. and Davies, P.S., Habitual physical activity and physical activity intensity: their relation to body composition in 5.0–10.5 year-old children, *Eur. J. Clin. Nutr.*, 58, 285, 2004.

Abrosimova, L.I. et al., Effect of motor activity on the physical work capacity of school children with excessive body weight, *Gig. Sanit.*, 8 Aug., 29, 1984 (in Russian).

Adeyanju, M. et al., A three-year study of obesity and its relationship to high blood pressure in adolescents, *J. Sch. Hlth.*, 57, 109, 1987.

Adeyemi, E., and Abdulle, A., A comparison of plasma leptin levels in obese and lean individuals in the United Arab Emirates, *Nutr. Res.*, 20, 157, 2000.

Aggoun, Y., et al., Arterial stiffness and endothelial dysfunction in obese children, *Arch. Mal. Coeur Vaiss.*, 95, 631, 2002.

Agostoni, C. et al., Dairy products and adolescent nutrition, *J. Int. Med. Res.*, 22, 67, 1994.

Agras, W.S. et al., Does a vigorous feeding style influence early development of adiposity? *J. Pediatr.*, 110, 799, 1987.

Agrelo, F. et al., Prevalence of thinness and excessive fatness in a group of school children in the city of Cordoba, Argentina, *Arch. Latinoam. Nutr.*, 38, 69, 1988 (in Spanish).

Aguirre, M. and Ruiz-Vadillo, V., Relationship between breakfast habits and overweight in a group of adolescents in San Sebastian, *Rev. Esp. Nutr. Communitaria*, 8, 24, 2002.

Ailhaud, G. and Guesnet, P., Fatty acid composition of fats is an early determinant of childhood obesity: a short review and an opinion, *Obes. Rev.*, 5, 21, 2004.

Alberton, A.M. et al., Nutrient intakes of 2- to 10-year-old American children: 10-year study, *J. Am. Diet. Assoc.*, 92, 1492, 1992.

Alcazar, M.L., Alvear, J., and Muzzo, S., Influence of nutrition on the bone development of children, *Arch. Latinoam. Nutr.*, 34, 298, 1984 (in Spanish).

Alexander, M.A., Sherman, J.B., and Clark, L., Obesity in Mexican-American preschool children — a population group at risk, *Pub. Hlth. Nurs.*, 8, 53, 1991.

Alexy, U., Fruit juice consumption and the prevalence of obesity and short stature in German preschool children: results of the DONALD Study, *J. Pediatr. Gastroenterol. Nutr.*, 29, 343, 1999.

Alexy, U. et al., Energy intake and growth of 3- to 36-month-old German infants and children, *Ann. Nutr. Metab.*, 42, 68, 1998.

Allison, D.B., Faith, M.S., and Gorman, B.S., Publication bias in obesity treatment trials? *Int. J. Obes. Metab. Disord.*, 20, 931, 1996.

Allison, D.B. et al., Race effects in the genetics of adolescents' body mass index, *Int. J. Obes. Relat. Metab. Disord.*, 18, 363, 1994.

Allison, D.B. et al., Is the intrauterine period really a critical period for the develop-ment of obesity? *Int. J. Obes. Relat. Metab. Disord.*, 19, 397, 1995.

Almeida, M.J., Fox, K.R. and Boutcher, S.H., Physical activity levels and fatness in male and female adolescents, in *Physical activity and obesity, 8th Int.Congress on obesity, Maastricht, The Netherlands, Aug. 26-29, 1998, Abstracts*, 35.

Alsaker, F.D., Pubertal timing, overweight, and psychological adjustment, *J. Early Adolesc.*, 12, 396, 1992.

Altabe, M. and Thompson, J.K., Size estimations versus figural ratings of body image disturbance: relation to body dissatisfaction and eating dysfunction, *Int. J. Eating Disord.*, 11, 397, 1992a.

Altabe, M. and Thompson, J.K., Body image changes during early adulthood, *Int. J. Eating Disord.*, 13, 323, 1992b.

Amador, M., Flores, P. and Pena, M., Normocaloric diet and exercise: a good choice for treating obese adolescents, *Acta Paediatr. Hung.*, 30, 123, 1990.

Amador, M. et al., Growth rate reduction during energy restriction in obese adoles-cents, *Exp. Clin. Endocrinol.*, 96, 73, 1990.

Ambrosius, W.T. et al., Relation of race, age, and sex hormone differences to serum leptin concentrations in children and adolescents, *Horm. Res.*, 49, 240, 1998.

Anavian, J. et al., Profiles of obese children presenting for metabolic evaluation, *J. Pediatr. Endocrinol. Metab.*, 14, 1145, 2001.

Andersen, A.E. and DiDomenico, L., Diet vs. shape content of popular male and female magazines: a dose–response relationship to the incidence of eating disorders? *Int. J. Eating Disord.*, 11 3, 1992.

Anderson, G.H., Sugars, sweetness, and food intake, *Am. J. Clin. Nutr.*, 62, 195S, 1995.

Anderson, P.M., Butcher, K.F. and Levine, P.B., Maternal employment and overweight children, *J. Hlth Econ.*, 22, 477, 2003.

Anding, J.D. et al., Blood lipids, cardiovascular fitness, obesity, and blood pressure: the presence of potential coronary heart disease risk factors in adolescents, *J. Am. Diet. Assoc.*, 96, 238, 1996.

Andre, J.L., Deschamps, J.P. and Gueguen, R., Relationship between blood pressure and weight characteristics in childhood and adolescence. I. Blood pressure, weight, and overweight, *Rev. Epidemiol. Santé Publique*, 30, 1, 1982.

Apter, D., Leptin in puberty, *Clin. Endocrinol.*, 47, 175, 1997.

Arashiro, R. et al., Effect of Trp6Arg mutation of the b 3 adrenergic receptor gene and c161T substitution of the peroxisome proliferator activated receptor g gene on obesity in Japanese children, *Pediatr. Int.*, 45, 135, 2003.

Araya, H.L. et al., Effect of protein and carbohydrate preloads on food and energy intakes in preschool children with different nutritional status, *Arch. Latinoam. Nutr.*, 45, 25, 1995 (in Spanish).

Archibald, E.H. et al., Changes in intraventricular septal thickness, left ventricular wall thickness and left ventricular volume in obese adolescents on a high protein weight reducing diet, *Int. J. Obes.*, 13, 265, 1989.

Argente, J. et al., Leptin plasma levels in healthy Spanish children and adolescents, children with obesity, and adolescents with anorexia nervosa and bulimia nervosa, *J. Pediatr.*, 131, 833, 1997a.

Argente, J. et al., Multiple endocrine abnormalities of the growth hormone and insulin-like growth factor axis in prepubertal children with exogenous obesity: effect of short- and long-term weight reduction, *J. Clin. Endocrin. Metab.*, 82, 2076, 1997b.

Arluk, S.L. et al., Childhood obesity's relationship to time spent in sedentary behavior, *Mil. Med.*, 168, 583, 2003.

Armstrong, J. and Reilly, J.J., Breastfeeding and lowering the risk of childhood obesity, *Lancet*, 359, 2003, 2002.

Asayama, K. et al., Relationships between biochemical abnormalities and anthropometric indices of overweight, adiposity and body fat distribution in Japanese elementary school children, *Int. J. Obes. Relat. Metab. Disord.*, 19, 253, 1995.

Asayama, K. et al., A new age-adjusted index of body fat distribution in children based on waist and hip circumferences and stature, *Int. J. Obes. Relat. Metab. Disord.*, 22, S11, 1998a.

Asayama, K. et al., A new mode of therapy for obese children in Japan, *Int. J. Obes. Relat. Metab. Disord.*, 22, S62, 1998b.

Asayama, K. et al., Relationship between an index of body fat distribution (based on waist and hip circumferences) and stature, and biochemical complications in obese children, *Int. J. Obes. Relat. Metab. Disord.*, 22, 1209, 1999.

Asayama, K. et al., Critical value for the index of body fat distribution based on waist and hip circumferences and stature in obese girls., *Int. J. Obes. Relat. Metab. Disord.*, 24, 1026, 2000.

Asayama, K. et al., Threshold values of visceral fat measures and their anthropometric alternatives for metabolic derangement in Japanese obese boys, *Int. J. Obes. Relat. Metab. Disord.*, 26, 208, 2002.

Ashton J.R., It is easier to change your own behaviour than to change somebody else's, *J. Epidemiol. Comm. Hlth.*, 58, 506, 2004.

Åstrand, P.O. and Rodahl, K. *Textbook of Work Physiology*, 2nd ed, McGraw-Hill, New York, 1977

Astrup, A., The role of energy expenditure in the development of obesity, *Int. J. Obes. Relat. Metab. Disord.*, 22, S68, 1998.

Astrup, A., Lunsgaard, C. and Stock, M.J., Is obesity contagious? *Int. J. Obes. Relat. Metab. Disord.*, 22, 375, 1999.

Attia, N. et al., The metabolic syndrome and insulin-like growth factor I regulation in adolescent obesity, *J. Clin. Endocrinol. Metab.*, 83, 1467, 1998.

Attie, I. and Brooks-Gunn, J., The development of eating problems in adolescent girls: a longitudinal study, *Dev. Psychol.*, 25, 70, 1989.

Bacardi-Gascon, M. et al., Validation of a semiquantitative food frequency questionnaire to assess folate status. Results discriminate a high-risk group of women residing on the Mexico–U.S. border, *Arch. Med. Res.*, 34, 325, 2003.

Bacon, J.G., Scheltema, K.E., and Robinson, B.E., Fat phobia scale revisited : The short form, *Int. J. Obes. Relat. Metab. Disord.*, 25, 252, 2001.

Balagopal, P. et al., Effect of lifestyle changes on whole-body protein turnover in obese adolescents, *Int. J. Obes. Relat. Metab. Disord.*, 27, 1250, 2003.

Ballor, D.L. et al., Resistance weight training during caloric restriction enhances lean body weight maintenance, *Am. J. Clin. Nutr.*, 47, 19, 1988.

Bandini, L.G., Schoeller, D.A. and Dietz, W.H., Energy expenditure in obese and nonobese adolescents, *Pediatr. Res.*, 27, 198, 1990.

Bandini, L.G. and Dietz, W.H., Myths about childhood obesity, *Pediatr. Ann.*, 21, 647, 1992.

Bandini, L.G. et al., Energy expenditure during carbohydrate overfeeding in obese and nonobese adolescents, *Am. J. Physiol.*, 256, E357, 1989.

430 · *Childhood Obesity: Prevention and Treatment*

Bandini, L.G. et al., Relationship of body composition, parental overweight, pubertal stage, and race-ethnicity to energy expenditure among premenarcheal girls, *Am. J. Clin. Nutr.*, 76, 1040, 2002.

Bandini, L.G. et al., Longitudinal changes in the accuracy of reported energy intake in girls 10–15 y of age, *Am. J. Clin. Nutr.*, 78, 480, 2004.

Baranowski, T. et al., Ethnicity, infant-feeding practices, and childhood adiposity, *J. Dev. Behav. Pediatr.*, 11, 234, 1990.

Baranowski, T. et al., Physical activity and nutrition in children and youth: an overview of obesity prevention, *Prev. Med.*, 31, S1, 2000.

Barbeau, P. et al., Correlates of individual differences in body composition changes resulting from physical training in obese children, *Am. J. Clin. Nutr.*, 69, 705, 1999.

Barker, D.J.P., *Mothers, Babies, and Diseases in Later Life*, BMJ Publishing Group, London, 1994.

Barker, D.J.P., Fetal undernutrition and obesity in later life, *Int. J. Obes. Relat. Metab. Disord.*, 22, S89, 1998.

Barker, D.J.P., The fetal and infant origin of adult diseases, *Br. Med. J.*, 301, 1111, 1990.

Barlett, H.L., Kenney, W.L. and Buskirk, E.R., Body composition and expiratory volume of pre-pubertal lean and obese boys and girls, *Int. J. Obes. Relat. Metab. Disord.*, 16, 653, 1992.

Barlow, S.E. and Dietz, W.H., Obesity evaluation and treatment: Expert Committee Recommendations, The Maternal and Child Health Bureau, Health Resources and Services Administration and the Department of Health and Human Services, *Pediatr.*, 102, E39, 1998.

Bar-Or, O., A commentary on children and fitness: a public health perspective, *Res. Q. Exerc. Sp.*, 58, 304, 1987.

Bar-Or, O. and Baranowski, T., Physical activity, adiposity, and obesity among adolescents, *Pediatr. Exerc. Sci.*, 6, 348, 1994.

Bar-Or, O., Obesity, in *Sports and Exercise for Children with Chronic Health Conditions*, Goldberg, B., Ed. Human Kinetics Publishers, Champaign, IL, 1995, Chap. 23.

Bar-Or, O. et al., Physical activity, genetic, and nutritional considerations in childhood weight management, *Med. Sci. Sports Exerc.*, 30, 2, 1998.

Barros, A.A. et al., Evaluation of the nutritional status of 1st-year school children in Campinas, Brazil, *Ann. Trop. Paediatr.*, 10, 75, 1990.

Bartkiw, T.P., Children's eating habits: a question of balance, *World Health Forum*, 14, 404, 1993.

Baughcum, A.E. et al., Maternal feeding practices and childhood obesity: a focus group study of low-income mothers, *Arch. Pediatr. Adolesc. Med.*, 152, 1010, 1998.

Baughcum, A.E. et al., Maternal feeding practices and beliefs and their relationship to overweight in early childhood, *J. Dev. Behav. Pediatr.*, 2001.

Bavdekar, A. et al., Insulin resistance syndrome in 8-year old Indian children: small at birth, big at 8 years, or both? *Diabetes*, 48, 2422, 1999.

Beckett, P.R., Wong, W.W., and Copeland, K.C., Developmental changes in the relationship between IGF-1 and body composition during puberty, *Growth Hormone IGF Res.*, 8, 283, 1998.

Becque, M.D. et al., Coronary risk incidence of obese adolescents: reduction by exercise plus diet intervention, *Pediatrics*, 81, 605, 1988.

Bedogni, G. et al., Association of waist circumference and body mass index with fasting blood insulin in severely obese children: a cross-sectional study, *Diab. Nutr. Metab. Clin. Exp.*, 15, 160, 2002.

Behnke, A.R., Feen, B.G. and Welham, W.C., The specific gravity of healthy men, *J. Am. Med. Assoc.*, 118, 495, 1942.

Bell, L., Chan, L. and Pencharz, P.B., Protein sparing diet for severely obese adolescents: design and use of an equivalency system for menu planning, *J. Am. Diet. Assoc.*, 85, 459, 1985.

Bell, S.K. and Morgan, S.B., Children's attitudes and behavioral intentions toward a peer presented as obese: does a medical explanation for the obesity make a difference? *J. Pediatr. Psychol.*, 25, 137, 2000.

Bellisle, F. et al., Obesity and food intake in children: evidence for a role of metabolic and/or behavioral daily rhythm, *Appetite*, 11, 111, 1988.

Bellisle, F. and Rolland-Cachera, M.F., How sugar-containing drinks might increase adiposity in children, *Lancet*, 357, 490, 2001.

Bellizzi, M.C. and Dietz, W.H., Workshop on childhood obesity: Summary of the discussion, *Am. J. Clin. Nutr.*, 70, 173S, 1999.

Bellone, S. et al., Circulating ghrelin levels as function of gender, pubertal status and adiposity in childhood, *J. Endocrinol. Invest.*, 25, RC13, 2002.

Bercedo-Sanz, A., et al., Television vewing habits in children in Cantabria (Spain), *An. Esp. Pediatr.*, 54, 1, 44, 2001.

Berenson, G.S. et al., Obesity and cardiovascular risk in children, *Ann. N.Y. Acad. Sci.*, 699, 93, 1993.

Berenson, G.S., Srinivasan, S.R. and Nicklas, T.A., Atherosclerosis: a nutritional disease of childhood, *Am. J. Cardiol.*, 82, 22T, 1998.

Berg, A. et al., Physical activity and eating behavior: strategies for improving the serum lipid profile of children and adolescents, *Wien Med. Wochenschr.*, 144, 138, 1994 (in German).

Bergel, E. et al., Perinatal factors associated with blood pressure during childhood, *Am. J. Epidemiol.*, 151, 594, 2000.

Bergmann, K.E. et al., Early determinants of childhood overweight and adiposity in a birth cohort study: role of breast-feeding, *Int. J. Obes. Relat. Metab. Disord.*, 27, 162, 2003.

Bergoni, A. et al., Italian multicenter study of liver damage in pediatric obesity, *Int. J. Obes. Relat. Metab. Disord.*, 22, S22, 1998.

Berkeling, B., Ekman, S., and Rössner, S., Eating behaviour in obese and normal weight 11-year-old children, *Int. J. Obes. Relat. Metab. Disord.*, 16, 355, 1992.

Berkowitz, R.I. et al., Physical activity and adiposity: a longitudinal study from birth to childhood, *J. Pediatr.*, 106, 734, 1985.

Bernard, L. et al., Overweight in Cree schoolchildren and adolescents associated with diet, physical activity, and high television viewing, *J. Am. Diet. Assoc.*, 95, 800, 1995.

Bernard, P.L.J. et al., Influence of obesity on postural capacities of teenagers. Preliminary study, *Ann. Readapt. Med. Phys.*, 46, 184, 2003.

Bernstein, N.R., Objective bodily damage: disfigurement and dignity, in *Body Images: Development, Deviance, and Change*, in Cash, T.F. and Pruzinsky, T., Eds., Guilford Press, New York, 1990, 131.

Beunen, G. and Thomis, M., Genetic determinants of sports participation and daily physical activity, *Int. J. Obes. Relat. Metab. Disord.*, 23, S55, 1999.

Bhargava, S.K. et al., Relation of serial changes in childhood body-mass index to impaired glucose tolerance in young adulthood, *N. Engl. J. Med.*, 350, 865, 2004.

Bianco, L. et al., Eating behavior in children and youth, *Int. J. Obes. Relat. Metab. Disord.*, 17, 34, 1993.

Bideci, A. et al., Serum levels of insulin-like growth factor-I and insulin-like growth factor binding protein-3 in obese children, *J. Pediat. Endocrinol. Nutr. Metab.*, 10, 295, 1997.

Birch, L.L. and Davison, K.K., Family environmental factors influencing the developing behavioral controls of food intake and childhood overweight, *Pediatr. Clin. North Am.*, 48, 893, 2001.

Birch, L.L. and Fisher, J.O., Mothers' child feeding practices influence daughters' eating and weight, *Am. J. Clin. Nutr.*, 71, 1054, 2000.

Birch, L.L. et al., Confirmatory factor analysis of the Child Feeding Questionnaire: a measure of parental attitudes, beliefs and practices about child feeding and obesity proneness, *Appetite*, 36, 201, 2001a.

Birch, L.L. et al., The variability of young children's energy intake, *N. Engl. J. Med.*, 24, 324, 1991b.

Birrer, R.B. and Levine, R., Performance parameters in children and adolescent athletes, *Sp. Med.*, 4, 211, 1987.

Blaak, E.E. et al., Total energy expenditure and spontaneous activity in relation to training in obese boys, *Am. J. Clin. Nutr.*, 55, 777, 1992.

Bláha, P. et al., The 5th nationwide anthropological study of children and adolescents held in 1991 (Czech republic) selected anthropometric characteristics, *Ceskoslovenská Pediatr.*, 48, 621, 1993 (in Czech).

Bláha, P., Lisá, L., and Krásnicanová, H., Czech obese children — the reduction treatment, *Int. J. Obes. Relat. Metab. Disord.*, 21, S123, 1997.

Bláha, P., Vígnerová, J., and Lisá, L., Czech population under new socio-economic conditions, in *9th European Congress on Obesity, 3-6 June 1999*, Milano, Italy, 1999,

Blair, S.N. et al., How much physical activity is good for health?, *Ann. Rev. Publ. Hlth.*, 13, 9, 1992.

Blanchard, M.S., Thermogenesis and its relationship to obesity and exercise, *Quest*, 34, 143, 1982.

Blecker, U. et al., Initial obesity level impacts long term weight maintenance in obese youth, *Int. J. Obes. Relat. Metab. Disord.*, 22, S63, 1998.

Boeck, M.A., Chen, C., and Cunningham-Rundles, S., Altered immune function in a morbidly obese pediatric population, *Ann. N.Y. Acad. Sci.*, 699, 253, 1993.

Bollen, P. et al., Intragastric balloon in the treatment of morbid obesity in adolescents: alternative treatment or gadget? *Int. J. Obes. Relat. Metab. Disord.*, 22, S33, 1998.

Bona, G. et al., The impact of gender, puberty and body mass on reference values for urinary growth hormone (GH) excretion in normal growing non-obese and obese children, *Clin. Endocrinol.*, 50, 775, 1999.

Bonat, S. et al., Self-assessment of pubertal stage in overweight children, *Pediatrics*, 110, 743, 2002.

Bondi, M. et al., Andromedullary response to caffeine in prepubertal and pubertal obese subjects, *Int. J. Obes. Relat. Metab. Disord.*, 23, 992, 1999.

Bonet-Serra, B. et al., Presence of genu valgum in obese children: cause or effect, *An. Pediatr.*, 58, 232, 2003.

Boot, A.M., Bouquet, J., Ridder, M.A.J., Krenning, E.P., de Muinck Keizer-Schrama, S.M.P.F., Determination of body composition measured by dual energy x-ray absorptiometry in Dutch children and adolescents, *Am. J. Clin. Nutr.*, 66, 232, 1997.

Booth, F.W. and Tseng, B.S., America needs to exercise for health, *Med. Sci. Sports Exerc.*, 27, 462, 1995.

Booth, M.L., Macaskill, P., and Baur, L.A., Sociodemographic distribution of measures of body fatness among children and adolescents in New South Wales, Australia, *Int. J. Obes. Relat. Metab. Disord.*, 23, 456, 1999.

Booth, M.L. et al., Change in the prevalence of overweight and obesity among young Australians, 1969-1997, *Am. J. Clin. Nutr.*, 77, 29, 2003.

Bordi, D. et al., Obesity, overweight and physical activity in elementary school children, *Minerva Pediatr.*, 47, 521, 1995.

Borms, J., The child and exercise: an overview, *J. Sports Sci.*, 4, 3, 1986.

Borra, S.T. et al., Food, physical activity and fun: inspiring American kids to more healthy lifestyles, *J. Am. Diet. Assoc.*, 95, 816, 1995.

Bosisio, E. et al., Ventilatory volumes, flow rates, transfer factor and its components (membrane component, capillary volume) in obese adults and children, *Respiration*, 45, 321, 1984.

Bouchard, C., Genetics of obesity and its prevention, in Nutrition and Fitness, in *World Rev. Nutr. Dietetics*, Simopoulos, A.P., Ed. Karger, Basel, 1993, 68.

Bouchard C., Genetic determinants of regional fat distribution, *Hum. Reprod.*, 12, S1, 1, 1997.

Bouchard, C. and Blair, S.N., Introductory comments for the consensus on physical activity and obesity, *Med. Sci. Sports Exerc.*, 31, S498, 1999.

Bougnères, P. et al., In vivo resistance of lipolysis to epinephrine. a new feature of childhood onset obesity, *J. Clin. Invest.*, 99, 2568, 1997.

Bourne, L.T. et al., Nutritional status of three 6-year-old African children in the Cape Peninsula, *East Afr. Med. J.*, 71, 695, 1994.

Bouvattier, C. et al., Hyperleptinaemia is associated with impaired gonadotrophin response to GnRH during late puberty in obese girls, not boys, *Eur. J. Endocrinol.*, 138, 653, 1998.

Braet, C., Van Winckel, M. and Van Leuwen, K., Follow-up results of different treatment programs for obese children, *Acta Paediatr.*, 86, 397, 1997.

Braet, C. et al., Inpatient treatment of obese children: a multicomponent programme without stringent calorie restriction, *Eur. J. Pediatr.*, 162, 391, 2003.

Brambilla, P.D. et al., Changes in dynamic respiratory volumes in obese children and adolescents related to weight loss and sex, *Minerva Pediatr.*, 44, 159, 1992 (in Italian).

Brambilla, P. et al., Waist circumference can predict visceral adiposity in obese adolescents, *Int. J. Obes. Relat. Metab. Disord.*, 21, S140, 1997.

Brambilla, P. et al., Persisting obesity starting before puberty is associated with stable intraabdominal fat during adolescence, *Int J. Obes. Relat. Metab. Disord.*, 23, 299, 1999.

Brandou, F. et al., Effects of two-month rehabilitation program on substrate utilization during exercise in obese adolescents, *Diabetes Metab.*, 29, 20, 2003.

Bray, G.A., The energetics of obesity, *Med. Sci. Sports Exerc.*, 15, 30, 1983.

Bray, G.A., Nutrient balance: new insights into obesity, *Int. J. Obes.*, 11, 83, 1987.

Brewis, A., Biocultural aspects of obesity in young Mexican schoolchildren, *Ann. J. Human. Biol.*, 15, 446, 2003.

Brock, K. et al., Is parental physical activity a predictor of prepubertal children's activity levels? *Int. J. Obes. Relat. Metab. Disord.*, 23, S118, 1999.

Brodie, D.A. and Slade, P.D., The relationship between body image and body fat in adult women, *Psychol. Med.*, 18, 623, 1988.

Brook, C.G.D., Evidence for a sensitive period in adipose-cell replication in man, *Lancet*, ii, 624, 1972.

Brook, C.G.D., Determination of body composition of children from skinfold measurement, *Arch. Dis. Child.*, 46, 182, 1975.

Brook, C.G.D., Lloyd, J.K. and Wolf, O.H., Relation between age of onset of obesity and size and number of adipose cells, *B.M.J.*, ii, 25, 1972.

Brooke, O.G. and Abernathy, E., Obesity in children, *Human Nutr.*, 39, 304, 1985.

Broussard, B.A. et al., Prevalence of obesity in American Indian and Alaska Natives, *Am. J. Clin. Nutr.*, 53, 1535, 1991.

Broussard, B.A. et al., Toward comprehensive obesity prevention programs in Native American communities, *Obes. Res.*, 3, 289, 1995.

Brownell, K.D., Dieting and the search for the perfect body: where physiology and culture collide, *Behav. Ther.*, 22, 1, 1991.

Brownell, K.D., and Kaye, F.S., A school-based behavior modification, nutrition education, and physical activity program for obese children, *Am. J. Clin. Nutr.*, 35, 277, 1982.

Brownell, K.D., Rodin, J. and Wilmore, J.H., Eating, body weight, and performance in athletes: an introduction, in *Eating, Body Weight, and Performance in Athletes*, Brownell, K.D., Rodin, J. and Wilmore, J.H., Eds., Lea & Febiger, London, 1992, 7.

Brownell, K.D., and Stunkard, A.J., Behavioral treatment of overweight children and adolescents, in *Obesity*, Stunkard, A.J., Ed. W.B. Saunders, Philadelphia, 1980.

Brožek, J. et al., Densitometric analysis of body composition: revision of some assumptions, *Ann. N.Y. Acad. Sci.*, 110, 113, 1963.

Bruce, B., and Agras, W.S., Binge eating in females: a population-based investigation, *Int. J. Eating Disord.*, 12, 365, 1992.

Bruch, H. *Eating Disorders*, Basic Books, New York, 1973.

Bryson, J.M., The future of leptin and leptin analogues in the treatment of obesity, *Diab. Obesity*, 2, 83, 2000.

Buchowski, M.S. and Sun, M., Energy expenditure, television viewing and obesity, *Int. J. Obes. Relat. Metab. Disord.*, 20, 236, 1996.

Bueno-Lozano, M., Balsamo, A., and Cacciari, E., Diet-induced changes as risk factors in obese children: arterial pressure, glycoregulation and lipid profile, *An. Esp. Pediatr.*, 35, 335, 1991 (in Spanish).

Bunt, J.C. et al., Weight, adiposity and physical activity as determinants, of an insulin sensitivity index in Pima Indian children, *Diabetes Care*, 26, 2524, 2003.

Burdette, H.L. et al., Association of maternal obesity and depressive symptoms with television-viewing time in low-income preschool children, *Arch. Paediatr. Adolesc. Med.*, 157, 894, 2003.

Burke, V., Beilin, L.J., and Dunbar, D., Family lifestyle and parental body mass index as predictors of body mass index in Australian children: A longitudinal study, *Int. J. Obes. Relat. Metab. Disord.*, 25, 147, 2001.

Burke, V. et al., Associations between blood pressure and overweight defined by new standards for body mass index in childhood, *Prev. Med.*, 38, 558, 2004.

Burniat, W., Childhood obesity : which specificities? *Int. J. Obes. Relat. Metab. Disord.*, 21, S136, 1997.

Burniat, W., Cole, C., Lissau, I., Poskitt, E., Eds., *Child and Adolescent Obesity*, Cambridge, Cambridge University Press, 2002.

Burniat, W. and Van Aelst, C., Evaluation of the food intake in 75 obese children successfully treated at least during 6 months, *Int. J. Obes. Relat. Metab. Disord.*, 17, 34, 1993.

Burns, R.B. *The Self Concept*, Longmans, London, 1979.

Burrows, A. and Cooper, M., Possible risk factors in the development of eating disorders in overweight pre-adolescent girls, *Int. J. Obes. Relat. Metab. Disord.*, 26, 1268, 2002.

Butte, N.F., The role of breastfeeding in obesity, *Pediatr. Clin. North Am.*, 48, 189, 2001.

Butters, J.W. and Cash, T.F., Cognitive-behavioral treatment of women's body-image dissatisfaction, *J. Consult. Clin. Psychol.*, 55, 889, 1987.

Byrne, N.M. and Hills, A.P., Should body-image scales designed for adults be used with adolescents? *Percept. Motor Skills*, 82, 747, 1996.

Byrne, N.M. and Hills, A.P., An evaluation of body image assessment protocols with implications for age and gender differences, in *Proc. Australasian Soc. Study Obesity*, Melbourne, 1993.

Byrne, N.M. and Hills, A.P., Assessment of eating practices in adolescence, *Proc. Nutr. Soc. (Australia)*, 19, 106, 1995.

Byrne, N.M. and Hills, A.P., Correlations of body composition and body-image assessments of adolescents, *Perceptual and Motor Skills*, 84, 1330, 1997.

Caballero, B. et al., Pathways: a school-based, randomized controlled trial for the prevention of obesity in American Indian schoolchildren, *Am. J. Clin. Nutr.*, 78, 904, 2003.

Caius, N. and Benefice, E., Food habits, physical activity and overweight among adolescents, *Rev. Epidemiol. Sante Publ.*, 50, 531, 2002.

Caldarone, G. et al., Nutrition and exercise in children, *Ann. Inst. Super. Sanita*, 31, 445, 1995.

Calderon, L.L. et al., Risk factors for obesity in Mexican-American girls: dietary factors, anthropometric factors, and physical activity, *J. Am. Phys. Assoc.*, 96, 1177, 1996.

Cameron, N., Changing prevalence of childhood obesity in developing countries, *Int. J. Obes. Relat. Metab. Disord.*, 22, S1, 1998.

Campaigne, B.N. et al., Indexes of obesity and comparisons with previous national survey data in 9- and 10-year-old black and white girls: the National Heart, Lung, and Blood Institute Growth and Health Study, *J. Pediatr.*, 124, 675, 1994.

Caprio, S. et al., Co-existence of severe insulin resistance and hyperinsulinaemia in preadolescent obese children, *Diabetologia*, 39, 1489, 1996a.

Caprio, S. et al., Hyperleptinemia: an early sign of juvenile obesity. Relations to body fat depots and insulin concentrations, *Am. J. Physiol.*, 271, E626, 1996b.

Carter, J.E.L. and Phillips, W.H., Structural changes in exercising middle aged males during a 2-year period, *J. Appl. Physiol.*, 27, 787, 1969.

Cash, T.F. and Green, T.F., Body weight and body image among college women: perception, cognition, and affect, *J. Personal. Assess.*, 50, 290, 1986.

Cashdan, E., A sensitive period for learning about food, *Hum. Nature*, 5, 279, 1994.

Caspersen, C.J., Nixon, P.A. and DuRant, R.H., Physical activity epidemiology applied to children and adolescents, *Exerc. Sport Sci. Rev.*, 26, 341, 1998.

Castro-Rodriguez, J.A. et al., Increased incidence of asthmalike symptoms in girls who become overweight or obese during the school years, *Am. J. Respir. Crit. Care Med.*, 163, 1344, 2001.

Ceratti, F. et al., Screening for obesity in a schoolchildren population of the 20th zone of Milan and a nutritional education intervention, *Epidemiol. Prev.*, 12, 1120, 1990 (in Italian).

Cezar, C. et al., Obese female adolescents in a followup of intervention with physical exercise and nutritional education, isolated and combined, *Int. J. Obes. Relat. Metab. Disord.*, 22, 1998.

Chalew, S.A. et al., Reduction of plasma insulin levels does not restore integrated concentration of growth hormone to normal in obese children, *Int. J. Obes. Relat. Metab. Disord.*, 16, 459, 1992.

Chalew, S.A. et al., The integrated concentration of cortisol is reduced in obese children, *J. Pediat. Endocrinol. Metab.*, 10, 287, 1997.

Challis, B.G. et al., A missense mutation disrupting a diabasic prehormone processing site in pro-opiomelanocortin (POMC) increases susceptibility to early-onset obesity through a novel molecular mechanism, *Hum. Mol. Genet.*, 11, 1997, 2002.

Chang, F.T., Hu, S.H., and Wang, R.S., The effectiveness of dietary instruction in obese children in southern Taiwan, *Kao Hsiung I Hsueh Tsa Chin*, 14, 528, 1998 (in Chinese).

Charzewska, J., and Figurska, K., Incidence of obesity in 7- to 8-year-old boys in Warsaw, *Pediatr. Pol.*, 58., 127, 1983.

Chay, O.M. et al., Obstructive sleep apnea in obese Singapore children, *Pediatr. Pulmonol.*, 29, 284, 2000.

Chen, W., Childhood obesity in Taiwan, *Chung Hua Min Kuo Hsiao Erh Ko I Hsueh Husi Tsa Chin.*, 38, 438, 1997.

Chen, W., Ku, F.D., and Wu, K.W., Parent-directed weight reduction program for obese children: model formulation and follow-up, *J. Formos. Med. Assoc.*, 92, 237, 1993 (in Chinese).

Chen, W. et al., Lack of association between obesity and dental caries in three-year-old children, *Acta Pediatr. Sin.*, 39, 109, 1998.

Chen, W. et al., An autosomal genome scan for loci influencing longitudinal burden of body mass index from childhood to young adulthood white sibships: the Bogalusa Heart Study, *Int. J. Obes. Relat. Metab. Disord.*, 28, 462, 2004.

Cheung, L., Do media influence childhood obesity?, *Ann. N.Y. Acad. Sci.*, 699, 104, 1993.

Chiloiro, M. et al., Play in obese and nonobese children in Southern Italy, *Int. J. Obes. Relat. Metab. Disord.*, 22, S10, 1998.

Chin, M.K. et al., Obesity, diet, exercise and weight control? A current review, *J.H.K. Med. Assoc.*, 44, 181, 1992.

Chinn, S. and Rona, R.J., Trends in weight-for-height and triceps skinfold thickness for English and Scottish children, 1972–1982 and 1982–1990, *Pediatr. Perinat. Epidemiol.*, 8, 90, 1994.

Chinn, S. and Rona, R.J., Can the increase in body mass index explain the rising trend in asthma in children? *Thorax*, 56, 845, 2001a.

Chinn, S. and Rona, R.J., Prevalence and trends in overweight and obesity in three cross sectional studies of British children, 1974-94, *B.M.J.*, 322, 24, 2001b.

Chitturi, S., Farell, G.C., and George, J., Non-alcoholic steatohepatitis in the Asia-Pacific region: future shock? *J. Gastroenterol. Hepatol.*, 19, 368, 2004.

Chiumello, G. and Poskitt, E.M.E., Prader-Willi and other syndromes, in *Child and Adolescent Obesity: Causes and Consequences*, Burniat et al., Ed., Cambridge University Press, Cambridge, UK, 2002, 171.

Chu, N.D. et al., Plasma TNF-R1 and insulin concentrations in relation to leptin levels among normal and overweight children, *Clin. Biochem.*, 35, 287, 2002.

Chu, N.F., Prevalence and trends of obesity among school children in Taiwan: the Taipei Children Heart Study, *Int. J. Obes. Relat. Metab. Disord.*, 25, 170, 2001.

Cirillo, G. et al., Molecular screening of the proopiomelanocortin (POMC) gene in Italian obese children; report of three new mutations. *Int. J. Obes. Relat. Metab. Disord.*, 25, 61, 2001.

Clement, K. and Ferre, P., Genetics and the pathophysiology of obesity, *Pediatr. Res.*, 53, 721, 2003.

Cohen, C.H., McMillan, C.S. and Samuelson, D.R., Long-term effects of a lifestyle modification exercise program on the fitness of sedentary, obese children, *J. Sports Med. Phys. Fitness*, 31, 183, 1991.

Cok, F., Body image satisfaction in Turkish adolescents, *Adolescence*, 25, 409, 1990.

Cole, T.J., Do growth charts need a face lift? *B.M.J.*, 308, 641, 1994.

Cole, T.J., Changing prevalence of childhood obesity in the Western world, *Int. J. Obes. Relat. Metab. Disord.*, 22, S1, 1998.

Cole, T.J., A chart to link child centiles of body mass index, weight and height, *Eur. J. Clin. Nutr.*, 56, 1194, 2002.

Cole, T.J., Assessing overweight and obesity in childhood, *Ital. J. Pediat.*, 29, 93, 2003.

Cole, T.J., Modelling postnatal exposures and their interactions with birth size. *J. Nutr.*, 134, 201, 2004.

Cole, T.J., Freeman, J.V., and Preece, M.A., Body mass index reference curves for the UK, 1990, *Arch. Dis. Child.*, 75, 25, 1995.

Cole, T.J. and Rolland-Cachera, M.F., Measurements and definition, in *Child and Adolescent Obesity*, Burniat, W. et al., Eds., Cambridge University Press, Cambridge, 2002, 3.

Cole, T.J. et al., Establishing a standard definition for child overweight and obesity: international survey, *B.M.J.*, 320, 1240, 2000.

Cole, T.J., Paul, A.A., and Whitehead, R.G., Weight references charts for British long-term breastfed infants. *Acta Paediatr.*, 91, 1296, 2002.

Coleman, K.J. et al., Relationships between TriTrac-R3D vectors, heart rate, and self-report in obese children, *Med. Sci. Sports Exerc.*, 29, 1535, 1997.

Comuzzie, A.G. et al., The genetic of obesity in Mexican American: the evidence for genome scanning efforts in the San Antonio family heart study, *Hum. Biol.*, 75, 635, 2003.

Considine, R.V., Weight regulation, leptin and growth hormone, *Horm. Res.*, 48, 116, 1997.

Cook, D.G. et al., Fibrinogen and factor VII levels are related to adiposity but not to fetal growth or social class in children aged 10–11 years, *Am. J. Epidemiol.*, 150, 727, 1999.

Cook, D.G. et al., C-reactive protein concentration in children: relationship to adiposity and other cardiovascular risk factors, *Atherosclerosis*, 149, 139, 2000.

Cooper, D.M. et al., Are obese children truly unfit? Minimizing the confounding effect of body size on the exercise response, *J. Pediatr.*, 335, 805, 1990.

Cooper, K.H., *Kid Fitness*, Bantam Books, New York, 1991.

Cordain, L. et al., Potassium content of the fat free body in children, *J. Sports Med. Phys. Fitness*, 29, 170, 1989.

Couch, S.C. et al., Rapid westernization of children's blood cholesterol in 3 countries: evidence for nutrient-gene interactions? *Am. J. Clin. Nutr.*, 72, 1266S, 2000.

Coutant, R. et al., Circulating leptin level and growth hormone response to stimulation tests in obese and normal children, *Eur. J. Endocrinol.*, 139, 591, 1998.

Covington, C., Childhood obesity: too much, too little, too late, *Issues Compr. Pediatr. Nurs.*, 19, iii, 1996.

Cowin, I. and Emmett, P., Cholesterol and triglyceride concentrations, birthweight and central obesity in pre-school children, *Int. J. Obes. Relat. Metab. Disord.*, 24, 330, 2000.

Cronk, C.E. et al., Longitudinal trends and continuity in weight/stature² from 3 months to 18 years, *Hum. Biol.*, 54, 729, 1982.

Crooks, D.L., Food consumption, activity and overweight among elementary school children in an Apalachian Kentucky community, *Am. J. Phys. Anthropol.*, 112, 159, 2000.

Csabi, G. et al., Presence of metabolic cardiovascular syndrome in obese children, *Eur. J. Pediatr.*, 159, 91, 2000.

Csabi, G.Y., Juricskay, S., and Molnar, D., Urinary cortisol to cortisone metabolites in hypertensive obese children, *J. Endocrinol. Invest.*, 23, 435, 2000.

Da Nascimento-Marreiro, D., Fisberg, M., and Fraciscato-Cozzolino, S.M., Zinc nutritional status in obese children and adolescents, *Biol. Trace. Elem. Res.*, 86, 107, 2002.

Dabelea, D. and Pettitt, D.J., Intrauterine diabetic environment confers risks for type 2 diabetes mellitus and obesity in the offspring, in addition to genetic susceptibility, *J. Pediatr. Endocrinol. Metab.*, 14, 1085, 2001.

Dahlström, S. et al., Atherosclerosis precursors in children: atherosclerosis precursors in Finnish children and adolescents. II. Height, weight, body mass index, and skinfolds and their correlation to metabolic variables, *Acta Paediatr. Scand.*, 318, 65, 1985.

Dai, S. et al., Longitudinal analysis of changes of indices of obesity from age 8 years to age 18 years, *Am. J. Epidemiol.*, 156, 720, 2002.

Danadian, K. et al., Lipolysis in African–American children: is it a metabolic risk factor predisposing to obesity?, *J. Clin. Endocrinol. Metab.*, 86, 3022, 2001.

Danforth, E. and Sims, E.A.H., Obesity and efforts to lose weight, *N. Engl. J. Med.*, 327, 1497, 1992.

Danielczyk, S. et al., Impact of parental BMI on the manifestation of overweight 5–7 year old children, *Eur. J. Nutr.*, 41, 132, 2002.

Daniels, S.R., Khoury, P.R., and Morrison, J.A., Utility of different measures of body fat distribution in children and adolescents, *Am. J. Epidemiol.*, 152, 1179, 2000.

Daniels, S.R. et al., Association of body fat distribution and cardiovascular risk factors in children and adolescents, *Circulation*, 99, 541, 1999.

Daniels, S.R. et al., Left atrial size in children with hypertension: the influence of obesity, blood pressure, and left ventricular mass, *J. Pediatr.*, 141, 186, 2002.

Darwish, O.K. et al., Aetiological factors of obesity in children, *Hum. Nutr. Clin. Nutr.*, 39, 131, 1985.

Davie, M.W.J. et al., Effect of high and low carbohydrate diets on nitrogen balance during calorie restriction in obese patients, *Int. J. Obes.*, 6, 457, 1982.

Davies, E. and Furnham, A., The dieting and body shape concerns of adolescent females, *J. Child Psychol. Psychiatr.*, 27, 417, 1986.

Davies, P.S., Energy requirements for growth and development in infancy, *Am. J. Clin. Nutr.*, Suppl. 68, S939, 1998.

Davies, P.S.W., Connolly, C., and Day, J.M.E., Energy expenditure in infancy and later body composition, *Int. J. Obes. Relat. Metab. Disord.*, 17, S35, 1993.

Davies, P.S.W., Day, J.M., and Lucas, A., Energy expenditure in early infancy and later body fatness, *Int. J. Obes. Relat. Metab. Disord.*, 15, 727, 1991.

Davies, P.S.W. et al., The prediction of total body water using bioelectrical impedance in children and adolescents, *Ann. Hum. Biol.*, 15, 237, 1988.

Davis, K. and Christoffel, K.K., Obesity in preschool and school-age children. Treatment early and often may be best, *Arch. Pediatr. Adolesc. Med.*, 148, 125, 1994.

Davis, K. et al., Early frequent treatment in prevention of childhood obesity. How we do it, *Ann. N.Y. Acad. Sci.*, 699, 260, 1993a.

Davis, K. et al., Obesity in preschool and school-age children. Early frequent treatment is best, *Ann. N.Y. Acad. Sci.*, 699, 262, 1993b.

Davis, K. et al., Primary prevention of obesity in American Indian children, *Ann. N.Y. Acad. Sci.*, 699, 167, 1993c.

Davison, K.K. and Birch, L.L., Child and parent characteristics as predictors of change in girls' body mass index, *Int. J. Obes. Relat. Metab. Disord.*, 25, 1834, 2001a.

Davison, K.K. and Birch, L.L., Weight status, parent reaction, and self-concept in five-year-old girls, *Pediatrics*, 107, 46, 2001b.

Davison, K.K. and Birch, L.L., Obesogenic families: parents' physical activity and dietary intake patterns predict girls' risk of overweight, *Int. J. Obes. Relat. Metab. Disord.*, 26, 1186, 2002.

Davison, K.K., Markey, C.N., and Birch, L.L., Etiology of body dissatisfaction and weight concerns among 5-year-old girls, *Appetite*, 35, 143, 2000.

De Bourdeaudhuij, I. et al., Effects of distraction on treadmill running time in severely obese children and adolescents, *Int. J. Obes. Relat. Metab. Disord.*, 26, 1023, 2002.

De la Eva, R.C. et al., Metabolic correlates with obstructive sleep apnoea in obese subjects, *J. Pediatr.*, 140., 654, 2002.

De Moura, E.C. et al., Childhood obesity: a new issue for public health in Brazil, *Int. J. Obes. Relat. Metab. Disord.*, 22, S3, 1998.

De Onis, M. and Blossner, N., Prevalence and trends of overweight among preschool children in developing countries, *Am. J. Clin. Nutr.*, 72, 1032, 2000.

De Ridder, C.M. et al., Body fat distribution in pubertal girls quantified by magnetic resonance imaging, *Int. J. Obes.*, 16, 443, 1992.

De Schepper, J., Van den Broeck, M., and Jonckheer, M.H., Study of lumbar spine bone mineral density in obese children, *Acta Paediatr.*, 84, 313, 1995.

De Simone, M. et al., Growth charts, growth velocity and bone development in childhood obesity, *Int. J. Obes. Relat. Metab. Disord.*, 19, 851, 1995.

Decaluwe, V. and Braet, C., Prevalence of binge-eating disorder in obese children and adolescents seeking weight-loss treatment, *Int. J. Obes. Relat. Metab. Disord.*, 27, 404, 2003.

Decaluwe, V., Braet, C., and Fairburn, C.C., Binge eating in obese children and adolescents., *Int. J. Eating Disord.*, 33, 78, 2003.

Decz, T., Molnar, D., and Koletzko, B., The effect of under- or overnutrition on essential fatty acid metabolism in childhood, *Eur. J. Clin. Nutr.*, 52, 541, 1998.

Deforche, B., De Bourdeaudhuij, I., and Hills, A.P., Changes in fat mass, fat-free mass and aerobic fitness in severely obese children and adolescents following a residential treatment programme, *Eur. J. Pediatr.*, 162, 616, 2003.

Deforche, B. et al., Physical fitness and physical activity in obese and nonobese Flemish youth, *Obes. Res.*, 11, 434, 2003.

Deforche, B. et al., Role of physical activity and eating behaviour in long-term weight-control in extremely obese children and adolescents. *Acta Paed. Scand.* (in press).

Deheeger, M., Rolland-Cachera, M.F., and Fontvieille, A.M., Physical activity and body composition in 10 year old French children: linkages with nutritional intake? *Int. J. Obes. Relat. Metab. Disord.*, 21, 372, 1997.

Dekkers, J.C. et al., Development of general and central obesity from childhood into young adulthood in African American and European American males and females with a family history of cardiovascular disease, *Am. J. Clin. Nutr.*, 79, 661, 2004.

Del Giudice, E.M. et al., Molecular screening of the proopiomelanocortin (POMC) gene in Italian obese children: report of three new mutations, *Int. J. Obes. Relat. Metab. Disord.*, 25, 61, 2001.

DeLany, J.P., Role of energy expenditure in the development of pediatric obesity, *Am. J. Clin. Nutr.*, 68, 950S, 1998.

DeLany, J.P., Harsha, D., and Bray, G.A., Parameters of energy metabolism predicting change in body fat over 2 years in boys, *Int. J. Obes. Relat. Metab. Disord.*, 22, S36, 1998.

DeLany, J.P. et al., Energy expenditure in lean and obese prepubertal children, *Obes. Res.*, 3, 67, 1995.

Delpeuch, F. and Maire, B., Obesity and developing countries of the south, *Med. Trp. (Mars.)*, 57, 380, 1997.

DeMeersman, R.E. et al., Maximal work capacity in prepubescent obese and nonobese females, *Clin. Pediatr.*, 24, 199, 1985.

Demerath, E.W. et al., Serum leptin concentration, body composition, and gonadal hormones, during puberty, *Int. J. Obes. Relat. Metab. Disord.* 23, 678, 1999.

Dennison, B.A., Fruit juice consumption by infants and children: a review, *J. Am. Coll. Nutr.*, 15, 4S, 1996.

Deurenberg, P., The dependency of bioelectrical impedance on intra- and extra-cellular water distribution, in *Recent Development in Body Composition Analysis: Methods and Applications*, Kral, J.G. and Van Itallie, T.B., Eds., Smith-Gordon/Nishimura, London, 1993, 43.

Devascar, S.U., Neurohumoral regulation of body weight gain, *Pediatr. Diabetes*, 2, 131, 2001.

Dhurandhar, N.V., and Kulkarni, P.R., Prevalence of obesity in Bombay, *Int. J. Obes. Relat. Metab. Disord.*, 16, 367, 1992.

Di Toro, A. et al., Unchanged iron and copper and increased zinc in the blood of obese children after two hypocaloric diets, *Biol. Trace Elem. Res.*, 57, 97, 1997.

Diamond, F. et al., Leptin binding activity (LBA) in plasma of nondiabetic and diabetic adolescents and obese children: relation to auxology and hormonal data, *J. Pediatr. Endocrinol. Metab.*, 13, 141, 2000.

Diehl, J.M., Attitudes to eating and body weight in 11- to 16-year-old adolescents, *Schweiz. Med. Wochenschr.*, 129, 162, 1999.

Dietz, W.H., Childhood obesity: susceptibility, cause, and management, *J. Ped.*, 103, 676, 1983.

Dietz, W.H., Jr., Prevention of childhood obesity, *Pediatr. Clin. North Am.*, 33, 823, 1986.

Dietz, W.H., You are what you eat? What you eat is what you are, *J. Adolesc. Health Care*, 11, 76, 1990.

Dietz, W., Physical activity and childhood obesity, *Nutrition*, 7, 295, 1991.

Dietz, W.H., Childhood obesity, in *Obesity*, Björntorp, P. and Brodoff, B.M., Eds., Lippincott, Philadelphia, 1992, 606.

Dietz, W.H., Therapeutic strategies in childhood obesity, *Horm. Res.*, 39, 86, 1993.

Dietz, W.H., Critical periods in childhood for the development of obesity, *Am. J. Clin. Nutr.*, 59, 955, 1994.

Dietz, W.H., Risk factors for childhood obesity, *Int. J. Obes. Relat. Metab. Disord.*, 22, S2, 1998a.

Dietz, W.H., Childhood origins of adult obesity, *Int. J. Obes. Relat. Metab. Disord.*, 22., S89, 1998b.

Dietz, W.H., Childhood weight affects adult morbidity and mortality, *J. Nutr.*, 128, 411S, 1998c.

Dietz, W.H., Overweight in childhood and adolescence, *N. Engl. J. Med.*, 350, 865, 2004.

Dietz, W.H. and Bellizzi, M.C., Introduction: the use of body mass index to asses obesity in children, *Am. J. Clin. Nutr.*, 70, 123S, 1999.

Dietz, W.H. and Hartung, R., Changes in height velocity of obese preadolescents during weight reduction, *Am. J. Dis. Ch.*, 139, 705, 1985.

Dietz, W.H. and Gortmaker, S.L., Do we fatten our children at the television set? Obesity and television viewing in children and adolescents, *Pediatrics*, 75, 807, 1985.

Dietz, W.H. and Gortmaker, S.L., TV or not TV: fat is the question, *Pediatrics*, 91, 499, 1993.

Dietz, W.M. and Gortmaker, S.L., Preventing obesity in children and adolescents, *Annu. Rev. Public Health.*, 22, 237, 2001.

Dietz, W.H. and Robinson, T.N., Assessment and treatment of childhood obesity, *Pediatr. Rev.*, 14, 337, 1993.

Dietz, W.H., Gross, W.L., and Kirkpatrick, J., Blount's disease (tibia vara): another skeletal disorder associated with childhood obesity, *J. Ped.*, 101, 735, 1982.

Ding, Z., Exercise prescription for obese children, *Chung Hua I Hsueh Tsa Chih Taipei*, 72, 131, 1992 (in Chinese).

DiPietro, L., Mossberg, H.O., and Stunkard, A.J., A 40-year history of overweight children in Stockholm: lifetime overweight, morbidity and mortality, *Int. J. Obes. Relat. Metab. Disord.*, 18, 585, 1994.

Doak, C.M. et al., Overweight and underweight coexist within households in Brazil, China and Russia, *J. Nutr.*, 130, 2965, 2000.

Docherty, D. and Bell, R., The relationship between flexibility and linearity measures in boys and girls 6–15 years, *J. Hum. Mvt. Stud.*, 11, 279, 1985.

Domargard, A. et al., Increased prevalence of overweight in adolescent girls with type I diabetes mellitus, *Acta Pediatr. Int. J. Pediatr.*, 88, 1223, 1999.

Donadian, K. et al., Lipolysis in African–American children: is it a metabolic risk factor predisposing to obesity? *J. Clin. Endocrinol. Met.*, 86, 3022, 2001.

Donelly, J.E. et al., Nutrition and physical activity program to attenuate obesity and promote physical and metabolic fitness in elementary school children, *Obes. Res.*, 4, 229, 1995.

Dorosty, A.R., Siassi, F., and Reilly, J.J., Obesity in Iranian children, *Arch. Dis. Child.*, 87, 388, 2002.

Dorosty, A.R. et al., Factors associated with early adiposity rebound, *Pediatrics*, 105, 1115, 2000.

Dosman, C.F., Senthilselvan, A., and Andrews, D., Psychiatric treatment: a risk factor for obesity? *Pediatr. Child. Hlth.*, 7, 76, 2002.

Dowda, M. et al., Environmental influences, aphysical activity and weight status in 8- to 16-year-olds, *Arch. Pediatr. Adolesc. Med.*, 155, 711, 2001.

Dowling, A.M., Steele, J.R., and Baur, L.A., Does obesity influence foot structure and plantar pressure patterns in prepubescent children? *Int. J. Obes. Relat. Metab. Disord.*, 25, 845, 2001.

Doxiadis, The city and the development of child, in *Proc. XII Internat. Congress of Pediatrics, Vol. I., Official Reports*, Mexico City, Mexico 1968, 10.

Drummer, G. et al., Pathogenic weight-control behaviours of young competitive swimmers, *Phys. Sports Med.*, 15, 75, 1987.

Dubern, B. et al., Mutational analysis of melanocortin-4 receptor, agouti-related protein, and α-melanocyte-stimulating hormone genes in severely obese children, *J. Pediatr.*, 139, 204, 2001.

Dupuis, J.M. et al., Self-training in the treatment of teenagers' obesity, *Arch. Pediatr.*, 7, 1185, 2000.

DuRant, R.H., Dover, E.V., and Alpert, B.S., An evaluation of five indices of physical working capacity in children, *Med. Sci. Sp. Exerc.*, 15, 83, 1983.

DuRant, R.H. et al., Association among serum lipid and lipoprotein concentration and physical activity, physical fitness, and body composition in young children, *J. Pediatr.*, 123, 185, 1993.

DuRant, R.H. et al., The relationship among television watching, physical activity, and body composition of young children, *Pediatrics*, 94, 449, 1994.

Durnin, J.V.G.A., Energy balance in childhood and adolescence, *Proc. Nutr. Soc.*, 43, 271, 1984.

Durnin, J.V.G.A. and Rahaman, M.M., The assessment of the amount of fat in the human body from skinfold thickness, *Br. J. Nutr.*, 21, 681, 1967.

Durnin, J.V.G.A. et al., A cross-sectional nutritional and anthropometric study with an interval of 7 years on 611 young adolescent children, *Br. J. Nutr.*, 32, 169, 1974.

Dwyer, J., Dietary assessments, in *Modern Nutrition in Health and Disease*, Shils, M.E., Olson, J.A., and Shike, M., Eds., Lea & Febiger, Philadelphia, 1994.

Dwyer, T. et al., Syndrome X in 8-y-old Australian children: stronger associations with current body fatness than with infant size or growth, *Int. J. Obes. Relat. Metab. Disord.*, 26, 1301, 2002.

Ebbelink, C.B. and Rodriguez, N.R., Effects of exercise combined with diet therapy on protein utilization in obese children, *Med. Sci. Sports Exerc.*, 31, 378, 1999.

Ebbelink, C.B. et al., A reduced glycemic load diet in the treatment of adolescent obesity, *Arch. Pediatr. Adolesc. Med.*, 157, 773, 2003.

Echwald, S.M. et al., Amino acid variants in the human leptin receptor: lack of association to juvenile onset of obesity, *Biochem. Biophys. Res. Commun.*, 233, 248, 1997.

Eck, L.H. et al., Children at familial risk for obesity: an examination of dietary intake, physical activity and weight status, *Int. J. Obes. Relat. Metab. Disord.*, 16, 71, 1992.

Edmunds, L. and Fox, K.R., A preliminary investigation into the physical activity and fatness of 9-year-old children at risk of obesity as adults, in *Physical Activity and Obesity, Satellite Symposium of the 8th Int. Congress on Obesity*, Maastricht, The Netherlands Aug. 26-29,1998, Book of abstracts, 27.

Eisenkolbl, J., Kartasurya, M., and Widhalm, K., Underestimation of percentage fat mass measured by bioelectrical impedance analysis compared to dual energy X-ray absorbtiometry method in obese children, *Eur. J. Clin. Nutr.*, 55, 423, 2001.

Eisenmann, J.C., Secular trends in variables associated with the metabolic syndrome of North American children and adolescents: a review and synthesis, *Am. J. Human Biol.*, 15, 786, 2003.

Eisenmann, J.C., Physical activity and cardiovascular disease risk factors in children and adolescents: an overview, *Can. J. Cardiol.*, 20, 295, 2004.

Eisenmann, J.C. et al., Growth and overweight of Navajo youth: secular changes from 1955 to 1997, *Int. J. Obes. Relat. Metab. Disord.*, 24, 211, 2000.

Eisenmann, J.C. et al., Growth status and obesity of Hopi children, *Am. J. Human Biol.*, 15, 741, 2003.

Ekelund, U.M., Yngve, A. and Sjostrom, M., The relationship between physical activity and body fat in adolescents, in *Physical Activity and Obesity, Satellite Symposium of the 8th Int. Congress on Obesity*, Maastricht, The Netherlands Aug. 26-29, 1998, 28 (Abstr.).

El Hazmi, M.A.F. and Warsy, A.S., The prevalence of obesity and overweight in 1–18-year-old Saudi children, *Ann. Saudi Med.*, 22, 303, 2002.

Elia, M., Body composition analysis: the evaluation of two component models, multi-component models, and bedside techniques? 11, 114, 1992.

Elia, M. and Ward, L.C., New techniques in nutritional assessment: body composition methods, *Proc. Nutr. Soc.*, 58, 33, 1999.

Eliakim, A., Nemet, D. and Wolach, B., Quantitative ultrasound measurements of bone strength in obese children and adolescents, *J. Pediatr. Endocrinol. Metab.*, 14, 159, 2001.

Eliakim, A. et al., The effect of a combined intervention on body mass index and fitness in obese children and adolescents: a clinical experience, *Eur. J. Pediatr.*, 161, 8, 449, 2002.

Elimam, A., Norgren, S., and Marcus, C., Effects of growth hormone treatment on the leptin system and body composition in obese prepubertal boys, *Acta Paediatr. Int. J. Paediatr.*, 90, 520, 2001.

Elliot, D.L. et al., Metabolic evaluation of obese and nonobese siblings, *J. Pediatr.*, 114, 957, 1989.

Ellis, K.J., Measuring body fatness in children and young adults: comparison of bioelectrical impedance analysis, total body electrical conductivity, and dual-energy X-ray absorptiometry, *Int. J. Obes. Relat. Metab. Disord.*, 20, 866, 1996.

Ellis, K.J. and Eastman, J.D. (Eds.), *Human Body Composition, In Vivo Methods, Models, and Assessment*, Plenum Press, New York, 1993.

Ellis, K.J. and Nicolson, M., Leptin levels and body fatness in children: effects of gender, ethnicity, and sexual development, *Pediatr. Res.*, 42, 484, 1997.

Ellis, K.J. et al., Accuracy of dual-energy X-ray absorptiometry for body composition measurements in children, *Am. J. Clin. Nutr.*, 60, 660, 1994.

Ellsworth, D.L. et al., Influence of the 3-adrenergic receptor Arg16Gly polymorphism on longitudinal changes in obesity from childhood through adulthood in biracial cohort: a Bogalusa Heart Study, *Int. J. Obes. Relat. Metab. Disord.*, 26, 928, 2002.

Elmadfa, I. et al., The Austrian study on nutritional status of 6- to 18-year-old pupils, *Bibl. Nutr. Dieta*, 51, 62, 1994.

Emmons, L., Dieting and purging behavior in black and white high school students, *J.A. Diet. Assoc.*, 92, 306, 1992.

Endo, H. et al., Beneficial effects of dietary intervention on serum lipid and apolipoprotein levels in obese children, *Am. J. Dis. Child.*, 146, 303, 1992.

Endo, K. et al., Association of Trp64Arg polymorphism of the β3-adrenergic receptor gene and no association of Gln223Arg polymorphism of the leptin receptor gene in Japanese schoolchildren with obesity, *Int. J. Obes. Relat. Metab. Disord.*, 24, 443, 2000.

Engel, G.M. and Staheli, L.T., The natural history of torsion and other factors influencing gait in childhood, *Clin. Orthop. Rel. Res.*, 99, 12, 1974.

Engstrom, E.M. and Anjos, L.A., Relationship between maternal nutritional status and obesity in Brazilian children, *Rev. Saude Publica*, 30, 233, 1996 (in Portuguese).

Enright, P.L. et al., Blood pressure elevation associated with sleep-related breath disorder in a community sample of white and Hispanic children: the Tucson Children's Assessment of Sleep Apnoea study, *Arch. Pediatr. Adolesc. Med.*, 157, 901, 2003.

Epstein, L.H., Methodological issues and ten-year outcomes for obese children, *Ann. N.Y. Acad. Sci.*, 699, 237, 1993.

Epstein, L.H., Exercise in the treatment of childhood obesity, *Int. J. Obes. Relat. Metab. Disord.*, 19, S117, 1995.

Epstein, L.H., Family-based behavioral intervention for obese children, *Int. J. Obes. Relat. Metab. Disord.*, 20, S14, 1996.

Epstein, L.H., Coleman, K.J., and Myers, M.D., Exercise in treating obesity in children and adolescents, *Med. Sci. Sports Exerc.*, 28, 428, 1996.

Epstein, L.H. and Goldfield, G.S., Physical activity in the treatment of childhood overweight and obesity: current evidence and research issues, *Med. Sci. Sports Exerc.*, 31, S533, 1999.

Epstein, L.H., Valoski, A. and McCurley, J., Effect of weight loss by obese children on long-term growth, *Am. J. Dis. Child.*, 147, 1076, 1993.

Epstein, L.H. et al., Effects of weight loss on fitness in obese children, *Am. J. Dis. Child.*, 137, 654, 1983.

Epstein, L.H. et al., Effect of diet and controlled exercise on weight loss in obese children, *J. Pediatr.*, 107, 358, 1985.

Epstein, L.H. et al., The effect of family variables on child weight change, *Hlth. Psychol.*, 5, 1, 1986a.

Epstein, L.H. et al., Effect of parent weight on weight loss in obese children, *J. Consult. Clin. Psychol.*, 54, 400, 1986b.

Epstein, L.H. et al., Long-term relationship between weight and aerobic-fitness change in children, *Hlth. Psychol.*, 7, 47, 1988.

Epstein, L.H. et al., The effect of weight control on lipid changes in obese children, *Am. J. Dis. Child.*, 143, 454, 1989a.

Epstein, L.H. et al., Resting metabolic rate in lean and obese children: relationship to child and parent weight and percent-overweight change, *Am. J. Clin. Nutr.*, 49, 331, 1989b.

Epstein, L.H. et al., Five-year follow-up study of family based behavioral treatments for childhood obesity, *J. Consult. Clin. Psychol.*, 58, 661, 1990.

Epstein, L.H. et al., Ten-year outcome of behavioral family-based treatment for childhood obesity, *Hlth. Psychol.*, 13, 373, 1994.

Epstein, L.H. et al., Do children lose and maintain weight easier than adults: a comparison of child and parent weight changes from six months to ten years, *Obes. Res.*, 3, 411, 1995a.

Epstein, L.H. et al., Effects of decreasing sedentary behavior and increasing activity on weight change in obese children, *Hlth. Psychol.*, 14, 109, 1995b.

Epstein, L.H. et al., Determinants of physical activity in obese children assessed by accelerometer and self-report, *Med. Sci. Sports Exerc.*, 28, 1157, 1996.

Epstein, L.H. et al., Effects of decreasing sedentary behaviors on activity choice in obese children, *Hlth. Psychol.*, 16, 107, 1997.

Epstein, L.H. et al., Treatment of pediatric obesity, *Pediatrics*, 101, 554, 1998.

Epstein, L.H. et al., Reinforcing value of physical activity as a determinant of child activity level, *Hlth. Psychol.*, 18, 599, 1999.

Epstein, L.H. et al., Decreasing sedentary behaviors in treating pediatric obesity, *Arch. Pediatr. Adolesc. Med.*, 154, 220, 2000.

Epstein, L.H. et al., Changes in eating disorder symptoms with pediatric obesity treatment, *J. Pediatr.*, 139, 58, 2001.

Erdeve, O. et al., Antioxidant superoxide dismutase activity in obese children, *Biol. Trace Elem. Res.*, 98, 219, 2004.

Ericson, S.J. et al., Are overweight children unhappy? Body mass index, depressive symptoms, and overweight concerns in elementary school children, *Arch. Pediatr. Adolesc. Med.*, 154, 931, 2000.

Eriksson, J. et al., Obesity from cradle to grave, *Int. J. Obes. Relat. Metab. Disord.*, 27, 722, 2003a.

Eriksson, J.G. et al., Early adiposity rebound in childhood and risk of Type 2 diabetes in adult life, *Diabetologia*, 46, 190, 2003b.

Ernst, N.D. and Obarzanek, E., Child health and nutrition: obesity and high blood cholesterol, *Prev. Med.*, 23, 427, 1994.

Escobar, O. et al., Hepatic clearence increases after weight loss in obese children and adolescents, *Am. J. Med. Sci.*, 317, 282, 1999.

Esposito-Del Puente, A. et al., High prevalence of overweight in a children population living in Naples (Italy), *Int. J. Obes. Relat. Metab. Disord.*, 20, 283, 1996.

Esquivel, M. et al., Nutritional status of preschool children in Ciudad de la Habana from 1972 to 1993, *Rev. Panam. Salud Publica*, 1, 349, 1997 (in Spanish).

Estelles, A. et al., Plasma PAI-1 levels in obese children: effect of weight loss and influence of PAI-1 promoter 4G/5gG genotype, *Thromb. Haemostat.*, 86, 647, 2001.

Etelson, D. et al., Childhood obesity: do parents recognize this health risk? *Obes. Res.*, 11, 1362, 2003.

Eto, C. et al., Validity of the body mass index and fat mass index as an indicator of obesity in children aged 3–5 years, *Physiol. Anthropol. Appl. Human.*, 23, 25, 2004.

Faith, M.S., Johnson, S.L., and Allison, D.B., Putting the behavior into the behavior genetics of obesity, *Behav. Genet.*, 27, 423, 1997.

Faith, M.S. et al., Effects of contingent television on physical activity and television viewing in obese children, *Pediatrics*, 107, 1043, 2001.

Faith, M.S. et al., Maternal-child feeding patterns and child body weight: findings from a population-based sample, *Arch. Pediatr. Adolesc. Med.*, 157, 926, 2003.

Faith, M.S. et al., Project Grow-2-Gether: a study of the genetic and environmental influences on child eating and obesity, *Twin. Res.*, 5, 472, 2002.

Faith, M.S. et al., Genetic–environmental architecture of percent body fat measured by bioimpedance analysis in a pediatric twin sample, *Int. J. Obes. Relat. Metab. Disord.*, 22, S13, 1998.

Falk, B. et al., The association between adiposity and the response to resistance training among pre- and early-pubertal boys, *J. Pediatr. Endocrinol. Metab.*, 15, 597, 2002.

Falkner, F., Obesity and cardiovascular disease risk factors in prepubescent and pubescent black and white females, *Crit. Rev. Food. Sci. Nutr.*, 33, 397, 1993.

Fallon, A. and Rozin, P., Sex differences in perceptions of desirable body shape, *J. Abnorm. Psychol.*, 94, 102, 1985.

Falorni, A. et al., Serum levels of type I procollagen C-terminal propeptide, insulin-like growth factor-I (IGF-I), and IGF binding protein-3 in obese children and adolescents: relationship to gender, pubertal development, growth, insulin and nutritional status, *Metab. Clin. Endocrinol.*, 46, 862, 1997a.

Falorni, A. et al., Leptin serum levels in normal weight and obese children and adolescents: relationships with age, sex, pubertal development, body mass index and insulin, *Int. J. Obes. Relat. Metab. Disord.*, 21, 881, 1997b.

Falorni, A. et al., Using obese-specific charts of height and height velocity for assessment of growth in obese children and adolescents during weight excess reduction, *Eur. J. Clin. Nutr.*, 53, 181, 1999.

Fanconi, G., Has malnutrition only bad consequences? What is the definition of health? in *Protein and Energy Malnutrition*, Von Muralt, A., Ed. Nestlé Foundation, Springer-Verlag, Berlin, 1969, 57.

Faozof, G., Saenz, S. and Gonzales, C., Television viewing and obesity in a sample of Argentinian children, *Int. J. Obes. Relat. Metab. Disord.*, 23, S45, 1999.

Farooqui, I.S. and O'Rahilly, S., Recent advances in the genetics of severe childhood obesity, *Arch. Dis. Child.*, 83, 31, 2000.

Farooqui, I.S. et al., Clinical spectrum of obesity and mutations in the melanocortin 4 receptor gene, *N. Engl. J. Med.*, 348, 1085, 2003.

Felson, D.T. et al., Obesity and knee osteoarthritis, *Ann. Intern. Med.*, 109, 18, 1988.

Feng, N. et al., Sequence variants of the POMC gene and their associations with body compoisiton in children, *Obes. Res.*, 11, 619, 2003.

Ferguson, M.A. et al., Fat distribution and hemostatic measures in obese children, *Am. J. Clin. Nutr.*, 67, 1136, 1998.

Ferguson, M.A. et al., Effects of exercise training and its cessation on components of the insulin resistance syndrome in obese children, *Int. J. Obes. Relat. Metab. Disord.*, 23, 889, 1999a.

Ferguson, M.A. et al., Effects of physical training and its cessation on the hemostatic system in obese children, *Am. J. Clin. Nutr.*, 69, 1130, 1999b.

Fernandes-do-Prado, L.B. et al., Body position and obstructive sleep apnea in children, *Sleep*, 25, 66, 2002.

Fernandez, A.C. et al., Correlation between percentage of fat and physical performance in obese children, *Int. J. Obes. Relat. Metab. Disord.*, 22, S12, 1998a.

Fernandez, A.C. et al., The lean body mass as determinant of physical performance in children, *Int. J. Obes. Relat. Metab. Disord.*, 22, S199, 1998b.

Ferrante, E. et al., Nutritional epidemiology during school age, *Ann. Inst. Super. Sanita*, 31, 435, 1995.

Ferrer-Gonzales, J. et al., The development of lipid and anthropometric parameters in the treatment of pre-pubertal obese patients, *An. Esp. Pediatr.*, 48, 267, 1998 (in Spanish).

Figueroa-Colon, R. et al., Body composition changes in obese children after a 10-week weight loss program using dual-energy X-ray absorptiometry measurements (DXA), *Int. J. Obes. Relat. Metab. Disord.*, 22, S12, 1998.

Figueroa-Colon, R. et al., Possibility of a clinic-based hypocaloric dietary intervention implemented in a school setting for obese children, *Obes. Res.*, 4, 419, 1996.

Figueroa-Colon, R. et al., Comparison of two hypocaloric diets in obese children, *Am. J. Dis. Child.*, 147, 160, 1993.

Figueroa-Munoz, J.I., Chinn, S. and Rona, R.J., Association between obesity and asthma in 4 11-year-old children in the UK, *Thorax*, 56, 133, 2001.

Fiorotto, M., Cochran, W.J., and Klish, W.J., Fat-free mass and total body water of infants estimated from total body electrical conductivity measurements, *Pediatr. Res.*, 22, 417, 1987.

Fisberg, M. et al., Body composition assessment by dual-energy X-ray absorptiometry in Brazilian school children with severe obesity, *Int. J. Obes. Relat. Metab. Disord.*, 22, S198, 1998.

Fisher, J.O. and Birch, L.L., Eating in the absence of hunger and overweight in girls from 5 to 7 y of age, *Am. J. Clin. Nutr.*, 6, 226, 2002.

Fisher, M. et al., Eating attitudes, health-risk behaviours, self-esteem, and anxiety among adolescent females in a suburban high school, *J. Adolesc. Hlth.*, 12, 377, 1991.

Fisher, S., The evolution of psychological concepts about the body, in *Body Images: Development, Deviance, and Change*, Cash, T.F. and Pruzinsky, T., Eds., Guilford Press, New York, 1990, 3.

Fisher, S.B and Cleveland, S.E., *Body Image and Personality*, 2nd ed, Dover, New York, 1968.

Flanery, R.C. and Kirschenbaum, D.S., Dispositional and situational correlates of long-term weight reduction in obese children, *Addict. Behav.*, 11, 249, 1986.

Fleta Zaragozano, J. et al., Assessment of the submandibular adipose skinfold for the determination of nutritional status in children and adolescents, *An. Esp. Pediatr.*, 47, 258, 1997.

Flodmark, C.E., How to influence the development of eating behaviors: implications for the prevention of obesity, *Int. J., Obes. Relat. Metab. Disord.*, 23, S6, 1999.

Flodmark, C.E. et al., Prevention of progression to severe obesity in a group of obese schoolchildren treated with family therapy, *Pediatrics*, 91, 880, 1993.

Florencio, T.M. et al., Obesity and undernutrition in a very-low-income population in the city of Maceio, northeastern Brazil, *Br. J. Nutr.*, 86, 277, 2001.

Flynn, J.M., Lou, J.E., and Ganley, T.J., Prevention of sports injuries in children, *Curr. Opin. Pediatr.*, 14, 6, 719, 2002.

Fogelholm, M. et al., Parent–child relationship of physical activity patterns and obesity, *Int. J. Obes. Relat. Disord.*, 23, 1262, 1999.

Fomon, S.J. et al., Body composition of reference children from birth to age 10 years, *Am. J. Clin. Nutr.*, 35, 1169, 1982.

Fontvieille, A.M., Kriska, A., and Ravussin, E., Decreased physical activity in Pima Indian compared with Caucasian children, *Int. J. Obes. Relat. Metab. Disord.*, 17, 445, 1993.

Forbes, G.B. *Human Body Composition: Growth, Aging, Nutrition, and Activity*, Springer-Verlag, New York, 1987.

Forbes, G.B., Diet and exercise in obese subjects: self-report versus controlled measurements, *Nutr. Rev.*, 51, 296, 1993.

Forbes, G.B., and Brown, M.R., Energy need for weight maintenance in human beings: effect of body size and composition, *J. Am. Diet. Assoc.*, 89, 499, 1989.

Foreyt, J.P. and Cousins, J.H., Primary prevention of obesity in Mexican American children, *Ann. J. Acad. Sci.*, 699, 137, 1993.

Foreyt, J.P. et al., A weight reduction intervention for Mexican Americans, *Am. J. Clin. Nutr.*, 53, S1639, 1991.

Fox, K.R., Childhood obesity and the role of physical activity, *J.R. Soc. Hlth.*, 124, 34, 2004.

Francis, C.C. et al., Body composition, dietary intake and energy expenditure in nonobese, prepubertal children of obese and nonobese biological mothers, *J. Am. Diet. Assoc.*, 99, 58, 1999.

Freedman, D.S., Clustering of coronary heart disease risk factors among obese children, *J. Pediatr. Endocrinol. Metab.*, 15, 1099, 2002.

Freedman, D.S. et al., Relation of circumferences and skinfold thicknesses to lipid and insulin concentrations in children: the Bogalusa Heart Study, *Am. J. Clin. Nutr.*, 69, 308, 1999.

Freedman, D.S. et al., Relationship of childhood obesity to coronary heart disease risk factors in adulthood: the Bogalusa Heart Study, *Pediatrics*, 108, 712, 2001a.

Freedman, D.S. et al., BMI rebound, childhood height and obesity among adults: the Bogalusa Heart Study, *Int. J. Obes. Relat. Metab. Disord.*, 25, 543, 2001b.

Freedman, D.S. et al., The relationship of obesity throughout life to carotid intima-media thickness in adulthood: the Bogalusa Heart Study., *Int. J. Obes. Relat. Metab. Disord.*, 28, 159, 2004.

Freeman, W. et al., Association between risk factors for coronary heart disease in schoolboys and adult mortality rates in the same localities, *Arch. Dis. Child.*, 65, 78, 1990.

Freeman-Fobbs, P., Feeding our children to death: the tragedy of childhood obesity in America, *J. Nat. Med. Assoc.*, 95, 119, 2003.

Frelut, M.L., From childhood obesity to adult obesity, *Cah. Nutr. Diet.*, 36, 123, 2001.

Frelut, M.L., Childhood obesity: from clinics to leptin, *Int. J. Obes. Relat. Metab. Disord.*, 21, S137, 1997.

Frelut, M.L. et al., Leptin plasma concentrations in morbidly obese children suggest heterogenous responsiveness. Impact of weight loss, *Int. J. Obes. Relat. Metab. Disord.*, 21, S142, 1997.

Frelut, M.L. et al., Changes in bone mineral density and vitamin status in obese adolescents during weight loss, *Int. J. Obes. Relat. Metab. Disord.*, 22, S33, 1998.

Freymond, D. et al., Energy expenditure during normo- and overfeeding in peripubertal children of lean and obese Pima Indians, *Am. J. Physiol.*, 257, E647, 1989.

Friedel, S. et al., Glucose transporter 4 gene: association studies pertaining to alleles of two polymorphisms in extremely obese children and adolescents and in normal and underweight control., *Ann. New York Acad. Sci.*, 967, 554, 2002.

Fripp, R.R. et al., Aerobic capacity, obesity, and atherosclerotic risk factors in male adolescents, *Pediatrics*, 75, 813, 1985.

Frisancho, A.R., Prenatal compared with parental origins of adolescent fatness, *Am. J. Clin. Nutr.*, 72, 1186, 2000.

Frittitta, L. et al., The Q121 PC-1 variant and obesity have additive and independent effect effects in causing insulin resistance, *J. Clin. Endocrinol. Metab.*, 86, 5888, 2002.

Frontini, M.G., Srinivasan, S.R., and Berenson, G.S., Longitudinal changes in risk variables underlying metabolic Syndrome X from childhood to young adulthood, in female subjects with a history of early menarche: the Bogalusa Heart Study, *Int. J. Obes. Relat. Metab. Disord.*, 27, 1398, 2003.

Frontini, M.G. et al., Comparison of weight-for-height indices as a measure of adiposity and cardiovascular risk from childhood to young adulthood: the Bogalusa Heart Study, *J. Clin. Epidemiol.*, 54, 817, 2001.

Frost, H.M., *The Physiology of Cartilaginous, Fibrous and Body Tissue: Orthopedic Lectures*, Charles C Thomas, Springfield, 1972.

Frost, H.M., A chondral modeling theory, *Calcified Tissue Int.*, 28, 181, 1979.

Frye, C. and Heinrich, J., Trends and predictors of overweight and obesity in East German children, *Int. J. Obes. Relat. Metab. Disord.*, 27, 963, 2003.

Fu, W.P.C. et al., Screening for childhood obesity: international vs. population-specific definitions. Which is more appropriate? *Int. J. Obes. Relat. Metab. Disord.*, 27, 1121, 2003.

Fuentes, R.M. et al., Familial aggregation of body mass index: a population-based family study in eastern Finland, *Horm. Metab. Res.*, 34, 406, 2002.

Fukushige, T. et al., Effect of age and overweight on the QT Interval and the prevalence of long OT syndrome in children, *Am. J. Cardiol.*, 89, 395, 2002.

Fung, K.P. et al., Effects of overweight on lung function, *Arch. Dis. Child.*, 65, 512, 1990.

Gadzhiev, A.A. et al., Acupuncture therapy of constitutional-exogenous obesity in children, *Probl. Endokrinol., (Mosk)*, 39, 21, 1993 (in Russian).

Gallistl, S. et al., Insulin is an independent correlate of plasma homocystein levels in obese children and adolescents, *Diabetes Care*, 23, 1348, 2000a.

Gallistl, S. et al., Correlation between cholesterol, soluble P-selectin, and D-dimer in obese children, *Blood Coagul. Fibrinolysis*, 11, 755, 2000b

Gallistl, S. et al., Inverse correlation between thyroid function and hemostatic markers for coronary heart disease in obese children and adolescents, *J. Pediatr. Endocrinol. Metab.*, 13, 1615, 2000c.

Gallistl, S. et al., Changes in serum interleukin-6 concentration in obese children and adolescents during a weight reduction program, *Int. J. Obes. Relat. Metab. Disord.*, 25, 1640, 2001a.

Gallistl, S. et al., Effects of short-term energy restriction and physical training on haemostatic risk factors for coronary heart disease in obese children and adolescents, *Int. J. Obes. Relat. Metab. Disord.*, 25, 529, 2001b.

Gallistl, S. et al., Determinants of homocysteine during weight reduction in obese children and adolescents, *Metab. Clin. Exp.*, 50, 1220, 2001c.

Galloway, P.J., Donaldson, M.D.C., and Wallace, A.M., Sex hormone binding globulin concentration as a prepubertal marker for hyperinsulinaemia in obesity, *Arch. Dis. Child.*, 85, 489, 2001.

Garfinkel, P.E. et al., Body dissatisfaction in bulimia nervosa: relationship to weight and shape concerns and psychological functioning, *Int. J. Eating Disord.*, 11, 151, 1992.

Garner, D.M. and Garfinkel, P.E., Body image in anorexia nervosa: measurement, theory, and clinical implications, *Int. J. Psychiatry Med.*, 11, 263, 1981.

Garrow, J.S., Effect of exercise on obesity, *Acta. Med. Scand.*, Suppl 711, 67, 1986.

Garrow, J.S., Health risks of obesity, in *Obesity*, British Nutrition Foundation, Blackwell Sciences, Oxford, 1999.

Garrow, J.S., Is it possible to prevent obesity? *Infusions Therapie*, 17, 28, 1990.

Gascón, F. et al., Sex hormone-binding globulin as a marker for hyperinsulinemia and/or insulin resistance in obese children., *Eur. J. Endocrinol.*, 143, 85, 2000.

Gately, P., Cooke, C.B. and Mackreth, P., A three-year follow up of an eight week diet and exercise programme on children attending a weight loss camp, Abstr., in *8th Int. Congress of Obesity, Satellite Symposium Physical Activity and Obesity*, Aug. 26–29, Maastricht, 1998, 38.

Gazzaniga, J.M. and Burns, T.L., Relationship between diet composition and body fatness, with adjustment for resting energy expenditure and physical activity, in preadolescents children, *Am. J. Clin. Nutr.*, 58, 21, 1993.

Geiss, H.C., Parhofer, K.G. and Schwandt, P., Parameters of childhood obesity and their relationship to cardiovascular risk factors in healthy prepubescent children, *Int. J. Obes. Relat. Metab. Disord.*, 25, 830, 2001.

Gelernter-Yaniv, L. et al., Associations between a polymorphism in the 11-beta hydroxysteroid dehydrogenase type I gene and body composition, *Int. J. Obes. Relat. Metab. Disord.*, 27, 983, 2003.

Gerald, L.B. et al., Social class, social support and obesity risk in children, *Child Care Hlth. Dev.*, 20, 145, 1994.

Gibney, M.J., Epidemiology of obesity in relation to nutrient intake, *Int. J. Obes. Relat. Disord.*, 19, S1, 1995.

Gilbert, T.J. et al., Obesity among Navajo adolescents. Relationship to dietary intake and blood pressure, *Am. J. Dis. Child.*, 146, 289, 1992.

Gilliland, F.D. et al., Obesity and the risk of newly diagnosed asthma in school-age children, *Am. J. Epidemiol.*, 158, 406, 2003.

Gillis, L.J. et al., Relationship between juvenile obesity, dietary energy and fat intake and physical activity, *Int. J. Obes. Relat. Metab. Disord.*, 26, 458, 2002.

Gillman, M.W. et al., Risk of overweight among adolescents who were breastfed as infants, *J.A.M.A.*, 285, 2461, 2001.

Giovannini, M. et al., Cholesterol and lipoprotein levels in Milanese children: relation to nutritional and familial factors, *J. Am. Coll. Nutr.*, 11, 28S, 1992.

Girardet, J.P. et al., Obesity in children: value of clinical evaluation criteria, *Ann. Pediatr. (Paris)*, 40, 297, 1993 (in French).

Glenny, A.M., et al., The treatment and prevention of obesity: a systematic review of the literature, *Int. J. Obes. Relat. Metab. Disord.*, 21, 715, 1997.

Glowinska, B., Urban, M., and Koput, A., Cardiovascular risk factors in children with obesity, hypertension and diabetes: lipoprotein(a) levels and body mass index correlate with family history of cardiovascular disease, *Eur. J. Pediatr.*, 161, 511, 2002.

Glowinska, B. et al., Endothelial dysfunction in children and adolescents with obesity and hypertension: assessment based on cell adhesion molecular levels, *Kardiol. Pol.*, 54, 35, 2001.

Gokbel, H. and Atas, S., Exercise-induced bronchospasm in nonasthmatic obese and nonobese children, *J. Sp. Med. Phys. Fitness*, 39, 361, 1999.

Golan, M. and Crow, S., Parents are key players in the prevention and treatment of weight-related problems, *Nutr. Rev.*, 62, 39, 2004.

Golan, M. and Weizman, A., Familial approach to the treatment of childhood obesity: conceptual model, *J. Nutr. Educ.*, 33, 102, 2001.

Golan, M., Weizman, A., and Fainaru, M., Impact of treatment for childhood obesity on parental risk factors for cardiovascular disease, *Prev. Med.*, 29, 519, 1999.

Golan, M. et al., Parents as exclusive agents of change in the treatment of childhood obesity, *Am. J. Clin. Nutr.,*, 67, 1130, 1998.

Goldfield, G.S. et al., Open-loop feedback to increase physical activity in obese children, *Int. J. Obes. Relat. Metab. Disord.*, 24, 888, 2000.

Gonzales Moran, I. et al., Circadian rhythms of cortisol and insulin in nutritional obesity in children, *An. Esp. Pediatr.*, 30, 79, 1989 (in Spanish).

Goran, M.I., Kaskoun, M., and Shuman, W.P., Intra-abdominal adipose tissue in young children, *Int. J. Obes. Relat. Metab. Disord.*, 19, 279, 1995.

Goran, M.I., Reynolds, K.D., and Lindquist, C.H., Role of physical activity in the prevention of obesity in children, *Int. J. Obes. Relat. Metab. Disord.*, 23, S18, 1999.

Goran, M.I. and Sun, M., Total energy expenditure and physical activity in prepubertal children: recent advances based on the application of the doubly labelled water method, *Am. J. Clin. Nutr.*, 68, S944, 1998.

Goran, M.I. and Treuth, M.B., Energy expenditure, physical activity, and obesity in children, *Pediatr. Clin. North. Am.*, 48, 931, 2001.

Goran, M.I. et al., Estimating body composition of young children by using bioelectrical resistance, *J. Appl. Physiol.*, 75, 1776, 1993.

Goran, M.I. et al., Energy expenditure in children of lean and obese parents, *Am. J. Physiol.*, 268, E917, 1995.

Goran, M.I. et al., Longitudinal changes in fatness in white children: no effect of childhood energy expenditure, *Am. J. Clin. Nutr.*, 67, 309, 1998.

Gordon, F.K. et al., High levels of childhood obesity observed among 3- to 7-year New Zealand Pacific children is a public health concern, *J. Nutr.*, 133, 3456, 2003.

Gortmaker, S.L., Dietz, W.H., and Cheung, L.W., Inactivity, diet, and the fattening of America, *J. Am. Diet. Assoc.*, 90, 1247, 1990.

Gortmaker, S.L. et al., Increasing pediatric obesity in the United States, *Am. J. Dis. Child.*, 141, 535, 1987.

Gortmaker, S.L. et al., Social and economic consequences of overweight in adolescence and young adulthood, *New Engl. J. Med.*, 329, 1008, 1993.

Goulding, A. et al., Overweight and obese children have low bone mass and area for their weight, *Int. J. Obes. Relat. Metab. Disord.*, 24, 627, 2000.

Goulding, A. et al., Spinal overload: a concern for obese children and adolescents, *Osteoporosis Int.*, 13, 835, 2002.

Goulding, A. et al., Dynamic and static tests of balance and postural sway in boys: effects of previous wrist bone fractures and high adiposity, *Gait Posture*, 17, 136, 2003a.

Goulding, A. et al., Body composition of 4- and 5-year-old New Zealand girls: a DXA study of initial adiposity and subsequent 4-year fat change, *Int. J. Obes. Relat. Metab. Disord.*, 27, 410, 2003b.

Gracey, M., Child health implications of worlwide urbanization, *Rev. Environ. Health*, 18, 51, 2003.

Gralen, S.J. et al., Dieting and disordered eating during early and middle adolescence: do the influences remain the same? *Int. J. Eating Disord.*, 9, 501, 1990.

Grant, A.M. et al., Thyroidal hormone metabolism in obesity during semi-starvation, *Clin. Endocrinol.*, 9, 227, 1978.

Gray, D.S. and Bray, G.A., Evaluation of the obese patient, in *Handbook of Eating Disorders, Part 2: Obesity*, Burrows, G.D., Beumont, P.J.V., and Casper, R.C., Eds., Elsevier, Amsterdam, 1988.

Greco, M. et al., Caloric intake and distribution of the main nutrients in a population of obese children, *Minerva Endocrinol.*, 15, 257, 1990.

Greecher, C.P., Physicians' perceptions of childhood and adolescent obesity, *Ann. N.Y. Acad. Sci.*, 29, 699, 1993.

Greene, L.C. et al., Comparison of total energy expenditure among children at low and high risk of obesity, *Int. J. Obes. Relat. Metab. Disord.*, 22, 1998.

Griffiths, M., Rivers, J.P., and Payne, P.R., Energy intake in children at high and low risk of obesity, *Hum. Nutr. Clin. Nutr.*, 41, 425, 1987.

Griffiths, M. et al., Metabolic rate and physical development in children at risk of obesity, *Lancet*, 336, 76, 1990.

Grugni, G. et al., Hyperuricemia and obesity in young female subjects, *Int. J. Obes. Relat. Metab. Disord.*, 22, S27, 1998.

Grund, A. et al., Functional, behavioral and sociodemographic characteristics of prepubertal children with obese and non-obese parents, *Aktuel Ernahr. Med.*, 26, 1, 2001a.

Grund, A. et al., Is TV viewing an index of physical activity and fitness and overweight in normal weight children? *Pub. Hlth. Nutr.*, 4, 1245, 2001b.

Guerra, A. et al., Influence of apolipoprotein E polymorphism on cardiovascular risk factors in obese children, *Ann. Nutr. Metab.*, 47, 49, 2003.

Guillaume, M., Differences in associations of fatness status, familial and nutritional factors with blood lipids between boys and girls, *Int. J. Obes. Relat. Metab. Disord.*, 22, S24, 1998.

Guillaume, M., Defining obesity in childhood: current practice, *Am. J. Clin. Nutr.*, 70, 126S, 1999.

Guillaume, M. et al., Prevalence of obesity in children in Belgian Luxembourg, *Int. J. Obes. Relat. Metab. Disord.*, 17, S36, 1993.

Guillaume, M. et al., Familial trends of obesity through three generations: the Belgian-Luxembourg Child Study, *Int. J. Obes. Relat. Metab. Disord.*, 19, S5, 1995.

Guillaume, M. et al., Physical activity, obesity, and cardiovascular risk factors in children. The Belgian Luxemburg Child Study II, *Obes. Res.*, 5, 549, 1997.

Guillaume, M., Lapidus, L. and Lambert, A., Obesity and nutrition in children. The Belgian Luxembourg Child Study IV, *Eur. J. Clin. Nutr.*, 52, 323, 1998.

Guillaume, M. and Lissau, I., Epidemiology, in *Child and Adolescent Obesity*, Burniat, W. et al., Eds., Cambridge University Press, Cambridge, 2002, 28.

Gunnarsdottir, I. and Thorsdottir, I., Relationships between growth and feeding in infancy and body mass index at the age of 6 years, *Int. J. Obes. Relat. Metab. Dis.*, 27, 1523, 2003.

Gunnell, D.J. et al., Childhood obesity and adult cardiovascular mortality: a 57-y follow-up study based on the Boyd Orr cohort, *Am. J. Clin. Nutr.*, 67, 1111, 1998.

Guo, S.S. and Chumlea, W.C., Tracking of body mass index in children in relation to overweight in adulthood, *Am. J. Clin. Nutr.*, 70, 145S, 1999.

Guo, S.S. et al., The prediction value of childhood body mass index values for overweight at age 35y, *Am. J. Clin. Nutr.*, 59, 810, 1994.

Guo, S.S. et al., Age- and maturity-related changes in body composition during adolescence into adulthood: the Fels Longitudinal Study, *Int. J. Obes. Relat. Metab. Disord.*, 21, 1167, 1997.

Guo, S.S. et al., Long-term changes in BMI during growth in relation to adulthood obesity and cardiovascular risk factors, *Int. J. Obes. Relat. Metab. Disord.*, 22, S25, 1998.

Guo, S.S. et al., Effect of lipoproteine lipase gene polymorphism on plasma lipid levels, BMI and subcutaneous fat distribution in simple obesity children, *Chin. J. Med. Genet.*, 17, 105, 2000.

Guo, S.S. et al., Predicting overweight and obesity in adulthood from body mass index values in childhood and adolescence, *Am. J. Clin. Nutr.*, 76, 653, 2002.

Gupta, N.K. et al., Is obesity associated with poor sleep quality in adolescents? *Am. J. Human Biol.*, 14, 762, 2002.

Gurney, M. and Gorstein, J., The global prevalence of obesity. An initial overview of available data, *World Health Statistics*, 41, 251, 1988.

Gustafson-Larson, A.M., and Terry, R.D., Weight-related behaviors and concerns of fourth-grade children, *J. Am. Diet. Assoc.*, 92, 818, 1992.

Gutin, B., Exercise, body composition, and health in children in exercise science and sports medicine, in *Exercise, Nutrition and Weight Control*, Lamb, D. and Murray, R., Eds., Cooper, Carmel, 1998, 295.

Gutin, B. and Manos, T.M., Physical activity in the prevention of obesity, *Ann. N.Y. Acad. Sci.*, 699, 115, 1993.

Gutin, B. et al., The dominance of body fat in explaining endurance performance of 11- to 12-year-old girls, *Res. Q.*, 49, 44, 1978.

Gutin, B. et al., Physical training improves body composition of black obese 7- to 11-year-old girls, *Obes. Res.*, 3, 305, 1995.

Gutin, B. et al., Effect of physical training on heart-rate variability in obese children, *J. Pediatr.*, 130, 938, 1997.

Gutin, B. et al., Effect of physical training and its cessation on components of the insulin resistance syndrome in obese children, *Int. J. Obes. Relat. Metab. Disord.*, 22, S23, 1998.

Gutin, B. et al., Effect of physical training and its cessation on percent fat and bone density of children with obesity, *Obes. Res.*, 7, 208, 1999a.

Gutin, B. et al., Plasma leptin concentrations in obese children, changes during 4-month period with and without physical training, *Am. J. Clin. Nutr.*, 69, 388, 1999b.

Guzzaloni, G. et al., Thyroid-stimulating hormone and prolactin response to thyrotropin-releasing hormone in juvenile obesity before and after hypocaloric diet, *J. Endocrinol. Invest.*, 18, 621, 1995.

Gwinup, G., Effect of exercise alone on weight of obese women, *Arch. Int. Med.*, 135, 676, 1975.

Hager, R.L., Tucker, L.A., and Seljaas, G.T., Aerobic fitness, blood lipids, and body fat in children, *Am. J. Pub. Hlth.*, 85, 1702, 1995.

Hainer, V. et al., The response to VLCD treatment in obese female identical twins, *Int. J. Obes. Relat. Metab. Disord.*, 19, 40, 1995.

Hainer, V. et al., Early postnatal nutrition in preterm infants and their anthropometric characteristics in later life, *Int. J. Obes. Relat. Metab. Disord.*, 23, S45, 1999.

Hainer, V. et al., Intrapair resemblance in very low calorie diet-induced weight loss in female obese identical twins, *Int. J. Obes. Relat. Metab. Disord.*, 24, 1051, 2000.

Hajniš, K., New growth norms for Czech and Slovak children and youth, *Anthrop. Anz.*, 51, 207, 1993 (in German).

Hajniš, K., and Petrásek, R., Body height, weight, and BMI in the Czech and Slovak population, *Homo*, 59, 163, 1999 (in German).

Hakanen, M. et al., Serum leptin concentration and dietary aspects in lean, normal weight and obese children during the first five years of life, *Int. J. Obes. Relat. Metab. Disord.*, 22, S27, 1998.

Halford, J.C. et al., Effect of television advertisements for foods on food consumption in children, *Appetite*, 42, 221, 2004a.

Halford, J.C. et al., Food advertisements induce food consumption in both lean and obese children, *Obes. Res.*, 12, 171, 2004b.

Halsall, D.J. et al., Uncoupling protein 3 genetic variants in human obesity: the c-55t promoter polymorphism is negatively correlated with body mass index in a UK Caucasian population, *Int. J. Obes. Relat. Metab. Disord.*, 25, 472, 2001.

Hammer, L.D., The development of eating behavior in childhood, *Pediatr. Clin. North Am.*, 39, 379, 1992.

Hammer, L.D. et al., Standardized percentile curves of body mass index for children and adolescents, *Am. J. Dis. Child.*, 145, 259, 1991.

Hara, M., Trends in obesity, *Nippon Rinsho*, 46, 2361, 1988.

Harada, K., Orino, T., and Takada, G., Body mass index can predict left ventricular diastolic filling in asymptomatic obese children, *Pediatr. Cardiol.*, 22, 273, 2001.

Hardman, A.E., Physical activity, obesity and blood lipids, *Int. J. Obes. Relat. Metab. Disord.*, 23, Suppl. 3, S64, 1999.

Hardy, R. et al., Birthweight, childhood growth, and blood pressure at 43 years: a British cohort, *Int. J. Epidemiol.*, 33, 121, 2004.

Hardy, S.C. and Kleinman, R.E., Fat and cholesterol in the diet of infants and young children: implications for growth, development, and long-term health, *J. Pediatr.*, 125, S69, 1994.

Hasanoglu, A. et al., Bone mineral density in childhood obesity, *J. Pediatr. Endocrinol. Metab.*, 13, 307, 2000.

Hasegawa, T. et al., Free form of insulin-like growth factor-1 in circulation is normal in children with simple obesity, *Hormone Res.*, 49, 51, 1998.

Hassink, S.G. et al., Placental leptin: an important new growth factor in intrauterine and neonatal development? *Pediatrics*, 100, E1, 1997.

Haszon, I. et al., Platelet aggregation, blood viscosity and serum lipids in hypertensive and obese children, *Eur. J. Pediatr.*, 162, 385, 2003.

Hauck, F.R. et al., Trends in anthropometric measurements among Mescalero Apache Indian preschool children 1968 through 1988, *Am. J. Dis. Child.*, 146, 1194, 1992.

Hawks, S.R. et al., A cross-cultural analysis of "motivation for eating" as a potential factor in the emergence of global obesity: Japan and the United States, *Hlth. Prom. Int.*, 18, 153, 2003.

Hayashi, T. et al., Echocardiographic and electrocardiographic measures in obese children after an exercise program, *Int. J. Obes.*, 11, 465, 1987.

He, O. et al., Blood pressure is associated with body mass index in both normal and obese children, *Hypertension*, 36, 165, 2000.

Heath, G.W., Pate, R.R., and Pratt, M., Measuring physical activity among adolescents, *Pub. Hlth. Report*, 108, 42, 1993.

Hebebrand, H. et al., Epidemic obesity: are genetic factors involved via increased rates of assortative mating? *Int. J. Obes. Relat. Metab. Disord.*, 24, 345, 2000.

Helland, I.B. et al., Leptin levels in pregnant women and newborn infants: gender differences and reduction during the neonatal period, *Pediatrics*, 101, E12, 1998.

Heptulla, R.A. et al., Augmentation of alimentary insulin secretion despite similar gastric inhibitory peptide (GIP) response in juvenile obesity, *Pediatr. Res.*, 47, 628, 2000.

Hermelo, M.P. et al., Changes in body composition and serum lipid fractions after four weeks of slimming treatment: results in nineteen obese male adolescents, *Acta Paediatr. Hung.*, 28, 29, 1987a.

Hermelo, M.P. et al., Slimming treatment and changes in serum lipid and lipoprotein in obese adolescents, *Exp. Clin. Endocrinol.*, 90, 347, 1987b.

Hernandez, B. et al., Overweight in 12–49-year-old women and children under 5 years of age in Mexico, *Salud Publica Mex.*, 38, 178, 1996.

Herpertz-Dahlmann, B. et al., Secular trends in body mass index measurements in preschool children from the City of Aachen, Germany, *Eur. J. Pediatr.*, 162, 104, 2003.

Heymsfield, S.B. et al., Chemical and elemental analysis of humans *in vivo* using improved body composition models, *Am. J. Physiol.*, 261, E103, 1991.

Heymsfield, S. et al., Multicompartment chemical models of human body composition: recent advance and potential implications, in *Body Composition Analysis: Methods and Applications, Int. Monographs on Nutrition, Metabolism and Obesity: 2*, Kral, J.G. and Van Hallie, T.B., Eds., Smith-Gordon/Nishimura, London, 1993, 75.

Hill, A.J. and Silver, E.K., Fat, friendless and unhealthy-9-year-old children's perception of body shape stereotype, *Int. J. Obes. Relat. Metab. Disord.*, 19, 423, 1995.

Hills, A.P., Effects of diet and exercise on body composition of pre-pubertal children, *J. Phys. Ed. Sp. Sci.*, 3, 22, 1991.

Hills, A.P., Education for preventing obesity, *J. Int. Counc. Hlth. Phys. Ed. Recr. Dance*, 30, 30, 1993.

Hills, A.P., Locomotor characteristics of obese children, in *Exercise and Obesity*, Hills, A.P. and Wahlqvist, M.L., Eds., Smith-Gordon, London, 1994.

Hills, A.P., Physical activity and movement in children: it's consequences for growth and development, *Asia-Pacific J. Clin. Nutr.*, 4, 43, 1995.

Hills, A.P. and Cambourne, B., Walking to school — a sustainable environmental strategy to prevent childhood obesity, *Aus. Epidemiol.*, 9, 2, 15, 2002.

Hills, A.P. and Byrne, N.M., Bioelectrical impedance: use and abuse, in *Nutrition and Physical Activity*, Coetsee, M.F. and Van Heerden, H.J., Eds., Proc. Int. Council Physical Activity Fitness Res., Itala, 1997a, 23.

Hills, A.P. and Byrne, N.M., Body composition and body image: implications for weight-control practices in adolescents, *Int. J. Obes.*, 21, S115, 1997b.

Hills, A.P. and Byrne, N.M., Exercise prescription for weight management, *Proc. Nutr. Soc.*, 57, 93, 1998a.

Hills, A.P. and Byrne, N.M., Body composition, body satisfaction, eating and exercise behaviour of Australian adolescents, in *Physical Fitness and Nutrition during Growth*, Pařízková, J. and Hills, A.P., Eds., Karger, Basel, 1998b, 44.

Hills, A.P. and Byrne, N.M., Exercise prescription, body satisfaction and exercise motivation of girls and boys, *Med. Sci. Sports Exer.*, 30, S120, 1998c.

Hills, A.P. and Byrne, N.M., The promotion of physical activity and the prescription of exercise in the obese, *J. Physiol. Biochem.*, 55, 107, 1999.

Hills, A.P. and Byrne, N.M., Exercise, daily physical activity, eating and weight disorders in children, in *Paediatric Exercise and Medicine*, Armstrong, N. and van Mechelen, W., Eds., Oxford University Press, Oxford, 2000.

Hills, A.P. and Byrne, N.M., Bioelectrical impedance and body composition assessment. *H.K.J. Sp. Med. Sp. Sc.*, 12, 81, 2001.

Hills, A.P., Byrne, N.M., and Pařízková, J., Methodological considerations in the assessment of nutritional status and physical activity of children and youth, in *Physical Fitness and Nutrition in Children and Youth in Different Environments*, Pařízková, J. and Hills, A.P., Eds., Karger, Basel, 1998.

Hills, A.P., Byrne, N.M. and Ramage, A.J., Submaximal markers of exercise intensity, *J. Sports Sci.*, 16, S71, 1998.

Hills, A.P. and Parker, A.W., Obesity management via diet and exercise intervention, *Child: Care, Hlth. Dev.*, 14, 409, 1988.

Hills, A.P. and Parker, A.W., Anthropometric and body composition assessment of obese children, *J. Sport Sci.*, 8, 175, 1990.

Hills, A.P. and Parker, A.W., Gait characteristics of obese pre-pubertal children: effects of diet and exercise on parameters, *Int. J. Rehabil. Res.*, 14, 348, 1991.

Hills, A.P. and Parker, A.W., Locomotor characteristics of obese children, *Child: Care, Hlth. Dev.*, 18, 29, 1992.

Hills, A.P. and Parker, A.W., Physical fitness of obese children, in *Physical Activity for a Better Lifestyle*, Rychtecky, A., Svoboda, B., and Tilinger, P., Eds., Proc. 6th ICHPER Eur. Congr., Prague, 1993a, 179.

Hills, A.P. and Parker, A.W., Electromyography of walking in obese children, *Electromyogr. Clin. Neurophysiol.*, 33, 225, 1993b.

Hills, A.P. and Wahlqvist, M.L., What is overfatness? in *Exercise and Obesity*, Hills, A.P. and Wahlqvist, M.L., Eds., Smith-Gordon, London, 1994, 1.

Hills, A.P., et al., Plantar pressure differences between obese and non-obese adults: a biomechanical analysis, *Int. J. Obes.*, 25, 1674, 2001.

Hills, A.P., et al., The biomechanics of adiposity: structural and functional limitations of obesity and implications for movement, *Obes. Rev.,* 3, 35, 2002.

Himes, J.H., Subcutaneous fat thickness as an indicator of nutritional status, in *Social and Biological Predictors of Nutritional Status, Physical Growth and Neurological Development,* Green, L.S. and Johnston, F.E., Eds., Academic Press, New York, 1980.

Hinney, A. et al., Absence of leptin deficiency mutation in extremely obese German children and adolescents, *Int. J. Obes. Relat. Metab. Disord.,* 21, 1190, 1997.

Hinney, A. et al., Ghrelin gene: identification of missense variants and a frameshift mutation in extremely obese children and adolescents and healthy normal weight students, *J. Clin. Endocrin. Metab.,* 87, 2716, 2002.

Hirasing, R.A. et al., Increased prevalence of overweight and obesity in Dutch children, and the detection of overweight and obesity using international criteria and new reference diagrams, *Med. Tijdschr. Geneeskd.,* 145, 1303, 2001.

Hirsch, J. and Knittle, J.L., Cellularity of obese and nonobese human adipose tissue, *Fed. Proc.,* 29, 1516, 1970.

Hiura, M. et al., Elevation of serum C-reactive protein levels is associated with obesity in boys, *Hypertens. Res.,* 26, 541, 2003.

Hjern, A. et al., Health and nutrition in newly resettled refugee children from Chile and the Middle East, *Acta Paediatr. Scand.,* 80, 859, 1991.

Ho, S.C., Risk factor of obesity among Hong Kong youths, *Pub. Hlth.,* 104, 249, 1990.

Ho, T.F. et al., Evaluation of lung function in Singapore obese children, *J. Singapore Paediatr. Soc.,* 31, 46, 1989.

Hodge, A.M. et al., Dramatic increase in the prevalence of obesity in Western Samoa over 13 year period 1978–1991, *Int. J. Obes. Relat. Metab. Disord.,* 18, 419, 1994.

Hodge, A.M. et al., Modernity and obesity in coastal and Highland Papua New Guinea, *Int. J. Obes. Relat. Metab. Disord.,* 19, 154, 1995.

Hölcke, M., Norgren, S., and Danielsson, P., Gastric banding in obese but otherwise healthy adolescents, *Int. J. Obes. Relat. Metab. Disord.,* 28, S1, 30, 2004.

Hoerr, S.L., Nelson, R.A., and Essex-Sorlie, D., Treatment and follow-up of obesity in adolescent girls, *J. Adolesc. Hlth. Care,* 9, 28, 1988.

Hoffman, D.J. et al., Why are nutritionally stunted children at increased risk of obesity? Studies of metabolic rate and fat oxidation in shantytown children from São Paolo, Brazil, *Am. J. Clin. Nutr.,* 72, 702, 2000.

Hoffman, R.P. and Armstrong, P.T., Glucose effectiveness, peripheral and hepatic insulin sensitivity, in obese and lean prepubertal children, *Int. J. Obes. Relat. Metab. Disord.,* 20, 521, 1996.

Hoffman, R.P. et al., Altered insulin resistance is associated with increased dietary weight loss in obese children, *Hormon. Res.,* 44, 17, 1995.

Holub, M. et al., Plasma leptin decreases in obese children undergoing weight reduction and binds to high-density lipoproteins, *Int. J. Obes. Relat. Metab. Disord.,* 22, S28, 1998.

Holub, M. et al., Relation of plasma leptin to lipoproteins in overweight children undergoing weight reduction, *Int. J. Obes. Relat. Metab. Disord.,* 23, 60, 1999.

Hongo, T. et al., Nutritional assessment of a group of Japanese elementary school children in Tokyo: with special emphasis on growth, anaemia, and obesity, *J. Nutr. Sci. Vitaminol.,* 38, 177, 1992.

Hood, M.Y. et al., Parental eating attitudes and the development of obesity in children. The Framingham Children's Study, *Int. J. Obes. Relat. Metab. Disord.,* 24, 1319, 2000.

Hoos, M.B. et al., Physical activity level measured by doubly labeled water and accelerometer in children, *Eur. J. Appl. Physiol.*, 89, 624, 2003.

Hoppe, C., Molgaard, C. and Michaelsen, K.F., Bone size and bone mass in 10-year-old Danish children: effect of current diet, *Osteoporos. Int.*, 11, 1024, 2000.

Hoppe, C. et al., High intakes of skimmed milk, but not meat, increase serum IGF-1 and IGFBP-3 in eight-year-old boys, *Eur. J. Clin. Nutr.*, March 31, 2004.

Hoppe, C. et al., Protein intake at 9 mo of age is associated with body size but not with body fat in 10-y-old Danish children, *Am. J. Clin. Nutr.*, 79, 494, 2004.

Hoppeler, H., Skeletal muscle substrate metabolism, *Int. J. Obes. Relat. Metab. Disord.*, 23, S7, 1999.

Howard, A.N., The historical development, efficiency and safety of very low calorie diets, *Int. J. Obes.*, 5, 195, 1981.

Hsu, H.S. et al., Colored striae in obese children and adolescents, *Chung Hua Min Kuo Hsiao Erh. Ko I Hsueh Hui Tsa Chih.*, 37, 349, 1996.

Huang, M.H., Yang, R.C., and Hu, S.H., Preliminary results of triple therapy for obesity, *Int. J. Obes. Relat. Metab. Disord.*, 20, 830, 1996.

Huang, P.C. and Chiang, A.N., Anthropometric survey of students and school children in Taipei and group treatment of selected obese students, *Taiwan I Hsueh Hui Tsa Chih*, 86, 65, 1987 (in Chinese).

Huang, Y.C., Wu, J.Y., and Yang, M.J., Weight-for-height reference and the prevalence of obesity for school children and adolescents in Taiwan and Fuchien Areas, *J. Chin. Med. Assoc.*, 66, 599, 2003.

Hui, L.L. et al., Risk factors for childhood overweight in 6- to 7-y-old Hong Kong children, *Int. J. Obes. Relat. Metab. Disord.*, 27, 1411, 2003.

Hulens, M. et al., Trends in BMI among Belgian children, adolescents, and adults from 1969 to 1996, *Int. J. Obes. Relat. Metab. Disord.*, 25, 395, 2001.

Humphries, M.C. et al., Relations of adiposity and effects of training on the left ventricle in obese youths, *Med. Sci. Sports Exerc.*, 34, 1428, 2002.

Hundred, P., Kitchiner, D. and Buchan, I., Prevalence of overweight and obese children between 1989 and 1998: population-based series of cross-sectional studies, *Br. J. Nutr.*, 322, 326, 2001.

Hunt, S.M. and Groff, J.L. *Advanced Nutrition and Human Metabolism*, West Publishing, Los Angeles, 1990.

Huttunen, N.P., Knip, M., and Paavilainen, T., Physical activity and fitness in obese children, *Int. J. Obes.*, 10, 519, 1986.

Hwang, H.W. et al., Metabolic disturbances in obese children: glucose, insulin levels and lipid profile, *Acta Paediatr. Taiwan*, 42, 2, 75, 2001.

Hypponen, E. et al., Obesity is associated with an increased risk of insulin-dependent diabetes mellitus in children, *Int. J. Obes. Relat. Metab. Disord.*, 22, S22, 1998.

Ibanez, L. et al., Fat distribution in non-obese girls with and without precocious pubarche: central adiposity related to insulinaemia and androgenaemia from puberty to postmenarche, *Clin. Endocrinol.*, 58, 372, 2003.

Ikeda, J.P. and Mitchell, R.A., Dietary approaches to the treatment of the overweight pediatric patient, *Pediatr. Clin. North. Am.*, 48, 955, 2001.

Ikezaki, A. et al., Fasting plasma ghrelin levels are negatively correlated with insulin resistance and PAI-1, but not with leptin in obese children and adolescents, *Diabetes*, 51, 3408, 2002.

Ilies, I., Mahunka, I., and Sari, B., Relationship between immunoreactive insulin and plasma somatomedin-C/insulin-like growth factor 1 concentration in childhood obesity, *Orv. Hetil.*, 135, 1633, 1994 (in Hungarian).

ILSI Europe, Healthy lifestyles nutrition and physical activity, ILSI Europe Concise Monogr. Ser., ILSI Europe, Brussels, 1998.

Ilyes, I., Nagy, E., and Sari, B., Value of the waist-ratio in adolescent obesity, *Orv. Hetil.*, 135, 1467, 1994 (in Hungarian).

Inman, V.T., Human locomotion, *Can. Med. Assoc. J.*, 94, 1047, 1966.

Inselma, L.S., Milanese, A., and Deurloo, A., Effect of obesity on pulmonary function in children, *Pediatr. Pulmonol.*, 16, 130, 1993.

Isasi, C.R. et al., Physical fitness and C-reactive protein level in children and young adults: the Columbia University BioMarkers Study, *Pediatrics*, 111, 332, 2003.

Isnard, P. et al., Binge eating and psychopathology in severely obese adolescents, *Int. J. Eating Disord.*, 34, 235, 2003.

Israel, A.C. and Ivanova, M.Y., Global and dimensional self-esteem in preadolescent and early adolescent children who are overweight: age and gender differences, *Int. J. Eating Disord.*, 31, 424, 2002.

Iwata, F. et al., Body fat ratios in urban Chinese children, *Pediatr. Int.*, 45, 190, 2003.

Jabbar, M. et al., Excess weight and precocious pubarche in children: alteration of the adrenocortical hormones, *J. Am. Coll. Nutr.*, 10, 289, 1991.

Jackson, R.T., Rashed, M., and Saad-Eldin, R., Rural urban differences in weight, body image, and dieting behavior among adolescent Egyptian schoolgirls, *Int. J. Food. Sci. Nutr.*, 54, 1, 2003.

Jacquet, D. et al., Ontogeny of leptin in human fetuses and newborns: effects of intrauterine growth retardation on serum leptin concentrations, *J. Clin. Endocrinol. Metab.*, 83, 1243, 1998.

Jaeger, U. and Kromeyer-Hauschild, K., Rapid increase in prevalence of obesity in former East German children after reunification, *Int. J. Obes. Relat. Metab. Disord.*, 23, S7, 1999.

Jaffe, M. and Kosakov, C., The motor development of fat babies, *Clin. Pediatr.*, 21, 619, 1982.

Jahss, M., *Disorders of the Foot*, W.B. Saunders, Philadelphia, 1982.

Jain, A. et al., Why don't low-income mothers worry about their preschoolers being overweight? *Pediatrics*, 107, 1138, 2001.

James, W.P.T., The future, in *Child and Adolescent Obesity*, Burniat, W. et al., Eds., Cambridge University Press, Cambridge, 2002, 389.

James, W.P.T. and Schofield, E.C. *Human Energy Requirements*, Oxford Medical Publications, Oxford University Press, Oxford, 1990.

James, W.P.T. et al., Preventing childhood obesity by reducing consumption of carbonated drinks: cluster randomised controlled trial, *B.M.J.*, Apr 23, 2004.

Janssen, I. et al., Associations between overweight and obesity with bullying behaviors in school-aged children, *Pediatrics.*, 113, 1187, 2004.

Jebb, S.A. and Elia, M., Techniques for the measurement of body composition: a practical guide, *Int. J. Obes. Relat. Metab. Disord.*, 17, 611, 1993.

Jerk, I. and Widhalm, K., Nutritional intake by obese adolescents, *Aktuel Ernahr. Med.*, 25, 118, 2000.

Jeszka, J., Regula, J., and Kostrzewa-Tarnowska, A., Effect of sex on the results of weight reduction program in obese adolescents, *Scand. J. Nutr.*, 43, S43, 1999.

Jiang, X., Srinivasan, S.R., and Berenson, G.S., Relation of obesity to insulin secretion and clearance in adolescents: the Bogalusa Heart Study, *Int. J. Obes. Relat. Metab. Disord.*, 20, 951, 1996.

Jimenez-Cruz, A., Bacardi-Gascon, M., and Spindler, A.A., Obesity and hunger among Mexican–Indian migrant children on the U.S.–Mexico border, *Int. J. Obes. Relat. Metab. Disord.*, 27, 740, 2003.

Jinabhai, C.C., Taylor, M., and Sullivan, K.R., Implications of the prevalence of stunting, overweight and obesity amongst South African primary school children: a possible nutritional transition? *Eur. J. Clin. Nutr.*, 57, 357, 2003.

Jirapinyo, P. et al., A summer camp for childhood obesity in Thailand, *J. Med. Assoc. Thai*, 78, 238, 1995.

Johansson-Kark, M., Rasmussen, F. and Hjern, A., Overweight among international adoptees in Sweden. A population-based study, *Acta Pediatr. Int. J. Pediatr.*, 91, 827, 2002.

Johnson, S.L. and Birch, L.L., Parent's and children's adiposity and eating style, *Pediatrics*, 94, 653, 1994.

Johnson, W.G. et al., Dietary and exercise interventions for juvenile obesity: long-term effect of behavioral and public health models, *Obes. Res.*, 5, 257, 1997.

Johnson-Down, L.O. et al., High prevalence of obesity in low income and multi-ethnic schoolchildren: diet and physical activity assessment, *J. Nutr.*, 127, 2310, 1997.

Jorgensen, M.E. et al., Obesity and central fat pattern among Greenland Inuit and general population of Denmark: relationship to metabolic factors., *Int. J. Obes. Relat. Metab. Disord.*, 27, 1507, 2003.

Jung, E. and Czajka-Narins, D.M., Birth weight doubling and tripling times: an updated look at the effects of birth weight, sex, race and type of feeding, *Am. J. Clin. Nutr.*, 42, 182, 1985.

Juricskay, Z. and Molnar, D., Steroid metabolism in obese children. I. The relationship between body composition and adrenal function, *Acta Paediatr. Hung.*, 29, 383, 1988a.

Juricskay, Z. and Molnar, D., Steroid metabolism in obese children. II. Steroid excretion of obese and normal weight children, *Acta Paediatr. Hung.*, 29, 395, 1988b.

Jurimae, T. et al., Relationships between bioelectric impedance and subcutaneous adipose tissue thickness measured by LIPOMETER and skin calipers in children, *Eur. J. Appl. Physiol.*, 90, 178, 2003.

Kabir, I. et al., Changes in body composition of malnourished children after dietary supplementation as measured by bioelectrical impedance, *Am. J. Clin. Nutr.*, 59, 5, 1994.

Kachele, V. et al., Cholecystolithiasis in children and adolescents: influence of obesity and other factors, *Monatsschr. Kinderheilkd.*, 148, 600, 2000.

Kahle, E.B. et al., Exercise adaptation responses for gastric inhibitory polypeptide (GIP) and insulin in obese children, *Diabetes*, 35, 579, 1986.

Kahle, E.B. et al., Association between mild, routine exercise and improved insulin dynamics and glucose control in obese adolescents, *Int. J. Sports Med.*, 17, 1, 1996.

Kain, J., Uauy, R., and Diaz, M., Increasing prevalence of obesity among school children in Chile, *Int. J. Obes. Relat. Metab. Disord.*, 22, S4, 1998.

Kalies, H., Lenz, J., and Von Kries, R., Prevalence of overweight and obesity and trend in body mass index in German pre-school children, 1982-1997, *Int. J. Obes. Relat. Metab. Disord.*, 26, 1211, 2002.

Kalker, U., Hovels, O., and Kolbe-Saborowski, H., Significance of gender of obese children and body weight of parents and siblings for the results of the treatment of obesity in childhood, *Monatsschr. Kinderheilkd*, 139, 24, 1991 (in German).

Kalra, P.S. and Kalra, S.P., Obesity and metabolic syndrom: long-term benefits of central leptin gene therapy, *Drugs Today*, 38, 745, 2002.

Kalvachová, B. et al., Summer-vacation hospitalization of obese children, *Cesk. Pediatr.*, 41, 275, 1986 (in Czech).

Kamachandran, A. et al., Prevalence of overweight in urban Indian adolescent school children, *Diabetes Res. Clin. Pract.*, 57, 185, 2002.

Kamar'yt, J. et al., Insulin, glucose, proteins, and amylase in the saliva of obese children, *Cesk. Pediatr.*, 44, 517, 1989.

Kamel, A. et al., Effects of growth hormone treatment in obese prepubertal boys, *J. Clin. Endocrinol. Metab.*, 85, 1412, 2000.

Kamoda, T. et al., The phosphorylation status of insulin-like growth factor-binding protein-1 in prepubertal obese children, *Eur. J. Endocrinol.*, 141, 585, 1999.

Kannel, W.B., Health and obesity: an overview, in *Health and Obesity*, Conn, H.L., De Felice, E.A., and Kuo, P., Eds., Raven Press, New York, 1983, 1.

Kannel, W.B. and Dawber, T.R., Atherosclerosis as a pediatric problem, *Peadiatrics*, 80, 544, 1972.

Kapalín, V., Evaluation of child's growth, in *Repetitorium of Medical Doctor*, Avicenum, Prague, 1967, 109 (in Czech).

Kaplan, A.S. et al., Resting energy expenditure in clinical pediatrics measured values versus prediction equations, *J. Pediatr.*, 127, 200, 1995.

Kaplan, T.A., Obesity in a high school football candidate: a case presentation, *Med. Sci. Sports Exerc.*, 24, 406, 1992.

Kaplan, T.A. and Montana, E., Exercise-induced bronchospasm in nonasthmatic obese children, *Clin. Pediat.*, 12., 220, 1993.

Kapoor, G. et al., Triceps skinfold thickness in adolescents, *Indian J. Med. Res.*, 94, 281, 1991.

Karbonits, M. et al., A variation in the ghrelin gene increases weight and decreases insulin secretion in tall, obese children, *J. Clin. Endocrinol. Metab.*, 67, 4005, 2002.

Kasa-Vubu, J.Z. et al., Incomplete modified fast in obese early pubertal girls leads to an increase in 24-hour growth hormone concentration and a lessening of the circadian pattern in leptin, *J. Clin. Endocrinol. Metab.*, 87, 1885, 2002.

Kashani, I.A. and Nader, P.R., The role of pediatrician in the prevention of coronary heart disease in childhood, *Jap. Heart J.*, 27, 911, 1986.

Kaskoun, M.C., Johnson, R.K., and Goran, M.I., Comparison of energy intake by semiquantitative food-frequency questionnaire with total energy expenditure by the doubly labelled water method in young children, *Am. Clin. Nutr.*, 60, 43, 1994.

Katch, V. et al., Oxygen uptake and energy output during walking of obese male and female adolescents, *Am. J. Clin. Nutr.*, 47, 26, 1988a.

Katch, V. et al., Basal metabolism of obese adolescents: inconsistent diet and exercise effects, *Am. J. Clin. Nutr.*, 48, 565, 1988b.

Katch, V.L. et al., Reduced short-term effects of a meal in obese adolescent girls, *Eur. J. Appl. Physiol.*, 65, 535, 1992.

Katzmarzyk, P.T., Hebebrand, H., and Bouchard, C., Spousal resemblance in the Canadian population: implications for the obesity epidemic, *Int. J. Obes. Relat. Metab. Disord.*, 26, 241, 2002.

Katzmarzyk, P.T. et al., The utility of the international child and adolescent overweight guidelines for predicting coronary heart disease risk factors, *J. Clin. Epidemiol.*, 56, 456, 2003.

Kawasaki, T. et al., The relationship between fatty liver and hyperinsulinaemia in obese Japanese children, *J. Pediatr. Gastroenterol. Nutr.*, 24, 317, 1997.

Kelley, C. et al., Dietary intake of children at high risk for cardiovascular disease, *J. Am. Diet. Assoc.*, 104, 222, 2004.

Kelley, G.A., Gender differences in the physical activity levels of young African–American adults, *J. Natl. Med. Assoc.*, 87, 545, 1995.

Kemm, J.R., Eating patterns in childhood and adult health, *Nutr. Hlth.*, 4, 205, 1987.

Kemper, H.C.G. et al., Tracking of health and risk indicators of cardiovascular diseases from teenager to adult: Amsterdam Growth and Health Study, *Prev. Med.*, 19, 642, 1990.

Kemper, H.C.G. et al., Lifestyle and obesity in adolescence and young adulthood: results from the Amsterdam Growth and Health Longitudinal Study (AGAHLS), *Int. J. Obes. Relat. Metab. Disord.*, 23, S34, 1999.

Kennedy, E. and Goldberg, J., What are American children eating? Implications for public policy, *Nutr. Rev.*, 53, 111, 1995.

Keys, A. and Brožek, J., Body fat in adult man, *Physiol. Rev.*, 33, 245, 1953.

Keys, A. et al., *Biology Of Human Starvation*, Vol. 2., University of Minnesota Press, Minneapolis, 1950.

Khan, F. et al., Impaired microvascular function in normal children: Effects of adiposity and poor glucose handling, *J. Physiol.*, 551, 705, 2003.

Kiess, W. et al., High leptin concentrations in serum of very obese children are further stimulated by dexamethasone, *Horm. Metab. Res.*, 28, 708, 1996.

Kiess, W. et al., Clinical aspects of obesity in childhood and adolescence: diagnosis, treatment and prevention, *Int. J. Obes. Relat. Metab. Disord.*, 25, S75, 2001.

Killen, J.D. et al., An attempt to modify unhealthful eating attitudes and weight regulation practices of young adolescent girls, *Int. J. Eating Disord.*, 13, 369, 1993.

Kim, H.K., Matsuura, Y. and Inagaki, A., Physical fitness and motor ability in obese boys 12 through 14 years of age, *Ann. Physiol. Anthropol.*, 12, 17, 1993 (in Japanese).

Kimm, S.Y.S., Obesity prevention and macronutrient intakes in children in the United States, *Ann. N.Y. Acad. Sci.*, 699, 70, 1993.

Kimm, S.Y.S., The role of dietary fiber in the development and treatement of childhood obesity, *Pediatr.*, 96, 1010, 1995.

Kimm, S.Y.S. and Obarzanek, E., Childhood obesity: A new pandemic of the new millennium, *Pediatrics*, 110, 1003, 2002

Kimm, S.Y.S. et al., Longitudinal changes in physical activity in a biracial cohort during adolescence, *Med. Sci. Sports Exerc.*, 32, 1445, 2000

Kimm, S.Y.S. et al., Decline in physical activity in black girls and white girls during adolescence, *New Engl. J. Med.*, 347, 709, 2002.

Kinra, S., Nelder, R.P., and Lewendon, G.J., Deprivation and childhood obesity: a cross sectional study of 20,973 children in Plymouth, United Kingdom, *J. Epidemiol. Comm. Hlth.*, 54, 456, 2000.

Kiortsis, D. N., Darach, J., and Turpin, G., Effects of low calorie diet on resting metabolic rate and serum tri-iodothyronine levels in obese children, *Eur. J. Pediatr.*, 158, 446, 1999.

Klein, K.O. et al., Effect of obesity on estradiol level, and its relationship to leptin, bone maturation and bone mineral density in children, *J. Clin. Endocrinol. Metab.*, 83, 3469, 1998.

Klein, S., The national obesity crisis: a call for action, *Gastroenterology*, 126(1), 6, 2004.

Klesges, R.C., Haddock, C.K., and Eck, L.H., A multimethod approach to the measurement of childhood physical activity and its relationship to blood pressure and body weight, *J. Pediatr.*, 116, 888, 1990.

Klesges, R.C., Shelton, M.L., and Klesges, L.M., Effects of television on metabolic rate: potential implications for childhood obesity, *Pediatrics*, 91, 281, 1993.

Klesges, R.C. et al., Accuracy of self-reports of food intake in obese and normal-weight individuals: effects of parental obesity on reports of children's dietary intake, *Am. J. Clin. Nutr.*, 48, 1252, 1988

Klesges, R.C. et al., Effects of obesity, social interactions, and physical environment on physical activity in preschoolers, *Hlth. Psychol.*, 9, 435, 1990.

Klesges, R.C. et al., A longitudinal analysis of accelerated weight gain in preschool children, *Pediatrics*, 92, 126, 1995.

Klish, W.J., Use of TOBEC instrument in the measurement of body composition in children, in *Recent Developments in Body Composition Analysis: Methods and Applications*, Kraal, J.G. and Van Itallie, T.B., Eds., Smith-Gordon/Nishimura, London, 1993, 111.

Klish, W.J., Childhood obesity: pathophysiology and treatment, *Acta Pediatr. Jpn.*, 37, 1, 1995.

Klish, W.J. et al., New method for the estimation of lean body mass in infants (EEME Instrument): validation in nonhuman models, *J. Pediatr. Gastroenterol.*, 3, 199, 1984.

Klisovic, D. and Landoll, J., Gain in body fat is inversely related to the nocturnal rise in serum leptin level in young females, *J. Clin. Endocrionl. Metab.*, 82, 1368, 1997.

Knerr, I. et al., Laparoscopically performed gastric binding in a 13-year old with morbid obesity and end stage renal insufficiency allows lifesaving weight loss and hemodialysis, *J. Pediatr. Endocrinol. Metab.*, 16, 1179, 2003.

Kniazev, I.A. et al., Effect of diet therapy on indicators of lipid metabolism in obese children, *Voprosy Pitan.*, Mar.-Apr., 1985 (in Russian).

Knip, M., Lautala, P. and Puukka, R., Reduced insulin removal and erythrocyte insulin binding in obese children, *Eur. J. Pediatr.*, 148, 233, 1988.

Knip, M. and Nuutinen, O., Long-term effects of weight reduction on serum lipids and plasma insulin in obese children, *Am. J. Clin. Nutr.*, 57, 490, 1993.

Knittle, J.L., Childhood obesity, *Bull. N.Y. Acad. Sci. Med.*, 47, 579, 1971.

Koehler, B. et al., Obesity in children from nurseries in the city of Katowice. Analysis of socioeconomic conditions and the nutrition of obese children, *Pediatr. Pol.*, 63, 159, 1988.

Koeppen-Schomerus, G., Wardle, J., and Plomin, R., A genetic analysis of weight and overweight in 4-year-old twin pairs, *Int. J. Obes. Relat. Metab. Disord.*, 25, 838, 2001.

Koff, E. and Rierdan, J., Perceptions of weight and attitudes toward eating in early adolescent girls, *J. Adolesc. Health*, 12, 307, 1991.

Koff, E., Rierdan, J., and Stubbs, M., Gender, body image, and self-concept in early adolescence, *J. Early Adolesc.*, 10, 56, 1990.

Kohno, T., Tanaka, H., and Honda, S., Therapeutic assessment of childhood obesity with body composition measured by bioelectrical impedance analysis, *Fukuoka Igaku Zasshi*, 85, 267, 1994 (in Japanese).

Kolb, L.C., Disturbances of the body-image, in *American Handbook of Psychiatry*, Reiser, M.F., Ed., Basic Books, New York, 1975, 810.

Koletzko, B. and Von Kries, R., Is there early childhood imprinting for later risk of obesity? *Monatsschr. Kinderheilkd.*, 149, 11, 2001.

Koletzko, B. et al., Obesity in children and adolescents worldwide: current view and future directions. Working group report of the first World Congress of Pediatric Gastroenterology, Hepatology and Nutrition, *J. Pediatr. Gastroenterol. Nutr.*, 35, S205, 2002.

Kolody, B. and Sallis, J.F., A prospective study of ponderosity, body image, self-concept, and psychological variables in children, *J. Dev. Behav. Pediatr.*, 16, 1, 1995.

Kopp, W. et al., Low leptin levels predict amenorrhea in underweight and eating disordered females, *Mol. Psychiatry*, 2, 335, 1997.

Korsten-Reck, U., Bauer, S. and Keul, J., Sports and nutrition? An outpatient program for adipose children (long-term experience), *Int. J. Sports Med.*, 15, 242, 1994.

Korsten-Reck, U. et al., Sport and diet? An ambulatory program for obese children, *Offentl. Gesundheitswes.*, 52, 441, 1990 (in German).

Korsten-Reck, U. et al., Prevention and therapy of obesity with diet and sports, an ambulatory therapy program for overweight children, *Wien. Med. Wochenschr.*, 140, 232, 1994 (in German).

Korsten-Reck, U. et al., Sports and nutrition. An outpatient program for obese children, *Int. J. Obes. Relat. Metab. Disord.*, 22, S63, 1998.

Kortzinger, I. and Mast, M., School-oriented intervention for the prevention of obesity as part of KOPS (Kiel Obesity Prevention Study), *Int. J. Obes. Relat. Metab. Disord.*, 21, 30, 1997.

Kotagal, S., Krahn, L.E., and Slocumb, N., A putative link between childhood narcolepsy and obesity, *Sleep Med.*, 5, 147, 2004.

Kovářová, M. et al., Bodily characteristics and lifestyle of Czech children aged 7.00 to 10.99 years, incidence of childhood obesity, *Centr. Eur. J. Pub. Hlth.*, 10, 169, 2002.

Kozlov, V.I. *Long Living in Abkhasia*, Nauka, Moscow, 1987 (in Russian).

Krahenbuhl, G.S. and Martin, S.L., Adolescent body size and flexibility, *Res. Q.*, 48, 797, 1977.

Krassas, G.E. et al., Prevalence and trends in overweight and obesity among children and adolescents in Thessaloniki, Greece, *J. Pediatr. Endocrinol. Metab.*, 14, 1319, 2001.

Kratzsch, J. et al., Increased serum GHBP levels in obese pubertal children and adolescents: relationship to body composition, leptin and indicators of metabolic disturbances, *Int. J. Obes. Relat. Metab.*, 21, 1130, 1997.

Kravets, E.B. and Kniazev, I.A., The effect of a hypocaloric diet enriched with polyunsaturated fatty acids on various indicators of cellular immunity in obese children, *Vopr. Pitan.*, 6, Nov.-Dec., 13, 1989.

Kromeyer-Hauschild, K. and Jaeger, U., Growth studies in Jena, Germany: changes in body size and subcutaneous fat distribution between 1975 and 1995, *Am. J. Hum. Biol.*, 10, 579, 1998.

Kromeyer-Hauschild, K. et al., Prevalence of overweight and obesity among schoolchildren in Jena (Germany), *Am. J. Clin. Nutr.*, 1999.

Kromeyer-Hauschild, K. et al., Percentiles of body mass index in children and adolescents evaluated from different regional German studies, *Monatsschr. Kkinderheilkd.*, 149, 807, 2001.

Krosnick, A., The diabetes and obesity epidemic among Pima Indians. *N.J. Med.* 97, 31, 2000.

Kunešová, M. et al., Simple anthropometric measurements: relation to body fat mass, visceral adipose tissue and risk factors of atherogenesis, *Sborník Lék.*, 96, 349, 1995.

Kuntzleman, C.T. and Reiff, G.G., The decline in American children's fitness level, *Res. Q. Exerc. Sport* , 63, 107, 1992.

Kushner, R.F. and Schoeller, D.A., Estimation of total body water by bioelectrical impedance analysis, *Am. J. Clin. Nutr.*, 44, 417, 1986.

Kuzuma, N. et al., Heart rate variability in normotensive healthy children with aging, *Clin. Exp. Hypertens.*, 24, 83, 2002.

L'Allemand, D., Mundt, A., and Gruters, A., Physical activity improves the outcome of a pediatric weight control program, *Int. J. Obes. Relat. Metab. Disord.*, 22, S3, S9, 1998.

L'Allemand, D. et al., Associations between body mass, leptin, IGF-1, and circulating adrenal androgens in children with obesity and and premature adrenarche, *Eur. J. Endocrinol.*, 146, 537, 2002.

Labarthe, D.R., Mueller, W.H., and Eissa, M., Blood pressure and obesity in childhood and adolescence: epidemiological aspects, *Ann. Epidemiol.*, 1, 337, 1991.

Lacar, E.S., Soto, X., and Riley, W.J., Adolescent obesity in a low-income Mexican American district in South Texas, *Arch. Pediatr. Adolesc. Med.*, 154, 837, 2000.

Laessle, R., Wurmser, H., and Pirke, K.M., Energy expenditure in preadolescent girls at high risk of obesity, *Int. J. Obes. Relat. Metab. Disord.*, 22, S37, 1998.

Laessle, R.G., Wurmser, M., and Pirke, K.M., Restrained eating and leptin levels in overweight preadolescent girls, *Physiol. Behav.*, 70, 45, 2000.

Lahlou, N. et al., Circulating leptin in normal children and during the dynamic phase of juvenile obesity: relation to body fatness, energy metabolism, caloric intake, and sexual dimorphism, *Diabetes*, 46, 989, 1997.

Lahlou, N. et al., Soluble leptin receptor in serum of subjects with complete resistance to leptin: relation to fat mass, *Diabetes*, 49, 1347, 2000.

Lahlou, N. et al., Mutations in the human leptin and leptin receptor genes as models of serum leptin receptor regulation, *Diabetes*, 51, 1980, 2002.

Lai, S.W. et al., Association between obesity and hyperlipidemia among children, *Yale J. Biol. Med.*, 74, 205, 2001.

Laitinen, J. et al., Unemployment and obesity among young adults in northern Finland 1966 birth cohort, *Int. J. Obes. Relat. Metab. Disord.*, 26, 1329, 2002.

Lamphiear, D.E. and Montoye, H.J., Muscular strength and body size, *Human Biol.*, 48, 147, 1976.

Langnase, K., Mast, M. and Muller, M.J., Social class differeces in overweight of prepubertal children in northwest Germany, *Int. J. Obes. Relat. Metab. Disord.*, 26, 566, 2002.

Lanouette, C.M. et al., Association between uncoupling protein 3 gene and obesity-related phenotypes in the Quebec Family Study, *Mol. Med.*, 7, 433, 2001.

Laubach, L.L. and McConville, J.T., The relationship of strength to body size and topology, *Med. Sci. Sp.*, 1, 189, 1969.

Lazarus, R. et al., Recommended body mass index cut-off values for overweight screening programmes in Australian children and adolescents: comparisons with North American values, *J. Pediatr. Child Hlth.*, 31, 143, 1995.

Lazarus, R. et al., Body mass index in screening for adiposity in children and adolescents: systematic evaluation using receiver operating characteristic curves, *Am. J. Clin. Nutr.*, 63, 500, 1996.

Le Fur, Le Stunff, C., and Bougnères, P., Increased insulin resistance in obese children who have both 972 IRS-1 and 1057 IRS-2 polymorphisms, *Diabetes*, 51, S303, 2002.

Le Stunf, C. and Bougnères, P., Early changes in postprandial insulin secretion, not in insulin sensitivity, characterize juvenile obesity, *Diabetes*, 43, 696, 1994.

Le Stunff, C., Fallin, D., and Bougneres, P., Paternal transmission of a very common class I INS VNTR alleles predisposes to childhood obesity, *Nat. Genet.*, 29, 96, 2001.

Le Veau, B.F. and Bernhardt, D.B., Developmental biomechanics, *Phys. Ther.*, 63, 2, 1984.

Lebedkova, S.E. et al., Effectiveness of treatment of obese children in a pioneer camp of a sanatorium type, *Pediatriia*, 8, 51, 1984 (in Russian).

Lecendreux, M. et al., Weight loss reduces sleep associated breathing disorders in morbidly obese children, *Int. J. Obes. Relat. Metab. Disord.*, 21, S141, 1997.

Lecerf, J.M., Labrunie, M., and Charles, M.A., Triglycerides increase and LpA1 decreases with weight in obese boys and with waist:hip ratio in obese girls, *Int. J. Obes. Relat. Metab. Disord.*, 22, S24, 1998.

Lecomte, E. et al., Segregation analysis of fat mass and fat-free mass with age- and sex-dependent effects: the Stanislas Family Study, *Genet. Epidemiol.*, 14, 51, 1997.

Ledovskaya, N.M., Experience in the assessment of physical activity in twins, in *Physical Activity in Man and Hypokinesia*, Slonim, A.D. and Smirnov, K.M., Eds., Academy of Sciences of USSR, Siberian Dept., Institute of Physiology, Novosibirsk, 1972, 30 (in Russian).

Lee, Y.S., Poh, L.K.S., and Loke, K.Y., A novel melanocortin 3 receptor gene (MC4R) mutation associated with severe obesity, *J. Clin. Endocrinol. Metab.*, 87, 1423, 2002.

Leger, J. et al., Magnetic resonance imaging evaluation of adipose tissue and muscle tissue mass in children with growth hormone (GH) deficiency, Turner's syndrome, and intrauterine growth retardation during the first year of treatment with GH, *J. Clin. Endocrinol. Metab.*, 78, 904, 1994.

Lehingue, Y. et al., Restoration of GH in urine during an in-patient slimming course in obese children, enhanced by physical activity, *Int. J. Obes. Relat. Metab. Disord.*, 22, S26, 1998.

Lehingue, Y. et al., Evolution of GH secretion in urine during an in-patient slimming course in obese children, *Int. J. Obes. Relat. Metab. Disord.*, 24, 363, 2000.

Lehrke, S. and Laessle, R.G., Multimodal treatment for obese children: outcome with respect to psychosocial criteria, *Verhaltenstherapie*, 12, 256, 2002.

Lemaire, B. and De Maegd, M., Les malnutritions dans le Tiers-Monde: prevalence de la malnutrition proteine-calorique, de l'anemie et du goitre dans, Imbo, Burundi (Afrique Centrale), *Colloque INSERM*, 136, 149, 1986.

Leung, A.K. and Robson, W.L., Childhood obesity, *Postgrad. Med.*, 87, 123, 1990.

Leung, S.S. et al., Weight-for-age and weight-for-height references for Hong Kong children from birth to 18 years, *I. Pediatr. Child Hlth.*, 32, 103, 1996.

Levent, E. et al., Stiffness of the abdominal aorta in obese children, *J. Pediatr. Endocrinol. Metab.*, 15, 405, 2002.

Levine, M.D. et al., Is family based behavioral weight control appropriate for severe pediatric obesity? *Int. J. Eating Disord.*, 30, 318, 2001.

Lev-Ran, A., Human obesity: an evolutionary approach to understanding our bulging waistline, *Diabetes Metab. Res. Rev.*, 17, 347, 2001.

Li, A.M. et al., The effects of obesity on pulmonary function, *Arch. Dis. Child.*, 88, 361, 2003.

Li, X., A study of intelligence and personality in children with simple obesity, *Int. J. Obes. Relat. Metab. Disord.*, 19, 355, 1995.

Liese, A.D. et al., Inverse association of overweight and breast feeding in 9- to 10-y-old children in Germany, *Int. J. Obes. Relat. Metab. Disord.*, 25, 1644, 2001.

Lifshitz, F. and Moses, N., Growth failure: a complication of dietary treatment of hypercholesterolemia, *Am. J. Dis. Child.*, 143, 537, 1989.

Lindgren, G. et al., Swedish population reference standards for height, weight and body mass index attained at 6 to 16 years (girls) or 19 years (boys), *Acta Paediatr.*, 84, 1019, 1995.

Lindsay, R.S. et al., Body mass index as a measure of adiposity in children and adolescents: relationship to adiposity by dual energy x-ray absorptiometry and to cardiovascular risk factors, *J. Clin. Endocrinol. Metab.*, 86, 4061, 2001.

Lioret, S. et al., INCA study: prevalence of childhood obesity, *Cah. Nutr. Diet.*, 36, 495, 2001.

Lísková, S., Hošek, P., and Stožický, F., The metabolic syndrome and cardiovascular risk factors in obese children, *Int. J. Obes. Relat. Metab. Disord.*, 22, S25, 1998.

Lissau, I. and Sorensen, T.I.A., Parental neglect during childhood and increased risk of obesity in young adulthood, *Lancet*, 343, 324, 1994.

Lissner, I. et al., Relations between leptin and body weight history in Swedish female populations, using serum stored 29 years, *Int. J. Obes Relat. Metab. Disord.*, 22, S37, 1998.

Litrell, M.A., Damhorst, M.L., and Littrell, J.M., Clothing interests, body satisfaction, and eating behavior of adolescent females: related or independent dimensions? *Adolescence*, 25, 77, 1990.

Livingstone, B., Epidemiology of childhood obesity in Europe, *Eur. J. Pediatr. Suppl.*, 159, S14, 2000.

Livingstone, M., Childhood obesity in Europe: a growing concern, *Public Health Nutr.*, 4, 109, 2001.

Lobstein, T., Baur, L., and Uauy, R., Obesity in children and young people: a crisis in public health, *Obes. Rev.*, 5, S1, 4, 2004.

Lobstein, T. and Frelut, M.L., Prevalence of overweight among children in Europe, *Obes. Rev.*, 4, 195, 2003.

Lobstein, T.J., James, W.P.T., and Cole, T.J., Increasing levels of excess weight among children in England, *Int. J. Obes. Relat. Metab. Disord.*, 27, 1136, 2003.

Locard, E. et al., Risk factors of obesity in a five-year-old population, parental versus environmental factors, *Int. J. Obes. Relat. Metab. Disord.*, 16, 721, 1992.

Locard, E. et al., Which anthropometric measurements are related with urine GH excretion restoration in obese children attending an in-patient slimming course? *Int. J. Obes. Relat. Metab. Disord.*, 22, S26, 1998.

Lohman, T.G., Measurement of body composition in children, *J. Phys. Ed. Recr. Dance*, 53, 67, 1982.

Lohman, T.G. *Advances in Body Composition Assessment*, Human Kinetics Publishers, Champaign, IL, 1993.

Lohman, T.G., Roche, A.F., and Martorell, R., Eds., *Anthropometric Standardization, Reference Manual*, Human Kinetics Publishers, Champaign, IL, 1988.

Longjohn, M.M., Chicago project uses ecological approach to obesity prevention, *Pediatr. Ann.*, 33, 62, 2004.

Loosemore, D.J. and Moriarty, D., Body dissatisfaction and body image distortion in selected groups of males, *Can. Council Hlth. Phys. Ed. Rec. J.*, Nov/Dec., 11, 1990.

Lopez-Benedicto, M.A. et al., Lipid, lipoproteins, apoproteins and physical exercise in young female athletes, *An. Esp. Pediatr.*, 28, 395, 1988 (in Spanish).

Lubrano-Berthelier, C. et al., Intracellular retention is a common characteristic of childhood obesity-associated MC4R mutations, *Hum. Mol. Genet.*, 12, 145, 2003.

Luciano, A., Bressan, F. and Zoppi, G., Body mass index reference curves for children aged 3–19 years from Verona, Italy, *Eur. J. Clin. Nutr.*, 51, 6, 1997.

Luciano, A. et al., Definition of obesity in childhood: criteria and limits, *Monerva Pediatr.*, 55, 453, 2003 (in Italian).

Ludwig, D.S., Peterson, K.E., and Gortmaker, S.L., Relations between consumption of sugar-sweetened drinks and childhood obesity: a prospective observational analysis, *Lancet*, 357, 505, 2001.

Lukas, A., Does early diet program future outcome? *Acta Paediatr. Scand.*, Suppl. 365, S58, 1990.

Lukaski, H.C. et al., Assessment of fat free mass using bioelectrical impedance measurements of the human body, *Am. J. Clin. Nutr.*, 41, 810, 1985.

Lukaski, H.C. et al., Validation of tetrapolar bioelectrical impedance method to assess human body composition, *J. Appl. Physiol.*, 60, 1327, 1986.

Luna, R. et al., High serum leptin levels in children with type 1 diabetes mellitus: contribution of age, BMI, pubertal development and metabolic status, *Clin. Endocrinol.*, 51, 603, 1999.

Luo, J. and Hu, F.B., Time trends of obesity in pre-school children in China from 1989 to 1887, *Int. J. Obes. Relat. Metab. Disord.*, 26, 553, 2002.

Lusky, A. et al., Relationship between morbidity and extreme values of body mass index in adolescents, *Int. J. Epidemiol.*, 25, 829, 1996.

Ma, Z. et al., Radioimmunoassay of leptin in human plasma, *Clin. Chem.*, 42, 942, 1996.

MacKeown, J.M. et al., Energy, macro- and micronutrient intake of 5-year-old urban black South African children in 1984 and 1995, *Pediatr. Perinatal Epidemiol.*, 12, 297, 1998.

Madeiros-Neto, G.A., Should drugs be used for treating obese children? *Int. J. Obes. Relat. Metab. Disord.*, 17, 363, 1993.

Maffeis, C., Role of energy metabolism in the pathophysiology of childhood obesity, *Int. J. Obes. Relat. Metab. Disord.*, 22, S89, 1998.

Maffeis, C., Aetiology of overweight and obesity in children and adolescents, *Eur. J. Pediatr. Suppl.*, 159, S35, 2000.

Maffeis, C., Pinelli, L., and Schutz, Y., Increased fat oxidation in prepubertal obese children: a metabolic defence against further weight gain? *J. Pediatr.*, 126, 15, 1995.

Maffeis, C., Pinelli, L., and Schutz, Y., Fat intake and adiposity in 8- to 11-yr-old obese children. *Int. J. Obes. Relat. Metab. Disord.*, 20, 170, 1996.

Maffeis, C., Schutz, Y., and Pinelli, L., Effect of weight loss on resting energy expenditure in obese prepubertal children, *Int. J. Obes. Relat. Metab. Disord.*, 16, 41, 1992a.

Maffeis, C., Schutz, Y., and Pinelli, L., Postprandial thermogenesis in obese children before and after weight reduction, *Eur. J. Clin. Nutr.*, 46, 577, 1992b.

Maffeis, C., Talamini, G., and Tato, L., Influence of diet, physical activity and parent's obesity on children's adiposity: a four-year longitudinal study, *Int. J. Obes. Relat. Metab. Disord.*, 22, 758, 1998.

Maffeis, C. and Tato, L., Long-term effects of childhood obesity on morbidity and mortality, *Horm. Res.*, 55, 42, 2001.

Maffeis, C., Zaffanello, M., and Schutz, Y., Relationship between physical inactivity and adiposity in prepubertal boys, *J. Pediatr.*, 131, 288, 1997.

Maffeis, C. et al., Energy expenditure during walking and running in obese and nonobese prepubertal children, *J. Pediatr.*, 123, 193, 1993a.

Maffeis, C. et al., Caloric intake, diet composition and habitual physical activity in obese children, *Int. J. Obes. Relat. Metab. Disord.*, 17, 37, 1993b.

Maffeis, C. et al., Energy intake and energy expenditure in free-living condition prepubertal obese and control subjects, *Int. J. Obes. Relat. Metab. Disord.*, 17, 37, 1993c.

Maffeis, C. et al., Meal-induced thermogenesis in lean and obese prepubertal children, *Am. J. Clin. Nutr.*, 57, 481, 1993d.

Maffeis, C. et al., Meal-induced thermogenesis in obese children with or without familial history of obesity, *Eur. J. Pediatr.*, 152, 128, 1993e.

Maffeis, C. et al., Parental and perinatal factors associated with childhood obesity in northeast Italy, *Int. J. Obes. Relat. Metab. Disord.*, 18, 301, 1994a.

Maffeis, C. et al., Maximal aerobic power during running and cycling in obese and non-obese children, *Acta Pediatr.*, 83, 113, 1994b.

Mafffeis, C. et al., Elevated energy expenditure and reduced energy intake in obese prepubertal children: paradox of poor dietary reliability in obesity ? *J. Pediatr.*, 124, 348, 1994c.

Maffeis, C. et al., Total energy expenditure and patterns of activity in 8–10-year-old obese and nonobese children, *J. Pediatr. Gastroenterol. Nutr.*, 23, 256, 1996.

Maffeis, C. et al., Leptin concentration in cord blood: relationship to gender and hormones, *Int. J. Obes. Relat. Metab. Disord.*, 22, S28, 1998.

Maffeis, C. et al., Fat oxidation and adiposity in prepubertal children: exogenous versus endogenous fat utilization, *J. Clin. Endocrinol. Metab.*, 84, 654, 1999a.

Maffeis, C. et al., Patterns of food intake and obesity in Italian children, *Int. J. Obes. Relat. Metab. Disord.*, 23, S44, 1999b.

Maffeis, C. et al., Distribution of food intake as a risk factor for childhood obesity, *Int. J. Obes. Relat. Metab. Disord.*, 24, 75, 2000.

Maffeis, C. et al., Meal-induced thermogenesis and obesity. Is fat meal a risk factor for fat gain in children? *J. Clin. Endocrinol. Metab.*, 86, 214, 2001.

Maffeis, C. et al., Insulin resistance and the persistence of obesity from childhood into adulthood, *J. Clin. Endocrinol. Metab.*, 87, 71, 2002.

Maffeis, C. et al., Waist circumference as a predictor of cardiovascular and metabolic risk factors in obese girls, *Eur. J. Clin. Nutr.*, 57, 566, 2003.

Magarey, A.M., Daniels, L.A., and Boulton, T.J.C., Prevalence of overweight and obesity in Australian children and adolescents: reassessment of 1985 and 1995 data against new standard international definitions, *Med. J. Aust.*, 174, 561, 2001.

Magarey, A.M. et al., Does fat intake predict adiposity in healthy children and adolescents age 2–15 y? A longitudinal analysis, *Eur. J. Clin. Nutr.*, 55, 471, 2001.

Magarey, A.M. et al., Predicting obesity in early adulthood from childhood and parental obesity, *Int. J. Obes. Relat. Metab. Disord.*, 27, 505, 2003.

Magnusson, P.K.E. and Rassmussen, F., Familial resemblance of body mass index and familial risk of high and low body mass index. A study of young men in Sweden, *Int. J. Obes. Relat. Metab. Disord.*, 26, 1225, 2002.

Mahan, L.K., Family-focused behavioral approach to weight control in children, *Pediatr. Clin. North Am.*, 34, 983, 1987.

Maillard, G. et al., Diet and adiposity indices in prepubertal children, *Int. J. Obes. Relat. Metab. Disord.*, 22, S204, 1998.

Malandry, D. et al., Interest in plastic surgery for weight loss sequellae in children, *Int. J. Obes. Relat. Metab. Disord.*, 22, S33, 1998.

Malecka-Tendera, E., and Molnar, D., Hormonal and metabolic changes, in *Child and Adolescent Obesity*, Burniat, W. et al., Eds., Cambridge University Press, Cambridge, 2002, 189.

Malecka-Tendera, E. et al., Relationship between lipid profile and body mass index in nonobese pubertal children, *Int. J. Obes. Relat. Metab. Disord.*, 21, S140, 1997.

Malecka-Tendera, E. et al., Overweight in adolescent girls with menstrual irregularities is a risk factor for polycystic ovary syndrome (PCOS), *Int. J. Obes. Relat. Metab. Disord.*, 22, S26, 1998.

Malina, R.M. et al., Fatness and physical fitness of girls 7 to 17 years, *Obes. Res.*, 3, 221, 1995.

Mallory, G.B., Jr., Fisher, D.H., and Jackson, R., Sleep-associated breathing disorders in morbidly obese children and adolescents, *J. Pediatr.*, 115, 892, 1989.

Malova, N.A., Simonova, L.A., and Fetisov, G.V., Hygienic rationale for diagnosis and correction of excessive body weight in schoolchildren with physical training, *Vestn. Ross. Akad. Med. Nauk.*, 51, 9, 1993 (in Russian).

Maramatsu, S. et al., A longitudinal study of obesity in Japan: relationship of body habitus between birth and age 17, *Int. J. Obes.*, 14, 39, 1990.

Marcus, C.L. et al., Evaluation of pulmonary function and polysomnography in obese children and adolescents, *Pediatr. Pulmonol.*, 21, 176, 1996.

Marelli, G. et al., Relation of body fat distribution to blood lipid pattern in severe childhood obesity, *Int. J. Obes. Relat. Metab. Disord.*, 17, 38, 1993.

Margetic, S. et al., Leptin: a review of its peripheral actions and interactions, *Int. J. Obes. Relat. Metab. Disord.*, 26, 1407, 2002.

Marinov, B., Kostianev, S., and Turnovska, T., Ventilatory efficiency and rate of percieved exertion in obese and non-obese children performing standardized exercise, *Clin. Physiol. Funct. Imaging*, 22, 254, 2002.

Martini, G. et al., Heart rate variability in childhood obesity, *Clin. Auton. Res.*, 11, 87, 2001.

Martos-Estepa, R. et al., High level of alanine aminotransferase and cholinesterase in obese obese pre-pubertal children: correlation with basal insulin concentration and anthropometric, *An. Esp. Pediatr.*, 53, 330, 2000.

Massé, G. and Moreigne, F. *Croissance et developpement de l'enfant a Dakar*, Centre International de l'Enfance, Paris, 1969.

Mast, M. et al., Gender differences in fat mass of 5–7 year old children, *Int. J. Obes. Relat. Metab. Disord.*, 22, 878, 1998.

Mast, M. et al., Inconsistencies in bioelectrical impedance and anthropometric measurements of fat mass in a field study of prepubertal children, *Br. J. Nutr.*, 87, 163, 2002.

Matiegka, J. *Somatology of School Children*, Czechoslovak Academy of Sciences and ARTS (CAVU), Prague, 1929 (in Czech).

Matkovic, V. et al., Gain in body fat is inversely related to the nocturnal rise in serum leptin level in young females, *J. Clin. Endocrinol. Metab.*, 82, 1368, 1997.

Mayer, J., *Health*, Van Nostrand, New York, 1974.

Mayer, J. et al., Exercise, food intake and body weight in normal rats and genetically obese adult mice, *Am. J. Physiol.*, 177, 544, 1954.

Maynard, L.M. et al., Maternal perception of weight status of children, *Pediatrics*, 111, 1226, 2003.

Maziekas, M.T. et al., Follow up exercise studies in paediatric obesity: implications for long term effectiveness, *Br. J. Sports Med.*, 37, 425, 2003.

McArdle, W.D., Katch, F.I., and Katch, V.L. *Exercise Physiology. Energy, Nutrition and Human Performance*, 3rd ed, Lea & Febiger, Philadelphia, 1991.

McCance, D.R. et al., Glucose, insulin concentrations and obesity in childhood and adolescence as predictors of NIDDM, *Diabetologie*, 37, 617, 1994.

McCarron, P., Smith, G.D., and Okasha, M., Secular changes in blood pressure in childhood, adolescence and young adulthood: systematic review of trends from 1948 to 1998, *J. Hum. Hypertens.*, 16, 677, 2002.

McCarthy, H.D., Ellis, S.M., and Cole, T.J., Central overweight and obesity in British youth aged 11–16 years: cross-sectional surveys of waist circumference, *B.M.J.*, 326, 624, 2003.

McDonald, K. and Thompson, J.K., Eating disturbance, body image dissatisfaction, and reasons for exercising: gender differences and correlational findings, *Int. J. Eating Disord.*, 11, 289, 1992.

McElroy, A. and Townsend, P.K. *Medical Anthropology in Ecological Perspective*, Westview Press, Harper Collins, 12, Boulder, 1996.

McGill, H.C., Childhood nutrition and adult cardiovascular disease, *Nutr. Rev.*, 55, S2, 1997.

McGloin, A.F. et al., Energy and fat intake in obese and lean children at varying risk of obesity, *Int. J. Obes. Relat. Metab. Disord.*, 26, 200, 2002.

McLeod, W.P., Hunter, S.C., and Etchison, B., Performance measurement and percent body fat in the high school athlete, *Am. J. Sp. Med.*, 11, 390, 1983.

McMurray, R.G. et al., Childhood obesity elevates blood pressure and total cholesterol independently of physical activity, *Int. J. Obes. Relat. Metab. Disord.*, 19, 881, 1995.

McNutt, S.W. et al., A longitudinal study of the dietary practices of black and white girls 9 and 10 years old at enrollment: the NHLBI Growth and Health Study, *J. Adolesc. Hlth. Care*, 20, 27, 1997.

Mei, Z. et al., Increasing prevalence of overweight among U.S. low-income preschool children: the Centers for Disease Control and Prevention of pediatric nutrition surveillance, 1983 to 1995, *Pediatrics*, 101, E12, 1998.

Mei, Z. et al., Validity of body mass index compared with other body composition screening indexes for the assessment of body fatness in children and adolescents, *Am. J. Clin. Nutr.*, 75, 978, 2002.

Menghetti, E. et al., Obesity and hypercholesterolemia in primary school in Rome, *Minerva Pediatr.*, 47, 303, 1995.

Menghetti, E.P. et al., The nutritional aspects and incidence of obesity and hypertension in groups of Roman adolescents, *Minerva Pediatr.*, 45, 177, 1993 (in Italian).

Metcalf, B.S., Voss, L.D., and Wilkin, T.J., Accelerometers identify inactive and potentially obese children., *Arch. Dis. Child.*, 87, 166, 2002.

Meyre, D. et al., A genome-wide scan for childhood obesity-associated traints in French families shows significant linkage on chromosome 6q22.31-q23.2, *Diabetes*, 53, 803, 2004.

Micheli, L.J., Overuse injuries in children's sports: the growth factor, *Orthop. Clin. North Am.*, 14, 337, 1983.

Mijailovic, V., Micic, D., and Mijailovic, M., Effects of childhood and adolescent obesity on morbidity in adult life, *J. Pediatr. Endocrinol. Metab.*, 14, 1339, 2001.

Mills, J.K. and Adrianopoulos, G.D., The relationship between childhood onset obesity and psychopathology in adulthood, *J. Psychol.*, 127, 547, 1993.

Miraglia-del-Giudice, E. et al., Low frequency of melanocortin-4 receptor (MC4R) mutations in a Mediterranean population with early-onset obesity, *Int. J. Obes. Relat. Metab. Disord.*, 26, 647, 2002a.

Miraglia-del-Giudice, E. et al., Inadequate leptin level negatively affects body fat loss during a weight reduction programme for childhood obesity, *Acta Pediatr. Int. J.*, 91, 132, 2002b.

Miraglia-del-Giudice, E. et al., Molecular screening of the ghrelin gene in Italian obese children: the Leu77Met variant is associated with an earlier onset of obesity, *Int. J. Obes. Relat. Metab. Disord.*, 28, 447, 2004.

Mirmiran, P., Mirbolooki, M., and Azizi, F., Familial clustering of obesity and the role of nutrition: Tehran Lipid and Glucose Study, *Int. J. Obes. Relat. Metab. Disord.*, 26, 1617, 2002.

Mirtipati, A. et al., Body mass index of preschool youth with high socioeconomic status in Chiang Mai, Thailand, *Int. J. Obes. Relat. Metab. Disord.*, 22, S4, 1998.

Misra, A., Revisions of cut-offs of body mass index to define overweight and obesity are needed for the Asian-ethnic groups, *Int. J. Obes. Relat. Metab. Disord.*, 27, 1294, 2003.

Miyzaki, Y. et al., Effects of hyperinsulinaemia on renal function and the pressor system in insulin-resistant obese adolescents, *Clin. Exp. Pharmacol. Physiol.*, 23, 287, 1996.

Mo, B. et al., The role of β-3- adrenergic receptor Trp/Arg mutation in childhood obesity, *Chin. J. Med. Genet.*, 18, 371, 2001.

Molleston, J.P. et al., Obese child with steatohepatitis can develop cirrhosis in childhood, *Am. J. Gastroenterol.*, 97, 2460, 2002.

Molnar, D., The effect of meal frequency on postprandial thermogenesis in obese children, *Pediatr. Padol.*, 27, 177, 1992.

Molnar, D., Development of physical activity behaviours: implications for prevention of obesity, *Int. J. Obes. Relat. Metab. Disord.*, 23, Suppl. 5, S7, 1999.

Molnar, D., Decsi, T., and Csábi, G., Multimetabolic syndrome in childhood obesity, *Int. J. Obes. Relat. Metab. Disord.*, 21, S141, 1997.

Molnar, D., Dober, I., and Soltesz, G., The effect of unprocessed wheat bran on blood glucose and plasma immunoreactive insulin levels during oral glucose tolerance test in obese children, *Acta Paediatr. Hung.*, 26, 75, 1985.

Molnar, D. and Malecka-Tendera, E., Drug therapy, in *Child and Adolescent Obesity*, Burniat, W. et al., Eds., Cambridge University Press, Cambridge, 2002, 345.

Molnar, D. and Schutz, Y., The effect of obesity, age, puberty and gender on resting metabolic rate in children and adolescents, *Eur. J. Pediatr.*, 156, 376, 1997.

Molnar, D. and Schutz, Y., Fat oxidation in nonobese and obese adolescents: effect of body composition and pubertal development, *J. Pediatr.*, 132, 98, 1998.

Molnar, D. et al., Measured and predicted resting metabolic rate in obese and nonobese adolescents, *J. Pediatr.*, 127,, 571, 1995.

Molnar, D. et al., Effect of weight reduction on plasma total antioxidative capacity in obese children, *Int. J. Obes. Relat. Metab. Disord.*, 22, S23, 1998.

Molnar, D. et al., Effectivity and safety of Letigen (caffeine/ephedrine): the first double blind placebo-controlled pilot study in adolescents, *Int. J. Obes. Relat. Metab. Dis.*, 23, S62, 1999.

Mondini, L. and Monteiro, C.A., The stage of nutrition transition in different Brazilian region, *Arch. Latinoam. Nutr.*, 47, 17, 1997.

Montague, C.T. et al., Congenital leptin deficiency is associated with severe early-onset obesity in humans, *Nature*, 387, 903, 1997.

Monteiro, P.O.A. et al., Birth size, early childhood growth, and adolescent obesity in Brazilian birth cohort, *Int. J. Obes. Relat. Metab. Disord.*, 27, 1274, 2003.

Montoye, H.J. et al., *Measuring Physical Activity and Energy Expenditure*, Human Kinetics Publishers, Champaign, IL, 1996.

Moore, D.B., Howell, P.B. and Treiber, F.A., Changes in overweight in youth over a period of 7 years; impact of ethnicity, gender and socioeconomic status, *Ethn. Dis.*, 12, 1, 2002.

Moore, L.L. et al., Preschool physical activity level and change in body fatness in young children: the Framingham Children's Study, *Am. J. Epidemiol.*, 142, 982, 1995.

Moore, L.L. et al., Does early physical activity predict body fat change throughout childhood? *Prev. Med.*, 37, 1, 10, 2003.

Moran, O. and Philip, M., Leptin: obesity, diabetes and other peripheral effects — a review, *Pediatr. Diabetes*, 4, 101, 2003.

Moreno, L.A. et al., Indices of body fat distribution in Spanish children aged 4.0 to 14.9 years, *J. Pediatr. Gastroenterol. Nutr.*, 25, 175, 1997.

Moreno, L.A. et al., Body fat distribution and postprandial lipidemia in obese adolescents, *Int. J. Obes. Relat. Metab. Disord.*, 22, S24, 1998.

Moreno, L.A. et al., Trends in body mass index and overweight prevalence among children and adolescents in the region of Aragon (Spain) from 1985 to 1995, *Int. J. Obes. Relat. Metab. Disord.*, 24, 925, 2000.

Moreno, L.A. et al., Postprandial triglyceridemia in obese and non-obese adolescents. Importance of body composition and fat distribution, *J. Pediatr. Endocrinol. Metab.*, 14, 193, 2001a.

Moreno, L.A. et al., Sociodemographic factors and trends on overweight prevalence in children and adolescents in Aragon (Spain) from 1985 to 1995, *J. Clin. Epidemiol.*, 54, 921, 2001b.

Moreno, L.A. et al., Leptin. A metabolic syndrome in obese and non-obese children, *Horm. Metab. Res.*, 34, 394, 2002.

Morgan, C.M. et al., Loss of control over eating, adiposity, and psychopathology in overweight children, *Int. J. Eating Disord.*, 31, 430, 2002.

Morrison, J.A. et al., Overweight fat patterning and cardiovascular diseases risk factors in black and white boys, *J. Pediatr.*, 135, 451, 1999.

Mossberg, H.O., 40-year follow-up of overweight children, *Lancet*, 2, 491, 1989.

Mossberg, H.O., Overweight in children and youths: a 40-year follow-up study, *Nord. Med.*, 106, 184, 1991.

Mo-suwan, L. and Gaeter, A.F., Risk factors for childhood obesity in a transitional society in Thailand, *Int. J. Obes. Relat. Metab. Disord.*, 20, 698, 1996.

Mo-suwan, L., Junjana, C., and Puetpaiboon, A., Increasing obesity in school children in a transitional society and the effect of the weight control program, *S.E. Asian J. Trop. Med. Pub. Hlth.*, 24, 590, 1993.

Mo-suwan, L. et al., Effects of controlled trial of a school-based exercise program on the obesity indices of preschool children, *Am. J. Clin. Nutr.*, 68, 1006, 1998.

Muecke, L. et al., Is childhood obesity associated with high-fat foods and low physical activity? *J. Sch. Hlth.*, 62, 19, 1992.

Muller, M.J. et al., Physical activity and diet in 5 to 7 years old children, *Public Health Nutr.*, 2, 443, 1999.

Muller, M.J. et al., Prevention of obesity: more than an intention. Concept and first results of the Kiel Obesity Prevention Study (KOPS), *Int. J. Obes. Relat. Metab. Disord.*, 25, S66, 2001.

Mumbiela Pons, V., Sanmartin Zaragoza, S., and Gonzales Alvarez, C., Obesity in childhood and food habits, *Rev. Enferm.*, 20, 11, 1997.

Murata, M., Nutrition for the young - its current problems, *Nutr. Health*, 8, 143, 1992.

Murata, M., Secular trends in growth and change in eating patterns of Japanese children, *Am. J. Clin. Nutr.*, 72, 1379S, 2000.

Musaiger, A.O. et al., Obesity among secondary school students in Bahrain, *Nutr. Health*, 9, 25, 1993.

Must, A., Dallal, G.E., and Dietz, W.H., Reference data for obesity: 85th and 95th percentiles of body mass index (wt/ht^2) and triceps skinfold thickness, *Am. J. Clin. Nutr.*, 53, 839, 1991.

Must, A. et al., Long-term morbidity and mortality of overweight adolescents. A follow-up of the Harvard Growth Study of 1922 to 1935, *N. Engl. J. Med.*, 327, 1350, 1992.

Mustillo, S. et al., Obesity and psychiatric disorder: Developmental trajectories, *Pediatrics*, 111, 851, 2003.

Nagai, N. and T., M., Effect of physical activity on autonomic nervous system function in lean and obese children, *Int. J. Obes. Relat. Metab. Disord.*, 28, 27, 2004.

Nagy, T.R. et al., Effects of gender, ethnicity, body composition, and fat distribution on serum leptin concentration in children, *J. Clin. Endocrinol. Metab.*, 82, 2148, 1997.

National Health and Medical Research Council (NHMRC), 1997 (+ clinical management docs, 2003) (Chap. 12)

Naziekas, M.T. et al., Follow up exercise studies in paediatric obesity: implications for long term effectiveness, *Br. J. Sports. Med.*, 37, 426, 2003.

Neel, J.V., The "thrifty genotype" in 1998, *Nutr. Rev.*, 57, S2, 1999.

Nelson, J.A., Chiasson, M.A., and Ford, V., Childhood overweight in a New York City WIC population, *Am. J. Pub. Hlth.*, 94, 458, 2004.

Neovius, M. et al., Discrepancies between classificiation systems of childhood obesity, *Obes. Res.*, 5, 105, 2004.

Neumark-Sztainer, D., Palti, H., and Butler, R., Weight concerns and dieting behaviors among high school girls in Israel, *J. Adolesc. Hlth.*, 16, 53, 1995.

Nguyen, N.V. et al., Fat intake and adiposity in children of lean and obese parents, *Am. J. Clin. Nutr.*, 63, 507, 1996.

Nichols, J.F., Bigelow, D.M., and Canine, K.M., Short-term weight loss and exercise training effects on glucose-induced thermogenesis in obese adolescent males during hypocaloric feeding, *Int. J. Obes.*, 13, 683, 1989.

Nicklas, T. and Johnson, R., ADA: Position of the American Dietetic Association: dietary guidelines for healthy children ages 2 to 11 years, *J. Am. Diet. Assoc.*, 104, 660, 2004.

Nicklas, T.A. et al., Eating patterns and obesity in children. The Bogalusa Heart Study, *Am. J. Prev. Med.*, 25, 9, 2003.

Nicklas, T.A. et al., Children's meal patterns have changed over 21-year period. The Bogalusa Heart Study. *J. Am. Diet. Assoc.*, 104, 753, 2004.

Nishina, M. et al., Relationship among systolic blood pressure serum insulin and leptin and visceral fat accumulation in obese children, *Hypertens. Res.*, 26, 281, 2003.

Noonan, S.S., Children and obesity: flunking the fat test, *N.J. Med.*, 94, 49, 1997.

Norgren, S. et al., Orlistat treatment in obese prepubertal children: a pilot study, *Acta Paediatr. Int. J. Paediatr.*, 92, 666, 2003.

Nova, A., Russo, A., and Sala, E., Long-term management of obesity in paediatric office practice: experimental evaluation of two different types of intervention, *Ambul. Child Health*, 7, 3–4, 239, 2001.

Nuutinen, O., Long-term effects of dietary counselling on nutrient intake and weight loss in obese children, *Eur. J. Clin. Nutr.*, 45, 287, 1991.

Nuutinen, O. and Knip, M., Long-term weight control in obese children: persistence of treatment outcome and metabolic changes, *Int. J, Obes. Relat. Metab. Disord.*, 16, 279, 1992a.

Nuutinen, O. and Knip, M., Predictors of weight reduction in obese children, *Eur. J. Clin. Nutr.*, 16, 785, 1992b.

Obarzanek, E. et al., Energy intake and physical activity in relation to indices of body fat: The National Heart, Lung and Blood Institute Growth and Health Study, *Am. J. Clin. Nutr.*, 60, 15, 1994.

Obrebowski, A., Obrebowska-Karsznia, Z., and Gawlinski, M., Smell and taste in children with simple obesity, *Int. J. Pediatr. Otorhinolaryngol.*, 55, 191, 2000.

Obuchowitz, A. and Obuchowitz, E., Plasma beta-endorphin and insulin concentrations in relation to body fat and nutritional parameters in overweight and obese prepubertal children, *Int. J. Obes. Relat. Metab. Disord.*, 21, 783, 1997.

Obuchowitz, A. and Szczepanski, Z., Evaluation of the biochemical indicators of risk of atherosclerosis in children with simple obesity, *Pediatr. Pol.*, 61., 409, 1986.

O'Dea, E.A. and Caputi, P., Association between socioeconomic status, weight, age and gender, and the body image and weight control practices of 6- to 19-year-old children and adolescents. *Health Educ. Res.* 16, 521, 2000.

Offman, H.J. and Bradley, S.J., Body image of children and adolescents and its measurement: an overview, *Can. J. Psychiat*, 37, 417, 1992.

Ogden, C.L. et al., Prevalence of overweight among preschool children in the United States, 1971 through 1994, *Pediatrics*, 99, 1098, 1997.

Ogle, G.D. et al., Body composition assessment by dual-energy x-ray absorptiometry in subjects aged 4–26 y, *Am. J. Clin. Nutr.*, 61, 746, 1995.

Olefski, J., Kolterman, O.G., and Scarlett, J., Insulin action and resistance in obesity and non-insulin-dependent type II diabetes mellitus, *Am. J. Physiol. Endocrinol. Metab.*, 6, E15, 1982.

Olmstead, M.P. et al., Psychoeducational principles in the treatment of bulimia and anorexia nervosa, in *Handbook of Psychotherapy for Anorexia Nervosa and Bulimia*, Garner, D.M. and Garfinkel, P.E., Eds., Guilford Press, New York, 1985, 513.

O'Loughlin, J. et al., A five-year trend of increasing obesity among elementary schoolchildren in multiethnic, low-income, inner-city neighborhoods in Montreal, Canada, *Int. J. Obes. Relat. Metab. Disord.*, 24, 1176, 2000.

Ong, K.K. and Dunger, D.B., Perinatal growth failure: the road to obesity, insulin resistance and cardiovascular disease in adults, *Bailliere's Best Practice and Research in Clinical Endocrinology and Metabolism*, 16, 191, 2002.

Ong, K.K.L. et al., Association between postnatal catch-up growth and obesity in childhood: prospective cohort study, *Br. Med. J.*, 320, 967, 2000.

Oppert, J.M. and Rolland-Cachera, M.F., Prevalence, evolution dans le temps et consequence économique de l'obesité, *Med. Sci.*, 11, 939, 1998.

O'Rahilly, S. Et al., Minireview: human obesity — lessons from monogenic disorders, *Endocrinology*, 144, 3757, 2003.

Oren, A. et al., Change in body mass index from adolescence to young adulthood and increased carotid intima-media thickness at 28 years of age: the Atherosclerosis Risk in Young Adults Study, *Int. J. Obes. Relat. Metab. Disord.*, 27, 1383, 2003.

Ortega, R.M. et al., Relationships between diet composition and body mass index in a group of Spanish adolescents, *Br. J. Nutr.*, 74, 765, 1995.

Ortega, R.M. et al., The food habits and energy and nutrient intake in overweight adolescents compared to those with normal weight, *An. Esp. Pediatr.* 44, 203, 1996 (in Spanish).

Ortega, R.M. et al., Differences in the breakfast habits of overweight/obese and normal weight schoolchildren, *Int. J. Vitam. Nutr. Res.*, 68, 125, 1998.

Oscai, L.B., The role of exercise in weight control, in *Exercise and Sports Sciences Reviews*, Wilmore, J.H., Ed. Academic Press, New York, 1973, 103.

Owens, S. et al., Visceral adipose tissue and cardiovascular risk factors in obese children, *J. Pediat.*, 133, 41, 1998.

Owens, S. et al., Effect of physical training on total and visceral fat in obese children, *Med. Sci. Sports. Exerc.*, 31, 143, 1999.

Paeratakul, S. et al., Fast-food consumption among U.S. adults and children: dietary and nutrient intake profile, *J. Am. Diet. Assoc.*, 103, 1332, 2003.

Palgi, Y. et al., Physiologic and anthropometric factors underlying endurance performance in children, *Int. J. Sports Med.*, 5, 67, 1984.

Pallaro, A. et al., Total salivary IgA, serum C3c and IgA in obese children, *Int. J. Obes. Relat. Metab. Disord.*, 22, S208, 1998.

Pallaro, A. et al., Total salivary IgA, serum C3c and IgA in obese school children, *J. Nutr. Biochem.*, 13, 539, 2002.

Palmert, M.R., Radovick, S.. and Beopple, P.A., The impact of reversible gonadal sex steroid suppression on serum leptin concentrations in children with central precocious puberty, *J. Clin. Endocrinol. Metab.*, 83, 1091, 1998.

Pantano, L.C. et al., Nutritional studies in a commune del Lazio. Anthropometric data and food consumption in childhood, *Minerva Pediatr.*, 44, 293, 1992 (in Italian).

Pařízková, J., Age trend in fatness in normal and obese children, *J. Appl. Physiol.*, 16, 173, 1961a.

Pařízková, J., Total body fat and skinfold thickness in children, *Metabolism*, 10, 794, 1961b.

Pařízková, J., The impact of age, diet and exercise on man's body composition, *Ann. N.Y. Acad. Sci.*, 110, 661, 1963a.

Pařízková, J., Morphologie du tissu gras, in *Problemes Actuels d'Endocrinologie et de Nutrition, L'Obésité*, Klotz, H. and Trémolières, J., Eds., Expansion Scientifique Française, Paris, 1963b, 271.

Pařízková, J., Longitudinal study of body composition and body build development in boys of various physical activity from 11 to 15 years of age, *Human Biol.*, 40, 212, 1968a.

Pařízková, J., Compositional growth in relation to metabolic activity, in *Proc. XIIth Int. Congr. Pediatrics, Opening Plenary Session, Dec. 2–7, 1968*, Mexico City, 1968b, 32.

Pařízková, J., Longitudinal study of the relationship between body composition and anthropometric characteristics in boys during growth and development, *Glasnik Antropoloskog Drusstvo Jugoslavii*, 7, 33, 1970.

Pařízková, J., Obesity and physical activity, in *Nutricia Symposium on Nutritional Aspects of Physical Performance*, De Wijn, J.F. and Binkhorst, R.A., Eds., Nutricia Ltd., Zoetermeer, 1972, 146.

Pařízková, J., Consequences of reduction treatment of child obesity in adult age, in *Proc. 1st Int. Congr. Obes., Recent Advances in Obesity Research*, London, Human Publishing, 1975, 293.

Pařízková, J., *Body Fat and Physical Fitness: Body Composition and Lipid Metabolism in Different Regimes of Physical Activity*, Martinus Nijhoff B.V. Medical Division, The Hague, 1977.

Pařízková, J., The impact of daily workload during pregnancy and/or postnatal life on the heart microstructure of rat male offspring, *Basic Res. Cardiol.*, 73, 433, 1978a.

Pařízková, J., Body composition and lipid metabolism in relation to nutrition and exercise, in *Nutrition, Physical Fitness and Health*, Pařízková, J. and Rogozkin, V.A., Eds., Series on Sport Sciences, Vol. 7, University Park Press, Baltimore, 1978b, 283.

Pařízková, J., Nutrition and work performance, in *Critical Reviews in Tropical Medicine*, Chandra, R.K., Ed. Plenum Press, New York, 1982a, 307.

Pařízková, J., Physical training and weight reduction in obese adolescents, *Ann. Clin. Res.*, 14, 63, 1982b.

Pařízková, J., Adaptation of functional capacity and exercise, in *Nutritional Adaptation in Man*, Blaxter, K. and Waterlow, J.C., Eds., John Libbey, London, Paris, 1985, Chap. 11:127.

Pařízková, J., Body composition and nutrition of different types of athletes, in *Proc. XIII Int. Congr. Nutr. 1985*, London, John Libbey, 1986, 309.

Pařízková, J., Age related changes in dietary intake related to work output, physical fitness and body composition, *Am. J. Clin. Nutr.*, 5, 962, 1989.

Pařízková, J., Human growth, physical fitness and nutrition under various environmental conditions, in *Human Growth, Physical Fitness and Nutrition*, Shephard, R.J. and Pařízková, J., Eds., Karger, Basel, 1991, 1.

Pařízková, J., Obesity and its treatment by diet and exercise, in *Nutrition and Fitness in Health and Disease*, Simopoulos, A.P., Ed. Karger, Basel, p. 78, 1993a.

Pařízková, J., Food choices in Czechoslovakia, *Appetite*, 21, 299, 1993b.

Pařízková, J., Obesity and physical fitness: an age-dependent functional and social handicap, in *Social Aspects of Obesity*, deGarine, I. and Pollock, N.J., Eds., Gordon and Breach Publishers, Australia, 1995, 163.

Pařízková, J., *Nutrition, Physical Activity, and Health in Early Life*, CRC Press, Boca Raton, 1996a.

Pařízková, J., How much energy is consumed and spent for optimal growth and development? *Nutrition*, 12, 820, 1996b.

Pařízková, J., Interaction between physical activity and nutrition early in life and their impact on later development, *Nutr. Res. Rev.*, 11, 71, 1998a.

Pařízková, J., Treatment and prevention of obesity by exercise in Czech children, in *Physical Fitness and Nutrition during Growth*, Pařízková, J. and Hills, A.P., Eds., Karger, Basel, 1998b, 145.

Pařízková, J., Early prevention and treatment of children's obesity, *Int. J. Obes. Relat. Metab. Disord.*, 22, S30, 1998c.

Pařízková, J., Effect of the interrelationships between diet and physical activity on aging, in Ecology of Aging, in *J. Human. Ecol. Special Issue*, Siniarska, A. and Wolanski, N., Eds., Kamla-Raj, New Delhi, 2000, Chap. 3.

Pařízková, J. and Carter, J.E.L., Influence of physical activity on stability of somatotypes in boys, *Am. J. Phys. Anthropol.*, 44, 327, 1976.

Pařízková, J. and Chin, M-K., Obesity prevention and health promotion during early periods of growth and development, *J. Exerc. Sci. Fitness*, 1, 1, 2003.

Pařízková, J. and Faltová, E,. Physical activity, body fat and experimental cardiac necrosis, *Brit. J. Nutr.*, 24, 3, 1970.

Pařízková, J. and Hainer, V., Exercise therapy in growing and adult obese, in *Current Therapy in Sports Medicine*, Walsh, R.P. and Shephard, R.J., Eds., Decker, Toronto, 1989, 22.

Pařízková, J. and Heller, J., Relationship of dietary intake to work output and physical performance in Czechoslovak adolescents adapted to various work loads, in *Human Growth, Physical Fitness and Nutrition*, Shephard, R.J. and Pařízková, J., Eds., Rager, Basel, 1991, 156.

Pařízková, J., Maffeis, C., and Poskitt, E.M.E., Management through activity, in *Child and Adolescent Obesity*, Burniat, W. et al., Eds., Cambridge University Press, Cambridge, 2002, 307.

Pařízková, J. and Novák, J., Dietary intake and metabolic parameters in adult men during extreme work load, in *World Rev. Nutr. Diet: Impacts on Nutrition and Health*, Simopoulos, A.P., Ed. Karger, Basel, 1991, 72.

Pařízková, J. and Poupa, O., Some metabolic consequences of adaptation to muscular work, *Brit. J. Nutr.*, 17, 341, 1963.

Pařízková, J. and Rolland-Cachera, M.F., High proteins early in life as a predisposition for late obesity and further health risks, *Nutrition*, 13, 818, 1997.

Pařízková, J. et al.., Growth, food intake, motor activity and experimental cardiac necrosis in early malnourished male rats, *Ann. Nutr. Metab.*, 26, 121, 1982.

Pařízková, J. et al., Body composition, food intake, cardiorespiratory fitness, blood lipids, and psychological development in highly active and inactive pre-school children, *Human Biol.*, 58, 261, 1986.

Pařízková, J. et al., Physiological capabilities of obese individuals and implications for exercise, in *Exercise and Obesity*, Hills, A.P., Wahlqvist, M., Eds., Smith-Gordon/Nishimura, London, 1995, 131.

Pařízková, J. et al., Body composition in obese subjects before and after weight reduction, *Biol. Hum. Anthropol.*, 21, 41, 2003.

Park, H.S. et al., Association with leptin, cardiovascular risk factors, and nutrition in Korean girls, *Int. J. Obes. Relat. Metab. Disord.*, 22, S27, 1998.

Park, M.J. et al., Serum levels of insulin-like growth factor (IGF-I), free IGF-I, IGF binding protein (IGFBP-1), IGFBP-3 and insulin in obese children, *J. Pediat. Endocrinol. Metab.*, 12, 139, 1999.

Parry-Jones, W.L., Obesity in childhood and adolescents, in *Handbook of Eating Disorders, Part 2: Obesity*, Burrows, G.D., Beumont, P.J.V., and Casper, R.C., Eds., Elsevier, Amsterdam, 1988.

Parsons, T.J., Power, C., and Manor, O., Infant feeding and obesity through lifecourse, *Arch. Dis. Child.*, 88, 793, 2002.

Pasquet, P. et al., Massive overfeeding and energy balance in men: the Guru Walla model, *Am. J. Clin. Nutr.*, 56, 483, 1992.

Pasquet, P. et al., Growth, maturation and nutrition transition: with special reference to urban populations in Central Africa, abstr., in *14th International Anthropological Congress of Ales Hrdlicka "World Anthropology at the Turn of Centuries,"* Aug. 31st–Sept. 4th, 1999, Prague-Humpolec, 1999, 115.

Pate, R.R., Physical activity assessment in children and adolescents, *Crit. Rev. Food Sci. Nutr.*, 33, 321, 1993.

Patterson, R.E. et al., Factors related to obesity in preschool children, *J. Am. Diet. Assoc.*, 86, 1376, 1986.

Pavlovic, M. et al., Nutrition and nutritional status in schoolchildren aged 10–18 from North Backa region in Yugoslavia, *Scand. J. Nutr.*, 43, S78, 1999a.

Pavlovic, M. et al., The prevalence of overweight and obesity in children and adolescents from North Backa Region in Yugoslavia, *Scand. J. Nutr.*, 43, S44, 1999b.

Paz-Cerezo, M. et al., Influence of energy expenditure on childhood obesity, *An. Pediatr.*, 58, 316, 2003.

Peja, M. and Velkey, L., The joint influence of diet and increased physical activity in obese children, *Acta Paediatr. Hung.*, 29, 373, 1988.

Pellegrini, A.D. and Smith, P.K., Physical activity play: the nature and function of a neglected aspect of playing, *Child Dev.*, 69, 607, 1998.

Pena, M. et al., Fiber and exercise in the treatment of obese adolescents, *J. Adolesc. Hlth. Care*, 10, 30, 1989.

Perez, B.M. and Landaeta-Jimenez, M., Relationship of weight and height with waist corcumference, body mass index and conicity index in adolescents, *Acta Med. Auxol.*, 33, 61, 2001.

Perrone, L. et al., Relationships among white blood cell count and anthropometric indexes of adiposity in obese children and adolescents, *Int. J. Obes. Relat. Metab. Disord.*, 22, S27, 1998a.

Perrone, L. et al., Anthropometric indexes and risk factors for atherosclerosis in obesity, *Int. J. Obes. Relat. Metab. Disord.*, 22, S25, 1998b.

Perusse, L. and Bouchard, C., Gene–diet interaction in obesity, *Am. J. Clin. Nutr.*, 72, 1285S, 2000.

Petersen, C., Childhood overweight: an epidemiological study from Hamburg, Germany (N = 32610), *Int. J. Obes. Relat. Metab. Disord.*, 22, S202, 1998.

Peterson, S. and Sigman-Grant, M., Impact of adopting lower-fat food choices on nutrient intake of American children, *Pediatrics*, 100, E4, 1997.

Petridou, E. et al., Blood lipids in Greek adolescents and their relationship to diet, obesity, and socioeconomic factors, *Ann. Epidemiol.*, 5, 286, 1995.

Petrolini, N., Iughetti, L. and Bernasconi, S., Difficulty in visual coordination as a possible cause of sedentary behaviour in obese children, *Int. J. Obes. Relat. Metab. Disord.*, 19, 928, 1995.

Pharaon, I., El Metn, J., and Frelut, M.L., Prevalence of obesity among Lebanese adolescent girls, *Int. J. Obes. Relat. Metab. Disord.*, 22, S7, 1998.

Pidlich, J. et al., The effect of weight reduction on the surface electrocardiogram: a prospective trial in obese children and adolescents, *Int. J. Obes. Relat. Metab. Disord.*, 21, 1018, 1997.

Pietrobelli, A. et al., Body mass index as a measure of adiposity among children and adolescents: a validation study, *J. Pediatr.*, 132, 204, 1998.

Pinelli, L. et al., Childhood obesity: results of a multicenter study of obesity treatment in Italy, *J. Pediatr. Endocrinol. Metab.*, 12, 795, 1999.

Pintor, C. et al., Adrenal androgens in obese boys before and after weight loss, *Horm. Metab. Res.*, 16, 544, 1984.

Plagemann, A. et al., Obesity and enhanced diabetes and cardiovascular risk in adult rats due to early postnatal overfeeding, *Exp. Clin. Endocrinol.*, 99, 154, 1992.

Plecas, D. et al., Prevalence of obesity among children under five in Federal Republic of Yugoslavia, *Int. J. Obes. Relat. Metab. Disord.*, 22, S6, 1998.

Polito, A., Pařízková, J., Toti, E., and Ferro-Luzzi, A., The measurement of body composition by infrared interactance: an evaluation, *Nutr. Res.*, 14, 1165, 1994.

Pongprapai, S., Mo-suwan, L., and Leelasamran, W., Physical fitness of obese schoolchildren in Hat Yai, southern Thailand, *S.E. Asian J. Trop. Med. Pub. Hlth.*, 25, 354, 1994.

Popkin, B.M., Richards, M.K., and Adair, L.S., Stunting is associated with childhood obesity: dynamic relationships, in *Human Growth in Context*, Johnston, F.E., Zemel, B., and Eveleth, P.B., Eds., Smith-Gordon/Nishimura, London, 1999, 321.

Popkin, B.M., Richards, M.K., and Montiero, C.A., Stunting is associated with overweight in children of four nations that are undergoing the nutrition transition, *J. Nutr.*, 126, 3009, 1996.

Popkin, B.M. and Udry, J.R., Adolescent obesity increases significantly in second and third generation of U.S. immigrants: The National Longitudinal Study of Adolescent Health, *J. Nutr.*, 128, 701, 1998.

Popkin, B.M. et al., Dietary and environmental correlates of obesity in a population study in China, *Obes. Res.*, 3, S135, 1995.

Poskitt, E., Obesity in the young child: whither and whence? *Acta Paediatr. Scand.*, Suppl. 323, 24, 1986.

Posner, B.M. et al., Secular trends in diet and risk factors for cardiovascular disease: The Framingham Study, *J. Am. Diet. Assoc.*, 595, 171, 1995.

Power, C. and Jafferis, B.J.M.N., Fetal environment and subsequent obesity: a study of maternal smoking, *Int. J. Epidemiol.*, 31, 413, 2002.

Power, C., Lake, J.K,. and Cole, T.J., Measurement and long-term health risks of child and adolescent fatness, *Int. J. Obes. Relat. Metab. Disord.*, 21, 507, 1997.

Power, C., Manor, O., and Matthews, S., Child to adult socioeconomic conditions and obesity in a national cohort, *Int. J. Obes.*, 27, 1081, 2003.

Power, C. and Moynihan, C., Social class and changes in weight for height between childhood and early adulthood, *Int. J. Obes. Relat. Metab. Disord.*, 12, 445, 1988.

Prentice, A.M., Stable isotopes in nutritional science and the study of energy metabolism, *Scand. J. Nutr.*, 43, 56, 1999.

Prentice, A. and Jebb, S., Obesity in Britain: gluttony or sloth? *B.M.J.*, 311, 437, 1995.

Prentice, A.M. et al., Are current dietary guidelines for young children a prescription for overfeeding? *Lancet*, 2, 1066, 1988.

Price, J.H. et al., Pediatricians' perceptions and practice regarding childhood obesity, *Am. J. Prev. Med.*, 5, 95, 1989.

Proctor, M.H. et al., Television viewing and change in body fat from preschool to early adolescence: The Framingham Children's Study, *Int. J. Obes. Relat. Metab. Disord.*, Jul; 27(7), 827, 2003.

Prokopec, M. and Bellisle, F., Adiposity in Czech children followed from 1 month of age to adulthood: analysis of individual BMI patterns, *Ann. Hum. Biol.*, 699, 253, 1993.

Prokopec, M. and Bellisle, F., Body mass index variations from birth to adulthood in Czech Youths, *Acta Med. Auxol.*, 24, 87, 1992.

Puhl, J. et al., Children's Activity Rating Scale (CARS): description and calibration, *Res. Q. Exerc. Sport*, 61, 26, 1990.

Raben, A. et al., Decreased activity of fat-oxidizing enzymes in muscle of obesity prone subjects, *Int. J. Obes. Relat. Metab. Disord.*, 21, S43, 1997.

Radetti, G. et al., Growth hormone bioactivity, insulin-like growth factors (IGFs) and IGF binding proteins in obese children, *Metab. Clin. Exper.*, 47, 1490, 1998a.

Radetti, G. et al., Insulin pulsatility in obese and normal prepubertal children, *Hormone Res.*, 50, 78, 1998b.

Rahman, S.M. et al., Energy intake and expenditure of obese and non-obese Bangladeshi children, *Bangladesh Med. Res. Counc. Bull.*, 28, 54, 2002.

Ramachandran, A., et al., Prevalence of overweight in urban Indian adolescent schoolchildren, *Diabetes Res. Clin. Pract.*, 73, 3, 185, 2002.

Ramos De Marins, V.M., et al., Overweight and risk of overweight in schoolchildren in the city of Rio de Janeiro, Brazil: prevalence and characteristics, *Ann. Trop. Paediatr.*, 22, 2, 137, 2002.

Rand, C.S. and MacGregor, A.M., Adolescents having obesity surgery: a 6-year follow-up, *South. Med. J.*, 87, 1208, 1994.

Ravens-Sieberer, U., Redegeld, M., and Bullinger, M., Quality of life after in-patient rehabilitation in children with obesity, *Int. J. Obes. Relat. Metab. Disord.*, 25, S63, 2001.

Ray, R., Lim, L.H., and Ling, S.L., Obesity in preschool children: an intervention programme in primary health care in Singapore, *Ann. Acad. Med. Singapore*, 23, 335, 1994.

Reilly, J.J. et al., An objective method for measurement of sedentary behavior in 3- to 4-year olds, *Obes. Res.*, 11, 1155, 2003.

Reilly, J.J. et al., Total energy expenditure and physical activity in young Scottish children: mixed longitudinal study, *Lancet*, 363, 182, 2004.

Reinehr, T. and Andler, W., Thyroid hormones before and after weight loss in obesity, *Arch. Dis. Child.*, 87, 320, 2002.

Reinehr, T. et al., Nutritional knowledge of obese compared to non-obese children, *Nutr. Res.*, 23, 645, 2003.

Reybrouck, T. et al., Cardiorespiratory function during exercise in obese children, *Acta Paediatr. Scand.*, 76, 342, 1987.

Reybrouck, T. et al., Exercise therapy and hypocaloric diet in the treatment of obese children and adolescents, *Acta Paediatr. Scand.*, 79, 84, 1990.

Reybrouck, T. et al., Assessment of cardiorespiratory exercise function in obese children and adolescents by body mass-independent parameters, *Eur. J. Appl. Physiol.*, 75, 478, 1997.

Rice, T. et al., Familial aggregation of body mass index and subcutaneous fat measures in the longitudinal Quebec Family Study, *Genet. Epidemiol.*, 16, 316, 1999.

Richards, L.H., Regina, C.C., and Larson, R., Weight and eating concerns among pre- and young adolescent boys and girls, *J. Adolesc. Hlth. Care*, 11, 203, 1990.

Richardson, L.P. et al., A longitudinal evaluation of adolescent depression and adult obesity, *Arch. Pediatr. Adolesc. Med.*, 157, 739, 2003.

Riddiford-Harland, D.L., Steele, J.R., and Storlien, L.H., Does obesity influence foot structure in prepubescent children? *Int. J. Obes. Relat. Metab. Disord.*, 24, 541, 2000.

Riezzo, G., Chiloiro, M., and Guerra, V., Electrogastrography in healthy children: evaluation of normal value, influence of age, gender and obesity, *Dig. Dis. Sci.*, 43, 1646, 1998.

Riganti, G. et al., Diet composition in obese children and obesity related diseases, *Int. J. Obes. Relat. Metab. Disord.*, 17, S39, 1993.

Rippe, J.M. and Hesse, S., The role of physical activity in the prevention and management of obesity, *J. Am. Diet. Assoc.*, 90, S31, 1998.

Riva, P. et al., Obesity and autonomi function in adolescence, *Clin. Exp. Hypertens.*, 23, 57, 2001.

Roberts, S.B., Abnormalities of energy expenditure and the development of obesity, *Obes. Res.*, 3, 155, 1995.

Roberts, S.B. et al., Energy expenditure and intake in infants born to lean and over-weight mothers, *New Engl. J. Med.*, 318, 727, 1988.

Robertson, S.M. et al., Factors related to adiposity among children aged 3 to 7 years, *J. Am. Diet. Assoc.*, 99, 938, 1999.

Robinson, T.N., Reducing children's television viewing to prevent obesity: a random-ized controlled trial, *J. Am. Med. Assoc.*, 282, 1561, 1999.

Robinson, T.N. et al., Does television viewing increase obesity and reduce physical activity? Cross-sectional and longitudinal analyses among adolescent girls, *Pediatrics*, 91, 273, 1993.

Rocandio, A.M., Ansotegui, L., and Arroyo, M., Comparison of dietary intake among overweight and non-overweight schoolchildren, *Int. J. Obes. Relat. Metab. Disord.*, 25, 1651, 2001.

Rocchini, A.P. et al., Insulin and blood pressure during weight loss in obese adoles-cents, *Hypertension*, 10, 267, 1987.

Rocchini, A.P. et al., Blood pressure in obese adolescents: effect of weight loss, *Pedi-atrics*, 82, 16, 1988.

Rocchini, A.P. et al., The effect of weight loss on the sensitivity of blood pressure to sodium in obese adolescents, *New Engl. J. Med.*, 31, 321, 1989.

Roche, A.F. *Growth, Maturation and Body Composition: the Fels Longitudinal Study, 1929–1991*, Cambridge University Press, Cambridge, 1992.

Roche, A.F., Heymsfield, S.B., and Lohmans, T.G. (Eds.), *Human Body Composition, Methods and Findings*, Human Kinetics Publishers, Champaign, IL, 1996.

Rodin, J. and Larson, L., Social factors and the ideal body shape, in *Eating, Body Weight, and Performance in Athletes*, Brownell, K.D., Rodin, J., and Wilmore, J.H., Eds., Lea & Febiger, London, 1992, 7.

Rodriguez, G. et al., Determinants of resting energy expenditure in obese and non-obese children and adolescents, *J. Physiol. Biochem.*, 58, 9, 2002.

Roemmich, J.N. et al., Pubertal alterations in growth and body composition. V. Energy expenditure, adiposity, and fat distribution, *Am. J. Endocrinol. Metab.*, 279, E1426, 2000.

Roemmich, J.N. et al., Pubertal alterations in growth and body composition. VI. Pubertal insulin resistance: relation to adiposity, body fat distribution and hormone release, *Int. J. Obes. Relat. Metab. Disord.*, 26, 701, 2002.

Rolland-Cachera, M.F., Onset of obesity assessed from the weight/stature^2 curve in children: the need for a clear definition, *Int. J. Obes. Relat. Metab. Disord.*, 17, 245, 1993.

Rolland-Cachera, M.F., Prediction of adult body composition from infant and child measurements, in *Body Composition Techniques in Health and Disease*, Davies, P.S.W. and Cole, T.J., Eds., Cambridge University Press, Cambridge, 1995, 100.

Rolland-Cachera, M.F., Obesity among adolescents: evidence for the importance of early nutrition, in *Human Growth in Context*, Johnston, F.E., Zemel, B. and Eveleth, P.B., Eds., Smith-Gordon/Nishimura, London, 1999, 245.

Rolland-Cachera, M.F. and Bellisle, F., No correlation between adiposity and food intake: why are working class children fatter? *Am. J. Clin. Nutr.*, 44, 779, 1986.

Rolland-Cachera, M.F. and Bellisle, F., Timing weight-control measures in obese children, *Lancet*, 335, 918, 1990.

Rolland-Cachera, M.F. and Bellisle, F., Nutrition, in *Child and Adolescent Obesity*, Burniat, W. et al., Eds., Cambridge University Press, Cambridge, 2002, 65.

Rolland-Cachera, M.F., Bellisle, F. and Sempé, M., The prediction in boys and girls of the weight/height^2 index and various skinfold measurements in adults: a two-decade follow-up study, *Int. J. Obes.*, 13, 305, 1989.

Rolland-Cachera, M.F. and Deheeger, M., Fatness development in children born in 1955 or 1985: two longitudinal studies, *Int. J. Obes. Relat. Metab. Disord.*, 21, S140, 1997.

Rolland-Cachera, M.F. and Deheeger, M., Correlations between anthropometric indicators of abdominal fat and fatness indices in children, *Int. J. Obes. Relat. Metab. Disord.*, 22, S11, 1998

Rolland-Cachera, M.F., Deheeger, M., and Bellisle, F., Nutrient balance and body composition, *Reprod. Nutr. Dev.*, 37, 727, 1997.

Rolland-Cachera, M.F., Deheeger, M., and Bellisle, F., Definition and prevalence of obesity in children, *Cah. Nutr. Diet.*, 36, 108, 2001.

Rolland-Cachera, M.F., Deheeger, M., and Guilloud-Bataille, M., Tracking the development of adiposity from one month of age to adulthood, *Ann. Hum. Biol.*, 14, 219, 1987.

Rolland-Cachera, M.F., Spyckerelle, Y., and Deschamps, P.J., Evolution of pediatric obesity in France, *Int. J. Obes. Relat. Metab. Disord.*, 16, S5, 1992

Rolland-Cachera, M.F. et al., Adiposity indices in children, *Am. J. Clin. Nutr.*, 36, 178, 1982.

Rolland-Cachera, M.F. et al., Adiposity rebound in children: a simple indicator for predicting obesity, *Am. J. Clin. Nutr.*, 39, 129, 1984.

Rolland-Cachera, M.F. et al., Adiposity development and prediction during growth in humans: a two-decade follow-up study, in *Obesity in Europe*, John Libbey, London, 1988, 73.

Rolland-Cachera, M.F. et al., Influence of body fat distribution during childhood on body fat distribution in adulthood: a two-decade follow-up study, *Int. J. Obes. Relat. Metab. Disord.*, 14, 473, 1990a.

Rolland-Cachera, M.F. et al., Body mass index variations: centiles from birth to 87 years, *Eur. J. Clin. Nutr.*, 45, 13, 1990b.

Rolland-Cachera, M.F. et al., Variations of the body mass index in the French population from 0 to 87 years, in *Obesity in Europe*, Ailhaud, G., et al., Eds., John Libbey, London, 1991, 113.

Rolland-Cachera, M.F. et al., Influence of macronutrients on adiposity development: a follow-up study of nutrition and growth from 10 months to 8 years of age, *Int. J. Obes. Relat. Metab. Disord.*, 19, 573, 1995.

Rollnick, S., Behaviour change in practice: targeting individuals, *Int. J. Obes. Relat. Metab. Disord.*, 20, S22, 1996.

Romanella, N.E. et al., Physical activity and attitudes in lean and obese children and their mothers, *Int. J. Obes.*, 15, 407, 1991.

Rose, H.E. and Mayer, J., Activity, caloric intake, fat storage, and the energy balance of infants, *Pediatrics*, 41, 18, 1968.

Rosen, J., Gross, J., and Vara, L., Psychological adjustment of adolescents attempting to lose or gain weight, *J. Consult. Clin. Psychol.*, 55, 742, 1987.

Rosen, J.C., Body-image disturbance in eating disorders, in *Body Images: Development, Deviance, and Change*, Cash, T.F. and Pruzinsky, T., Eds., Guilford Press, New York, 1990, 190.

Rosskamp, R., Becker, M., and Zallet, M., Circulating somatostatin concentrations in childhood. Studies in normal weight and obese children and patients with growth hormone deficiency, *Monatsschr. Kinderheilkd.*, 134, 849, 1986.

Rössner, S., Television viewing, life style and obesity, *J. Intern. Med.*, 229, 301, 1991.

Rössner, S., Childhood obesity and adulthood consequences, *Acta Pediatr.*, 87, 1, 1998.

Rovillé-Sausse, F., Increase of the body mass of children born to Maghrebi immigrant parents, *Int. J. Obes. Relat. Metab. Disord.*, 22, S7, 1998.

Rowland, T.W., *Exercise and Children's Health,* Human Kinetics Publishers, Champaign, IL, 1990, 129.

Rowland, T.W., Effects of obesity on aerobic fitness in adolescent females, *Am. J. Dis. Child.*, 145, 764, 1991.

Rowlands, A.V. et al., Physical activity levels of Hong Kong Chinese children: relationship with body fat, *Pediatr. Exerc. Sci.*, 14, 286, 2002.

Rueda-Maza, C.M. et al., Total and exogenous carbohydrate oxidation in obese prepubertal children, *Am. J. Clin. Nutr.*, 64, 844, 1996.

Rummukainen, I. and Rasanen, L., Overweight and pubertal maturation in adolescent girls living in the Arctic region of Finland, *Scand. J. Nutr.*, 43, S41, 1999.

Ruxton, C.H.S. et al., Changes in height, weight and body fat in pre-pubescent Scottish children, *Int. J. Obes. Relat. Metab. Disord.*, 22, S5, 1998.

Rychlewski, T. et al., Complex evaluation of body reaction in obese boys with systematic physical exertion and a low energy diet, *Pol. Arch. Med. Wewn.*, 96, 344, 1996.

Saar, K. et al., Genome scan for childhood and adolescent obesity in German families, *Pediatrics*, 111, 321, 2003.

Sahota, P. et al., Apples: a school-based intervention to reduce obesity risks, *Int. J. Obes. Relat. Metab. Disord.*, 22, S62, 1998.

Sahota, P. et al., Randomised controlled trial of primary school based intervention to reduce risk factors for obesity, *Br. Med. J.*, 323, 1029, 2001.

Saito, K. and Tatsumi, M., Effect of dietary therapy in a school health program for obese children, *Nippon Koshu Eisei Zasshi*, 41, 693, 1994.

Saitoh, H. et al., Serum concentrations of insulin, insulin-like growth factor (IGF-1), IGF binding protein (IGFBP)-1 and -3 and growth hormone binding protein in obese children: fasting IGFBP-1 is suppressed in normoinsulinemic obese children, *Clin. Endocrinol.*, 48, 487, 1998.

Sakamoto, N. et al., A social epidemiologi study of obesity among preschool children in Thailand, *Int. J. Obes. Relat. Metab. Disord.*, 25, 389, 2001.

Salas-Salvado, J. et al., Influence of adiposity on the thermic effect of food and exercise in lean and obese adolescents, *Int. J. Obes. Relat. Disord.*, 17, 717, 1993.

Salbe, A.D., Nicolson, M., and Ravussin, E., Total energy expenditure and the level of physical activity correlate with plasma leptin concentrations in five-year-old children, *J. Clin. Invest.*, 99, 592, 1997.

Salbe, A.D. et al., Low levels of physical activity in 5-year-old children, *J. Pediatr.*, 131, 423, 1997.

Salbe, A.D. et al., Low levels of physical activity and time spent viewing television at 9 years of age predict weight gain 8 years later in Pima Indian children, *Int. J. Obes. Relat. Metab. Disord.*, 22, S10, 1998.

Sallis, J.F., A commentary on children and fitness: a public health perspective, *Res. Q. Exer. Sp.*, 58, 326, 1987.

Sallis, J.F., Self-report measures of children's physical activity, *J. School Hlth.*, 61, 215, 1991.

Sallis, J.F., Epidemiology of physical activity and fitness in children and adolescents, *Crit. Rev. Food Sci. Nutr.*, 33, 403, 1993.

Sallis, J.F. et al., Family variables and physical activity in preschool children, *J. Dev. Behav. Pediatr.*, 9, 57, 1988.

Sallis, J.F. et al., Project SPARK. Effects of physical education on adiposity in children, *Ann. N.Y. Acad. Sci.*, 699, 127, 1993.

Salvatoni, A. et al., Is blood pressure more related to insulin sensitivity or to body weight? *Int. J. Obes. Relat. Metab. Disord.*, 21, S140, 1997.

Sampei, M.A. et al., Comparison of the body mass index to other methods of body fat evaluation in ethnic Japanese and Caucasian adolescent girls, *Int. J. Obes.*, 25, 3, 400, 2001.

Sanchez-Carracedo, D., Saldana, C., and Domenech, J.M., Obesity, diet and restrained eating in a Mediterranean population, *Int. J., Obes. Relat. Metab. Disord.*, 20, 943, 1996.

Sardinha, L.B. et al., Receiver operating characteristic analysis of body mass index, triceps skinfold thickness, and arm girth for obesity screening in children and adolescents, *Am. J. Clin. Nutr.*, 70(6):1090, 1999.

Saris, W.H., Habitual physical activity in children: methodology and findings in health and disease, *Med. Sci. Sports. Exerc.*, 18, 253, 1986.

Sartorio, A. et al., Reference values for urinary growth hormone excretion in normally growing nonobese and obese children, *Int. J. Obes. Relat. Metab. Disord.*, 23, S118, 1999.

Sasaki, J. et al., A long-term aerobic exercise program decreases the obesity index and increases the high density lipoprotein cholesterol concentration in obese children, *Int. J. Obes.*, 11, 339, 1987.

Satter, E.M., Internal regulation and the evolution of normal growth as the basis for prevention of obesity in children, *J. Am. Diet Assoc.*, 96, 860, 1996.

Savoye, M. et al., Importance of plasma leptin in predicting future weight gain in obese children: a two-and-a-half-year longitudinal study, *Int. J. Obes. Relat. Metab. Disord.*, 26, 942, 2002.

Savva, S.C. et al., Obesity in children and adolescents in Cyprus. Prevalence and predisposing factors, *Int. J. Obes. Relat. Metab. Disord.*, 26, 1036, 2002.

Sawada, Y., On the body composition of obese children and in particular, sexual, age, and regional differences of skinfold thickness, *J. Hum. Ergol.*, 7, 103, 1978.

Sawaya, A.L. et al., Mild stunting is associated with higher susceptibility to the effects of high fat diets: studies in a shantytown population in São Paulo, Brazil, *J. Nutr.*, 128, S415, 1998.

Scaglioni, S. et al., The role of childhood diet in preventing adult obesity, *Int. J. Obes. Relat. Metab. Disord.*, 23, S6, 1999.

Scaglioni, S. et al., Early macronutrient intake and overweight at five years of age, *Int. J. Obes. Relat. Metab. Disord.*, 24, 777, 2000.

Schaefer, F. et al., Usefulness of bioelectric impedance and skinfold measurements in predicting fat-free mass derived from total body potassium in children, *Pediatr. Res.*, 35, 617, 1994.

Schaefer, F. et al., Body mass index and percentage fat mass in healthy German school children and adolescents, *Int. J. Obes. Relat Metab. Disord.*, 22, 461, 1998.

Schauble, N. et al., No evidence for involvement of the promoter polymorphism: 866 G/A of the UCP2 gene in childhood-onset obesity in humans, *Exp. Clin. Endocrinol. Diabetes*, 111, 73, 2003.

Scheuring, A.J.W. et al., Exercise and the regulation of energy intake, *Int. J. Obes. Relat. Metab. Disord.*, 23, S1, 1999.

Schilder, P. *The Image and Appearance of the Human Body: Studies in the Constructive Energies of the Psyche*, International Universities Press, New York, 1950.

Schlicker, S.A., Borra, S.T., and Regan, C., The weight and fitness of United States children, *Nutr. Rev.*, 52, 11, 1994.

Schmidinger, H. et al., Potential life-threatening cardiac arrythmias associated with conventional hypocaloric diet, *Int. J. Cardiol.*, 14, 55, 1987.

Schoeller, D.A., Limitations in the assessment of dietary energy intake by self-report, *Metabolism*, 44, 18, 1995.

Schoeller, D.A. et al., Energy requirements of obese children and young adults, *Proc. Nutr. Soc.*, 47, 241, 1988.

Schonegger, K. and Widhalm, K., Relationship between body fat measured by TOBEC and BMI in obese children and adolescents, *Int. J. Obes. Relat. Metab. Disord.*, 22, S12, 1998.

Schonfeld, W.A., Body image disturbance in adolescence, *Arch. Gen. Psychiatry*, 15, 6, 1966.

Schonfeld-Warden, N. and Warden, C.H., Pediatric obesity. An overview of etiology and treatment, *Pediatr. Clin. North Am.*, 44, 339, 1997.

Schontz, F.C. *Perceptual and Cognitive Aspects of Body Experience*, Academic Press, New York, 1969

Schutz, Y., The role of physical inactivity in the etiology of obesity, *Ther. Umsch.*, 46, 281, 1989.

Schutz, Y. et al., Whole-body protein turnover and resting energy expenditure in obese, prepubertal children, *Am. J. Clin. Nutr.*, 69, 857, 1999.

Schwingshandl, J. and Borkenstein, M., Changes in lean body mass in obese children during weight reduction program: effect of short term and long term outcome, *Int. J. Obes. Relat. Metab. Disord.*, 19, 752, 1995.

Schwingshandl, J. et al., Effect of an individualised training programme during weight reduction on body composition, *Arch. Dis. Child.*, 81, 426, 1999.

Segal, K.R. et al., Lean body mass estimated by bioelectrical impedance analysis: a four site cross-validation study, *Am. J. Clin. Nutr.*, 47, 7, 1988.

Sekine, M. et al., A dose–response relationship between short sleeping hours and childhood obesity: results of the Toyama birth cohort study, *Child Care Health Dev.*, 28, 163, 2002.

Seliger, V. et al., Activity patterns, smoking habits and somatometric variables of the Czechoslovak population, *Eur. J. Appl. Physiol.*, 39, 165, 1978.

Shalitin, S. and Phillip, M., Role of obesity and leptin in the pubertal process and pubertal growth, *Int. J. Obes. Relat. Metab. Disord.*, 27, 869, 2003.

Shea, S. et al., The rate of increase in blood pressure in children 5 years of age is related to changes in aerobic fitness and body mass index, *Pediatrics*, 94, 465, 1994.

Shear, C.L. et al., Secular trends of obesity in early life: the Bogalusa Heart Study, *Am. J. Pub. Hlth.*, 78, 75, 1988.

Shekhavat, P.S. et al., Neonatal cord blood leptin: its relationship to birth weight, body, mass index, maternal diabetes, and steroids, *Pediatr. Res.*, 43, 338, 1998.

Shephard, R.J. *Body Composition in Biological Anthropology, Cambridge Studies in Biological Anthropology 6*, Cambridge University Press, Cambridge, 1991.

Sichieri, R., Siqueira, K.S., and Moura, A.S., Obesity and abdominal fatness associated with undernutrition early in life in a survey in Rio de Janeiro, *Int. J. Obes. Relat. Metab. Disord.*, 24, 614, 2000.

Siegfried, W. et al., Follow-up of severely obese adolescents after long-term inpatient treatment, *Int. J. Obes. Relat. Metab. Disord.*, 22, S63, 1998.

Siervogel, R.M. et al., Patterns of changes in weight/stature^2 from 2 to 18 years: findings from long-term serial data for children in the Fels longitudinal study, *Int. J. Obes. Relat. Metab. Disord.*, 15, 479, 1991.

Sigman-Grant, M., Zimmerman, S., and Kris-Etherton, P.M., Dietary approaches for reducing fat intake of preschool-age children, *Pediatrics*, 91, 955, 1993.

Silberstein, L. et al., Behavioural and psychological implications of body dissatisfaction: do men and women differ? *Sex Roles*, 19, 219, 1988.

Simmons, R.G., Blyth, D.A., and McKinney, K.L., The social and psychological effects of puberty on white females, in *Girls at Puberty: Biological and Psychosocial Perspectives*, Brooks-Gunn, J. and Petersen, A.C., Eds., Plenum, New York, 1983, 229.

Simon, J.A. et al., Correlates of high-density lipoprotein cholesterol in black and white girls: the NHLBI Growth and Health Study, *Am. J. Public Health*, 85, 1698, 1995.

Simons-Morton, B.G. et al., Children's frequency of participation in moderate to vigorous physical activities, *Res. Q. Exer. Sport*, 61, 307, 1990.

Sinaiko, A.R. et al., Insulin resistance syndrome in childhood: associations of the euglycemic insulin clamp and fasting insulin with fatness and other risk factors, *J. Pediatr.* 139, 700, 2001.

Singhal, A. et al., Programming of lean body mass: a link between birth weight, obesity, and cardiovascular disease? *Am. J. Clin. Nutr.*, 77, 726, 2003.

Sinha, R. et al., Assessment of skeltal muscle triglyceride content by 1H nuclear mgnetic resonance spectroscopy in lean and obese adolescents: relationship to insulin sensitivity, total body fat, and central adiposity, *Diabetes*, 51, 1022, 2002.

Skamenová, B. and Pařízková, J., Assessment of disproportional (spiderlike) and diffuse type of obesity by measurement of the total and subcutaneous body fat, *Čas. Lěkčes.*, CII, 142, 1963 (in Czech).

Skinner, J.S. *Exercise Testing and Exercise Prescription for Special Cases*, Lea & Febiger, Philadelphia, 1987.

Sklad, M., Similarity of movements in twins, *Wychowanie Fyziczne i Sport*, 3, 119, 1972.

Slade, P.D. and Russell, G.F.M., Awareness of body dimensions in anorexia nervosa: cross-sectional and longitudinal studies, *Psycholog. Med.*, 3, 188, 1973.

Smiciklas-Wright, H. et al., Foods commonly eaten in the United States. 1989–1991 and 1994–1996: are portion sizes changing? *J. Am. Diet. Assoc.*, 103, 41, 2003.

Smith, J.C. et al., Use of body mass index to monitor treatment of obese adolescents, *J. Adolesc. Hlth.* 20, 466, 1997.

Smolak, L., Levine, M.P., and Gralen, S., The impact of puberty and dating on eating problems among middle school girls, *J. Youth Adolesc.*, 22, 355, 1993.

Sohlström, A., Wahlund, L.O., and Forsum, E., Adipose tissue distribution as assessed by magnetic resonance imaging and total body fat by magnetic resonance imaging, underwater weighing and body-water dilution in healthy women, *Am. J. Clin. Nutr.*, 58, 830, 1993.

Somerville, S.M., Rona, R.J., and Chinn, S., Obesity and respiratory symptoms in primary school, *Arch. Dis. Child.*, 59, 940, 1984.

Šonka, J. et al., Hormonal and metabolic adaptation to a reducing regimen in children, *Acta Univ. Carolinae*, 39, 33, 1993.

Sorensen, T.I.A., Role of genes in the global epidemic of obesity, *Scand. J. Nutr.*, 43, 15S, 1999.

Sorensen, T.I.A. and Lund-Sorensen, I.L., Genetic–epidemiological studies of causes of obesity, *Nord. Med.*, 106, 182, 1991 (in Danish).

Sorof, J. and Daniels, S., Obesity hypertension in children: a problem of epidemic proportions, *Hypertension*, 40, 441, 2002.

Sorof, J.M. et al., Isolated systolic hypertension, obesity, and hyperkinetic hemodynamic states in children, *J. Pediatr.*, 140, 660, 2002.

Sothern, M.S. et al., An effective multidisciplinary approach to weight reduction in youth, *Ann. N.Y. Acad. Sci.*, 699, 292, 1993.

Sothern, M. et al., The impact of mild, moderate and severe obesity on upper and lower bone mineral content, lean and fat body mass, *Int. J. Obes. Relat. Metab. Disord.*, 22, S198, 1998.

Sothern, M.S. et al., Motivating the obese child to move: the role of structured exercise in pediatric weight management, *South. Med. J.*, 92, 577, 1999.

Sothern, M.S. et al., Inclusion of resistance exercise in a multidisciplinary outpatient treatment program for preadolescent obese children, *South. Med. J.*, 92, 585, 1999.

Sothern, M.S. et al., Lipid profiles of obese children and adolescents before and after significant weight loss: differences according to sex, *South. Med. J.*, 93, 278, 2000.

Sothern, M.S. et al., Safety, feasibility, and efficacy of a resistance training program in preadolescent obese children, *Am. J. Med. Sci.*, 319, 370, 2000.

Southam, M.A. et al., A summer day camp approach to adolescent weight loss, *Adolescence*, 19, 855, 1984.

Specker, B.L. et al., Total bone mineral content and tibial cortical bone measures in preschool children, *J. Bone Miner. Res.*, 16, 12, 2298, 2001.

Spieth, L.E. et al., A low-glycemic index diet in the treatment of pediatric obesity, *Arch. Pediatr. Adolesc. Med.*, 154, 947, 2000.

Spring, B. et al., Obesity: idealized or stigmatized? Sociocultural influences on the meaning and prevalence of obesity, in *Exercise and Obesity*, Hills, A.P. and Wahlqvist, M.L., Eds., Smith-Gordon, London, 1994, 49.

Šprynarová, S. *Biological Basis of Physical Fitness*, Universita Karlova, Prague, 1984 (in Czech).

Srinivasan, S.R., Mayers, L., and Berenson, G.S., Rate of change in adiposity and its relationship to concomitant changes in cardiovascular risk variables among biracial (black–white) children and young adults: the Bogalusa Heart Study, *Metab. Clin. Exp.*, 50, 299, 2001.

Srinivasan, S.R., Moyers, L., and Berenson, G.S., Predictability of childhood adiposity and insulin for developing insulin resistance syndrome (syndrome X) in young adulthood: the Bogalusa Heart Study, *Diabetes*, 51, 204, 2002.

Stallings, V.A. et al., One-year follow-up of weight, total body potassium, and total nitrogen in obese adolescents treated with the protein sparing modified fast, *Am. J. Clin. Nutr.*, 48, 91, 1988.

Stallings, V.A. and Pencharz, P.B., The effect of high protein low-calorie diet on the energy expenditure of obese adolescents, *Eur. J. Clin. Nutr.*, 46, 897, 1992.

Stang, J., Bayerl, C.T., Position of the American Dietetic Association: child and adolescent food nutrition programs, *J. Am. Diet. Assoc.*, 103, 7, 887, 2003.

Stanimirova, N., Petrova, C., and Stanimirov, S., Frequency and characteristics of obesity during the different periods of childhood, *Int. J. Obes. Relat. Metab. Disord.*, 17, S39, 1993.

Stanton, R. and Hills, A.P., *A Matter of Fat*, University of NSW Press, Sydney, 2004.

Stefan, N. et al., Plasma adiponectin concentrations in children: relationships with obesity and insulinemia, *J. Clin. Endocrinol. Metab.*, 87, 4652, 2002.

Stehling, O. et al., Leptin reduces juvenile fat stores by altering the circadian cycle of energy expenditure, *Am. J. Physiol.*, 271, R1170, 1997.

Stein, D.M. and Riechert, P., Extreme dieting behaviors in early adolescence, *J. Early Adolesc.*, 10, 108, 1990.

Steinbeck, K.S. et al., Leptin as a predictor of weight gain in prepubertal children, *Int. J. Obes. Relat. Metab. Disord.*, 22, S200, 1998.

Steinbeck, K.S. et al., Low-density lipoproteine subclasses in children under 10 years of age, *J. Pediatr. Child Health*, 37, 550, 2001.

Stensel, D.J., Lin, F.P., and Nevill, A.M., Resting metabolic rate in obese and nonobese Chinese Singaporean boys aged 13–15 y, *Am. J. Clin. Nutr.*, 74, 369, 2001.

Stephen, A.M. and Sieber, G.M., Trends in individual fat consumption in the UK 1900-1985, *Br. J. Nutr.*, 71, 775, 1994.

Stern, J.S., Is obesity a disease of inactivity? in *Eating and its Disorders*, Stunkard, A.J. and Stellar, E., Eds., Raven Press, New York, 1983.

Sterpa, A. et al., Changes of the lipid and protein profile in the obese child in diet therapy (with and without added fiber), *Pediatr. Med. Chir.*, 7, 419, 1985.

Stettler, N. et al., Prevalence and risk factors for overweight and obesity in children from Seychelles, a country in rapid transition: the importance of early growth, *Int. J. Obes. Relat. Metab. Disord.*, 26, 214, 2002.

Stevens, J., Ethnic-specific revisions of body mass index cut-offs to define overweight and obesity in Asians are not warranted, *Int. J. Obes. Relat. Metab. Disord.*, 27, 1297, 2003.

Stevens, J. et al., Comparison of attitudes and behaviors related to nutrition, body size, dieting, and hunger in Russia, black–American, and white–American adolescents, *Obes. Res.*, 5, 227, 1997.

Stewart, K.J. et al., Physical fitness, physical activity, and fatness in relation to blood pressure and lipids in preadolescent children. Results from the FRESH Study, *J. Cardiopulm. Rehabil.*, 15, 122, 1995.

Štich, V. et al., Endurance training increases the β-adrenergic lipolytic response in subcutaneous adipose tissue in obese subjects, *Int. J. Obes. Relat. Metab. Disord.*, 23, 374, 1999.

Stichel, H., D'Allemand, D., and Gruters, A., Thyroid function and obesity in children and adolescents, *Horm. Res.*, 54, 14, 2000.

Stock, M. and Rothwell, N. *Obesity and Leanness*, John Wiley, London, 1982.

Stolley, M.R. et al., Hip-Hop to health Jr., an obesity prevention program for minority preschool children baseline: baseline characteristics of participants, *Prev. Med.*, 36, 320, 2003.

St-Onge, M.P., Keller, K.L., and Heymsfield, S.B., Changes in childhood food consumption patterns: a cause for concern in light of increasing body weight, *Am. J. Clin. Nutr.*, 78, 1068, 2003.

Story, M. et al., The epidemic of obesity in American Indian communities and the need for childhood obesity-prevention programs, *Am. J. Clin. Nutr.*, 69, 747S, 1999.

Strauss, R.S., Comparison of serum concentration of alpha-tocopherol and beta-carotene in a cross-sectional sample of obese and nonobese children (NHANES III), *J. Pediatr.*, 124, 160, 1999.

Strauss, R.S., Effects of intrauterine environment on childhood growth, *Br. Med. Bull.*, 53, 81, 1997.

Strauss, R.S. and Knight, J., Influence of the home environment on the development of obesity in children, *Pediatrics*, 103, E851, 1999.

Strauss, R.S. and Mir, H.M., Smoking and weight loss attempts in overweight and normal-weight adolescents, *Int. J. Obes. Relat. Metab. Disord.*, 25, 1381, 2001.

Strauss, R.S. and Pollack, H.A., Social marginalization of overweight children, *Arch. Pediatr. Adolesc. Med.*, 157, 746, 2003.

Streigel-Moore, R.H. et al., A prospective study of disordered eating among college students, *Int. J. Eating Disord.*, 8, 499, 1989.

Stunkard, A.J., Obesity: risk factors, consequences and control, *Med. J. Aust.*, 148, S21, 1988.

Stunkard, A.J., Perspectives on human obesity, in *Perspectives in Behavioral Medicine: Eating, Sleeping and Sex*, Stunkard, A.J. and Baum, A., Eds., Hillsdale, NJ, 1989, 9.

Stunkard, A.J., Faith, M.S., and Allison, K.C., Depression and obesity, *Biol. Psychiatry*, 54, 330, 2003.

Stunkard, A.J. and Messick, S., The three-factor eating questionnaire to measure dietary restraint, disinhibition and hunger. *J.Psychosom. Res.* 29, 71, 1985.

Stunkard, A.J. et al., Weights of parents and infants: is there a relationship?, *Int. J. Obes. Relat. Metab. Disord.*, 23, 159, 1999.

Sturney, P. and Slade, P.D., Body image and obesity, a critical psychological perspective, in *Handbook of Eating Disorders, Part 2*, Burrows, G.D., Beumont, P.J.V., and Casper, R.C., Eds., Elsevier, Amsterdam, 1988.

Subash, B.D. and Chuttani, C.S., Indices of nutritional status derived from body weight and height among school children, *Ind. J. Pediatr.*, 45, 289, 1978.

Subramanyam, V., Jayashree, R., and Rafi, M., Prevalence of overweight in affluent adolescent girls in Chennai in 1981 and 1998, *Indian Pediatr.*, 40, 775, 2003a.

Subramanyam, V., Jayashree, R., and Rafi, M., Prevalence of overweight and obesity in affluent adolescent girls in Chennai in 1981 and 1998, *Indian Pediatr.*, 40, 332, 2003b.

Sudi, K.M. et al., Insulin and insulin resistance index are not independent determinants for the variation in leptin in obese children and adolescents, *J. Pediatr. Endocrinol. Metab.*, 13, 923, 2000a.

Sudi, K.M. et al., No relationship between leptin and cortisol in obese children and adolescents, *J. Pediatr. Endocrinol. Metab.*, 13, 913, 2000b.

Sudi, K.M. et al., The relationship between different subcutaneous adipose tissue layers, fat mass and leptin in obese children and adolescents, *J. Pediatr. Endocrinol. Metab.*, 13, 505, 2000c.

Sudi, K.M. et al., Relationship between different subcutaneous adipose tissue layers, fat mass, and leptin in response to short-term energy restriction in obese girls, *Am. J. Hum. Biol.*, 12, 803, 2000d.

Sudi, K.M. et al., Relationship between plasminogen activator inhibitor-1 antigen, leptin, and fat mass in obese children and adolescents, *Metab. Clin. Exp.*, 49, 890, 2000e.

Sudi, K.M. et al., No evidence for leptin as an independent associate of blood pressure in childhood and juvenile obesity, *J. Pediatr. Endocrinol. Metab.*, 13, 513, 2000f.

Sudi, K.M. et al., Interrelationship between estimates of adiposity and body fat distribution with metabolic and haemostatic parameters in obese children, *Metab. Clin. Exp.*, 50, 681, 2001a.

Sudi, K.M. et al., The influence of weight loss on fibrinoplytic and metabolic parameters in obese children and adolescents, *J. Pediatr. Endocrinol. Metab.*, 14, 85, 2001b.

Sudi, K.M. et al., The effects of changes in body mass and subcutaneous fat on the improvement in metabolic risk factors in obese children after short-term weight loss, *Metab. Clin. Exp.*, 50, 1323, 2001c.

Sugimori, H. et al., Temporal course of the development of obesity in Japanese obese children: a cohort study based on the Keio Study, *J. Pediat.*, 134, 749, 1999.

Sundaram, K.R., Ahuja, R.K., and Ramachandran, K., Indices of physical build, nutrition and obesity in school children, *Indian J. Pediatr.*, 55, 889, 1988.

Sung, R.Y.T. et al., Measurement of body fat using leg to leg bioimpedance, *Arch. Dis. Child.*, 85, 263, 2001.

Sung, R.Y.T. et al., Effects of dietary intervention and strength training on blood lipid level in obese children, *Arch. Dis. Child.*, 86, 407, 2002.

Sunnegardh, J. et al., Physical activity in relation to energy intake and body fat in 8- and 13-year-old children in Sweden, *Acta Paediatr. Scand.*, 75, 955, 1986.

Suskind, R.M. et al., Recent advances in the treatment of childhood obesity, *Ann. N.Y. Acad. Sci.*, 699, 181, 1993.

Suskind, R. et al., Recent advances in the treatment of childhood obesity, *Pediatr. Diabetes*, 1, 23, 2000.

Suttapreyasri, D. et al., Weight-control training models for obese pupils in Bangkok, *J. Med. Assoc. Thai.*, 73, 394, 1990.

Su-Youn-Nam, and Marcus, C., Growth hormone and adipocyte function in obesity, *Horm. Res.*, 53, 87, 2000.

Suzuki, M. and Tatsumi, M., Effect of therapeutic exercise on physical fitness in a school health program for obese children, *Nippon Koshu Eisei Zasshi*, 40, 17, 1993 (in Japanese).

Sveger, T. et al., Apolipoproteins A-I and B in obese children, *J. Pediatr. Gastroenterol. Nutr.*, 9, 497, 1989.

Swinburn, B. and Ravussin, E., Energy balance or fat balance? *Am. J. Clin. Nutr.*, 57, S766, 1993.

Takadoro, M. et al., Analysis of beta3-adrenergic receptor gene polymorphism using noninvasive samples obtained at scheduled infant health checkups, *Environ. Health. Prev. Med.*, 4, 190, 2000.

Takahashi, E. et al., Influence factors on the development of obesity in 3-year-old children based on the Toyama study, *Prev. Med.*, 28, 293, 1999.

Takamura, M. et al., Change in infantile obesity among the population of Beijing in 1997: comparison with the data of major Chinese cities in 1985, 1986, *Int. J. Obes. Relat. Metab. Disord.*, 22, S204, 1998.

Tamiya, N., Study of physical fitness in children, and its application to pediatric clinics and sports medicine, *Hokkaido Igaku Zasshi*, 66, 849, 1991 (in Japanese).

Tamura, A., Mori, T., and Komiyama, A., Unfavorable lipid profiles in mild obesity with excess body fat percentage, *Pediatr. Int.*, 42, 8, 2000.

Tamura, A. et al., Preperitoneal fat thickness in childhood obesity: association with serum insulin concentration, *Pediatr. Int.*, 42(2), 155, 2000.

Tanaka, T. et al., Association between birthweight and body mass index at 3 years of age, *Pediatr. Int.*, 43, 641, 2001.

Tang, R.B. et al., Pulmonary function during exercise in obese children, *Chin. Med. J. Taipei*, 64, 403, 2001.

Tang, R.B. et al., Cardiopulmonary response in obese children using treadmill exercise testing, *Chin. Med. J. Taipei*, 65, 79, 2002.

Tanner, J.M., Whitehouse, R.H., and Takaishi, M., Standards from birth to maturity for height, weight, height velocity and weight velocity: British children, *Arch. Dis. Childh.*, 41, Part I, 1966.

Tanoffsky-Kraff, M. et al., Eating-disordered behaviors, body fat, and psychopathology in overweight and normal-weight children, *J. Consult Clin. Psychol.*, 72, 53, 2004.

Tao, X.Y. and Segaloff, D.L., Functional characterization of melanocortin-4 receptor mutations associated with childhood obesity, *Endocrinology*, 144, 4544, 2003.

Taras, H.L. et al., Television's influence on children's diet and physical activity, *J. Dev. Behav. Pediatr.*, 10, 176, 1989.

Tasevska, N. et al., Prevalence of overweight and obesity in school-aged children, *Scand. J. Nutr.*, 43, S46, 1999.

Taubes, G., As obesity rates rise, experts struggle to explain why, *Science*, 280, 1367, 1998.

Taylor, R.W. et al., Gender differences in body fat content are present well before puberty, *Int. J., Obes. Relat. Metab. Disord.*, 21, 1082, 1997.

Taylor, R.W. et al., Body fat percentages measured by dual-energy x-ray absorptiometry corresponding to recently recommended body mass cutoffs for overweight and obesity in children and adolescents aged 3–18 y, *Am. J. Clin. Nutr.*, 76, 1416, 2002.

Taylor, R.W. et al., Identifying adolescents with high percentage body fat: a comparison of BMI cutoffs using age and stage of pubertal development compared with BMI cutoff using age alone, *Eur. J. Clin. Nutr.*, 57, 764, 2003.

Taylor, W. and Baranowski, T., Physical activity, cardiovascular fitness, and adiposity in children, *Res. Q.Exerc. Sport*, 62, 157, 1991.

Terrier, P., Aminian, K., and Schutz, Y., Can accelerometry accurately predict energetic cost of walking in uphill and downhill conditions? *Int. J. Obes. Relat. Metab. Disord.*, 23, 1999.

Tershakovec, A.M., Weller, S.C., and Gallagher, P.R., Obesity, school performance and behavior of black, urban elementary school children, *Int. J. Obes. Relat. Metab. Disord.*, 18, 323, 1994.

Tershakonec, A.M. et al., Age, sex, ethnicity, body composition, and resting energy exoenditure of obese African American and white children and adolescents, *Am. J. Clin. Nutr.*, 75, 867, 2002a.

Tershakovec, A.M. et al., Persistent hypercholesterolemia is associated with the development of obesity among girls: the Bogalusa Heart Study, *Am. J. Clin. Nutr.*, 76, 730, 2002b.

Thakur, N. and D'Amico, F., Relationship of nutrition knowledge and obesity in adolescence, *Fam. Med.*, 31, 122, 1999.

Theriot, J.A. et al., Childhood obesity: a risk factor for omental torsion, *Pediatrics*, 112, e460, 2003.

Thomas-Dobersen, D.A., Butler-Simon, N., and Fleshner, M., Evaluation of a weight management intervention program in adolescents with insulin-dependent diabetes mellitus, *J. Am. Diet. Assoc.*, 93, 535, 1993.

Thompson, J.K., Larger than life, *Psychol. Today*, April 20 and 28, 1986.

Thompson, J.K., Penner, L.A., and Altabe, M., Procedures, problems, and progress in the assessment of body images, in *Body Images: Development, Deviance, and Changes*, Cash, T.F. and Pruzinsky, T., Eds., Guilford Press, New York, 1990, 21.

Thompson, J.K. and Thompson, C.M., Body size distortion and self-esteem in asymptomatic, normal weight males and females, *Int. J. Eating Disord.*, 5, 1061, 1986.

Thompson, J.L., Energy balance in young athletes, *Int. J. Sport. Nutr.*, 8, 160, 1998.

Thompson, O.M. et al., Food purchased away from home as a predictor of change in BMI z-score among girls, *Int. J. Obes. Relat. Metab. Disord.*, 28, 282, 2004.

Thomsen, B.I., Ekstrom, C.T., and Sorensen, T.I.A., Development of the obesity epidemic in Denmark: cohort, time and age effects among boys born 1930–1975, *Int. I. Obes. Relat. Metab. Disord.*, 23, 693, 1999.

Thoren, C. et al., The influence of training on physical fitness in healthy children with chronic diseases, in *Current Aspects of Perinatology & Physiology of Children*, Linnewaeh, C., Ed. Springer, Berlin, 1973.

Thornton, B. and Ryckman, R.M., Relationship between physical attractiveness, physical effectiveness, and self-esteem: a cross-sectional analysis among adolescents, *J. Adolesc.*, 14, 85, 1991.

Tichet, J. et al., Android fat distribution by age and sex. The waist–hip ratio, *Diabet. Metab.*, 19, 273, 1993.

Torok, K. and Molnar, D., Physical fitness in obese adolescents with multimetabolic syndrome, *Int. J. Obes. Relat. Metab. Disord.*, 23, Suppl. 5, S118, 1999.

Toschke, A.M. et al., Overweight and obesity in 6- to 14-year old children in 1991: protective effect of breast-feeding, *J. Pediatr.*, 141, 764, 2002.

Toschke, A.M. et al., Early intrauterine exposure to tobacco-inhaled products and obesity, *Am. J. Epidemiol.*, 156, 1068, 2003.

Tounian, P. et al., Resting energy expenditure and food-induced thermogenesis in obese children, *J. Pediatr. Gastroenterol. Nutr.*, 16, 451, 1993.

Tounian, P. et al., Presence of increased stiffness of the common carotid artery and endothelial dysfunction in severely obese children: a prospective study, *Lancet*, 358, 1400, 2001.

Tounian, P. et al., Resting energy expenditure and substrate utilization rate in children with constitutional leanness or obesity, *Clin. Nutr.*, 22, 353, 2003.

Toyran, M., Ozmert, E., and Yurdakok, K., Television viewing on physical health of schoolage children, *Turk. J. Pediatr.*, 44, 194, 2002.

Travers, S.H. et al., Insulin-like growth factor binding protein-I levels are strongly associated with insulin sensitivity and obesity in early pubertal children, *J. Clin. Endocrinol. Metab.*, 83, 1935, 1998.

Tremblay, A., Doucet, E., and Imbeault, P., Physical activity and weight maintenance, *Int. J. Obes. Relat. Metab. Disord.*, 23, S50, 1999.

Tremblay, M.S. and Willms, J.D., Is the Canadian childhood obesity epidemic related to physical inactivity? *Int. J. Obes.*, 27, 1100, 2003.

Tremblay, A. et al., Long-term adiposity changes are related to a glucocorticoid receptor polymorphism in young females, *J. Clin. Endocrinol. Metab.*, 88, 3141, 2003

Treuth, M.S., Butte, N.F., and Herrick, R., Skeletal muscle energetics assessed by 31P-NMR in prepubertal girls with a familial predisposition to obesity, *Int. J. Obes. Relat. Metab. Disord.*, 25, 1300, 2001.

Treuth, M.S. et al., Fitness and energy expenditure after strength training in obese prepubertal girls, *Med. Sci. Sports Exerc.*, 30, 1130, 1998.

Treuth, S.M. et al., Familial resemblance of body composition in prepubertal girls and their biological parents, *Am. J. Clin. Nutr.*, 74, 529, 2001.

Troiano, R.P. et al., Overweight prevalence and trend for children and adolescents, *Arch. Pediatr. Adolesc. Med.*, 149, 1085, 1995.

Trost, S.G. et al., Physical activity and determinants of physical activity in obese and non-obese children, *Int. J. Obes. Relat. Metab. Disord.*, 25, 822, 2001.

Trost, S.G., et al., Physical activity in overweight and nonoverweight preschool children, *Int. J. Obes. Relat. Metab. Disord.*, 27, 7, 834, 2003.

Trudeau, F. et al., BMI in the Trois-Rivieres study: child–adult and child–parent relationships, *Ann. J. Human. Biol.*, 15, 187, 2003.

Tsukuda, T. et al., Relationship of childhood obesity to adult obesity: a 20-year longitudinal study from birth in Ishikawa Prefecture, Japan, *Nippon Koshu EiseiZasshi*, 50, 1125, 2003 (in Japanese).

Tsukuda, T. and Shiraki, K., Excessive food aversion, compulsive exercise and decreased height gain due to fear of obesity in a prepubertal girl, *Psychother. Psychosom.*, 62, 203, 1994.

Tucker, L.A., Seljaas, G.T., and Hager, R.L., Body fat percentage of children varies according to their diet composition, *J. Am. Diet. Assoc.*, 97, 981, 1997.

Tudor-Locke, C., Ainsworth, B.E., and Adair, L.S., Physical activity and inactivity in Chinese school-aged youth: the China Health and Nutrition Survey, *Int. J. Obes. Relat. Metab. Disord.*, 27, 1093, 2003.

Tudor-Locke, C. et al., Comparison of pedometer and accelerometer measures of free-living physical activity, *Med. Sci. Sports Exerc.*, 34, 2045, 2002a.

Tudor-Locke, C. et al., Omission of active commuting to school and the prevalence of children's health-related physical activity levels: the Russian Longitudinal Monitoring Study, *Child Care Hlth. Dev.*, 28, 507 2002b.

Tulio, S., Egle, S., and Greilly, B., Blood pressure response to exercise of obese and lean hypertensive and normotensive male adolescents, *J. Hum. Hypertens.*, 9, 953, 1995.

Turconi, G. et al., Adolescent Body Mass Index data: what differences result us from different reference standard curves? *Ann. Ig.*, 5, 601, 2003 (in Italian).

Turnbull, A. et al., Changes in body mass index in 11–12-year-old children in Hawkes Bay, New Zealand (1989-2000), *J. Pediatr. Child Health*, 40, 33, 2004.

Turnin, M.C. et al., Learning good eating habits by playing computer games at school: perspectives for education of obese children, *Int. J. Obes. Relat. Metab. Disord.*, 22, S62, 1998.

Tyrell, V.J. et al., Foot-to-foot bioelectrical impedance analysis: a valuable tool for the measurement of body composition in children, *Int. J. Obes. Relat. Metab. Disord.*, 25, 273, 2001.

Ulanova, L.N. et al., Role of therapeutic physical exercise in the combined treatment of children with obesity, *Pediatriia*, 4, 66, 1985 (in Russian).

Unger, R., Kreeger, L., and Christoffel, K.K., Childhood obesity. Medical and familial correlates and age of onset, *Clin. Pediatr.*, 29, 368, 1990.

Urbina, E.M. et al., Association of fasting blood sugar level, insulin level, and obesity with left ventricular mass in healthy children and adolescents. The Bogalusa Heart Study, I, *Am. Heart J.*, 138, 122, 1999.

Urhammer, S.A. et al., Studies of the synergistic effect of the Trp/Arg64 polymorphism of the β3-adrenergic receptor gene and the -3826 A-®G variant of the uncoupling protein-1 gene on features of obesity and insulin resistance in a population-based sample of 379 young Danish subjects, *J. Clin. Endocrionl. Metab.*, 85, 3151, 2000.

Utter, J. et al., Couch potatoes and French fries: are sedentary behaviors associated with body mass index, physical activity, and dietary behaviors among adolescents? *J. Am. Diet. Assoc.*, 103, 1298, 2003.

Uysal, F.K. et al., Breast milk leptin: its relationship to maternal and infant adiposity, *Clin. Nutr.*, 21, 157, 2002.

Vague, J., Degree of masculine differentiation of obesities: a factor determining predisposition to diabetes, atherosclerosis, gout and uric calculus disease, *Am. J. Clin. Nutr.*, 4, 20, 1956.

Valle, M. et al., Infantile obesity: a situation of atherothrombotic risk? *Metab. Clin. Exp.*, 49, 672, 2000.

Valli-Jaakola, K.M. et al., Identification and characterization of melanocortin-4 receptor gene mutations in morbidly obese Finnish children and adults, *J. Clin. Endocrinol. Metab.*, 89, 940, 2004.

Valoski, A. and Epstein, L.H., Nutrient intake of obese children in a family-based behavioral weight control program, *Int. J. Obes.*, 14, 667, 1990.

Vamberová, M., Pařízková, J., and Vanková, M., Vegetative reaction to optimal work load as related to body weight and composition in adolescent boys and girls, *Physiol. Bohemoslov.*, 20, 415, 1971.

Van Baak, M.A., Exercise training and substrate utilization in obesity, *Int. J. Obes. Relat. Metab. Disord.*, 23, S3, S11, 1999.

Van Gaal, L.F. et al., Clinical endocrinology of human leptin, *Int. J. Obes. Relat. Metab. Disord.*, 23, 29, 1999.

Van Mil, E.G.A.H., Goris, A.H.C., and Westerterp, K.R., Physical activity and the prevention of childhood obesity: Europe versus the United States, *Int. J. Obes. Relat. Metab. Disord.*, 23, S41, 1999.

Van Poppel, G. et al., Socioeconomic differences in nutrition and nutritional status in 10–11-year-old boys, *Ned. Tijdschr. Geneeskd.*, 133, 1223, 1989 (in Dutch).

Vanderschueren-Lodeweyck, M., The effect of simple obesity on growth and growth hormone, *Horm. Res.*, 40, 23, 1993.

Vander-Wal, J.S. and Thelen, M.H., Eating and body image concerns among obese and average-weight children, *Addict Behav.*, 25, 775, 2000.

Vandewater, E.A., Shim, M.S., and Caplowitz, A.G., Linking obesity and activity level with children's television and video game use, *J. Adolesc.*, 27, 71, 2004.

Vanhala, M. et al., Relation between obesity from childhood to adulthood and the metabolic syndrome: population-based study, *B.M.J.*, 317, 319,1998.

Vara, L. and Agras, S., Caloric intake and activity levels are related in young children, *Int. J. Obes.*, 13, 613, 1989.

Vasunaga, T. et al., Nutrition related hormonal changes in obese children, *Endocr. J.*, 45, 221, 1998.

Vedhuis, J.D. and Iranmanesh, A., Physiological regulation of the human growth hormone (GH), insulin-like growth factor type I (IGF-I) axis: predominant impact of age, obesity, gonadal function and sleep, *Sleep*, 19, S221, 1996.

Vermorel, M. et al., Variability of physical activity and energy expenditure in adolescents: which consequences on occurrence of obesity? *Int. J. Obes. Relat. Metab. Disord.*, 22, S8, 1998.

Verrotti, A. et al., Leptin levels in non-obese and obese children and young adults with type I diabetes mellitus, *Eur. J. Endocrinol.*, 139, 49, 1998.

Vido, L. et al., Childhood obesity treatment: double blind trial on dietary fibres (gluconnan) versus placebo, *Pediatr. Padol.*, 28, 133, 1993.

Vígnerová, J. et al., Social inequality and obesity in Czech school children, *Econ. Hum. Biol.*, 2, 107, 2004.

Vígnerová, J., Lhotská, L., and Bláha, P., Proposed standard definition for child overweight and obesity, *Cent. Eur. J. Publ. Hlth.*, 9, 145, 2001.

Vígnerová, J. et al., Growth of Czech child population 0–18 years compared to the World Health Organization Growth Reference, *Am. J. Hum. Biol.*, 9, 459, 1997.

Vignolo, M. et al., Variability of height and skeletal maturation in simple obesity, *Int. J. Obes. Relat. Metab. Disord.*, 22, S14, 1998.

Visali, N. et al., Obesity in childhood. Update in one district of Rome, *Int. J. Obes. Relat. Metab. Disord.*, 22, S5, 1998.

Vitolo, M.R. et al., Group treatment for post-pubertal obese adolescents, *Int. J. Obes. Relat. Metab. Disord.*, 22, S257, 1998.

Vol, S., Tichet, J. and Rolland-Cachera, M.F., Trends in the prevalence of obesity between 1980 and 1996 among French adults and children, *Int. J. Obes. Relat. Metab. Disord.*, 22, S210, 1998.

Volta, C. et al., Growth hormone response to growth hormone-releasing hormone (GHRH), insulin, clonidine and arginine after GHRH pretreatment in obese children: evidence of somatostatin increase, *Eur. J. Endocrinol.*, 132, 716, 1995.

Von Kries, M. et al., Is obesity a risk factor for childhood asthma? *Allergy Eur. J. Allergy Clin. Immunol.*, 56, 318, 2001.

Von Kries, R. et al., Does breast-feeding protect against childhood obesity? *Adv. Exp. Ned. Biol.*, 478, 29, 2000.

Von Kries, R. et al., Maternal smoking during pregnancy and childhood obesity, *Am. J. Epidemiol.*, 156, 954, 2002a.

Von Kries, R. et al., Reduced risk for overweight and obesity in 5- and 6-y-old children by duration of sleep: a cross-sectional study, *Int. J. Obes. Relat. Metab. Disord.*, 26, 710, 2002b.

Wabitsch, M., The obese child: the need for a specific approach; treatment compounds: an update, *Int. J. Obes. Relat. Metab. Disord.*, 21, S139, 1997.

Wabitsch, M., Overweight and obesity in European children: definition and diagnostic procedures, risk factors and consequences for later health outcome, *Europ. J. Pediatr.*, 159, S8, 2000.

Wabitsch, M. et al., Association of insulin-like growth factors and their binding proteins with anthropometric parameters in obese adolescent girls, in *Obesity in Europe 1993*, Eds., Ditschuneit, H. et al., John Libbey, London, 155.

Wabitsch, M. et al., Insulin-like growth factors and their binding proteins before and after weight loss and their associations with hormonal and metabolic parameters in obese adolescent girls, *Int. J. Obes. Relat. Metab. Disord.*, 20, 1073, 1996.

Wabitsch, M. et al., Contribution of androgens to the gender difference in leptin production in obese children and adolescents, *J. Clin.*, 100, 808, 1997a.

Wabitsch, M. et al., Role of insulin-like growth factor I (IGF I) in growth and metabolism of human adipose tissue, *Eur. J. Pediatr.*, 156, 170, 1997b.

Wabitsch, M. et al., More and more children and adolescents are overweight. How can we stop the "obesity epidemic"? *MMW Fortschr. Med.*, 144, 99, 2002.

Wadden, T.A. et al., Dissatisfaction with weight and figure in obese girls; discontent but not depression, *Int. J. Obesity*, 13, 89, 1989.

Wadden, T.A. et al., Obesity in black adolescent girls: a controlled clinical trial of treatment by diet, behavior modification, and parental support, *Pediatrics*, 85, 345, 1990.

Wade, A.J., Marbut, M.M., and Round, J.M., Muscle fibre type and etiology of obesity, *Lancet*, 335, 805, 1990.

Wake, M., Hesketh, K., and Waters, E., Television, computer use and body mass index in Australian primary school children, *J. Paediatr. Child Hlth.*, 39, 130, 2003.

Wake, M. et al., Parent-reported health status of overweight and obese Australian primary school children: a cross-sectional population survey, *Int. J. Obes. Relat. Metab. Disord.*, 26, 717, 2002.

Walberg, J. and Ward, D., Physical activity and childhood obesity, *J. Phys. Educ., Recr., Dance*, 12, 82, 1985.

Walker, S.P. et al., The effects of birth weight and postnatal linear growth retardation on body mass index, fatness and fat distribution in mid- and late childhood, *Pub. Hlth. Nutr.*, 5, 391, 2002.

Wandel, M., Nutrition-related diseases and dietary change among Third World immigrants in northern Europe, *Nutr. Hlth.*, 9, 117, 1993.

Wang, Y., Ge, K. and Popkin, B.M., Why do some overweight children remain overweight, whereas others do not? *Pub. Hlth. Nutr.*, 6, 549, 2003.

Wang, Y.F., Monteiro, C., and Popkin, B.M., Trends of obesity and underweight in older children and adolescents in the United States, Brazil, China and Russia, *Am. J. Clin. Nutr.*, 75, 971, 2002.

Wang, Z.M., *Human Body Composition Models and Methodology: Theory and Experiment*, thesis. Landbouw Universiteit Wageningen, Grafisch Service Centrum Van Gils B.V., Wageningen, 1997.

Wang, Z., Patterson, C., and Hills, A.P., Association between overweight or obesity, household income and parental BMI in Australian youth: an analysis of the Australian National Health and Nutrition Survey, 1995, *Asia–Pac. J. Clin. Nutr.*, 11, 3, 200, 2002.

Wang, Z., Patterson, C., and Hills, A.P., A comparison of self-reported and measured height, weight and BMI in Australian adolescents, *Aust. N.Z.J. Pub. Hlth.*, 26, 473, 2002.

Wang, Z., Patterson, C., and Hills, A.P., The relationship between BMI and intake of energy and fat of Australian youth: a secondary data analysis of the Australian National Nutrition Survey 1995, *Nutr. Dietet.*, 60, 1, 23, 2003.

Wang, Z., et al., Influences of ethnicity and socioeconomic status on the body dissatisfaction and eating behaviour of Australian children and adolescents, *Eating Behav.*, 2004 (in press).

Ward, D.S. and Bar-Or, O., Role of the physician and physical education teacher in the treatment of obesity at school, *Pediatrician*, 13, 44, 1986.

Ward, D.S. et al., Physical activity and physical fitness in African–American girls with and without obesity, *Obes. Res.*, 5, 572, 1997.

Ward, L.C. et al., Reliability of multiple frequency bioelectrical impedance analysis: an intermachine comparison, *Am. J. Hum. Biol.*, 9, 63, 1997.

Wardle, J. et al., Food and activity preferences in children of lean and obese parents, *Int. J. Obes. Relat. Metab. Disord.*, 25, 971, 2001a.

Wardle, J. et al., Development of the children's eating behavior Questionnaire, *J. Child. Psychol. Psychiatry*, 42, 963, 2001b.

Warren, J.M. et al., Evaluation of a pilot school programme aimed at the prevention of obesity in children, *Health Promot. Int.*, 18, 287, 2003.

Warsburger, P. et al., Conceptualisation and evaluation of a cognitive-behavioural training programme for children and adolescents obesity, *Int. J. Obes. Relat. Metab. Disord.*, 25, S93, 2001.

Waterland, R.A. et al., Calibrated-orifice nipples for measurement of infant nutritive sucking, *J. Pediatr.*, 132, 523, 1998.

Waterlow, J.C., Observations on the variability of creatinine excretion, *Hum. Nutr. Clin. Nutr.*, 40c, 125, 1994.

Waterlow, J.C. et al., The presentation and use of height and weight data for comparing the nutritional status of groups of children under the age of 10 years, *Bull. W.H.O.*, 55, 489, 1977.

Watson, A.W.S. and O'Donovan, D.J., Factors relating to the strength of female adolescents, *J. Appl. Physiol.*, 43, 834, 1977.

Wattigney, W.A. et al., Increasing obesity impact on serum lipids and lipoproteins in young adults, *Arch. Intern. Med.*, 151, 2017, 1991.

Wear, C.L.M., Relationship of physique and developmental level to physical performance, *Res. Q.*, 33, 615, 1962.

Wearing, S. et al., The arch index: a measure of flat or fat feet? *Foot Ankle Int.* (in press).

Weder, A.B. et al., The antihypertensive effects of calorie restriction in obese adolescents: dissociation of effects on erythrocyte countertransport and cotransport, *J. Hypertens.*, 2, 507, 1984.

Wells, J.C.K. and Fuller, N.J., Precision of measurement and body size in whole-body air-displacement plethysmography, *Int. J. Obes. Relat. Metab. Disord.*, 25, 1161, 2001.

Wells, J.C.K. et al., The contribution of fat and fat-free tissue to body mass index in contemporary children and the reference child, *Int. J. Obes. Relat. Metab. Disord.*, 26, 1323, 2002.

Wertheim, E.H. et al., Psychosocial predictors of weight loss behaviors and binge eating in adolescent girls and boys, *Int. J. Eating Disord.*, 12, 151, 1992.

Westenhoefer, J., Establishing dietary habits during childhood for long-term weight control, *Ann. Nutr. Metab.*, 46 (Suppl. 1), 18, 2002.

Westerterp, K.R., Obesity and physical activity, *Int. J. Obes. Relat. Metab. Disord.*, 23, S59, 1999.

Wetzel, N.V., Growth, in *Medical Physics*, Year Book Publishers, Chicago, 1942, 513.

Weyer, C. et al., Exaggerated pancreatic polypeptide secretion in Pima Indians: can an increased parasympathetic drive to the pancreas contribute to hyperinsulinemia, obesity, and diabetes in humans? *Metab. Clin. Exp.*, 50, 223, 2001.

Weyhreter, H. et al., Evaluation of an outpatient treatment program for obese children and adolescents, *Klin. Pediatr.*, 215, 57, 2003.

Whitaker, R.C. et al., Gestational diabetes and the risk of offspring obesity, *Pediatrics*, 101, E9, 1998.

Whiting, S.J., Obesity is not protective for bones in childhood and adolescence, *Nutr. Rev.*, 60, 27, 2002.

Widdowson, E.M., W., Nutritional individuality, *Proc. Nutr. Soc.*, 21, 121, 1962.

Widdowson, E.M., Changes in pigs due to undernutrition before birth, and for one, two, and three years afterwards, and the effects of rehabilitation, in *Advances in Experimental Medicine and Biology: Nutrition and Malnutrition, Identification and Measurement*, Roche, A.F. and Falkner, F., Eds., Plenum Press, New York and London, 1974, 165.

Widdowson, E.M., How much food does man require? An evaluation of human energy needs, *Experientia*, 44, 11, 1983.

Widhalm, K., Obesity in childhood-diagnosis and therapy, *Pediatr. Padol.*, 20, 403, 1985 (in German).

Widhalm, K., Fat nutrition during infancy and childhood, in *Bibl. Nutr. Diet — Nutrition in Pregnancy and Growth*, Porrini, M. and Walter, P., Eds., Karger, Basel, 1996, 116.

Widhalm, K., Prevention of morbid obesity in adolescents: a new pediatric clinical syndrome? *Int. J. Obes. Relat. Metab. Disord.*, 23, S7, 1999.

Widhalm, K. and Schonegger, K., BMI: does it really reflect body fat mass? *J. Pediatr.*, 134, 522, 1999.

Widhalm, K., Sinz, S., and Egger, E., Prevalence of obesity in Viennese school children: a longitudinal study of 900 11–18-y-old children and adolescents, *Int. J. Obes. Relat. Metab. Disord.*, 22, S5, 1998.

Widhalm, K.M. and Zwiauer, K.F., Metabolic effects of a very low calorie diet in obese children and adolescents with special reference to nitrogen balance, *J. Am. Coll. Nutr.*, 6, 467, 1987.

Widhalm, K., Zwiauer, K., and Eckharter, I., External stimulus dependence in food intake of obese adolescents: studies using a food dispenser, *Klin. Pediatr.*, 202, 168, 1990 (in German).

Widhalm, K. et al., Does BMI reflect body fat in obese children and adolescents? A study using the TOBEC method, *Int. J. Obes. Relat. Metab. Disord.*, 25, 279, 2001.

Wiecha, J.L. and Casey, V.A., High prevalence of overweight and short stature among Head Start children in Massachusetts, *Pub. Hlth. Rep.*, 109, 767, 1994.

Wilkin, T.J. et al., The relative contributions of birth weight, weight change, and current weight to insulin resistance in contemporary 5-year-olds: the EarlyBird study, *Diabetes*, 51, 3468, 2002.

Williams, C. L., Importance of dietary fiber in childhood, *J. Am. Diet. Assoc.*, 95,1140, 1995.

Williams, C.L., Bollella, M., and Carter, B.J., Treatment of childhood obesity in pediatric practice, *Ann. N.Y. Acad. Sci.*, 699, 207, 1993.

Williams, S., Obesity at age 21: the association with body mass index in childhood and adolescence and parents' body mass index. A cohort study of New Zealanders born in 1972–1973, *Int. J. Obes. Relat. Metab. Disord.*, 25, 158, 2001.

Williams, S., Davie, G., and Lam, F., Predicting BMI in young adults from childhood data using two approaches to modelling adiposity rebound, *Int. J. Obes. Relat. Metab. Disord.*, 23, 348, 1999.

Williams, S. and Dickson, N., Early growth, menarche and adiposity rebound, *Lancet*, 359, 580, 2002.

Williamson, D.A., Assessment of eating disorders, in *Obesity, Anorexia, and Bulimia Nervosa*, Elmsford, Pergamon Press, New York, 1990.

Williamson, D.A. et al., Psychopathology of eating disorders: a controlled comparison of bulimic, obese, and normal subjects, *J. Consult. Clin. Psychol.*, 53, 161, 1985.

Williamson, D.A. et al., Development of a simple procedure for assessing body image disturbances, *Behav. Assess.*, 11, 433, 1989.

Wilmore, J.H., Body composition in sport and exercise. Directions for future research, *Med. Sci. Sports Exerc.*, 1521, 1983.

Wilmore, J.H., Eating and weight disorders in the female athlete, *Int. J. Sport Nutr.*, 1, 104, 1991.

Wiseman, C. et al., Cultural expectations of thinness in women: an update, *Int. J. Eating Disord.*, 11, 85, 1992.

Wisemandle, W., Siervogel, R.M., and Guo, S.S., Childhood levels of weight, stature, and body mass index for individuals with early and late onset of overweight, *Int. J. Obes. Relat. Metab. Disord.*, 22, S3, 1998.

Wit, J.M. et al., Obese children and their treatment, *Tijdschr. Kindergeneeskd.*, 55, 191, 1987.

Wolf, A.M. et al., Activity, inactivity, and obesity: racial, ethnic, and age differences among schoolgirls, *Am. J. Pub. Hlth.*, 83, 1625, 1993.

Wolfe, W.S. et al., Overweight schoolchildren in New York State: prevalence and characteristics, *Am. J. Pub. Hlth.*, 84, 807, 1994.

Woolley, S.C. and Woolley, O.W., Should obesity be treated at all? in *Health and Obesity*, Conn, H.L., De Felice, E.A., and Kuo, P., Eds., Raven Press, New York, 1983, 185.

Woringer, W. and Schutz, Y., What is the evolution of the body mass index (BMI) in Swiss children from five to sixteen years, measured one decade apart? *Int. J. Obes. Relat. Metab. Disord.*, 22, S209, 1998.

Woringer, V. and Schutz, Y., Obesity in Switzerland: percentiles of body mass index of a cohort of children and adolescents born in 1980 in Lausanne and differences with the Swiss percentiles calculated for boys and girls in 1955, *Soz. Prev. Med.*, 48, 121, 2002.

World Health Organization, *Energy and Protein Requirements,* report of a joint FAO/ WHO/UNU Expert Consultation, Rome 1981, Technical Report Series, No. 724, WHO, Geneva, 1985, 180.

World Health Organization MONICA Project, Geographical variation in the major risk factors of coronary heart diseases in men and women age 35–64 years, *World Health Statistics Q.*, 41, 115, 1988.

World Health Organization, *Prevention in Childhood and Youth of Adult Cardiovascular Diseases: Time for Action,* report of a WHO Expert Committee, WHO Technical Report Series, No. 792, WHO, Geneva, 1990.

World Health Organization, *Diet, Nutrition and the Prevention of Chronic Diseases,* WHO Technical Report Series, No. 797, WHO, Geneva 1990.

World Health Organization, *WHO Global Database on Child Growth and Malnutrition.* Compiled by M. de Onis and M. Blossner, WHO, Geneva 1997.

World Health Organization, *Obesity: Preventing and Managing the Global Epidemic,* WHO Consultation on Obesity, 3-5 June, 1997, Geneva, WHO, 1998.

Wright, C.M. et al., Implications of childhood obesity for adult health: findings from thousand families cohort study, *B. M. J.*, 323, 1280, 2001.

Wu, D.M. et al., Familial resemblance of adiposity-related parameters. Results from a health check-up population in Taiwan, *Eur. J. Epidemiol.*, 18, 221, 2003.

Xinli, W. et al., Association of a mutation in the β3 adrenergic receptor gene with obesity and response to dietary intervention in Chinese children, *Acta Pediatr. Int. J. Pediatr.*, 90, 1233, 2001.

Yajnik, C.S., Early life origins of insulin resistance and type 2 diabetes in India and other Asian countries, *J. Nutr.*, 134, 205, 2004.

Yakinci, C. et al., Autonomic nervous system functions in obese children, *Brain. Dev.*, 22, 151, 2000.

Yamamoto, A. et al., Serum lipid levels in elementary and junior high school children and their relationship to obesity, *Prog. Clin. Biol. Res.*, 255, 107, 1988.

Yanovski, J.A. et al., Association between uncoupling protein 2, body composition, and resting energy expenditure in lean and obese African American, white, and Asian children, *Am. J. Clin. Nutr.*, 71, 1404, 2000.

Yanovski, J.A. and Yanovski, S.Z., Treatment of pediatric and adolescent obesity, *J.A.M.A.*, 289, 1851, 2003.

Yasunaga, T. et al., Nutrition related hormonal changes in obese children, *Endocr. J.*, 45, 221, 1998.

Yiannakou, P. et al., Evaluation with the multifrequencies bioimpedance method of body water in the male prepubertal obese child, *Int. J. Obes. Relat. Metab. Disord.*, 22, S13, 1998.

Ylitalo, V.M., Treatment of obese schoolchildren with special reference to the mode of therapy, cardiorespiratory performance and the carbohydrate and lipid metabolism, *Acta Paediatr. Scand. Suppl.*, 290, 1, 1981.

Ylitalo, V.M., Treatment of obese schoolchildren, *Klin. Pediatr.*, 194, 310, 1982.

York, D. and Bouchard, C., How obesity develops: insights from the new biology, *Endocrine*, 13, 143, 2000.

Yoshiike, N. et al., Descriptive epidemiology of body mass index in Japanese adults in a representative sample from the National Nutrition Survey 1990–1994, *Int. J. Obes. Relat. Metab. Dis.*, 22, 684, 1998.

Yoshinaga, M. et al., Rapid increase in the prevalence of obesity in elementary school children, *Int. J. Obes. Relat. Metab. Disord.*, 28, 494, 2004.

Yoshino, Y. et al., Comparison of body compositions between Korean and Japanese schoolchildren? How different lifestyles may relate to these body compositions, *Int. J. Obes. Relat. Metab. Disord.*, 22, S13, 1998.

Young-Hyman, D. et al., Evaluation of the insulin resistance syndrome in 5- to 10-year-old overweight/obese African-American children, *Diabetes Care*, 24, 1359, 2001.

Yussef, A.A. et al., Time course of adiposity and fasting insulin from childhood to young adulthood in offspring of parents with coronary artery disease: the Bogalusa Heart Study, *Ann. Epidemiol.*, 12, 553, 2002.

Zamboni, G. et al., Mineral metabolism in obese children, *Acta Paediatr. Scand.*, 77, 741, 1988.

Zametkin, A.J. et al., Psychiatric aspects of child and adolescent obesity: a review over the past 10 years, *J. Am. Acad. Child Adolesc. Psychiatry*, 43, 151, 2004.

Zanconato, S. et al., Gas exchange during exercise in obese children, *Eur. J. Pediatr.*, 148, 614, 1989.

Zanelli, R. et al., Hyperinsulinism as a marker in obese children, *Am. J. Dis. Child.*, 147, 837, 1993.

Zellner, K., Kromeyer, K., and Jaeger, U., Growth studies in Jena, Germany: historical background and secular changes in stature and weight in children 7–14 years, *Am. J. Hum. Biol.*, 8, 371, 1996.

Zephier, E., Himes, J.H., and Story, M., Prevalence of overweight and obesity in American Indian school children and adolescents in the Aberdeen area: a population study, *Int. J. Obes. Relat. Metab. Disord.*, 23, S28, 1999.

Zhai, F.Y., et al., Validation of lipids on body mass index reference recommendations, Obesity Working Group, International Life Sciences Association, China, *Zhonghua Liu Xing Bing Xue Za Zhi*, 25, 117, 2004 (in Chinese).

Zhang, H. and Li., Y., Harmfulness of obesity in children to their health, *Chung Hua Yu Fang I Hsueh Tsa Chih* 30, 77, 1996 (in Chinese).

Zhang, Y.Y. et al., Positional cloning of the mouse obese gene and its human homolog, *Nature*, 372, 425, 1994.

Zoppi, G. et al., Obesity in pediatrics: statistical analysis of school performance of obese children, *Pediatr. Med. Chir.*, 17, 559, 1995 (in Italian).

Zurlo, F., Ferraro, R.T., and Fontvieille, A.M., Spontaneous physical activity and obesity: cross-sectional and longitudinal studies in Pima Indians, *Am. J. Physiol.*, 263, E296, 1992.

Zwiauer, K.W., K., Effect of 2 different reducing diets on the concentration of HDL cholesterol in obese adolescents, *Klin. Pediatr.*, 199, 392, 1987 (in German).

Zwiauer, K.F.M., Treatment of childhood obesity: which approach? *Int. J. Obes. Relat. Metab. Disord.*, 22, S2, 1998.

Zwiauer, K.F.M., Prevention and treatment of overweight and obesity in children and adolescents, *Eur. J. Ped. Suppl.*, 159, S56, 2000.

Zwiauer, K., Kerbl, B., and Widhalm, K., No reduction of high density lipoprotein 2 during weight reduction in obese children and adolescents, *Eur. J. Pediatr.*, 149, 192, 1989..

Zwiauer, K.F. and Widhalm, K.M., The development of obesity in childhood, *Klin. Pediatr.*, 196, 327, 1984 (in German).

Zwiauer, K. et al., 24 hours electrocardiographic monitoring in obese children and adolescents during 3 weeks of low calorie diet (500 kcal), *Int. J. Obes.*, 13, 101, 1989.

Zwiauer, K. et al., Effect of body fat distribution on resting energy expenditure and diet-induced thermogenesis in adolescents, *Int. J. Obes. Relat. Metab. Disord.*, 17, S41, 1993.

Zwiauer, K.F.M. et al., Clinical features, adverse effects and outcome, in *Child and Adolescent Obesity*, Burniat, W. et al., Eds., Cambridge University Press, Cambridge, 2002, 131.

Index

Index

A

Milton Keynes UK
Ingram Content Group UK Ltd.
UKHW021925071024
449327UK00022B/1705